GABRIELA SCHMIDT-WYKLICKY

Ernst Fuchs (1851–1930)

and the Worldwide Renown of the Vienna School of Ophthalmology
around 1900

GABRIELA SCHMIDT-WYKLICKY

Ernst Fuchs (1851–1930)

and the Worldwide Renown of the Vienna School of Ophthalmology around 1900

A documentary biography

Translated from the German by Otmar Binder

AUSTRIAN ACADEMY OF SCIENCES PRESS

Published with the support of the Fuchs-Stiftung zur Förderung der Augenheilkunde

Published with the support of Austrian Science Fund (FWF) PUB 917-Z

This publication has undergone the process of anonymous, international peer review.

Peer review is an essential part of the Austrian Academy of Sciences Press evaluation process. Before any book can be accepted for publication, it is assessed by international specialists and ultimately must be approved by the Austrian Academy of Sciences Publication Committee.

The paper used in this publication is DIN EN ISO 9706 certified and meets the requirements for permanent archiving of written cultural property.

ISBN 978-3-7001-9158-2

Typeset by Rudi Krammer, Vienna; PER MEDIEN & MARKETING GmbH, Germany
Printed and bound by Print Alliance, Bad Vöslau
https://epub.oeaw.ac.at/9158-2
https://verlag.oeaw.ac.at
Made in Europe

In memoriam Helmut Wyklicky (1921–2007)

Table of Contents

Appendix

Ernst Fuchs and Ophthalmology in the United States

A uniquely charismatic teacher and researcher, Ernst Fuchs made significant contributions over several decades to the development of ophthalmological training and to research on the physiology and the diseases of the eye in the United States. Contacts with American colleagues he had established at the very beginning of his medical career matured into lifelong, close, and mutually beneficial friendships. This monograph, based as it is throughout on authentic source material, offers a detailed insight into how this was achieved.

Responding to the request of a group of American medical doctors, who had come to Vienna to complete their training as eye specialists, Fuchs, himself at that stage no more than an assistant at the Vienna University Eye Clinic under Professor Ferdinand Ritter von Arlt (1812–1887), set up an innovative and highly successful crammer course. In what was a historic first in the history of the Vienna Medical Faculty, he initiated – some years before his own habilitation in 1880 – specialist courses for English-speaking physicians. After a trial run in German in 1878 the Faculty acceded to the express wishes of its target audience and held the courses in English from 1879 onwards. Lasting several weeks, they covered select chapters of ophthalmology, such as physiological optics (refraction, accommodation) and the pathological anatomy of the eye. Given that at that time academic institutions in the United States suitable for the training of ophthalmologists were, if not totally non-existent, at least few and far between, it came as no surprise that these postgraduate courses in Vienna were in great demand throughout the last third of the nineteenth and the first two decades of the twentieth century. At that time, Vienna was, in Fuchs's own words, the "Mecca" of American ophthalmologists. Participants of these summer courses came from all over the Anglophone world, but as Americans tended to predominate, they were soon referred to as *Amerikanerkurse*. After Fuchs had been awarded the chair at the Second University Eye Clinic in Vienna (1885), the courses were held by his assistants and continued to attract an ever greater number of participants (see Ch. 2). Back in the USA, graduates often attained leading positions in the clinics and academic institutions specialising in ophthalmology that sprang up across the country. They frequently modelled their new work places on Fuchs's clinic in Vienna, replicating the setting where they had gained their own expertise. They made specialist training available for ophthalmologists nationwide. A case in point is Adolph Barkan (1845–1935), one of Fuchs's first private students in Vienna, who pioneered modern ophthalmology at San Francisco's Stanford University. In 1911, Barkan was the first to invite Fuchs to the United States to deliver the prestigious Lane Lectures (see Chapters 2 and 11).

Fuchs's textbook on ophthalmology was studied throughout the world. The first of eighteen German editions up until 1945 was published in 1889. Ten English editions followed between 1892 and 1933, and there were subsequent translations into French, Italian, Spanish, Russian, Japanese, and Chinese. The science was profound, but it was his talent for addressing the needs of students and medical specialists alike that allowed him to set his seal on the teaching of ophthalmology for more than half a century. The textbook paved the way for the tenets upheld by the Vienna School of Ophthalmology as represented by Ernst Fuchs to be spread all over the world. As a classic textbook the work was awarded the title of the Bible of Ophthalmology in the United States (see Ch. 6).

During the three decades (1885 to 1915) Fuchs was at the head of the Second University Eye Clinic, trainees from the States were constant visitors, taking part in the everyday life of the clinic and making their own contributions to its research work.

The First World War, with Austria-Hungary and the United States fighting on different sides, put an end to the previously intense relationship between German speaking and American ophthalmologists. Given his immense prestige in specialist circles, Ernst Fuchs was uniquely qualified to revive this relationship. In contrast to other German speaking ophthalmologists, who continued to be ostracised, Fuchs was invited in 1921 to give courses at leading US universities on the pathological anatomy and the histology of the eye and to give presentations to specialist associations. Former students of his and friends in the US medical establishment hosted him on his eighteen months long lecture tour.

In recognition of his outstanding achievements, several US specialist associations made him an honorary member. Prestigious awards Fuchs received in the United States include the Lucien Howe Medal of the American Ophthalmological Society in 1924 and the Leslie Dana Gold Medal for Outstanding Achievements in the Prevention of Blindness in 1929.

The author hopes that this carefully tailored analysis will appeal to its target audience in the USA and worldwide.

Preface

When Ernst Fuchs was awarded a chair in Vienna in 1885, the Second Vienna Medical School had already reached the apex of its achievements. The First Vienna Medical School, with its critical milestones – the introduction of clinical tuition and the dissection of cadavers – had been founded in the era of Maria Theresa by the monarch's court physician Gerard van Swieten (1700–1772). It had put in-vivo diagnostics on a more assured footing by virtue of percussion and auscultation. Pathologist Carl Freiherr von Rokitansky (1804–1878) made a seminal contribution to the verification of results obtained by clinician Joseph Škoda (1805–1881) and his students. Percussion and auscultation made it possible to assess the status of interior organs acoustically in terms of shape, size and function. The two techniques were of particular use in the context of chest diseases to localise pathological processes. Comparison between the physical findings obtained from the living patient and the results of autopsy helped to hone clinical diagnosis.

Surgery, too, had progressed by leaps and bounds since the second half of the nineteenth century. In 1881, Theodor Billroth (1829–1894) succeeded in removing a pyloric carcinoma, a signal achievement. Under the maxim of "cleanliness to a fault", he campaigned for the replacement of the antiseptic approach by an aseptic one. Local anaesthesia (Carl Koller, 1884) came to supplement general anaesthesia, which was already well established by that time. The differentiation of general medicine into a raft of specialties – dermatology, otology, laryngology, orthopedics, gynaecology, etc. – was imminent, causing Hermann Nothnagel (1841–1905) to claim for internal medicine at least the rank of "prima inter pares".

In addition to his revered teachers Ferdinand von Arlt (1812–1887) and Billroth, Fuchs was on friendly terms with pathologist Hans von Chiari (1851–1916), a contemporary with whom he had attended a grammar school in Vienna run by Benedictine monks, the Schottengymnasium, and with gynaecologist Rudolf Chrobak (1843–1910) and psychiatrist Julius Wagner

Ritter von Jauregg (1857–1940). Billroth had not only been his teacher but had accepted Fuchs as a trainee surgeon. Fuchs had also retained special respect since his student days for physiologist Ernst Wilhelm Ritter von Brücke (1819–1892) and histologist Carl Wedl (1815–1891). The influence of these two men on the student's methodological-experimental work was profound and will be considered below in greater detail.

During the three decades Fuchs was active in Vienna, several ground-breaking innovations were achieved in new specialties by exponents of the Vienna Medical School: in the newly established field of immunology, Clemens Freiherr von Pirquet (1874–1929) laid the foundations of allergology and pushed this discipline in the last years of his life as far as the postulate of "auto aggression" carried out by endogenous metabolites. In his study of the agglutination reaction, which is primarily associated with infectious diseases and had first been flagged by hygienist Max von Gruber (1853–1927), Karl Landsteiner (1868–1943) was the first to show in 1901 that human blood comes in different types. Guido Holzknecht (1872–1931) fought for the use of X-rays and for their improved clinical-therapeutic application. In his search for a therapy for progressive paralysis Julius Wagner Ritter von Jauregg (1857–1940) discovered the efficacy of a malaria therapy built on deliberately induced fever bouts to stabilise a pathology that had been considered incurable until then.

This is a thumb nail sketch of what medical science looked like when Ernst Fuchs was active at Vienna's Allgemeines Krankenhaus. Because of the multiple layers both of innovative research and the art of clinical therapy, Vienna around 1900 was frequently referred to as the "Mecca of medicine".

Helmut Wyklicky †

Introduction

During the almost half century spanned by Ernst Fuchs's scientific activities he was one of the foremost representatives of his discipline. It would be difficult to name another ophthalmologist in either the German-speaking countries or the wider world who contributed as much to the development of ophthalmology as a science. He grounded ophthalmological nosology in pathological changes of the anatomy and defined a great number of new disease entities, many of which bear his name to this day. This remains Ernst Fuchs's lasting achievement. Furthermore, he was a charismatic teacher. Running to many editions and published in translations into most major languages, his textbook, considered the "Bible of Ophthalmology" for half a century, was in use all over the world.

Initiated by Fuchs in 1879, tutorials in English in the summer months thereafter became an annual fixture. This summer school enabled Fuchs to bring together a great number of students from all over the world at his clinic. Fired up by his inspired teaching and the courses given by assistants whom Fuchs painstakingly trained for the task, these students took the Vienna Ophthalmological School back to their own countries, often founding eye clinics modelled on the principles taught by Fuchs. The outbreak of the First World War put an end to this fruitful process.

In the decade and a half between his voluntary retirement in 1915 and his death in 1930, Fuchs travelled all the continents apart from Australia to stay in touch with his former students. In this way he made the Vienna Ophthalmological School, as the Viennese historian of medicine, Erna Lesky (1911–1986) so aptly – if in Latin – put it, the "magistra ophthalmologiae totius mundi", the teacher of ophthalmology for the entire globe. It is therefore no surprise that Fuchs was acclaimed as the leading eye specialist of his time both in many appraisals during his lifetime and in obituaries carried by all the major specialist journals.

This biography is based on Fuchs's two autobiographies. When towards the end of his active professional life he was about to be made an honorary member of the Austrian Academy of Sciences, he was asked to present a CV. This hitherto unpublished autograph, a sort of thumb-nail sketch of a self-portrait, forms the first chapter of this work. A second, more detailed autobiography, also dating to 1926, was published in 1946 by his son Adalbert (1887–1973), himself an eye specialist, in conjunction with pages from Fuchs's diaries. Entitled *Wie ein Augenarzt die Welt sah* [The World as Seen by an Eye Specialist], it reflects all the exigencies of postwar publishing in its outward form.

On the occasion of the 150th anniversary of the foundation of the First University Eye Clinic in Vienna in 1962, an exhibition at the Institute for the History of Medicine of Vienna University at the Josephinum paid a fitting tribute to the achievements that Fuchs, himself one of Arlt's disciples, had to his credit. The exhibition benefited from the largesse of Fuchs's descendants, who made a great number of highly significant, previously unknown documents and other objects available. Another exhibition at the Josephinum, this time in celebration of the 100th anniversary of the Second University Eye Clinic in 1983, again showcased Ernst Fuchs's scientific achievements. The exhibition was accompanied by an illustrated volume in German and English by Helmut Wyklicky, entitled *Zur Geschichte der Augenheilkunde in Wien. 100 Jahre II. Universitäts-Augenklinik* [Aspects of the History of Ophthalmology in Vienna. The first one hundred years of the Second University Eye Clinic].

When in 1992 the clinics relocated from the historical buildings of the Allgemeines Krankenhaus in Alserstraße/Spitalgasse to the new buildings off the Währinger Gürtel, the author of this monograph was put in charge by the Federal Ministry of Education and Research of a project designed to ensure the safekeeping of museum-grade objects from the old buildings. This ensured that, during the five years that followed, documents, pictures and other objects of historical interest were among the material retrieved from the two eye clinics to be given a new lease of life. These relics comprised several important aides-mémoire with a bearing on Ernst Fuchs, pulled together presumably by his student Josef Meller (1874–1968), who eventually became the director of the *Parallelklinik*. Most of these aides-mémoire were previously unpublished photos of Ernst Fuchs in the company of assistants at his clinic and of students from abroad both during the summer schools mentioned above and his frequent trips abroad. This new material prompted the author to start work on a comprehensive biography of Ernst Fuchs against the backdrop of the history of medicine. Again, the Fuchs family were most generous in allowing the author use of the richly stocked family archive. The upshot was that a wealth of original documents and pictures was assembled, providing a valuable complement to the archival holdings kept at what was then referred to as the Institut für Geschichte der Medizin at the Josephinum [Institute for the History of Medicine, today: Sammlungen der Medizinischen Universität Wien – Collections of the Medical University of Vienna]. The author's own acquisitions broadened this collection by adding a great number of happy finds made in antiquarian bookshops, such as original documents, autographs, pictures, special prints of Fuchs's original publications, first editions of his *Lehrbuch*, which has been translated into seven languages, and relevant secondary literature – all of them indispensable to base the present biography of Ernst Fuchs on authentic and scientifically impeccable source material.

In the United States of America, too, the memory of Ernst Fuchs has been kept alive to this day. In the course of the annual conference of the American Society for Cataract and Refractory Surgery held in Boston in 1999, an Ophthalmology Hall of Fame was founded, and at the next conference Ernst Fuchs was inducted into this Hall of Fame of the history of ophthalmology as one of the leading eye specialists in the world. On that festive occasion, Günther Grabner, then the Director of the Landesaugenklinik Salzburg, himself an exponent of the Vienna Ophthalmological School, delivered the keynote speech.

At the instigation of Prof. Grabner, the Fuchs Stiftung zur Förderung der Augenheilkunde [Fuchs Foundation for the Promotion of Ophthalmology] was called into being at the Landesaugenklinik Salzburg in the autumn of 2001. The author of this monograph has herself been co-opted in an advisory capacity to the Foundation's Board of Governors. This is especially relevant to the objective explicitly stated in the foundation deed of cultivating "the memory of Prof. Dr Ernst Fuchs and the Second Eye Clinic of the Medical University of Vienna, which he was in charge of". On 11 October 2001 the author was given the privilege of outlining the lasting merits of this outstanding Austrian ophthalmologist in a keynote speech given to the formal founding meeting of the Fuchs Stiftung in Salzburg. After several lengthy delays, the time has now come to fulfil the wish of the Fuchs Stiftung for a comprehensive biographical sketch of the life and work of its patron.

A research project like this cannot be realised without unstinting spiritual, specialist and material support from many sympathetic and patient helpers. My special thanks therefore go out to Ernst Fuchs's extremely gracious descendants (subsumed here under "Family archive") and to Günther Grabner. Heartfelt thanks belong to my late teacher and husband Helmut Wyklicky, who accompanied my work as an inspiring and encouraging adviser. I want to dedicate this book to him, a book to which he himself wrote a foreword shortly before his death.

Several archives, libraries and academic institutions, both in Austria and abroad, have been instrumental in my archival research. I owe them a special debt of gratitude. Let me here list the persons in charge of them in alphabetical order:

Manfred Anselgruber, M. A. (archivist, Schottengymnasium, Vienna)
Bruno Bauer †, M. A., and staff (Library of the Medical University of Vienna)
Dr. Heinrich Berg and staff (City Archive Vienna)
Colleen Bradley-Sanders (archivist of the Medical Library of New York University)
Prof. Dr. Christiane Druml (Collections of the Medical University, Vienna)
University Lecturer Dr. Peter Goller (archivist of the University of Innsbruck)
Hofrat Dr. Michael Göbl (Austrian State Archives/Haus-Hof-und Staatsarchiv, Vienna)
Marie-Élisabeth Henneau (archivist of the University of Liège)
Dr. Susanne Kühberger (Austrian State Archives/Allgemeines Verwaltungsarchiv, Vienna)
Hofrat Thomas Maisel, M. A., University Lecturer Hofrat Dr. Kurt Mühlberger, University Lecturer Dr. Johannes Seidl and staff (Vienna University Archive)
Friedrich Ribar, M. A., Dr. Hermann Zeitlhofer and staff (Library of the Gesellschaft der Ärzte in Wien)
Dr. Stefan Sienell (archivist of the Academy of Sciences, Vienna)
Hofrat Dr. Gerald Theimer and staff (Austrian State Archives/Allgemeines Verwaltungsarchiv, Vienna)

I would like to thank Brigitte Maurer and Karl Stöckl at the former Bildarchiv des Instituts für Geschichte der Medizin der Universität Wien [Pictorial Archive of the Institute for the History of Medicine of the University of

Vienna] as well as curators Dr. Ruth Koblizek (Picture Collection) and Monika Grass, M. A. (Autograph Archive) of the Collections of the Medical University of Vienna, and last but not least, their present director, Prof. Dr. Christiane Druml.

Hassan Alabass spurred me on to finish the manuscript of this monograph; I would like to offer him special thanks. The lively exchange of ideas with my former colleague at the Institute, University Lecturer Dr. Helmut Gröger, consistently gave me the benefit of his specialist expertise and advice, for which I am deeply grateful. The care, patience, and professional expertise Otmar Binder, M. A. (London), and copy-editor David Sinclair-Jones, M. A. (Oxon.), brought to the task of rendering the German manuscript into English are much appreciated, and I would like to express my profound gratitude to both.

Wherever applicable in an English translation, the original spelling of German quotations has been retained to add to the flavour of authenticity. This becomes something of a problem where Fuchs's spelling of proper names and of the names of cities and places is concerned. To name but one example: in 1949, the official spelling of the French name of the city called Lüttich in German and Luik in Dutch, where Ernst Fuchs served as Chair of Ophthalmology between 1881 and 1885, was changed from Liége, with an acute accent on the first -e-, to Liège with a grave accent.

The Fuchs Stiftung in Salzburg and the FWF in Vienna have provided generous funding for this monograph and its translation, for which I would like to thank them. My thanks also go out to the publishers, the Austrian Academy of Sciences Press, and all their staff who contributed to the realisation of this project.

Abstract

In the early 1900s, Ernst Fuchs (1851–1930) established the Vienna School of Ophthalmology at the top of the international league table in his specialty and was himself considered to be the world's leading ophthalmologist. He came from the school of Ferdinand Ritter von Arlt (1812–1887), who, in the middle years of the nineteenth century, had joined with Carl von Rokitansky (1804–1878) and Josef Škoda (1805–1881) to found the Second Vienna Medical School. Fuchs graduated from Vienna University in 1874, "habilitated" in ophthalmology as Arlt's assistant in 1880 and took charge of the University Eye Clinic of Liège between 1881 and 1885. At the age of thirty-four, Fuchs was recalled to Vienna to become director of the Second University Eye Clinic. Appointed the youngest chair ever at the Medical Faculty of Vienna University, Fuchs devoted himself to his innovative research and teaching activities for three decades, until his resignation in 1915. He broke new ground in several respects both as an academic teacher and researcher. When he was still an assistant at the University Eye Clinic under Arlt, he established antisepsis as pioneered by British surgeon Joseph Lister (1827–1912) in operations and wound treatment. Even before his own "habilitation", in 1878, he taught a private course for American trainee doctors in English. A premiere in the history of Vienna University, this developed into a regular range of courses from 1879, attracting hundreds of doctors from English-speaking countries every year to Vienna to undergo ophthalmological training in a dedicated post-graduate programme.

Fuchs's greatest achievement lay in setting up ophthalmology on the entirely new basis of pathological anatomy. His histological research enabled him to delimit roughly thirty new diseases that bear his name to this day. This was made possible by his vast collection of histological preparations, at the time the largest collection of this kind in the world with more than 40,000 specimens. This collection has survived and is today part of the Sammlungen der Medizinischen Universität Wien. In 1888 Fuchs co-founded the *Wiener klinische Wochenschrift* and made it, among other things, the official mouthpiece of the Gesellschaft der Ärzte. His *Lehrbuch*, first published in German in 1889, went through eighteen editions in German, the last one published in 1945. Translated, sometimes several times, into English, French, Italian, Spanish, Russian, Chinese and Japanese, it became the dominant textbook of this specialty for more than fifty years. Its importance is aptly summed up in its sobriquet, "the Bible of Ophthamology". In 1909, Fuchs inaugurated the worldwide first trachoma ward in a university eye clinic. He was an indefatigable traveller and visited all the world's continents with the exception of Australia. A charismatic teacher, he was invited by his former students and by colleagues to deliver lectures and teach courses all over the world. His sojourns in the United States, Japan, China and South East Asia during the period between the autumn of 1921 and the spring of 1923 are showcased here.

What is of special interest in this bird's eye view of Ernst Fuchs's scientific oeuvre is the question of what intellectual capabilities and work techniques led him to become the innovative researcher he was. Special attention is paid to the faithful reconstruction of the multifaceted observations and the research activities that allowed Fuchs to delimit a multitude of new pathologies.

1. Autobiography

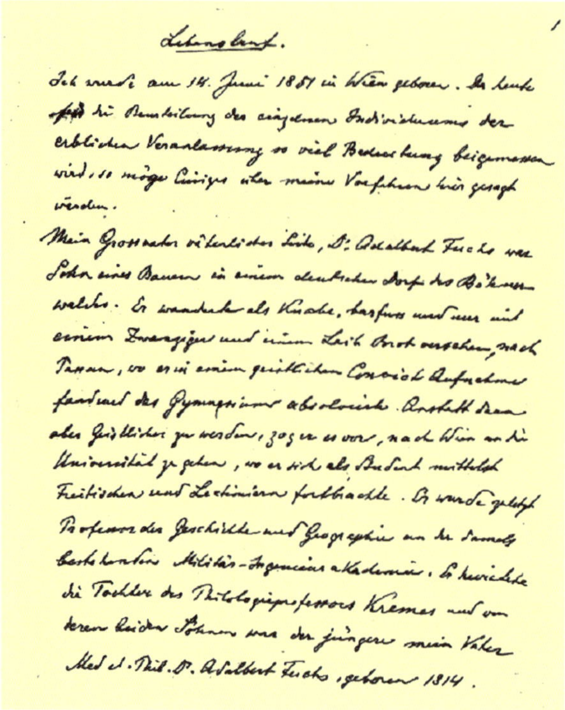
1

Lebenslauf.

Ich wurde am 14. Juni 1851 in Wien geboren. Da heute oft die Beurteilung des einzelnen Individuums der erblichen Veranlassung so viel Bedeutung beigemessen wird, so möge Einiges über meine Vorfahren hier gesagt werden.

Mein Grossvater väterlicher Seite, Dr. Adalbert Fuchs war Sohn eines Bauern in einem deutschen Dorfe des Böhmerwaldes. Er wanderte als Knabe, barfuss und nur mit einem Zwanziger und einem Laib Brot versehen, nach Passau, wo er in einem geistlichen Convict Aufnahme fand und das Gymnasium absolvierte. Anstatt dann aber Geistlicher zu werden, zog er es vor, nach Wien an die Universität zu gehen, wo er sich als Student mittelst Freitischen und Lectionen fortbrachte. Er wurde später Professor der Geschichte und Geographie an der damals bestehenden Militär-Ingenieur-Akademie. Er heiratete die Tochter des Philosophieprofessors Kremes und von deren beiden Söhnen war der jüngere mein Vater Med. et Phil. Dr. Adalbert Fuchs, geboren 1814.

Fig. 1.

Curriculum vitae[1]

I was born in Vienna on 14 June 1851.[2] *As a great deal of weight is attached today to heredity in the assessment of the individual, a few words about my ancestors will not go amiss.*
My grandfather on my father's side, Dr. Adalbert Fuchs,[3] *came from a family of farmers in a German-speaking village in the Bohemian woods.*[4] *From that village he walked barefoot to Passau as a boy, with all of twenty Gulden between him and destitution and nothing more than a loaf of bread to keep him going. He was taken in by a Catholic boarding school. Having obtained his school leaving certificate, he decided against the priesthood and enrolled at the university in Vienna, where he maintained himself by giving lessons and with the help of free meals. He then became a teacher of history and geography at the Militär-Ingenieurakademie* [Academy of Military Engineers], *which was still going in those days.*
He married the daughter of a teacher of philosophy called Kremes,[5] *and the younger of their two sons,*[6] *Dr. med. et phil. Adalbert Fuchs, born in 1814, was my father.*

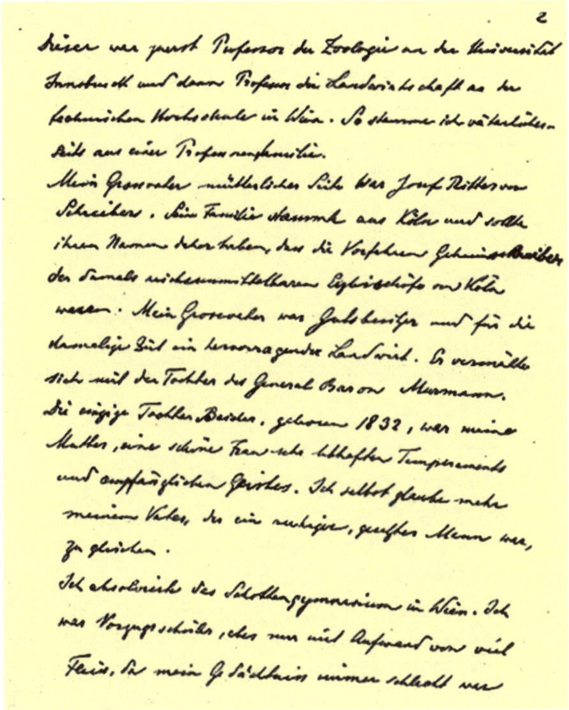

2

Dieser war zuerst Professor der Zoologie an der Universität
Innsbruck und dann Professor der Landwirtschaft an der
technischen Hochschule in Wien. So stamme ich väterlicher-
seits aus einer Professorenfamilie.
Mein Grossvater mütterlicher Seite war Josef Ritter von
Schreibers. Seine Familie stammt aus Köln und sollte
ihren Namen daher haben, dass die Vorfahren Geheimschreiber
der damals reichsunmittelbaren Erzbischöfe von Köln
waren. Mein Grossvater war Gutsbesitzer und für die
damalige Zeit ein hervorragender Landwirt. Er vermählte
sich mit der Tochter des General Baron Murmann.
Die einzige Tochter Beider, geboren 1832, war meine
Mutter, eine schöne Frau sehr lebhaften Temperaments
und empfänglichen Geistes. Ich selbst glaube mehr
meinem Vater, der ein ruhiger, gesetzter Mann war,
zu gleichen.
Ich absolvierte das Schottengymnasium in Wien. Ich
war Vorzugsschüler, aber nur mit Aufwand von viel
Fleiss, da mein Gedächtnis immer schlecht war

Fig. 2.

After a spell as Professor of Zoology at the University of Innsbruck, Adalbert was appointed Chair of Agriculture at Vienna's Technical University. On my father's side, I therefore come from a family of university professors.
My grandfather on my mother's side was Josef Ritter von Schreibers.[7] *His family originally hailed from Cologne and their name can be traced to their ancestors' connection to the private secretaries of the archbishops of Cologne, who at that stage enjoyed imperial immediacy* [a privileged constitutional and political status rooted in German feudal law]. *Being an outstanding agriculturalist by the standards of the time, my grandfather managed his estate himself. He married the daughter of General Baron Murmann.*[8] *Their only daughter, born in 1832, was my mother,*[9] *a beautiful woman with a very lively temper and an outgoing disposition. I myself believe that I take more after my quiet, staid father.*
I obtained my school leaving certificate from the Schottengymnasium in Vienna.[10] *I was near the top of my form, a position I had to work very hard for, as my memory has always been rather poor.*

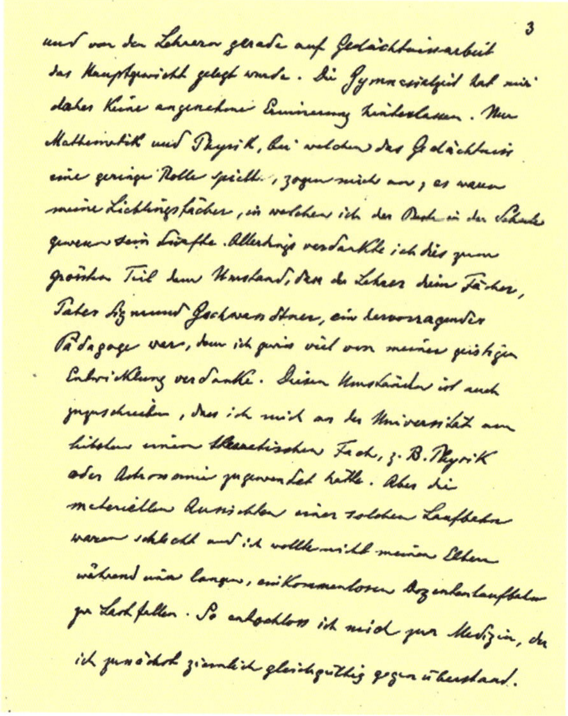

3

und von den Lehrern gerade auf Gedächtnisarbeit das Hauptgewicht gelegt wurde. Die Gymnasialzeit hat mir daher keine angenehme Erinnerung hinterlassen. Nur Mathematik und Physik, bei welchen das Gedächtnis eine geringe Rolle spielt, zogen mich an, es waren meine Lieblingsfächer, in welchen ich der Beste in der Schule gewesen sein dürfte. Allerdings verdankte ich dies zum größten Teil dem Umstand, daß der Lehrer dieser Fächer, Pater Sigmund Gschwandtner, ein hervorragender Pädagoge war, dem ich ganz viel von meiner geistigen Entwicklung verdanke. Diesem Umstande ist auch zuzuschreiben, daß ich mich an der Universität am liebsten einem theoretischen Fach, z. B. Physik oder Astronomie zugewendet hätte. Aber die materiellen Aussichten einer solchen Laufbahn waren schlecht und ich wollte nicht meinen Eltern während einer langen, einkommenlosen Dozentenlaufbahn zur Last fallen. So entschloss ich mich zur Medizin, der ich zunächst ziemlich gleichgültig gegenüberstand.

Fig. 3.

As a rule, it was feats of memory that counted most in the eyes of the teachers. Grammar school has therefore not left me with particularly pleasant memories. The only subjects that attracted me were mathematics and physics, where memory only plays a minor role; they were my favourite subjects and I was probably second to no other pupil at the school. However, I owed this largely to the fact that the man who taught these subjects, Pater Sigmund Gschwandtner,[11] *was an exceptionally gifted teacher, whom I have to thank in great part for my intellectual development. His influence can also be seen in my initial inclination towards physics, astronomy or some other theoretical course of study at university. However, the material prospects for such a career were poor and I did not want to be a burden on my parents during a long period of study with no income attached. This is why I decided in favour of medicine, a course of study of little real interest to me to begin with.*

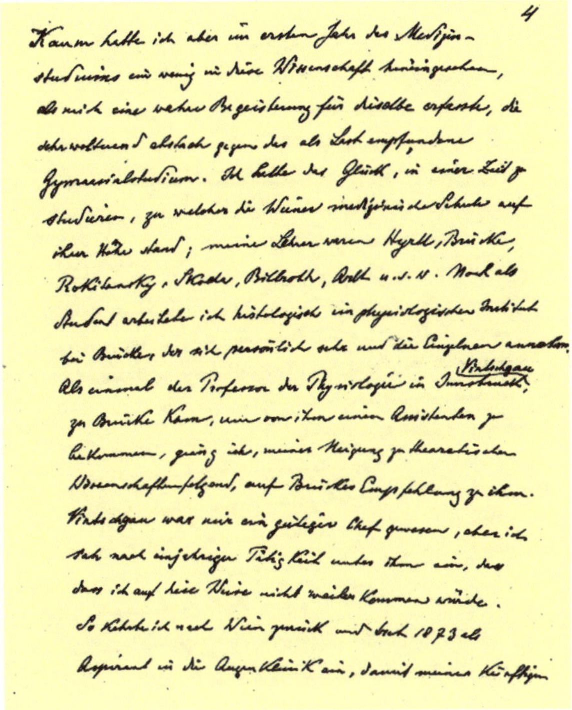
4

Kaum hatte ich aber im ersten Jahr des Medizin-
studiums ein wenig in diese Wissenschaft hineingesehen,
als mich eine wahre Begeisterung für dieselbe erfasste, die
sehr wohltuend abstach gegen das als Last empfundene
Gymnasialstudium. Ich hatte das Glück, in einer Zeit zu
studieren, zu welcher die Wiener medizinische Schule auf
ihrer Höhe stand; meine Lehrer waren Hyrtl, Brücke,
Rokitansky, Skoda, Billroth, Arlt u.s.w. Noch als
Student arbeitete ich histologisch im physiologischen Institut
bei Brücke, der sich persönlich sehr um die Einzelnen annahm.
Als einmal der Professor der Physiologie in ~~Innsbruck~~ Vintschgau
zu Brücke kam, um von ihm einen Assistenten zu
bekommen, ging ich, meiner Neigung zu theoretischen
Wissenschaften folgend, auf Brückes Empfehlung zu ihm.
Vintschgau war mir ein gütiger Chef gewesen, aber ich
sah nach einjähriger Tätigkeit unter ihm ein, dass
ich auf diese Weise nicht weiter kommen würde.
So kehrte ich nach Wien zurück und trat 1873 als
Aspirant in die Augenklinik ein, damit meinen künftigen

Fig. 4.

When I actually took stock of medicine during my first year at university, I was gripped by genuine enthusiasm. This was in contrast with my time at the grammar school, which had been little more than drudgery. I was fortunate to be studying at a time when the Vienna Medical School[12] *was at its peak; my teachers were Hyrtl,*[13] *Brücke,*[14] *Rokitansky,*[15] *Škoda,*[16] *Billroth,*[17] *Arlt,*[18] *etc. As a student I did histological work at the Institute of Physiology under Brücke, who personally took care of every individual student. When the Professor of Physiology at Innsbruck University, Vintschgau,*[19] *contacted Brücke in his search for an assistant, Brücke recommended me; I accepted the offer, in the hope that it would allow me to indulge my interest in theoretical science. Vintschgau proved a kindly superior but after a year I realised that I was not making any progress. I therefore returned to Vienna and in 1873 I joined the Eye Clinic as an aspirant* [a doctoral candidate], *thereby committing to my future*

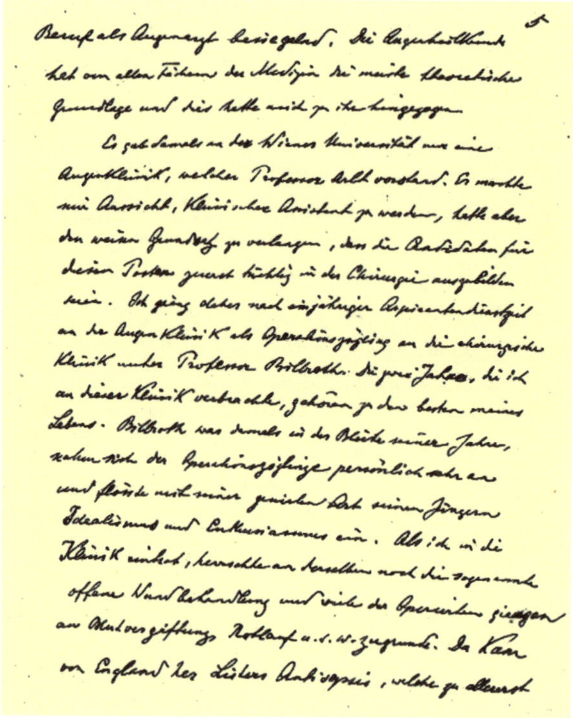
5
Beruf als Augenarzt besiegelt. Die Augenheilkunde
hat von allen Fächern der Medizin die meiste theoretische
Grundlage und dies hatte mich zu ihr hingezogen.
Es gab damals an der Wiener Universität nur eine
Augenklinik, welcher Professor Arlt vorstand. Er machte
mir Aussicht, klinischer Assistent zu werden, hatte aber
den weisen Grundsatz zu verlangen, dass die Anwärter für
diesen Posten zuerst tüchtig in der Chirurgie ausgebildet
sein. Ich ging daher nach einjährigem Aspirantendienst
an der Augenklinik als Operationszögling an die chirurgische
Klinik unter Professor Billroth. Die zwei Jahre, die ich
an dieser Klinik verbrachte, gehören zu den besten meines
Lebens. Billroth war damals in der Blüte seiner Jahre,
nahm sich der Operationszöglinge persönlich sehr an
und flösste mit seiner genialen Art seinen Jüngern
Idealismus und Enthusiasmus ein. Als ich in die
Klinik eintrat, herrschte an derselben noch die sogenannte
offene Wundbehandlung und viele der Operierten gingen
an Blutvergiftung, Rotlauf u.s.w. zugrunde. Da kam
von England her Listers Antisepsis, welche zu allererst

Fig. 5.

as an eye specialist. Of all medical disciplines, ophthalmology is most strongly grounded in theory and this is why I found it so attractive.
There was at that time only one Eye Clinic at the University of Vienna, presided over by Professor Arlt. He offered me the chance to become a clinical assistant so long as I was willing to undergo thorough training as a surgeon. So after my year as an aspirant in the Eye Clinic I joined Professor Billroth's surgical clinic as a trainee surgeon.[20] *The two years I spent at this clinic are among the best in my life. Billroth was then at the height of his powers. He took a personal interest in his trainee surgeons and his genius inspired these disciples of his with idealism and enthusiasm. When I joined the clinic, what was known as open wound treatment was still predominant and many operation patients died of blood poisoning, erysipelas, and other such conditions. Then Lister's*[21] *antisepsis arrived from England,*[22] *to be*

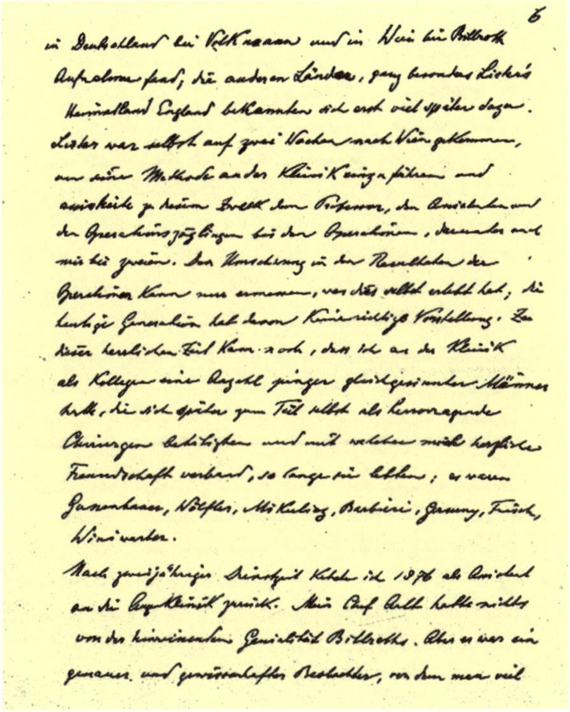
6
in Deutschland bei Volkmann und in Wien bei Billroth
Aufnahme fand; die anderen Länder, ganz besonders Lister's
Heimatland England bekannten sich erst viel später dazu.
Lister war selbst auf zwei Wochen nach Wien gekommen,
um seine Methode an der Klinik einzuführen und
assistierte zu diesem Zweck dem Professor, den Assistenten und
den Operationszöglingen bei den Operationen, darunter auch
mir bei zweien. Den Umschwung in den Resultaten der
Operationen kann nur ermessen, wer dies selbst erlebt hat; die
heutige Generation hat davon keine richtige Vorstellung. Zu
dieser herrlichen Zeit kam noch, dass ich an der Klinik
als Kollegen eine Anzahl junger gleichgesinnter Männer
hatte, die sich später zum Teil selbst als hervorragende
Chirurgen betätigten und mit welchen mich herzliche
Freundschaft verband, so lange sie lebten; es waren
Gussenbauer, Wölfler, Mikulicz, Barbieri, Gersuny, Frisch,
Winiwarter.
Nach zweijähriger Dienstzeit kehrte ich 1876 als Assistent
an die Augenklinik zurück. Mein Chef Arlt hatte nichts
von der hinreissenden Genialität Billroths. Aber er war ein
genauer und gewissenhafter Beobachter, von dem man viel

Fig. 6.

accepted first by Volkmann[23] in Germany and by Billroth in Vienna; other countries, especially Lister's own native country, England, did not follow until much later. Lister himself had come to Vienna for two weeks[24,25] to acquaint the clinic with his method. For this purpose, he assisted the professor, the assistants and the trainee surgeons, including me twice, in operations. The overwhelming turnaround in results can only be appreciated by those with direct experience; today's generation cannot possibly understand.[26] This wonderful time was made even more splendid by the fact that I was working at the clinic with a number of like-minded young colleagues, some of whom were themselves to go on to become outstanding surgeons and remain connected to me by ties of cordial, lifelong friendship. Amongst these I count Gussenbauer,[27] Wölfler,[28] Mikulicz,[29] Barbieri,[30] Gersuny,[31] Frisch,[32] and Winiwarter.[33]

Having completed my two-year period of service, I returned to Vienna's Eye Clinic in 1876 as a clinical assistant. Arlt, my superior, lacked Billroth's infectious ingenuity.[34] He was, however, a precise and conscientious observer, from whom a lot

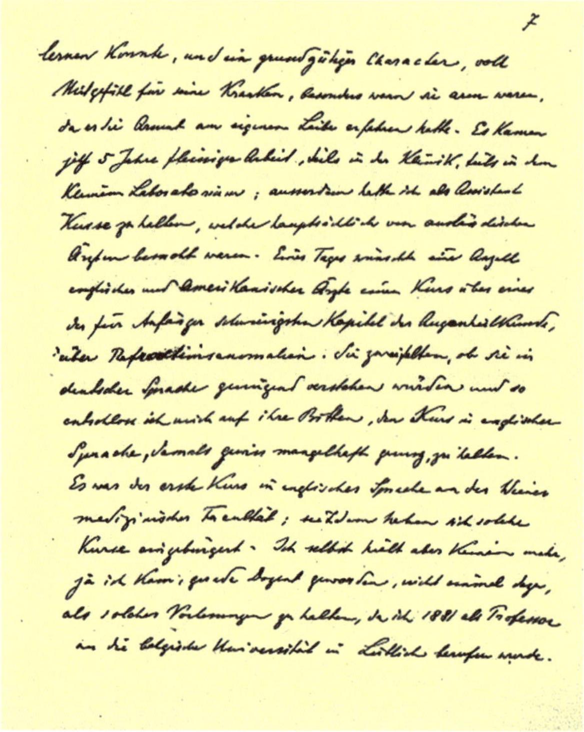

7

lernen konnte, und ein grundgütiger Character, voll
Mitgefühl für seine Kranken, besonders wenn sie arm waren,
da er die Armut am eigenen Leibe erfahren hatte. Es kamen
jetzt 5 Jahre fleissiger Arbeit, theils in der Klinik, theils in dem
kleinen Laboratorium; ausserdem hatte ich als Assistent
Kurse zu halten, welche hauptsächlich von ausländischen
Ärzten besucht waren. Eines Tages wünschte eine Anzahl
englischer und amerikanischer Ärzte einen Kurs über eines
der für Anfänger schwierigsten Kapitel der Augenheilkunde,
über Refraktionsanomalien. Sie zweifelten, ob sie in
deutscher Sprache genügend verstehen würden und so
entschloss ich mich auf ihre Bitten, den Kurs in englischer
Sprache, damals gewiss mangelhaft genug, zu halten.
Es war der erste Kurs in englischer Sprache an der Wiener
medizinischen Fakultät; seitdem haben sich solche
Kurse eingebürgert. Ich selbst hielt aber keinen mehr,
ja ich kam, gerade Dozent geworden, nicht einmal dazu,
als solcher Vorlesungen zu halten, da ich 1881 als Professor
an die belgische Universität in Lüttich berufen wurde.

Fig. 7.

could be learnt, and was a man notable for his kindness, full of sympathy for his patients, especially if they happened to be poor, having himself learnt the lesson of poverty the hard way. What followed now were five years of demanding work, partly at the Clinic, partly in the small lab. In addition, my duties as a clinical assistant included giving courses which were mainly frequented by medical doctors from abroad. One day a group of English and American doctors expressed interest in a course in an area of ophthalmology that is one of the most difficult for beginners, the anomalies of refraction. They doubted that their German was good enough for them to be able to follow. I therefore decided to give the course in English, even though my command of that language was at that time by no means perfect. This was the first course given in English at Vienna's Medical Faculty; since then they have become a fixture.[35] *I myself did not give any more such courses and, what is more, though I had just been appointed lecturer,*[36] *I was not to have the chance to make further use of my new skill: in 1881 I was given a chair at the Belgian University of Liège.*[37]

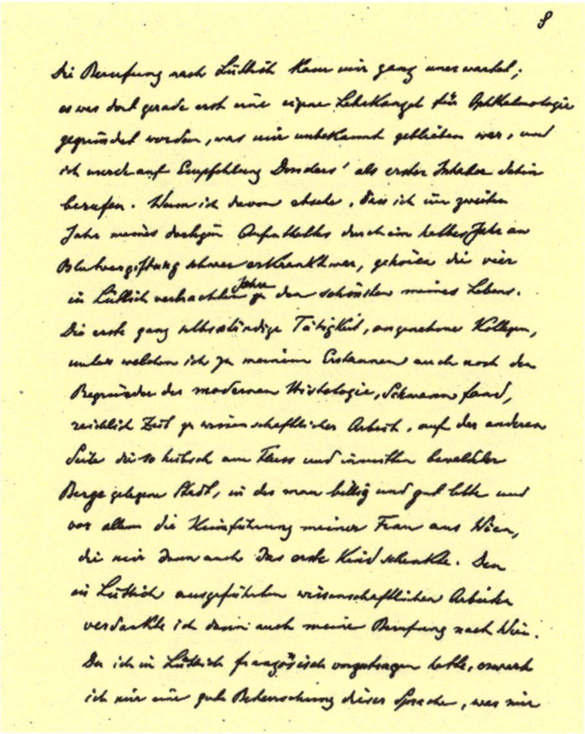
8
Die Berufung nach Lüttich kam mir ganz unerwartet;
es war dort gerade erst eine eigene Lehrkanzel für Ophthalmologie
gegründet worden, was mir unbekannt geblieben war, und
ich wurde auf Empfehlung Donders' als erster Inhaber dahin
berufen. Wenn ich davon absehe, dass ich im zweiten
Jahre meines dortigen Aufenthaltes durch ein halbes Jahr an
Blutvergiftung schwer erkrankt war, gehören die vier
in Lüttich verbrachten Jahre zu den schönsten meines Lebens.
Die erste ganz selbständige Tätigkeit, angenehme Kollegen,
unter welchen ich zu meinem Erstaunen auch noch den
Begründer der modernen Histologie, Schwann, fand,
reichlich Zeit zu wissenschaftlicher Arbeit, auf der anderen
Seite die so hübsch am Fluss und inmitten bewaldeter
Berge gelegene Stadt, in der man billig und gut lebte und
vor allem die Heimführung meiner Frau aus Wien,
die mir dann auch das erste Kind schenkte. Den
in Lüttich ausgeführten wissenschaftlichen Arbeiten
verdankte ich dann auch meine Berufung nach Wien.
Da ich in Lüttich französisch vorgetragen hatte, erwarb
ich mir eine gute Beherrschung dieser Sprache, was mir

Fig. 8.

The call to Liège came completely out of the blue. The chair of ophthalmology had been established there only very recently. I had not been aware of this, but at Donders'[38] *recommendation I was appointed as its first occupant. Even taking into account six months of serious illness from blood poisoning in the second year of my stay,*[39] *the four years I spent in Liège must rank among the best in my life. For the first time I was solely responsible for all that I did; I had pleasant colleagues, among whom I found to my astonishment Schwann,*[40] *the founder of modern histology, I had plenty of time for scientific work, and the very location of the city, situated as it is on the banks of the river, surrounded by wooded hills, where it is easy to live well at moderate expense, was a joy to me. Most importantly of all, there was the reunion with my wife, who joined me from Vienna, and then made me the gift of our first child.*[41] *It is to the scientific work I did in Liège that I owe the call to Vienna. As I had to give my lectures in Liège in French, I acquired a good command of this language, which*

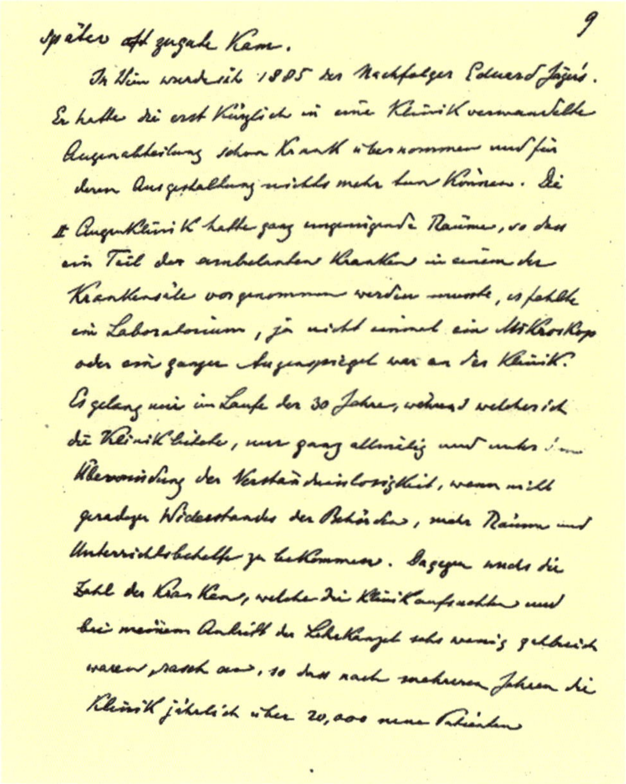
später oft zugute kam. 9
In Wien wurde ich 1885 der Nachfolger Eduard Jägers.
Er hatte die erst kürzlich in eine Klinik verwandelte
Augenabteilung schon krank übernommen und für
deren Ausgestaltung nichts mehr tun können. Die
II. Augenklinik hatte ganz ungenügende Räume, so dass
ein Teil der ambulanten Kranken in einem der
Krankensäle vorgenommen werden musste, es fehlte
ein Laboratorium, ja nicht einmal ein Mikroskop
oder ein ganzer Augenspiegel war an der Klinik.
Es gelang mir im Laufe der 30 Jahre, während welcher ich
die Klinik leitete, nur ganz allmälig und unter [illegible]
Überwindung der Verständnislosigkeit, wenn nicht
geradezu Widerstandes der Behörden, mehr Räume und
Unterrichtsbehelfe zu bekommen. Dagegen wuchs die
Zahl der Kranken, welche die Klinik aufsuchten und
bei meinem Antritt der Lehrkanzel sehr wenig zahlreich
waren, rasch an, so dass nach mehreren Jahren die
Klinik jährlich über 20,000 neue Patienten

Fig. 9.

stood me in good stead later on.
In Vienna I succeeded Eduard Jäger[42] *in 1885. By the time he took over the Eye Department, which had been transformed into a clinic only a short time before, he was already seriously ill, which rendered him unable to do anything towards its proper appointment. The rooms that housed the Second Eye Clinic were totally inadequate, leaving some outpatients to be treated in one of the* [other] *wards. Not only was there no laboratory, there was not so much as a microscope or a fully functioning ophthalmoscope to be found anywhere in the clinic. During the thirty years I was head of the clinic I managed only gradually to overcome the lack of understanding, if not the downright obstinacy of the authorities and to acquire more space and more teaching aids. Conversely, the number of patients turning to the Clinic for help, of whom there had only been very few at the time I became chair, grew rapidly so that after a few years the clinic was welcoming more than 20,000 new patients every year, and*

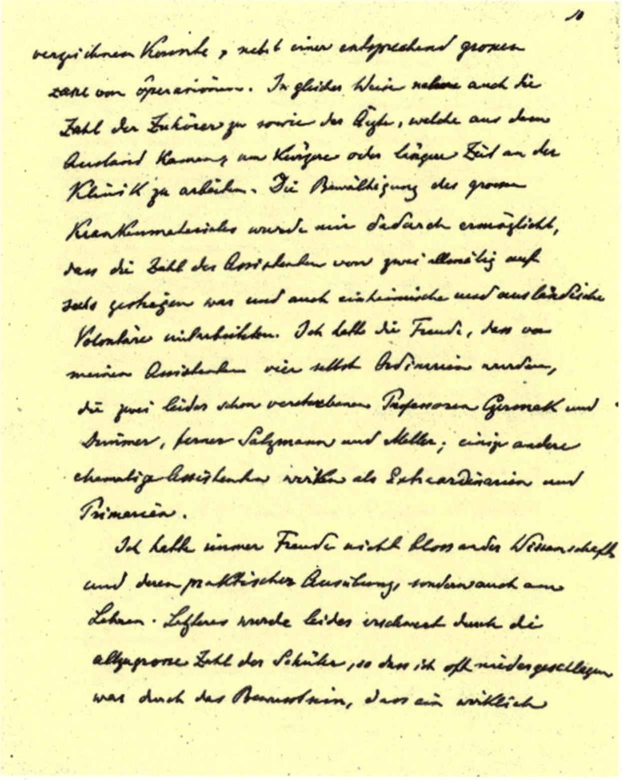
10
vergrösserten Klinik, nebst einer entsprechend grossen
Zahl von Operationen. In gleicher Weise nahm auch die
Zahl der Zuhörer zu sowie der Ärzte, welche aus dem
Ausland kamen, um kürzere oder längere Zeit an der
Klinik zu arbeiten. Die Bewältigung des grossen
Krankenmaterials wurde nur dadurch ermöglicht,
dass die Zahl der Assistenten von zwei allmälig auf
sechs gestiegen war und auch einheimische und ausländische
Volontäre mitarbeiteten. Ich hatte die Freude, dass von
meinen Assistenten vier selbst Ordinarien wurden,
die zwei leider schon verstorbenen Professoren Czermak und
Dimmer, ferner Salzmann und Meller; einige andere
ehemalige Assistenten wirken als Extraordinarien und
Primarien.

Ich hatte immer Freude nicht bloss an der Wissenschaft
und deren praktischer Ausübung, sondern auch am
Lehren. Letzteres wurde leider erschwert durch die
allzugrosse Zahl der Schüler, so dass ich oft niedergeschlagen
war durch das Bewusstsein, dass ein wirklich

Fig. 10.

conducting a correspondingly great number of operations. Similarly, the number of students and the number of medical doctors who had come from abroad to work at the clinic for a shorter or longer spell was growing all the time. Coping with this massive influx was made possible by a gradual increase in the number of assistants from two to six and by both Austrian and foreign volunteers undertaking additional work. To my great joy, four of my assistants went on to become full professors: Professors Czermak[43] and Dimmer,[44] both of whom have since regretfully passed away, and Salzmann[45] and Meller.[46] Others of my former assistants are now active as associate professors and chief physicians.

I have always taken great pleasure not only in science and its practical application but also in teaching. The latter was unfortunately made more difficult by the excessive number of students so that I often felt downcast, knowing in my heart that truly

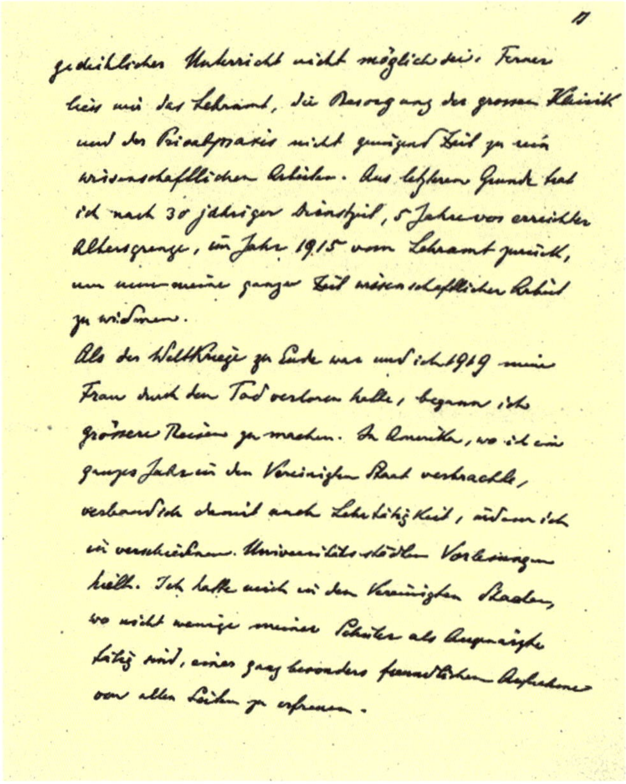
17

gedeihlicher Unterricht nicht möglich sei. Ferner
ließ mir das Lehramt, die Besorgung der grossen Klinik
und der Privatpraxis nicht genügend Zeit zu rein
wissenschaftlichen Arbeiten. Aus letzterem Grunde trat
ich nach 30jähriger Dienstzeit, 5 Jahre vor erreichter
Altersgrenze, im Jahr 1915 vom Lehramt zurück,
um nun meine ganze Zeit wissenschaftlicher Arbeit
zu widmen.
Als der Weltkrieg zu Ende war und ich 1919 meine
Frau durch den Tod verloren hatte, begann ich
grössere Reisen zu machen. In Amerika, wo ich ein
ganzes Jahr in den Vereinigten Staaten verbrachte,
verband ich damit auch Lehrtätigkeit, indem ich
in verschiedenen Universitätsstädten Vorlesungen
hielt. Ich hatte mich in den Vereinigten Staaten,
wo nicht wenige meiner Schüler als Augenärzte
tätig sind, einer ganz besonders freundlichen Aufnahme
von allen Seiten zu erfreuen.

Fig. 11.

instructive classes were not possible in such circumstances. Furthermore, teaching and attending to both the large clinic and my private practice did not leave me enough time for purely scientific work. It was with the idea of devoting all my time to scientific work that I resigned from the clinic in 1915, after thirty years' service but with five years still to go before the prescribed retirement age.
Following the death of my wife in 1919, shortly after the end of the World War,[47] *I began to spend longer spells travelling abroad. In America, where I spent an entire year in the United States, I combined this with teaching, lecturing in various university cities.*[48] *In the States, where a great number of my students are now active as eye specialists, I was given an especially friendly reception by all concerned.*

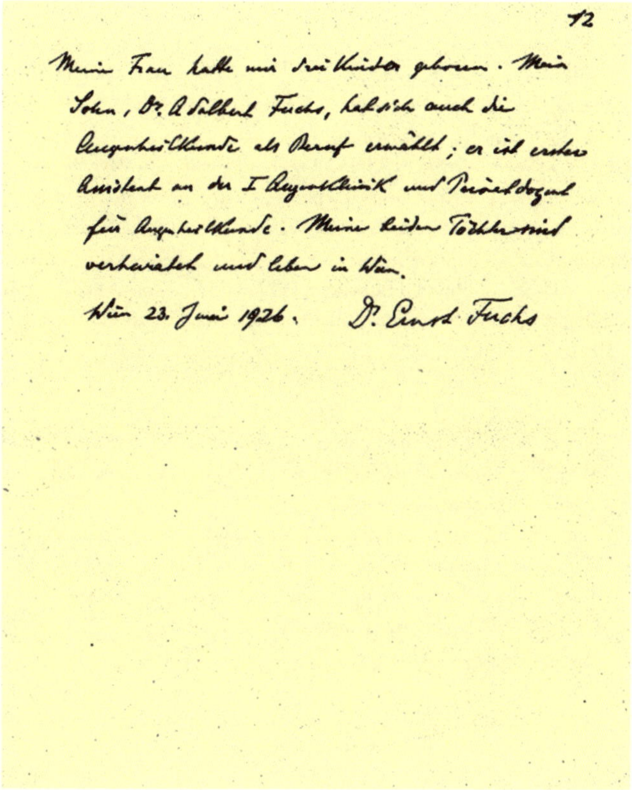
12

Meine Frau hatte mir drei Kinder geboren. Mein Sohn, Dr. Adalbert Fuchs, hat sich auch die Augenheilkunde als Beruf erwählt; er ist erster Assistent an der I Augenklinik und Privatdozent für Augenheilkunde. Meine beiden Töchter sind verheiratet und leben in Wien.

Wien 23. Juni 1926. Dr. Ernst Fuchs

Fig. 12.

My wife presented me with three children. My son, Dr. Adalbert Fuchs,[49] *has also chosen ophthalmology as a profession; he is First Assistant at the First Eye Clinic and Private Lecturer in Ophthalmology. My two daughters*[50] *are married and live in Vienna.*

Vienna, 23 June 1926. *Dr. Ernst Fuchs*

Notes

1 Facsimile & transcription of this autograph of Ernst Fuchs's own account of his life, dating from 25 June 1926. (Library and Archive of the Austr. Acad. of Sciences). I am indebted to the Presidium of the Austrian Academy of Sciences for the permission to publish this document for the first time.

2 Adalbert FUCHS (ed.), Ernst FUCHS. *Wie ein Augenarzt die Welt sah. Selbstbiographie und Tagebuchblätter*. Urban & Schwarzenberg, Vienna 1946, p. 21.

3 Adalbertus Fux (Fuchs) (22 March 1779 –12 Dec. 1854). Cf.: Ahnenpass of Wilhelm Raimund Hofbauer, Dr. med. habil., Vienna IX, Spitalgasse 17, p. 20. Original in the Family archive. Wilhelm Hofbauer (1911–1969), Ernst Fuchs's grandson, was a dermatologist. See: Personalakt Wilhelm Hofbauer. Archiv d. Univ. Wien [= UA Wien], fols. 1–205.

4 Rabits/Rabitz nr. Winterberg (today Vimperk/Czech Republic). The distance is roughly 80 km. See: FUCHS, *Augenarzt* (as in FN 2), p. 15, FN 1.

5 Theresia Ferdinanda Fuchs, née Cremes (11 March 1785–5 April 1839). Marriage 8 Nov. 1813 Wien Innere Stadt, RC Parish St. Augustin, Tom. VIII, fol. 133. See: Ahnenpass Hofbauer (as in FN 3), p. 20.

6 The elder son Carl (Edl. v.) Fuchs (d. 1 Aug. 1881) was also a medical doctor (Dr. med. et chir., Mag. obstetr.). The younger son, Adalbert Nikolaus Fuchs (5 June 1814–7 Jan. 1886) was the father of the ophthalmologist Ernst Josef Fuchs. See: Ahnenpass Hofbauer (as in FN 3), p. 14, and Family archive. See Ch. 2.

7 Josef Ludwig Ritter v. Schreibers (9 Sept. 1793 – 15 Feb. 1874). Cf.: Ahnenpass Hofbauer (as in FN 3), p. 21; Raimund HOFBAUER, *Der Edelhof zu Kritzendorf.* Version dated 10 March 1996, accessible at: http://www.komitee-kritzendorf.com/dorfmuseum-kritzendorf/archiv/44-archivtexte. See Ch. 2.

8 Anna Maria, geb. Murmann v. Marchfeld (24 May 1808 – 2 Oct. 1881). Marriage 12 Feb. 1829/Nieder-Hollabrunn. See: Ahnenpass Hofbauer (as in FN 3), p. 21.

9 Isabella Anna Fuchs, née v. Schreibers (2 Aug. 1832 – 15 Feb. 1902). Marriage 10 Sept. 1850/Kritzendorf. See: Ahnenpass Hofbauer (as in FN 3), S. 14.

10 For the four years of primary school and the first two years of grammar school Ernst and brother Wilhelm were schooled at home. In the autumn of 1860 Ernst was enrolled at the Gymnasium Unsere liebe Frau zu den Schotten, a grammar school run by the Benedictine order in what is today Vienna's 1st District. Their father had attended the same school. Cf.: FUCHS, *Augenarzt* (as in FN 2), p. 22. See Ch. 2.

11 The spelling of this scholar's first and second names varied during his lifetime and in later years. The following variants can be found: "Sigmund Gschwandtner", in: *Schriften des Vereins zur Verbreitung naturwissenschaftlicher Kenntnisse in Wien*. 1. vol., year 1860/61. Carl Gerold's Sohn, Vienna 1862, p. XVII; "Sigismund Gschwandner", in: Albert HÜBL, *Geschichte des Unterrichtes im Stifte Schotten in Wien. Herausgegeben anläszlich der Zentenarfeier des k. k. Schottengymnasiums*. Carl Fromme, Vienna 1907, pp. 186–188; Hans CHIARI, *Eine Erinnerung an Prof. Sigismund Gschwandner*, in: Heinrich Ritter v. WITTEK (ed.), *Festgabe zum 100jährigen Jubiläum des Schottengymnasiums gewidmet von ehemaligen Schottenschülern*. Wilhelm Braumüller, Vienna 1907, pp. 36–38; "Sigismund Gschwandtner", in: FUCHS, *Augenarzt* (as in FN 2), p. 28: *"The best among them was Sigismund Gschwandtner, who taught mathematics and physics. Those were my favourite subjects and I was his favourite student."*

Sigismund (Matthias) Gschwandner (1824–1896): attended Vienna's Schottengymnasiums, 1844 joined the Benedictine Order at the Schottenstift, 1845 PhD Vienna Univ., 1849 priestly ordination. 1850–1880 teacher of mathematics, physics and philosophical propaedeutics at the Schottengymnasium (headmaster 1886–1895). As a teacher, he drew on his thorough grounding in the sciences. Cf.: Leo SANTIFALLER/ Eva OBERMAYER-MARNACH (eds.), *Österreichisches Biographisches Lexikon 1815–1950* [ÖBL]. Herausgegeben von der Österreichischen Akademie der Wissenschaften. Hermann Böhlaus Nachfolger, Graz/Cologne 1957ff.

12 Cf.: Erna LESKY, *Die Wiener Medizinische Schule im 19. Jahrhundert*. 2nd ed. Böhlau, Graz/Cologne 1978.

13 Joseph Hyrtl (1810–1894). Originally from Eisenstadt, then part of Hungary. Grad. of Vienna Univ. (Dr. med. 1835). 1837–1845 Full Prof. of Anatomy at Prague Univ. and 1845–1874 at Vienna Univ. 1850 Foundation of the Museum of Comparat. Anat., enlargement of the Museum of Hum. Anat. Outstanding didactic skills, which enabled him to pass on his profound knowledge to his students to prepare them for the medical profession. At his instigation, topographical anatomy was made part of the med. curriculum. Introduction of corrosion and injection techniques to diversify anatom. preparations. Rector of Vienna Univ. 1864/65. Hon. doctorates awarded by the Univ. of Leipzig and Moscow. Vehemently opposed to materialism as an ideology. Remarkable social commitment (establishment of an orphanage and children's home in Perchtoldsdorf and of a church in Mödling). Support for gifted medical students in need through a bequest of 400,000 Gulden. Cf.: Felix CZEIKE, *Historisches Lexikon Wien in 5 Bänden*. Vol. 3. Kremayr & Scheriau, Vienna 1994; Ludwig EISENBERG, *Das geistige Wien. Künstler-und Schriftsteller-Lexikon*. Vol. 2. *Medicinisch-naturwissenschaftlicher Theil*. C. Daberkow, Vienna 1893; Hans-Heinz EULNER, *Die Entwicklung der medizinischen Spezialfächer an den Universitäten des deutschen Sprachgebietes* [= Studien zur Medizingeschichte des neunzehnten Jahrhunderts, vol. IV]. Ferdinand Enke, Stuttgart 1970; Werner E. GERABEK, Bernhard D. HAAGE, Gundolf KEIL, Wolfgang WEGNER (eds.), *Enzyklopädie Medizingeschichte*. Walter de Gruyter, Berlin 2005; ÖBL (as in FN 11); August HIRSCH (ed.), *Biographisches Lexikon der hervorragenden Aerzte aller Zeiten und Völker*. Urban & Schwarzenberg, Vienna/ Leipzig 1886 [Reprint Martino Publishing, Mansfield 2002]; Julius PAGEL (ed.), *Biographisches Lexikon hervorragender Ärzte des neunzehnten Jahrhunderts. Mit einer historischen Einleitung*. Urban & Schwarzenberg, Berlin/Vienna 1901 [Reprint Karger, Leipzig 1989]; LESKY, *Wien. Med. Schule* (as in FN 12), pp. 240–246; Rudolf-Josef GASSER, *Der Anatom Joseph Hyrtl 1810–1894*. Wilhelm Maudrich, Vienna/Munich/ Bern 1991. See Ch. 2.

14 Ernst Wilhelm Ritter von Brücke (1819–1892). Originally from Stralsund, studied at the Univ. of Berlin and Heidelberg (Dr. med. et chir. 1842, Berlin), 1843 Assist. at the Museum of Comparat. Anat. and prosector at the Anat. Inst. of Berlin Univ. under the direction of the outstanding natural scientist Johannes Müller (1801–1858). 1844 Habilitation in Physiol., 1846 Professor of Anat. at the Akad. f. bild. Künste in Berlin. 1847 Assoc. Prof. of Physiol. and General Pathol. at Königsberg Univ. At Hyrtl's instigation (cf. FN 13) 1849–1890 Full Prof. of Physiol. and Microscop. Anat. [i.e. Histology] at Vienna Univ. The most well-rounded physiol. of his time. 1868/69 the first Protestant (Augsb. Conf.) dean of Vienna's Med. Faculty. 1879/80 Rector of

Vienna Univ. Cf. CZEIKE; EISENBERG 2; EULNER; GERABEK et al.; HIRSCH (as in FN 13); ÖBL (as in FN 11); PAGEL (as in FN 13); LESKY, *Wien. Med. Schule* (as in FN 12), pp. 258–268. See Ch. 2.

15 Carl (Karl) Freiherr von Rokitansky (1804–1878). Originally from Königgrätz/Bohemia (today Hradec Králové/Czech Republic). Studied at the Univ. of Prague and Vienna (Dr. med. 1828). Started out as unsalaried prosector, from 1831 assist. at the Pathol.-Anat. Inst. of Vienna Univ. 1834 Assoc Prof., 1844–1875 Full Prof. of Pathol. Anat. From 1843 influential medical adviser at the Minist. f. Cultus u. Unterricht. Dean of the Med. Fac. of Vienna Univ. 1849/1850, 1856/1857, 1859/1860, 1862/1863). 1852/1853 Rector of Vienna Univ., Real Member of the Austr. Acad. of Sciences [ÖAW], Vicepres. 1866–1869, Pres. 1869/1870. As the proponent of pathomorphol. on a descriptive basis he laid the foundations, together with clinician Joseph Škoda (see below) and dermatologist Ferdinand Ritter v. Hebra (1816–1880, cf. FN 163), for the Second Vienna Medical School. By rejecting natural philosophy and jointly grounding pathol. anat. and clin. medicine on a scientific basis, the Second Viennese Medical School achieved worldwide recognition. Radical proponent of the freedom of scientific research. Cf.: CZEIKE; EISENBERG 2; EULNER; GERABEK et al. (as in FN 13); HIRSCH (as in FN 13); *Neue Deutsche Biographie* [= NDB]. Ed. by the Historical Commission of the Academy of Sciences and Humanities, vol. 8. Duncker & Humblot, Berlin; ÖBL (as in FN 11)*)*; PAGEL (as in FN 13); Constant von WURZBACH, *Biographisches Lexikon des Kaiserthums Oesterreich, enthaltend die Lebensskizzen der denkwürdigen Personen, welche seit 1750 in den oesterreichischen Kronländern geboren wurden oder darin gelebt und gewirkt haben*. Verlag d. Univ.-Buchdruckerei L. C. Zamarski, Vienna 1856–1891 (60 vols); LESKY, *Wien. Med. Schule* (as in FN 12), pp. 129–141; Max NEUBURGER, "Rokitansky als Vorkämpfer der mechanistischen Forschungsmethode und der idealistischen Weltanschauung", in: *Wien. klin. Wochenschr.* 47 (1934), p. 359; Helmut RUMPLER, Helmut DENK (eds.), *Carl Freiherr von Rokitansky 1804–1878. Pathologe, Politiker, Philosoph, Gründer der Wiener Medizinischen Schule des 19. Jahrhunderts*. Vienna, Böhlau 2005; Gabriela SCHMIDT, "Rokitansky als Pathophilosoph", in: *Sudhoffs Archiv* 89 (2005), pp. 170–195; Felicitas SEEBACHER, *"Freiheit der Naturforschung!"*. Carl Freiherr von Rokitansky und die Wiener Medizinische Schule: Wissenschaft und Politik im Konflikt. Math.-Naturwiss. Kl. d. ÖAW/Kommission f. Gesch. d. Naturwissensch., Math. u. Med. No. 56, Vienna 2006.

16 Joseph Škoda (1805–1881). Originally from Pilsen/Bohemia (today Plžen/Czech. Republic). Studied at Vienna Univ. (Dr. med. 1831). Trained as a med. clinician (Internal Med.) at Vienna's Allgem. Krankenhaus. 1839 Publication of his seminal *Abhandlung über Perkussion und Auskultation* [Treatise on Percussion and Auscultation] as the basis of physical examination at the sickbed. 1840 first successful therapeut. pleural puncture together with the surgeon Franz Schuh (1804–1865). 1841 Chief physician of a ward dedicated to diseases of the chest, 1846 Full Prof. at the 1st Med. Clinic (1846–1871). Founder of the Second Vienna Med. School together with Rokitansky (see above). Cf.: CZEIKE; EISENBERG 2; EULNER; GERABEK et al.; HIRSCH (as in FN 13); ÖBL (as in FN 11)*;* PAGEL (as in FN 13); Erna LESKY, *Joseph Skoda*, in: *Wiener klinische Wochenschrift* 68 (1956), pp. 726–729; LESKY, *Wien. Med. Schule* (as in FN 12), pp. 142–152.

17 Theodor Billroth (1829–1894). Originally from Bergen on Rügen, the German Baltic island. Studied at the Univ. of Greifswald, Göttingen and Berlin (Dr. med. 1852). 1853–1860 Assist. under Bernhard v. Langenbeck (1810–1887) at Berlin's Chir. Univ.-Klinik. 1856 Habilitation in Pathol. Anat. and Surgery. 1860–1867 Full Prof. of Surgery at Zurich. Univ., 1867–1894 Full Prof. at the 2nd Surg. Univ. Clinic in Vienna. 1873 first successful laryngectomy. 1881 first successful human gastropylorectomy. Pioneer of modern abdominal surgery. CZEIKE; EISENBERG 2; EULNER; GERABEK et al.; HIRSCH (as in FN 13); ÖBL (as in FN 11); PAGEL (as in FN 13); LESKY, *Wien. Med. Schule* (as in FN 12), pp. 435–447; W. KOZUSCHEK, D. LORENZ, H. THOMAS (eds.), *Theodor Billroth – Ein Leben für die Chirurgie. Mit Beiträgen zur Entwicklung der Magenchirurgie.* Karger, Basel 1992; Helmut WYKLICKY, *Unbekanntes von Theodor Billroth. Eine Dokumentation in Fragmenten.* Verlag d. ÖAW, Vienna 1993. See Ch. 2.

18 Ferdinand Arlt Ritter v. Bergschmidt (1812–1887). Originally from Obergraupen nr. Teplitz-Schönau/Bohemia (today Horní Krupka/Czech. Republic). Studied at Prague Univ. (Dr. med. 1839), 1840–1842 Assist. at the Univ. Eye Clinic Prague under Johann Nepomuk Fischer (1777–1847). 1846 Habilitation in Otology; 1847 Habilitation in Pathol. Anat. of the Eye at Prague Univ. 1848 Master of Ophthalmol. of Vienna Univ. 1849–1856 Full Prof. at Prague Univ. and 1856–1883 at Vienna's Univ. Eye Clinic. 1854 Discovery of the causes of near-sightedness (the lengthening of the sagittal axis of the eye [bulbus]). He put academic ophthalmol. in Vienna firmly on the basis of the pathol.-anat. clinic as conceived by Rokitansky and Škoda. For the first time, ophthalmol. nosology, terminology and the description of pathological changes in the eye were organised in strict accordance with the new system of pathol. anatomy. Cf.: CZEIKE; EISENBERG 2; EULNER; GERABEK et al.; HIRSCH (as in FN 13); ÖBL (as in FN 11); PAGEL (as in FN 13); Julius HIRSCHBERG, "Geschichte der Augenheilkunde", in: Theodor SAEMISCH (ed.), GRAEFE-SAEMISCH *Handbuch der gesamten Augenheilkunde.* 2nd ed., vol. 15/2. Julius Springer, Berlin 1918 [= Reprint vol. VI. Georg Olms, Hildesheim/New York 1977], § 1226–34, pp. 352–376; Jean-Paul WAYENBORGH, IBBO *International Biography and Bibliography of Ophthalmologists and Vision Scientists.* With the Co-Operation of Saiichi Mishima and C. Richard Keeler [= *Hirschberg History of Ophthalmology. The Monographs*, Vol. 7]. Oostende 2001; LESKY, *Wien. Med. Schule* (as in FN 12), pp. 220–226; Gabriela SCHMIDT-WYKLICKY, Helmut GRÖGER, "Ferdinand Ritter von Arlt. Vorstand der Universitäts-Augenklinik in Wien von 1856 bis 1883. Eine Würdigung zum 200. Geburtstag", in: *Spektrum der Augenheilkunde* [= *Spektrum Augenheilk.*] 26 (2012), pp. 290–295.

19 Maximilian Ritter v. Vintschgau zu Altenburg u. Hohenhaus (1832–1913). Cf.: HIRSCH; PAGEL (as in FN 13). See Ch. 2.

20 See Ch. 2.

21 Fuchs did not distinguish here between England and Great Britain. Joseph Lister did come from England originally, but he launched his epochal innovation from Scotland.

22 Joseph Lister (1827–1912), born in Essex. Studied medicine in London (1852 Bachelor of Medicine). 1855 Member of the Royal College of Surgeons in Edinburgh. 1860 Prof. of Surg. at Glasgow Univ., 1869 at Edinburgh Univ.; 1877 Prof. of Clin. Surgery at King's College London. 1891 Director of the British Institute of Medicine. Father of

antisepsis on the basis of carbolic acid. Cf.: GERABEK et al.; HIRSCH; PAGEL (as in FN 13). See Ch. 2.

23 Richard v. Volkmann (1830–1889). Studied at the Univ. of Halle, Gießen and Berlin (Dr. med. 1854). Special. in surgery at Halle Univ. (Habilitation 1857, 1863 Associate Prof., 1867 Full Prof. and Dir. of the Surg. Univ. Clinic). Cf.: GERABEK et al.; HIRSCH; PAGEL (as in FN 13); Richard von VOLKMANN, "Ueber den antiseptischen Occlusivverband und seinen Einfluss auf den Heilungsprocess der Wunden", in: *Sammlung klinischer Vorträge* No. 96. Breitkopf & Härtel, Leipzig 1875. Cf. the two letters from Volkmann to Billroth, dated 16 Feb. 1873 and 29 Oct. 1875, in: Isidor FISCHER (ed.), *Theodor Billroth und seine Zeitgenossen. In Briefen an Billroth. Aus dem Archiv der Gesellschaft der Ärzte in Wien.* Urban & Schwarzenberg, Berlin/Vienna 1929, pp. 33–34.

24 Cf.: LESKY, *Wien. Med. Schule* (as in FN 12), p. 439; FUCHS, *Augenarzt* (as in FN 2), pp. 53, 58 and 332.

25 Joseph LISTER, "A Method of Antiseptic Treatment of Wounded Soldiers in the Present War", in: *British Medical Journal* [BMJ] 2 (1870), pp. 243–244. Cf.: Ruth BRUNN-FAHRNI, "Joseph Listers antiseptische Wundbehandlung", in: *Ciba-Zeitschrift* No. 117. Basel, Oct. 1949, pp. 4311–16; BRUNN-FAHRNI, "Die Listersche Wundbehandlung in der zeitgenössischen Chirurgie", ibid., pp. 4317–19.

26 Ernst FUCHS, "Erinnerungen", in: *Wiener medizinische Wochenschrift* [*Wien. med. Wochenschr.*] 75 (1925), pp. 2475–77.

27 Carl (Karl) Gussenbauer (1842–1903). Studied at Vienna Univ. (Dr. med. 1867, Dr. chir. 1868). Trainee surgeon at the 2nd Surg. Univ. Clinic under Theodor Billroth. 1872 Assist., 1875 Full Prof. of Surgery at Liège Univ. 1878 Call to Prague Univ. (1886 Rector). 1894 Full Prof. as Billroth's successor at the 2nd Surg. Univ. Clinic in Vienna (1902 Rector). Significant contribution to the first laryngectomy by Billroth 1874 and to the development of the first artific. larynx. Cf.: CZEIKE; HIRSCH (as in FN 13); NDB (as in FN 15), ÖBL (as in FN 11); PAGEL (as in FN 13); LESKY, *Wien. Med. Schule* (as in FN 12), pp. 447–449; Obituaries: *Zentralbl. Chir.* 29 (1903) (R. Gersuny); *Wien. klin. Wochenschr.* 26 (1903), pp. 757–758, 903, 930.

28 Anton Frh. v. Wölfler (1850–1917). Studied at Vienna Univ. (Dr. med. 1874). Special. as surgeon under Billroth (1876 assist., 1880 habilitation). Significant contribution to the first successful human gastropylorectomy by Billroth in 1881. Other key areas of activity: thyroid surgery. 1886 Full Prof. of Surgery at Graz Univ., 1895–1917 Full Prof. Univ. Prague. Cf.: CZEIKE; EULNER (as in FN 13); Isidor FISCHER (ed.), 2. u. 3. Aufl. Zweiter Band. Urban & Schwarzenberg, Munich–Berlin 1962; PAGEL (as in FN 13); LESKY, *Wien. Med. Schule* (as in FN 12); Obituary: *Wien. med. Wochenschr.* 68 (1917), cols. 417–418; Franz SPÄTH, "Zur Geschichte der Chirurgie an der Karl-Franzens-Universität Graz", in: Walter HÖFLECHNER (ed.), *Publikationen aus dem Archiv der Universität Graz 18.* Graz 1986; Andreas HÖFERLIN, *Der Chirurg Anton Wölfler (1850–1917). Sein Leben und sein Werk mit besonderer Berücksichtigung seiner Arbeiten zur Schilddrüsenchirurgie.* Med. Diss. Univ. Mainz 1989.

29 Johann Mikulicz v. Radecki (1850–1905). Originally from Czernowitz/Bukovina (today Tscherniwzi/Western Ukraine). Studied at Vienna Univ. (Dr. med. 1875), then assist. under Billroth at the 2nd. Surg. Univ. Clinic (Habilitation 1880). 1882 Full Prof. of Surgery at Krakow Univ., 1887 at Königsberg Univ. and 1890–1895 at Breslau

Univ. Seminal contributions to wound treatment; innovations in the areas of surgic. anaesthesia and struma surgery; developed the first fit-for-purpose oesophago- and gastroscope for human use. Cf.: FISCHER (as in FN 28); GERABEK et al. (as in FN 13); NDB (as in FN 15), ÖBL (as in FN 11); PAGEL (as in FN 13).

30 Domenico Barbieri (1845–1906). Private assist. under Billroth. Billroth entrusted to his "faithful Domenico" the anaesthesia during his first gastropylorectomy in Vienna on 29 Jan. 1881 and Barbieri performed the same function during operations Billroth carried out abroad. As a token of respect f. Billroth Barbieri made a bequest of 300,000 kronen in support of needy students at Vienna's two university clinics for surgery. Cf.: Obituaries, in: *Wien. klin. Wochenschr.* 19 (1906), p. 53 (Alexander Fraenkel); BMJ, Feb. 24, 1906, p. 454; "Barbieri Endowment at Vienna", in: *Journal of the American Medical Association* [JAMA], Feb. 17, 1906, p. 522.

31 Robert Gersuny (1844–1924). Studied at the Univ. of Prague and Vienna (Dr. med. 1866). Junior doctor at Prague's General Hospital. 1869 Trainee surgeon at the 2nd Surg. Univ. Clinic under Billroth in Vienna (from 1872 private assist.). 1882 Head Surgeon at Vienna's Rudolfinerhaus, founded by Billroth, 1894 Dir. after Billroth's death. 1880–1893 Head Surgeon at the Karolinen Children's Hospital. Cf.: CZEIKE; EISENBERG 2 (as in FN 13); FISCHER (as in FN 28); ÖBL (as in FN 11); PAGEL (as in FN 13); Obituary: *Wien. med. Wochenschr.* 74 (1924), col. 2434; *Wien. klin. Wochenschr.* 37 (1924), pp. 1197ff.

32 Anton Ritter v. Frisch (1849–1917). At Billroth's suggestion special. in bacteriol. (wound infect.). 1882 Habilitation in Surgery at Vienna Univ. Chief physician at the surgical ward of Vienna's Allgemeine Poliklinik. Under Billroth's influence pioneering work in the new discipline of urology. 1889 Dir. of the Urol. Dept. at the Poliklinik as the successor of Robert Ultzmann (1842–1889). Cf.: CZEIKE (as in FN 13); FISCHER (as in FN 28); ÖBL (as in FN 11); PAGEL (as in FN 13); LESKY, *Wien. Med. Schule* (as in FN 12), pp. 464–465.

33 Alexander Ritter von Winiwarter (1848–1917). Studied at Vienna Univ. (Dr. med. 1870). Trainee surgeon at the 2nd Surg. Univ. Clinic under Theodor Billroth. Chief physician for Surgery at the Kronprinz-Rudolf-Kinderspital. 1876 Habilitation. Together with Carl Gussenbauer (cf. FN 27) significant contribution to the first successful human gastropylorectomy performed by Billroth in 1881. 1878–1917 Full Prof. at Liège Univ. as the successor of Gussenbauer. Cf.: CZEIKE (as in FN 13); FISCHER (as in FN 28); PAGEL (as in FN 13).

34 The appreciation of Arlt that Fuchs formulated in his obituary took a significantly more nuanced form: Ernst FUCHS, "Ferdinand Ritter von Arlt †", in: *Wiener medicinische Blätter* [Wien. med. Bl.] 10 (1887), pp. 317–321.

35 See Ch. 2.

36 Ibid.

37 See Ch. 3.

38 Frans (Franciscus) Cornelis Donders (1818–1889). Intern at the Groot Rijks Hospitaal ter Instructie in Utrecht, 1835–1840 Studied medicine at Utrecht Univ., then two-year stint as medical officer. Graduation from Leiden Univ. From 1842 Lecturer in Anat. and Physiol. at the Groot Rijks Hospitaal ter Instructie in Utrecht (1848 Associate Prof.). Seminal research in physiol. optics. 1852 Full Prof. of Ophthalmol. at Utrecht Univ. Until 1862 active as an ophthalmic medical practitioner. 1858 Foundation of

the Nederlandsch Gasthuis voor oglijders, where he taught Clin. Ophthalmology, attracting many students both from Holland and abroad. 1855 foundation of the *Arch. f. Ophthalmol.* [Graefes Archiv] together with Albrecht v. Graefe (cf. FN 235) and Arlt (cf. FN 18). Pioneering work above all in research on accommodation and refraction (main work: *On the Anomalies of Accommodation and Refraction of the Eye*, 1864; *Die Anomalien der Akkomodation und der Refraktion*, 1866). 1866 Inauguration of the physiol. lab built according to Donders' specification at Utrecht Univ. Cf.: Daniel M. ALBERT, Diane D. EDWARDS (eds.), *The History of Ophthalmology*. Blackwell Science, Cambridge 1996; Daniel M. ALBERT, Paul HENKIND [= ALBERT/HENKIND], *Men of Vision. Lives of Notable Figures in Ophthalmology*. Gryphon Editions, New York 1993, pp. 142–160; George GORIN, *History of Ophthalmology*. Publish or Perish, Wilmington 1982, pp. 139–142; GERABEK et al.; HIRSCH (as in FN 13); HIRSCHBERG, *Geschichte der Augenheilkunde* (as in FN 18), vol. 15/1 [= Reprint vol. VI], § 1038–49, pp. 174–208; IBBO (as in FN 18); PAGEL (as in FN 13). See Ch. 2.

39 Cf.: FUCHS, *Augenarzt* (as in FN 2), pp. 73–74.

40 Theodor Schwann (1810–1882), Studied at the Univ. of Bonn, Würzburg and Berlin (above all with the outstanding physiol. Johannes Müller (cf. FN 134). 1839 Prof. of Anat. at Louvain Univ. 1848–1880 Full Prof. of Physiol. and Comp. Anat. at Liège Univ. Cf.: GERABEK et al.; HIRSCH (as in FN 13); Fritz KRAFT (ed.), *Grosse Naturwissenschaftler. Biographisches Lexikon. Mit einer Bibliographie zur Geschichte der Naturwissenschaften.* 2nd ed. Verlag d. Vereins dt. Ing., Düsseldorf 1986; PAGEL (as in FN 13); *Manifestations en l'honneur de M. le professeur Th. Schwann.* Liège, 23 juin 1878. See Ch. 3.

41 See Ch. 3.

42 Eduard Jaeger Ritter v. Jaxtthal (1818–1884). See the detailed discussion of Jaeger and his achievements in Ch. 4.

43 Wilhelm Czermak (1856–1906). Originally from Brünn/Moravia (then part of the Austro-Hung. Monarchy, today Brno/Czech. Republic). Studied at Graz Univ. (Dr. med. 1882). Ophthalmolog. specialis. and habil. 1886 ibid. From 1887 assist. at the 2nd Univ. Eye Clinic in Vienna under Fuchs. 1892 tit. Associate Prof. and call to Innsbruck Univ. (Full Prof. 1894/95), 1895–1906 Full Prof. at Prague Univ. Cf.: EISENBERG 2; EULNER (as in FN 13); FISCHER (as in FN 28); HIRSCHBERG, *Geschichte der Augenheilkunde* (as in FN 18), vol. 15/2 [= Reprint vol. VI], § 1221, pp. 347–348; ÖBL (as in FN 11) (Čermák); PAGEL (as in FN 13); IBBO (as in FN 18).

44 Friedrich Dimmer (1855–1926). Originally from Prague. Studied at the Univ. of Prague and Vienna (Dr. med. 1878). Student of Arlt, Jaeger and Fuchs. 1885 Habilitation at the 2nd Univ. Eye Clinic under Fuchs, Full Prof. at all four Austrian Univ. Eye Clinics: Innsbruck 1895, Graz 1900, First Eye Clinic Vienna 1910–1915, Second Eye Clinic Vienna 1915–1926. Brother-in-law of Ernst Fuchs. Main areas of activity: anat. and physiol. of the macula lutea, refining photographic techniques of the ocular fundus. Cf.: CZEIKE; EISENBERG 2; EULNER (as in FN 13); *Spezialfächer*; FISCHER (as in FN 28); HIRSCHBERG, *Geschichte der Augenheilkunde* (as in FN 18), vol. 15/2 [= Reprint vol. VI], § 1255, p. 435; IBBO (as in FN 18); ÖBL (as in FN 11); PAGEL (as in FN 13); Helmut GRÖGER, Gabriela SCHMIDT-WYKLICKY, "Friedrich Dimmer. Vorstand beider Universitäts-Augenkliniken in Wien: I. Augenklinik 1910

bis 1915. II. Augenklinik 1916 bis 1926", in: *Spektrum der Augenheilkunde* [Spektrum Augenheilk.] 26 (2012), pp. 325–329.

45 Maximilian Salzmann (1862–1954). Studied at Vienna Univ. (Dr. med. 1887). Assist. at the 2nd Univ. Eye Clinic in Vienna under Fuchs. Habilitation 1895, tit. Associate Prof. 1906, Full Prof. of Ophthalmol. at Graz Univ. 1911–1935. Cf.: CZEIKE; EISENBERG 2; EULNER (as in FN 13); FISCHER (as in FN 28); HIRSCHBERG, *Geschichte der Augenheilkunde* (as in FN 18), vol. 15/2 [= Reprint vol. VI], § 1255, pp. 435–436; IBBO (as in FN 18); Peter C. KRONFELD, "Maximilian Salzmann", in: *Am. J. Ophthalmol.* 36 (1953), p. 128–129; Obituaries, in: *Am. J. Ophthalmol.* 38 (1954), pp. 738–740 (Dewey Katz); *Arch. Ophthalmol.* 52 (1954), pp. 808–809 (A. B. Reese); Appreciations: H. S. SUGAR, "Maximilian Salzmann. Ophthalmic pioneer and artist", in: *Survey of Ophthalmology* [= Surv. Ophthalmol.] 26 (1981), pp. 28–30; Wolfgang FASCHINGER, "Zum 150. Geburtstag von Maximilian Salzmann (1862–1954)", in: *Spektrum Augenheilk.* 27 (2013), pp. 153–156.

46 Josef Meller (1874–1968). Studied at Vienna Univ. (Dr. med. 1898). Ophthalmolog. specialisation at the 2nd Univ. Eye Clinic under Ernst Fuchs (1907 Habilitation, 1912 tit. Associate Prof.), 1915–1918 Full Prof. at Innsbruck Univ., 1919–1944 Full Prof. at the 1st Univ. Eye Clinic Vienna. Cf.: EULNER (as in FN 13); FISCHER (as in FN 28); HIRSCHBERG, *Geschichte der Augenheilkunde* (as in FN 18), vol. 15/2 [= Reprint vol. VI], § 1257, pp. 440–441; IBBO (as in FN 18); F. A. J., "Professor Dr. Josef Meller (Vienna)", in: *British Journal of Ophthalmology* [= Brit. J. of Ophthalmol.] 33 (1949), pp. 653–654; Helmut GRÖGER, Gabriela SCHMIDT-WYKLICKY, "Josef Meller. Vorstand der I. Universitäts-Augenklinik in Wien 1919 bis 1944", in: *Spektrum Augenheilk.* 26 (2012), pp. 332–335.

47 Julia-Rosina (known as Julie) Fuchs died on 12 June 1919. Cf.: Family archive, Ahnenpass Hofbauer (as in FN 3), p. 11. See Ch. 3.

48 For more details, see Ch. 11.

49 Adalbert (known as Bertl) Fuchs (13 Dec. 1887–12 Nov. 1973). Cf. FN 807.

50 The elder daughter, Rosa (1884–1965), married the Viennese medical doctor Raimund Wilhelm Hofbauer (17 Aug. 1866 – 9 May 1931) in 1901. The couple took up residence in Hainburgerstraße 20 in Vienna's third district. Cf.: UA Wien. Personalakt Wilhelm Hofbauer [son of Raimund Wilhelm Hofbauer], fol. 47 (Questionnaire/Form 2, signed by Dr. Wilhelm Hofbauer on 15 April 1943) and fol. 66 (Marriage certificate). The younger, Elisabeth (known as Lily), (28 Dec. 1885 – 21 Feb. 1945), was married to Lothar Schrutka Edl. v. Rechtenstamm (25 June 1881- 21 Feb. 1945), Full Prof. of mathematics at Vienna's Technical University. They were both killed in a bombing raid on Vienna. Cf.: Family archive; ÖBL (as in FN 11). Their son was the astronomer Guntram Schrutka-Rechtenstamm (1910–1995). Cf.: Obituary, in: *Mitteil. Astronom. Gesellsch.* 79 (1996), p. 9 (Hermann Haupt).

2. Family Background and Training

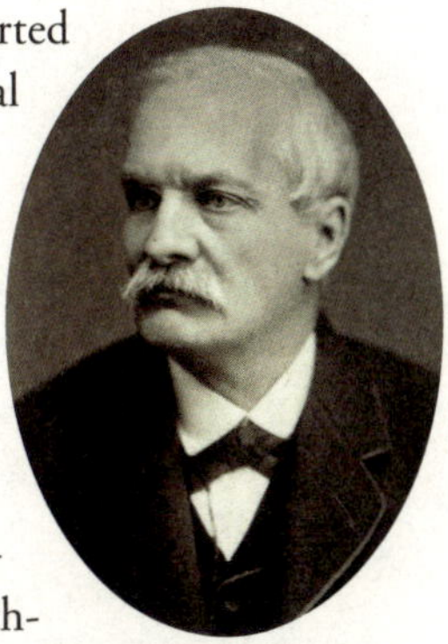

Fig. 13. Adalbert Fuchs

Fuchs's paternal grandfather and his father undoubtedly exerted a powerful formative influence on him. In his intellectual predisposition and in his interests he combined the humanistic and the scientific preoccupations of these two men.

Adalbert(us) Fuchs (1779–1854)

Ernst Fuchs's paternal grandfather, Adalbert Fuchs (Fig. 13), taught history and geography at the K. K. [Imperial-Royal] Ingenieurakademie[51] in what was then Vienna's suburb Laimgrube;[52] the academy was quartered in the northwestern part of the Stiftskaserne,[53] a barracks that exists to this day. Adalbert was a civilian member of the predominantly military teaching staff.[54] The subjects of history and geography – the latter going under the term *Erdbeschreibung* at that time – were part of the curriculum for the first and second forms. Adalbert Fuchs lived with his family close to the Stiftskaserne in the neighbouring suburb of Mariahilf, at No. 27[55] in a house called "Zum Goldenen Einhorn".[56]

Adalbert Nikolaus Fuchs (1814–1886)

Following in the footsteps of his brother Karl (1812–1881),[57] [58] his senior by two years, Ernst Fuchs's father Adalbert Nikolaus Fuchs (1814–1886)[59] (Fig. 14) decided to study medicine. Having caught tuberculosis in the process, he took up residence with a friend of the family, Ernst Ritter von Czaderski,[60] the owner of an estate in what used to be the Austrian Crownland of Galicia. In the two years Adalbert Nikolaus spent in Galicia he developed a pronounced taste for and interest in agriculture.[61]

Fig. 14. Adalbert Nikolaus Fuchs

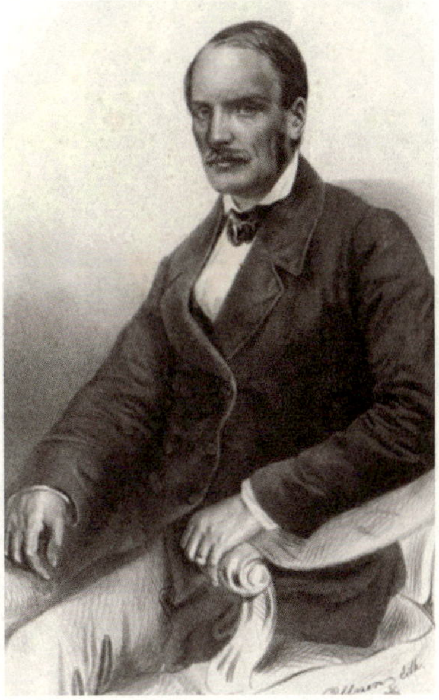

In 1839 he graduated in medicine from Vienna University and obtained a Master of Obstetrics in 1840 from the same university.[62] He then became a trainee surgeon in Vienna's Allgemeines Krankenhaus. Having completed his medical training, however, Adalbert Nikolaus proceeded to study zoology rather than setting up a medical practice. The reason for this was that he was now aiming for an academic career in agriculture, which was then part of the university's philosophical faculty, and a degree in zoology was a precondition for that. Attached since 1841 to the Department of General Natural History and Agronomy of Vienna University, Adalbert Nikolaus, who had not yet defended his doctoral thesis, applied unsuccessfully in July 1842 for the chair of Natural History and Agronomy at Olmütz University (today Olomouc/Czech Republic).[63]

Having been awarded a doctorate (Dr phil)[64] by Vienna University on 18 July 1843, Adalbert Nikolaus Fuchs was commissioned to teach Natural History at a grammar school in Tarnow/Austrian Galicia (today Tarnów/ Poland) in January 1844 as part of the course then known as Philosophical Propaedeutics.[65] When Polish was made the language of instruction at Galicia's grammar schools after the revolution of 1848, Adalbert Nikolaus was forced to give up his position in Tarnow. Only a year later he received a call to take up the post of Professor of Zoology (and Botany) at the newly re-established Philosophical Faculty of Innsbruck University. He was appointed Dean of the University in what was only his second year. He rendered outstanding services to the University's Botanical Garden[66] by having the cultivated plants rearranged according to what was referred to as the natural system.[67] When he received a call to the Chair of Agronomy at the Polytechnisches Institut (then Am Glacis No. 28; today Karlsplatz 13 in Vienna's 4th District, from 1872 Technische Hochschule, today Technische Universität) in Vienna, Adalbert Nikolaus returned to his native city in 1850.[68]

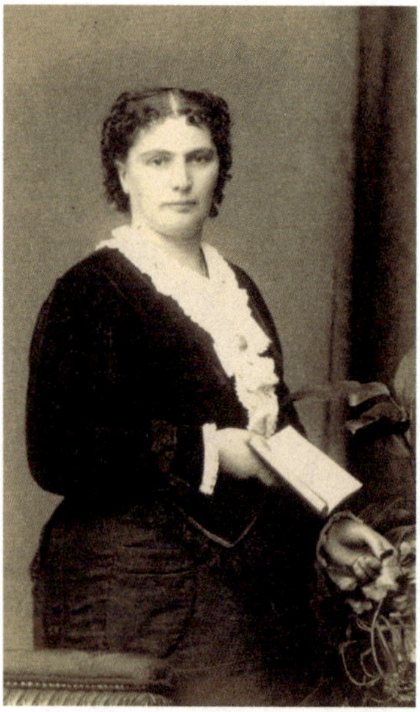

Fig. 15. Isabella Anna von Schreibers

A few months after his return to Vienna, he married Isabella Anna von Schreibers (1832–1902)[69] (Fig. 15) on 10 September 1850 in Kritzendorf. The bride's father, Joseph Ludwig Ritter von Schreibers (1793–1874),[70] was a close relative of the botanist, chemist and medical doctor Joseph Franz Freiherr von Jacquin (1766–1839), whose father, Nikolaus Joseph Freiherr von Jacquin (1727–1817), had founded the University's Botanical Garden[71] in Vienna in 1754. Joseph Ludwig Ritter von Schreibers was an eminent agronomist and jurist. Having sold the domain of Nieder-Hollabrunn, which he had owned between 1819 and 1840, he purchased the Edelhof estate in Kritzendorf near Vienna[72] in 1841. When the young Professor of Agronomy Adalbert Nikolaus Fuchs visited the Edelhof with a group of his students, he had his first meeting with the owner's daughter, Isabella Anna von Schreibers, who was destined to become his wife.

The newly-weds moved to Josephigasse/Josefsgasse No. 80, "Zum Mohren",[73] today Mariahilfer Straße 9, in the immediate vicinity of the Stiftskaserne[74] and in the parish of *Zum heiligen Joseph ob der Laimgrube*. Here their first son was born on 14 June 1851 and christened Ernst Josef on 23 June 1851.[75] Ernst's godfather was his grandfather on his mother's side.

As a charismatic teacher, Adalbert Nikolaus Fuchs built a reputation for himself both with his colleagues and the scientific community at large and had several scientific achievements to his credit. He made it a rule to supplement his lectures with hands-on excursions not only to the vicinity of Vienna but also to Bohemia, Moravia and Hungary.[76] Later on, Ernst was often allowed to accompany him on these study trips to model farms.[77]

Adalbert Nikolaus Fuchs built up a multifaceted, comprehensive collection of teaching aids for the Polytechnikum. Appointed Rector for the academic year 1869/70,[78] he had the courtyards transformed into gardens to provide live demonstration objects for natural history lectures. Over and above his academic duties after his "habilitation" in Agriculture and Forestry at Vienna University, he served from 1855 for many years as Permanent Secretary of the K. K. Landwirthschafts-Gesellschaft[79] under its patron, Crown Prince Rudolf. The high-profile feats he accomplished in this capacity included the organisation of the festivities marking the 50th anniversary of the foundation of this association[80] and the agricultural exhibitions in 1862, 1866[81] and from 1881 to 1884.

Furthermore, Adalbert Nikolaus made a significant contribution to the successful development of the viniculture school in Klosterneuburg (today: Höhere Bundeslehranstalt und Bundesamt für Wein- und Obstbau Klosterneuburg),[82] founded in 1860 at the instigation of the Landwirthschafts-Gesellschaft. In 1884 he reached the normal retirement age of 70. His request for retirement, submitted to the then Minister für Cultus und Unterricht, Sigmund Conrad Freiherr von Eybesfeld (1821–1898),[83] was passed on to Emperor Franz Joseph and honoured, with his achievements being acknowledged in detail.[84] After his retirement the family took up permanent residence in the

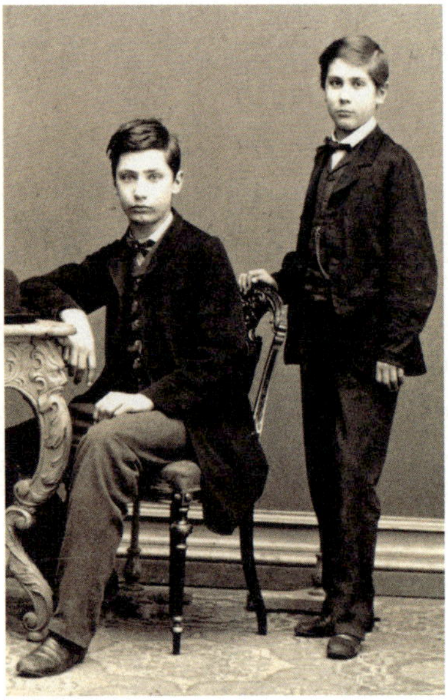

Fig. 16. Ernst (seated) and his brother Karl Wilhelm

Edelhof. Adalbert Nikolaus, who had been awarded the Knight's Cross of the Imperial Order of Franz Joseph as early as 1866 and given the title *K. K. Hofrat*, died there in 1886.[85]

At the beginning of Adalbert Nikolaus' professional career, the family lived in Mariahilf, as has already been said. In 1852, one year after the birth of their first son, Ernst, they moved to the Bärenmühle,[86] next to the Naschmarkt and only a stone's throw from the Polytechnikum,[87] the workplace of Ernst's father.

Wilhelm Fuchs (1853–1897)

The Fuchses' second son, Karl Wilhelm, was born in the Bärenmühle on 27 September 1853. (Fig. 16) Nicknamed Willus, Wilhelm followed the family tradition of attending the Schottengymnasium. He continued his studies at the Law Faculty of Vienna University[88] and received a doctorate utriusque iuris on 23 March 1875 sub auspiciis imperatoris.[89] He spent the summer term of 1875 at Heidelberg University and the winter term of 1875/76 at the University of Berlin. Having completed his court practice in the spring of 1876, he "habilitated" in 1877 at Vienna University as private lecturer in Austrian substantive private law.[90] On 9 August 1884 he married Stefanie, née Straub. A daughter, Adalberta, was born to them on 22 July 1886.[91] In 1893, Wilhelm (Fig. 17) was forced to suspend his teaching activities, probably due to poor health.[92] The untimely death[93] of this gifted jurist took place on 17 July 1897. He was a few months short of his forty-fourth birthday.[94]

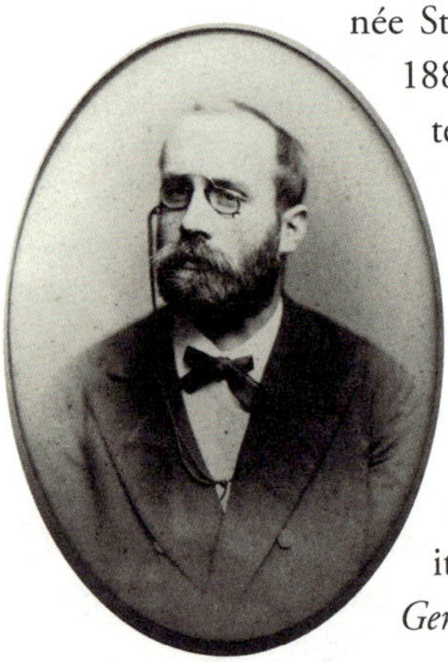

Fig. 17. Wilhelm Fuchs

Even though he was only active as a legal scholar for a relatively short time, Wilhelm Fuchs published several monographs on matrimonial law topics that are still cited today in studies of Austria's legal history.[95] As his brother Ernst saw it, the reason why he was in such great demand as a *Hof- und Gerichtsadvokat* was simple:

He had discovered that Catholics were entitled to remarry after a divorce if they were citizens of Transylvania, which was then part of Hungary. It was because of these 'Transylvanian marriages' that his practice had such a numerous clientele. [96]

Ernst Fuchs's Childhood and Youth

Even in his old age Ernst Fuchs loved to reminisce about the childhood he and brother Wilhelm had spent in the Bärenmühle, which remained operational until 1856, and in the park-like open spaces of the Glacis,[97] when the Innere Stadt was still ringed by a fortified wall:[98]

The Bärenmühle was at that time still a real mill, complete with water wheel, and the millstream, which had not yet been roofed over at that time, flowed along the narrow Mühlgasse; at night, you could hear the whistling of the countless rats from the millrace. Below our windows on one side was the highly frequented Naschmarkt and on the other side the Wien river, whose steep banks were densely wooded. As boys we used to spend a lot of our time down by the river, especially in winter for skating. In both directions the Glacis extended as far as the Danube, on one side more or less as far as the Aspern bridge, on the other to the Brigitta bridge. It was possible for us to play in the meadows wherever we wanted, and in that respect children were better off then than they are now, when they are made to keep strictly to the pathways in public parks.[99]

His way to the Schottengymnasium, which Ernst Fuchs attended from 1860, led him through the historic heart of Vienna's inner city. Ernst held two of his classmates in particularly high esteem, Eugen Böhm von Bawerk (1851–1914) and Friedrich Freiherr von Wieser (1851–1926); both were to become ministers of the crown.[100] Four of his other classmates, in addition to himself, became university professors, including pathologist Hans von Chiari (1851–1916)[101] and gynaecologist Friedrich Schauta (1849–1919).[102] Historian and publicist Heinrich Friedjung (1851–1920),[103] and hygienist and immunologist Max Ritter von Gruber (1853–1927),[104] a classmate of Ernst's brother Wilhelm, became especially close friends of his.[105]

Ernst Fuchs was a hard-working student. He was most conscientious about his academic duties and steeled himself early to a habit of strict discipline.[106] He held his teacher of mathematics and physics, P. Sigismund Gschwandner,[107] who has already been mentioned, in special veneration, and claimed to have been Gschwandner's favourite student. The extent to which this teacher's personality and didactic methods schooled his charges is attested by Hans Chiari's moving words.[108] Fuchs's annual school reports for the *Oberstufe*, the four final years of grammar school, bear out, in accordance with his autobiographical notes, that he worked hard consistently,[109] with

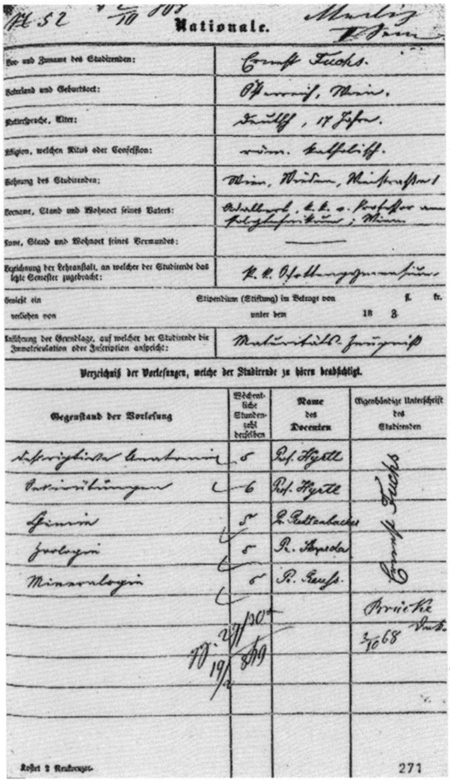
Nationale.

Ernst Fuchs

Verzeichniß der Vorlesungen, welche der Studirende zu hören beabsichtigt.

Gegenstand der Vorlesung | Name des Docenten

271

Fig. 18. University enrolment of Ernst Fuchs in the winter term of 1868–1869

the last one containing the remark *"1. Klasse mit Vorzug"* [First class with distinction].[110] Fuchs took his school-leaving exam[111] on 29 July 1868.

Fuchs kept his link to the Schottengymnasium alive for at least the next four decades. Following family tradition, his son Adalbert, born in 1887, attended the same school and, in 1907, Fuchs was asked, alongside other renowned alumni, for a contribution to a publication designed to commemorate the centenary of the school's foundation. Fuchs provided the account of an expeditionary trip across Asia Minor he had undertaken in 1906, following in the footsteps of Socrates' disciple Xenophon.[112]

Studying Medicine at the Universities of Vienna and Innsbruck

Faced with the question of what course of study to choose, young Ernst initially inclined towards physics and astronomy. His father, fearing that neither course of study would provide a graduate with what it took to support a family, wanted him to become an engineer – hardly surprising, given that he himself taught at the Technische Hochschule. Ernst even started preparing for the admission exam by taking private lessons in the obligatory subject of descriptive geometry.[113] In the end, however, he decided to follow the example of some of his former classmates and opted for medicine, at that stage without any great enthusiasm, as he himself admitted in retrospect.[114] He enrolled at the Medical Faculty of Vienna University for the winter term of 1868/69.[115] (Fig. 18) Alongside scientific foundation courses in chemistry, zoology and mineralogy, the focus in this first term was on lectures on descriptive anatomy and the practice of dissection[116] under Hyrtl.[117] In the second term, descriptive anatomy was continued, supplemented by topographical anatomy. Here Hyrtl put his ingenuity on full display and left a lasting impression on Fuchs:

Hyrtl was rhetorically brilliant and the very model of a polymath and he did not disdain letting his light shine in his lectures so that we were all completely fascinated by him. He awakened my interest in medicine and I spent every spare moment in the dissecting room.[118]

As the students made further progress in anatomy, the chemistry course continued and botany was added as a new subject.[119]

Even though Fuchs was still a neophyte in all matters concerning science, he soon felt like striking out into work of his own devising, perhaps following the predisposition so strongly marked in his family. In order to acquire the methodological-practical foundations required for this, he chose the laboratory established by physiologist Ernst Wilhelm Ritter von Brücke,[120] who had transplanted German laboratory medicine[121] to Vienna and, as a pioneer of the physiology of the senses, especially in the field of physiological optics,[122] already had a number of outstanding achievements to his credit. In an 1845 study on eyeshine in vertebrates,[123] Brücke had shown for the first time how to study the ocular fundus in candle light with the help of a tube.[124] It is well known that this achievement of his paved the way for Hermann von Helmholtz's (1821–1894)[125] invention of the ophthalmoscope as a practical tool in 1850/51.[126] In 1846, Brücke discovered the part of the ciliary muscle that still bears his name.[127] His *Anatomische Beschreibung des menschlichen Augapfels* was published one year later.[128] His *Vorlesungskompendium,*[129] a pedagogical aid for attendees of his lectures published towards the end of Fuchs's time at the university, devoted a great deal of space to the physiology of the senses. In addition to the microstructure of the eye, Brücke dealt in detail with the act of seeing in general and with seeing colours in particular.
As a macro-morphologist, the anatomist Hyrtl, who had originally been the driving force behind getting Brücke to swap Königsberg for Vienna, soon found himself at loggerheads with Brücke the physiologist, who habitually referred to his own discipline as "higher anatomy". Acquiring all the traits of deep-seated personal enmity, this scholars' dispute was fought out in public and gained legendary status.[130]

Even in his old age Fuchs retained vivid memories of the contrasting characters of these two exceptional scholars, whose different approaches had made so deep an impression on him, especially at the beginning of his studies, and had helped determine the direction his career would take:

The second year of the study of medicine brought physiology under Brücke. The change from Hyrtl was absolute. No rhetoric whatever; purely objective, but very clear oral presentation, from the moment in his very first lecture when he told us something that is common knowledge but was nevertheless new to us at the time: that according to Kant[131] *our knowledge of things is confined to what our senses tell us about them and that we have no way of knowing for sure that there is an actual substrate out there. This drove me straight to the pages of Kant himself, quite an undertaking for me at the time, as well as to the English philosopher John Stuart Mill,*[132] *who, in contrast, proved eminently readable.*
Between Hyrtl and Brücke a bitter enmity had sprung up for a reason that was positively risible. It was at Hyrtl's instigation that Brücke had received the call that brought him from Königsberg to Vienna; he had made a name for himself through the discovery of the ciliary muscle and other notable feats. In Vienna he announced his lecture series as "Physiology and Higher Anatomy", taking the latter to refer to histology, a subject that Hyrtl did not lecture on (similarly, Brücke was the only one to lecture on physiological chemistry). Hyrtl took it extremely badly that there was supposed to be a "higher" version of his beloved anatomy. Brücke's lectures were a source of delight for me no less than Hyrtl's, if in an entirely different way. They presented a purely intellectual challenge, and were an altogether different experience from the florid and usually highly entertaining lectures provided by Hyrtl. It was most unfortunate that Brücke fossilized before his time and went on to repeat his lectures verbatim for many years.[133]

Hyrtl and Brücke were also very different in their respective ideologies. Hyrtl rejected the materialist approach to an understanding of nature and humanity, whereas Brücke was a self-confessed supporter of this philosophical school. Around the middle of the nineteenth century materialism had begun to supersede natural philosophy, which had been predominant in science teaching in Vienna up until that time.[134] During his time as a student in Berlin under Johannes Müller[135] and others, such as Helmholtz and Emil Heinrich du Bois-Reymond (1818–1896), later the founder of Experimental Electrophysiology and co-founder in the German-speaking world of physiology as a scientific discipline, scientific materialism primarily based on physics and chemistry had come into being and was making great strides:

Brücke and I have conspired to make the truth generally known that no forces are active in the organism other than the common physical-chemical ones; and to make sure in those cases where these forces are not yet sufficient as an explanation that either ways and means are found to show the specific efficacy of these forces in such cases or to assume the presence of new forces, which must be acting similarly to those known in Physics and Chemistry, are inherent to matter and can be shown to consist only of repellent or attracting components.[136]

One must beware of reading Brücke's part in that conspiracy – presented here in rather stark terms – as one-sided limitation on his part. Such a stance would hinder the appreciation of its fruitful effect on the multifaceted, scientific-experimental basic research carried out in the Second Vienna Medical School, which paved the way for future developments. Sketching in almost five decades later the overall context that is required for a deeper understanding, Brücke's successor, Si(e)gmund Exner von Ewarten (1846–1926),[137] had this to say on the position his teacher maintained at the time:

When the dictum that all of life rested on chemical and physical laws kept exercising minds and the cell law traced all of life back to the feats of individual cells, people were emboldened to hope that cellular chemistry and physics were allowing them to tackle the riddle of cellular life and, by the same token, of life itself. How much unresearchable chemistry or physics was supposed to be folded into such a minuscule object? […]
Such efforts are being continued to this day; even now there is a belief in certain quarters that the identification of a chemical reaction that is supposed to be unique to living – as opposed to dead – protoplasm has moved us closer to solving the riddle of life […].
Here too we see how Ernst von Brücke, one of the foremost proponents of the cell theory, views such overzealous pursuit of his own ideas with cool detachment and his trademark circumspection. Having boldly advanced into this territory and conquered it, he did not take a single step forward in the rush that he was later forced to retract.[138]

Belonging to the Kantian school of thought, Viennese pathologist Carl von Rokitansky[139] vehemently pleaded that materialism[140] should be restricted to its role as a method of scientific research and not be embraced as an ideology.[141] This, then, was the prevailing philosophical field of tension within the Vienna Medical School and the theoretical foundations of medicine in research, tuition and practice when Ernst Fuchs started out on his research.

Fuchs was to retain vivid memories of his beginnings in Brücke's lab for a long time to come:

I had heard that some protegés – Fleischl,[142] *Exner, Paneth,*[143] *Frisch,*[144] *Obersteiner,*[145] *etc – were allowed to work histologically with Brücke. These people projected the idea that special dispensation was required for this. By chance I learnt from one of my completely penniless fellow students that he had been admitted without any fuss at all.* [...] *So I called on Brücke. The only condition he imposed on every candidate was that he attend a histological course under Wedl,*[146] *who was at that time Associate Professor of Histology. This was a hands-on course designed to introduce students to histological techniques. We made preparations of muscles and tendons, slicing desiccated skin or soft organs with a razor. The latter we sandwiched between elder pith, which we had to procure ourselves. The only available colouring was carmine.* [...]
The few students that practised histology under Brücke worked in the lecture hall at times when there were no lectures, some of them on windowsills, others on benches, where the light was very poor. The technique was no great improvement on Wedl but we studied many more different types of tissue and Brücke himself moved around in the lecture hall, looking into each microscope and dispensing advice. By doing so, he devoted a great deal of time to practical teaching. The more advanced among the students were given special tasks. After some time, he came up with one for me: the question to be studied was whether the [fallopian] *tubes were making any special movements during conception, for instance by blood being pumped into their vessels, and I was to study this under increased pressure, by injecting the vessels that supply the tubes. I did this with inner genitalia that I had procured from the dissecting room, with the result that I fell ill with a slight infection which made me bedridden, albeit not for long. This made me give up on this particular task.*[147] [Fig. 19]

Fuchs did the practical course under Wedl that Brücke demanded in his third semester, in the autumn of 1869/70.[148]

After obtaining his doctorate from the University of Vienna in 1841, Wedl had gone to France and England in 1844 on a study trip. Back in Vienna, he began to examine pathologically altered tissue. Encouraged by Rokitansky, he followed up his habilitation in Histology in 1849 (1853 Assoc. Prof., 1872 Full Prof.) by publishing, in 1854, *Grundzüge der pathologischen Histologie,*[149] a comprehensive monograph on the fundamental characteristics of diseased tissue.[150] In the same year, and in the immediate vicinity of the workplaces of Hyrtl and Brücke, in a building that used to house the K. K. Gewehrfabrik,[151] the first University Institute of Histology was created for Wedl.[152] A contemporary report describes this teaching venue for the theoretical subjects of Vienna's Medical Faculty, which was considered inadequate even by the standard of the time, as follows:

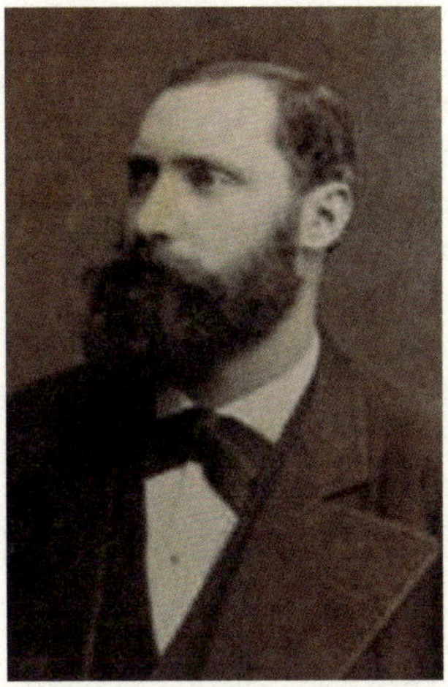

Fig. 19. Ernst Fuchs as a student in Brücke's lab

The appointments of the lecture halls, the dissecting room and the laboratories located in this building are not fit for purpose and their acute shortcomings have repeatedly been flagged. In consequence, some improvements have been made recently in respect of the lighting of the anat[omical] *lecture hall and the ventilation of the dissecting room, but the main evil, the lack of quiet, persists – the building also houses the k.k. Police Barracks. Radical improvement will arguably have to await the construction of a new university building, whose building plot has now at long last been agreed. The courtyard building houses the Institute of Physiology with Prof. Brücke at its head. Here anatom*[ical]*-physiol*[ogical] *work is carried out every day for as long as daylight lasts, partly by medical doctors, partly by people from outside. It is the birthplace of many an important discovery, and Prof. Brücke encourages his students with his friendly, outgoing manner and his kind advice concerning the choice of study objectives.*

[…]

The second floor of the wing that extends as far as the Währinger Gasse houses Prof. Wedl's Institute of Histology, which, while not spacious, is nevertheless welcoming and well suited for microscopic work. Here work is carried out on an ongoing basis in the field of physiolog[ical], *patholog*[ical] *and comparative histology; researchers from abroad and locals use this laboratory, whose director is as much distinguished by his sober approach to research as by his genial personality.*[153]

As an extracurricular course, Wedl's histological *"Propädeutikum"*[154] required the payment of a fee amounting to 5 fl. a month for students and 10 fl. for postgraduates.[155]

Particular and enduring recognition is owed to Wedl for his well-informed, nuanced treatment of the pathological anatomy and histology of the human eye.[156] He proceeded along lines comparable to the intentions of the Director of the Ophthalmological Clinic, Ferdinand R. v. Arlt.[157] (Fig. 20) As Director of the Eye Clinic of Prague University[158] Arlt had begun prising ophthalmology loose from its ancient roots in humoral pathology and natural philosophy and grounding it in the fruitful soil of pathological anatomy.[159] It was only logical for Arlt's habilitation at Prague University in 1847 to be focused on the pathological anatomy of the eye.[160] His memoirs feature the following admission, which is doubly important in view of the future development ophthalmological research underwent in Ernst Fuchs's hands, away from macropathology and towards the pathohistology of the eye:

I was prevented from mastering the use of the microscope first by the lack of the requisite tuition, then by a lack of time; I have never managed to do autonomous research in that field, regardless of how highly I rated its importance. There was, however, still a great deal to be done in those days for the macroscopic anatomy of the eye.[161]

Acting on that assessment in 1862, Arlt commissioned the physician, medical draughtsman, modeller and cartoonist Anton Elfinger (1821–1864),[162] who, among other things, had been in charge of the illustrations for the *Atlas der Hautkrankheiten* by Ferdinand Hebra (1816–1880),[163] to make a drawing of a cross-section of the human eye from Arlt's own preparations.[164]

The fruit of the collaboration between the theoretician Wedl and the ophthalmic clinician Carl Stellwag von Carion (1823–1904),[165] their comprehensive *Atlas der pathologischen Histologie des Auges,*[166] dedicated to their mentor Rokitansky, had appeared as early as 1861. The extremely accurate drawings of the tissue sections are the work of Carl Heitzmann (1836–1896),[167] who, like Elfinger, had worked as a draughtsman for Hebra and later emigrated to the United States, where he built up a reputation as a dermatologist.

Wedl revived this collaboration with Stellwag and his assistant two decades later.[168] His interest in ophthalmopathology was to bear fruit once more a quarter of a century after the publication of his first atlas. In 1886, Wedl and one of Stellwag's students, Emil Bock (1857–1916),[169] published a comprehensive treatment of the pathological anatomy of the eye,[170] supplemented by an atlas.[171] The extent to which they had every reason to believe that they were entering terra incognita is apparent from the following passage taken from the Introduction:

A systematic treatment of the pathological anatomy of the eye, as we will concede quite happily, can at present be no more than an attempt. This aspect has only been pursued through case studies for a few decades; furthermore, in view of theories moving now this way, now that, the basic tenets of general pathology are a long way away from providing a firm basis for the pathology of a medical speciality to build on.[172]

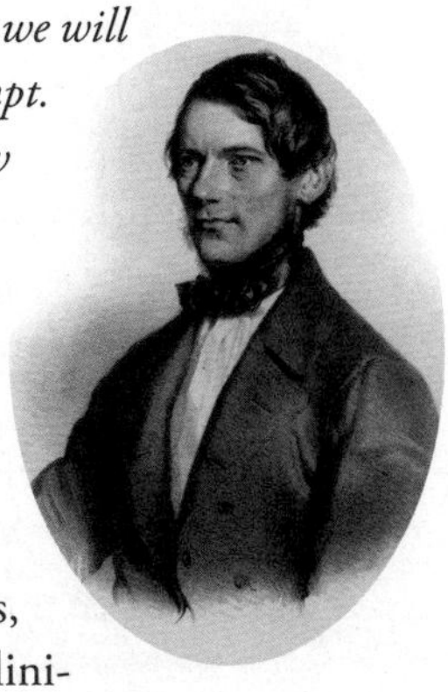

Fig. 20.
Ferdinand Arlt

That said, Wedl had nevertheless provided with these works a theoretical foundation of sorts. His student Ernst Fuchs, combining with characteristic ingenuity microscopic and clinical research, made use of this foundation to confirm the worldwide leading position of ophthalmopathology as conceived by the Second Vienna Medical School at the turn of the century.[173]

Even after Fuchs had acquired the expertise and the skills at Brücke's laboratory that he required for scientific work he continued to work there during the remainder of his studies.[174] In the summer term of 1872, his eighth university semester, he attended Brücke's lecture series "Über Stimme und Sprache" [Voice and Language] in addition to the obligatory courses.[175]

Ernst Fuchs as a Temporary Assistant at Innsbruck University

Having formed a highly favourable opinion of Ernst Fuchs, whom he had had occasion to observe at close quarters over several years, Brücke recommended him in the spring of 1873 to one of his former students, Maximilian Ritter von Vintschgau,[176] for the position of assistant at Innsbruck University's Medical Faculty, which had been newly established in 1869.[177] In those days it was not unusual for specially talented students who had trained under a distinguished professor to be appointed assistants even before they had obtained their doctorate. As a matter of fact, shortly before Vintschgau, the former Arlt assistant Otto Becker (1828–1890),[178] since 1868 Chair at the newly founded University Eye Clinic at Heidelberg,[179] where he was to make significant contributions to research on pathological ocular anatomy over the next two decades, had already asked Brücke to help him find an assistant. Brücke had named Fuchs at the time, but the latter had not yet warmed to the idea of making a career of ophthalmology.[180] The excellent training he had received in Brücke's lab and his resulting expertise encouraged Ernst Fuchs to go along with Brücke's next recommendation and he switched to Innsbruck University during his ninth semester.

On 15 February 1873, the assistant at Vintschgau's Institute of Physiology, Michael Josef Dietl (1847–1887),[181] notified the Dean of his intention to resign from his post at the end of March 1873.[182] Twenty-two-year-old Ernst Fuchs submitted his application for this soon-to-be-vacant post on 11 March 1873. The following passage from his letter of application speaks to the academic maturity Fuchs had attained already:

The applicant is encouraged to apply for this post, even though he has not yet graduated, by the fact that he has worked in the physiological laboratory of his distinguished teacher, Hofrath Brücke, since the second year of his medical studies. The undersigned would like to add that he is proficient in French and English and that his father, a professor at the Imperial Royal Technical University in Vienna, has given his consent to this application.[183]

Only five days later Vintschgau notified the professorial council of Innsbruck's Medical Faculty of his decision:

For the soon-to-be-vacant position of assistant at the Department of Physiology at this medical faculty two applicants have come forward, namely Hr. Ernest Fuchs, med. stud. in the ninth semester at the University of Vienna [and] *Hr. Ant. Tinzl,*[184] *med. stud. in the ninth semester at the University of Innsbruck.*
Seeing that Herr E. Fuchs has passed both the three preliminary exams in Mineralogy, Botany and Zoology and the First Medical Rigorosum with distinction and that, according to the testimony of Herr Hofrath Prof. v. Brücke, he has been doing microscopic work at the Institute of Physiology of Vienna University since the beginning of the summer semester of 1870 with great diligence and excellent results, and seeing furthermore that Herr Ant. Tinzl only has to his credit that he has passed the three preliminary exams, in Botany and Zoology with the grade Sufficient, in Mineralogy with the grade Excellent, the undersigned would like to propose Herr Ernest Fuchs, med. stud in the ninth semester at the University of Vienna, for the position of temporary assistant at the Department of Physiology of this University.[185]

Once the consent of the Ministerium für Cultus und Unterricht in Vienna had been obtained,[186] Ernst Fuchs was appointed temporary assistant at the Department of Physiology of Innsbruck University for a two-year term; a resolution of 22 March 1873 confirmed this.[187] From the start of the summer term of 1873,[188] Fuchs, who had been notified of his first university post one day after the decision had been taken by Innsbruck's professorial council,[189] received the same salary as his predecessor, 600 gulden, paid in twelve monthly instalments.[190] During his time as assistant-cum-student in Innsbruck,[191] Fuchs attended lectures on such topics as "The Medical Clinic" and "Surgical Operation Practice"[192] delivered, respectively, by Anton von Tschurtschenthaler (1815–1900)[193] and Karl Wilhelm Ritter von Heine (1838–1877).[194] Ernst Fuchs remained active as Vintschgau's temporary assistant in the winter term 1873–74[195] and was still listed in that function in the summer term of 1874.[196] Fuchs himself explained this:

In order to obtain my Absolutorium, I had to enrol at Innsbruck before the summer term was over. [197]

Fuchs owed the first stimulating impulse in the direction of his future specialisation in ophthalmology to his time in Innsbruck. While Arlt's "Theoretisch-praktischer Unterricht in der Augenheilkunde" [Theoretical-practical lectures in ophthalmology], which he had attended in his seventh term in Vienna,[198] had left him cold,[199] this new experience almost amounted to an initiation, and in describing it Fuchs departs significantly from his otherwise sober and matter-of-fact diction:

In the meantime the ophthalmologist Mauthner[200] *had come; I had not enrolled for his lectures but Plenk,*[201] *one of my colleagues and Mauthner's assistant, taught me* [who to use] *the ophthalmoscope and I will never forget the moment when the papilla became visible to me for the first time like the full moon in the night sky.*[202]

At the end of April 1873 Fuchs applied for permission to take the 2nd *Rigorosum* at the end of his stay at Innsbruck University.[203] On 24 May 1873 the then Minister für Cultus und Unterricht, Minister-President-to-be Karl Ritter von Stremayr (1823–1904), granted the necessary dispensation to allow Fuchs to take the 2nd and 3rd *Rigorosa* at Innsbruck University.[204] On 25 July 1873, Fuchs passed one of them, No. 2, at the Medical Faculty of Innsbruck University – again with distinction.[205]

Return to Vienna and Finals

Fuchs gave notice to Vintschgau on 15 November 1873 and submitted his request to be allowed to take the 3rd *Rigorosum* at the University of Vienna less than a week later, on 21 November 1873.[206] In his memoir, Fuchs explains this decision as follows:

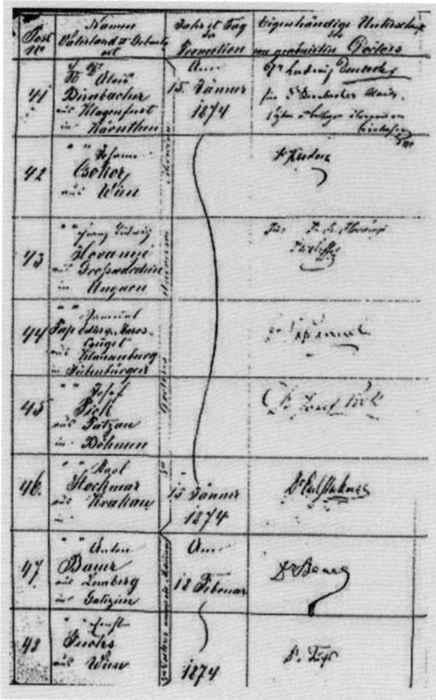

Fig. 21. Fuchs's graduation documented in the last column

I had found out in the meantime that the highest position I could hope for in Innsbruck was that of an Associate Professor, which would not enable me to make ends meet. My father, too, felt that I should opt for a specialty that would allow me to earn a living. After my return to Innsbruck at the end of the holidays I gave notice to my boss for the end of the year – to his great consternation, for it was not easy to find assistants in the theoretical disciplines. I returned to Vienna in the Christmas vacation. I had the additional motivation of wanting to take my last Rigorosum in Vienna in order to obtain my doctorate from Vienna University. I prepared for the exam and passed the third Rigorosum in early 1874 with distinction, like the first two. I was awarded my doctorate in February.[207] (Fig. 21)

Ophthalmological Special Training at the University Eye Clinic in Vienna

Having obtained my doctorate, I joined the hospital[208] *as an aspirant and chose Arlt's clinic.*[209] *Less than a year before I had declined the offer of an assistantship at the clinic in Heidelberg.*[210]

As Arlt took surgical skills for granted in his assistants, these had to make sure they obtained the requisite qualification before they definitively joined his clinic. Fuchs therefore enrolled *ex propriis* (i. e., at his own expense) as trainee surgeon under Theodor Billroth from November 1874 to the end of December 1875.[211] This gave Ernst Fuchs a ringside seat from which to observe at first hand the change from open to closed wound treatment thanks to Lister's antiseptic method, leading to a dramatic reduction in wound infections.[212]

Pioneer of Skiing

In his time as a temporary assistant to the physiologist Maximilian von Vintschgau in Innsbruck,[213] Fuchs had developed a passion for mountaineering and high-altitude climbing and had become surefooted in even the most difficult terrain. In the vacations following the winter term of 1875, Billroth student Carl Gussenbauer[214] invited him to join him for a trip to Sweden and Norway.[215] In those countries Fuchs saw people skiing, skied himself and bought a pair of "snow shoes", as skis were called at the time. He brought them and the "snow-shoe sport" back to Vienna,[216] from where skiing soon spread to all of Austria. Though rarely now accredited as such,[217] Fuchs is therefore a pioneer of skiing in Austria, as is stressed in a recent Anglo-American appreciation of his achievements:

Following a trip to Scandinavia in 1875, Fuchs brought back a pair of 'snow-shoes', as they were called at the time, thus introducing skiing to Vienna.[218]

Fuchs's assistantship at Arlt's clinic lasted from 1876 to 1880, an exceptionally long stay by the standard prevailing there at the time:

It was a matter of principle with Arlt to keep his assistants for no longer than two, at most, three years, because he felt that in view of the then current status of science this was enough to ensure a thorough training and that there were hardly any eye specialists in the country, for instance, not even in Brno. Totally unselfishly, he wanted to provide the country with ophthalmologists, even though he did so to the detriment of his own practice. I was the first assistant he kept for longer, because being old already he did not want to change his first assistant before his own resignation.[219]

After Hubert Sattler (1844–1928)[220] had resigned from his assistantship under Arlt, Fuchs was appointed assistant at the clinic, initially from 1 March 1876 to the end of February 1878. On the occasion, Arlt described Fuchs in words radiating benevolence:

He is arguably known to all professors who have been in contact with him as a young man who is as gifted as he is diligent and reputable.[221]

Writing about it many years later,[222] Fuchs got muddled about the holders and the order of assistantships at Arlt's clinic:

After my two years of surgical training I would have liked to continue as a surgeon but the decision had already been made that I was to accept the assistantship under Arlt that was due to fall vacant after Bergmeister's departure;[223] *Kerschbaumer*[224] *had succeeded Sattler.*[225]

Fuchs's annual salary was now 700 fl,[226] which enabled him to set up his own household. Until then, he had been living in his parents' home in the Bärenmühle.[227] Now Fuchs moved into the clinic, as was usual at that time:

I was assigned two small rooms above the Eye Clinic; the room below contained the library that I was to be in charge of and a large part of which I read during my time as an assistant. I did not move in for several weeks, because the bed, which was part of the furniture the assistants' rooms were supplied with by the hospital, was much too short and the director refused to supply another one. I did not move in until the director had changed his mind.
The assistants were on duty every other day. [...]
In Arlt's clinic I was assigned the two larger rooms; even though Kerschbaumer was my senior, he had to his annoyance been given the two smaller hospital rooms, presumably because Arlt had noticed that he was lacking in diligence.[228]

At the Eye Clinic Fuchs made an outstanding contribution by introducing asepsis, which he himself had learnt from Billroth. The application of carbolic acid pioneered by Lister had to be modified for ophthalmology, as the spray had to be dispensed with. Lint,[229] which had been in general use in wound dressing until then, was replaced by cotton wool.[230]

After Fuchs had published his first scientific paper as Arlt's assistant on Herpes iris conjunctivae in 1876[231] – the initial description of this disease pattern[232] – he devoted himself to the study of experimental keratitis[233] and frog's blood.[234] What is remarkable about these papers is that, even though they were Fuchs's first publications, they were readily accepted by two – then as well as now – leading specialist journals of ophthalmology and pathological anatomy. To continue laying the foundation for his academic career as an ophthalmologist, Fuchs methodically honed his expertise and gained access to the relevant expert circles. The most prestigious ophthalmologic forum in the German speaking world at the time was the Deutsche Ophthalmologische Gesellschaft (DOG)[235] in Heidelberg. The DOG had been founded in 1863 at the instigation of Albrecht von Graefe (1828–1870),[236] with significant input from Arlt, as the first ophthalmological association, and it has been organising scientific conferences in Heidelberg almost annually ever since. On the occasion of the 10th Conference (17–19 August 1877), 26-year-old Ernst Fuchs was made a member of this prestigious association, which in itself speaks volumes.[237] This was the prelude to a friendship that was to develop between Fuchs and the host of the Heidelberg conferences, Becker.[238]

Under the aegis of his teacher Arlt in Vienna, Becker had zealously been conducting pathological research and had made tissue sections of enucleated eyes. During his assistantship at the First University Eye Clinic in Vienna he was thus able to create the foundation for what was to become the unique histological collection Fuchs later built up at "his" Second University Eye Clinic.[239]

Fuchs's assistantship at Arlt's clinic was due to end in late February 1878. On 14 February 1878, Fuchs therefore submitted a request to the Professorial Council to have his assistantship prolonged by another two years.[240] Arlt expressed his support for this request in a refreshingly personal manner by adding the handwritten remark on Fuchs's form two days later: *"I warmly support this request."*[241] Fuchs's term was prolonged for another two years, until the end of February 1880.[242]

In addition to clinical work, Fuchs's duties as assistant under Arlt included holding courses, which were initially focused on the use of the ophthalmoscope. There was a very strong demand for these courses on the part of students and medical doctors from abroad.[243] The most prominent non-ophthalmologists among the participants were the future Breslau dermatologist Albert Neisser (1855–1916)[244] and the internal clinician Adolf von Strümpell (1853–1925).[245] The latter reminisces in his memoirs about the manifold impressions he received during his stay in Vienna in 1877.[246]

The 1878 Study Trip

In January 1878 Fuchs applied to the medical Professorial Council for the Universitäts-Jubiläums-Reisestipendium [University Jubilee travel grant] with a view to broadening his specialist training.[247] To justify his application, Fuchs spoke candidly about the plans he had for his academic future:

The undersigned is planning, if the Professorial Council deem him worthy when the time comes, to establish himself as a lecturer in ophthalmology at the University of Vienna. He feels there is no better way to prepare for this, in addition to

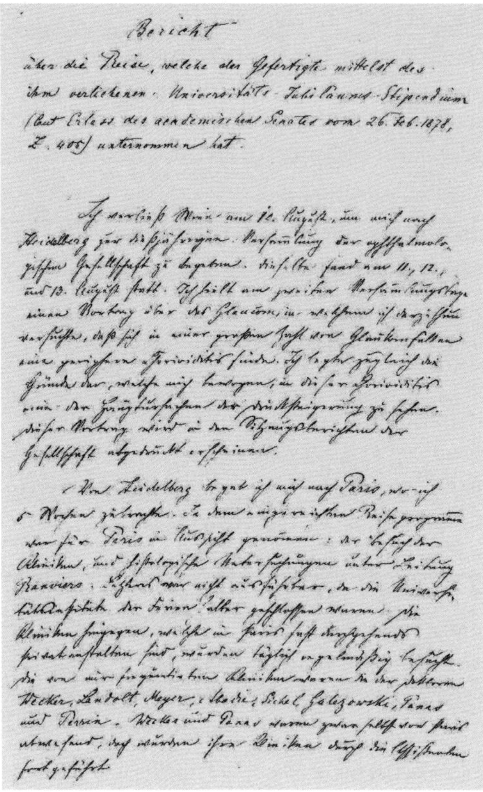
Bericht
über die Reise, welche der Gefertigte mittelst des ihm verliehenen Universitäts-Jubiläums-Stipendiums (laut Erlass des academischen Senates vom 26. Feb. 1878, Z. 405) unternommen hat.

Fig. 22. Ernst Fuchs's report on his 1878 study trip

diligent work at this clinic, than to spend some time at clinics abroad, to get to know the methods of tuition and practice that are being cultivated there. The need for this is perhaps felt in no other speciality as acutely as it is in ophthalmology, where the different schools coexist with little in common in their terminology, therapy and operation technique.[248]

The travel grant awarded to Fuchs on 6 March 1878[249] enabled him to visit several European eye clinics between August and October 1878. Fuchs's final travel report (Fig. 22), reprinted for the first time in full in the German edition of this book, reads in English as follows:

Report on a study trip, which the University Jubilee Grant awarded to the undersigned (according to the decree of the Academic Senate of 26. Feb. 1878, No. 405) allowed him to undertake.

I left Vienna on 10 August for Heidelberg to attend this year's Conference of the Ophthalmological Society, which took place on 11, 12, and 13 August. On the second day, I delivered a paper on glaucoma, in which I tried to show that in a great number of cases glaucoma is associated with peripheral chorioiditis. I set out the reasons that lead me to believe that this chorioiditis is one of the main causes for the increase in pressure. The paper will be reprinted in the proceedings of the Society's conference.[250]

From Heidelberg I travelled to Paris, where I spent five weeks. In the itinerary I had submitted the programme for Paris consisted in visits to clinics and histological studies under the guidance of Ranvier.[251] *The latter proved impossible, as university institutes were closed for the vacation. The clinics, which in Paris are almost invariably private institutions, were visited on a daily basis. I frequented those of the doctors Wecker,*[252] *Landolt,*[253] *Meyer,*[254] *Abadie,*[255] *Sichel,*[256] *Galezowski,*[257] *Panas,*[258] *and Perrin.*[259] *Wecker and Panas had both left Paris, but their clinics were kept going by their assistants.*

Of the observations I made in the clinics mentioned above, the following deserve special attention: with regard to cataract extraction, almost all of the doctors I have mentioned more or less agree on one and the same method. It is roughly identical with the formation of a flap cut in the scleral border as described by Wecker. Those, like Landolt, who want to avoid an iridectomy, cut the incision downward to be able to access the wound more easily. On the whole, the results of this method are reputedly satisfactory.
With regard to operations in general I observed similar methods and indications to the ones in use in the Vienna School. What I would like to mention is that, in cases of dacryo-cysto-blennorrhoea where tearing persists in spite of protracted probe treatment, Abadie opts for the extirpation of the lacrimal gland.
With respect to therapy, French doctors show a strong inclination to treat acute conjunctival catarrhs with warm poultices. For afflictions of the lacrimal sac they very often resort to injections of astringent fluids. In the treatment of corneal ulcers, eserine[260] *plays an important role; there is, however, no unanimous agreement on the efficacy of this substance. In cases of glaucoma, pilocarpine*[261] *is deployed as a miotic in addition to eserine;*[262] *this is especially true of Meyer.*
Non-recent corneal opacity is almost universally treated with vaporisation. A vaporiser is activated by a spirit flame and a thin, warm jet is directed at the cornea, while patients are holding their eyelids apart. Excluding cases of recent inflammation, the reaction is minimal and clarification is said to take place very quickly.
I found several new apparatuses in use, especially in Landolt's clinic. His perimeter differs from Förster's[263] *by having a broader arc. The mark is moved by hand. Landolt also uses this perimeter for the measurement of squint angles. The patient sits in front of the perimeter in such a position that the misaligned eye is at the centre of the perimeter arc. The other eye is fixated on a point in the direction of the perimeter's zero point, but further away. Now the examiner moves a candle flame along the perimeter arc until, focusing across the flame, its reflection becomes visible at the centre of the cornea. The angle measured in this way corresponds to the squint angle. This method can be modified by putting the candle flame once and for all at the zero point of the perimeter arc and by making the eye follow the arc until the picture of the flame is again visible at the centre of the misaligned eye's cornea. The angle measured in this way represents double the squint deviation.*
To make focusing on the reflection on the cornea easier, Nicati[264] *has mounted binoculars which can be shifted along the perimeter arc. The perimeter can be*

used not only for the measurement of squint angles but also for measurement of the visual field.
In order to calibrate an exact measure of the capacity for colour perception numerically, Landolt uses the following apparatus: a Maxwell[265] *disc has colour applied to it in sectors, whose angles get ever smaller towards the periphery. Turn the disc and you get all the different shadings of the chosen colour, in accordance with the diminishing size of the sectors. To make them stand out against an absolutely black background, the disc is mounted at the back of a box lined with black velvet. To make only one nuance or select nuances of the chosen colour visible as required, a lid can be put on the box, which has openings according to the individual sectors.*
A very useful device for the demonstration of ophthalmoscopic images is Abadie's tripod ophthalmoscope. It comprises all the necessary apparatuses for the creation of an inverted image (mirror, convex lens, chin support and fixation mark) on four stand-alone tripods. This makes focussing on the ocular fundus much quicker and easier than is possible with either the Liebreich[266] *or the Ruete*[267] *tripod ophthalmoscopes.*
The number of newly designed ophthalmoscopes is great, but nearly all of them rely on the same principle: to create a great number of lens values by combining lenses mounted in two discs that rotate on top of each other. The most commonly used of these ophthalmoscopes are those designed by Landolt, Wecker and Meyer. They differ from each other by minor variations in the mechanism.
The World Exhibition had little to offer of interest to the ophthalmologist. The most outstanding optical instruments, the majority of which were on display in the showcase of Cretès,[268] *have just been mentioned. What stood out in addition was the excellently crafted metrical trial lens cases by Cretès.*
On 19 September I travelled to London, where I paid visits to Moorfields,[269] *St. Thomas, St. Bartholomew's, Guy's, London, Middlesex, University College and King's College Hospital.*[270] *In these hospitals, Doctors Critchett,*[271] *Streatfield,*[272] *Wharton Jones,*[273] *Couper,*[274] *Hutchinson,*[275] *Nettleship,*[276] *Adams,*[277] *Soelberg Wells,*[278] *Higgins,*[279] *Dunnage,*[280] *Tay,*[281] *and Amphlett work as physicians. The appointments of English hospitals can only be called excellent, both in the hospital rooms and the examination and the treatment of out-patients in the dedicated spaces. Particularly in the organisation of the ophthalmoscope rooms there is much that merits copying.*
The volume of patient material is colossal. In 1877, 20,730 eye patients were treated in Moorfields Hospital's outpatient clinic alone.
Concerning operation technique, it is worth noting that for the extraction of senile

cataract a linear incision in the cornea is nearly always used, roughly similar to Lebrun's[282] *method. To this, Critchett adds Gräfe's*[283] *method as an alternative. He proceeds from the assumption that some eyes fare better with a scleral incision, others maybe with an incision in the cornea. In cases where, for instance, he has lost one eye through a corneal incision, he will operate on the other with a scleral incision, and vice versa. When he operates on both eyes simultaneously, he uses a different method for each eye, just to be on the safe side.*
For soft and liquid cataracts suction is used. Suction is effected either by mouth or with a syringe. Partial cataracts of young patients, e.g. squint cataracts, are prepared for suction by previous discission. The lens fibre mass is churned up as thoroughly as possible, which promptly causes it to swell extensively; it can then be sucked out after 2–3 days.
In cases of secondary cataract and of membranous cataracts in general the needle operation is usually carried out by inserting two needles simultaneously.
Tenotomy is usually carried out subconjunctivally by making a horizontal incision in the conjunctiva along the inferior edge of the tendon. According to Soelberg Wells, however, even with this method a subsidence of the caruncle can only be prevented if a conjunctival suture is applied afterwards. The advantage claimed for the subconjunctival method does therefore seem to be somewhat problematic.
With regard to theory it is worth noting that for certain forms of scrofulous conjunctivitis, particularly those that go hand in hand with the lively formation of vessels (e.g. keratitis fascicularis); a seton,[284] *applied to the temple, is very often used here.*
The common occurrence of keratitis parenchymatosa is surprising. It is associated with malformations of the teeth, of the nose, scars in the corners of the mouth, deafness, indolent bone swellings and other symptoms of hereditary syphilis.[285] *What is apparently less well known is the presence of chorioiditis in this disease. Isolated, mostly richly pigmented plaques are found in the periphery of the ocular fundus. As these can only be identified after the corneal disease has run its full course, they have presumably been mostly overlooked.*
Very common are those cases of amblyopia[286] *that, while displaying only scant ophthalmological abnormality, are characterised by the roughly equal affection of both eyes, improved acuity of vision in dimmed light and central scotoma for the colour red. Arlt first separated off this disease as a discrete group under the name of retinitis nyktalopica.*[287] *In our time, Leber*[288] *has attempted to link it to retrobulbar neuritis. The English ophthalmologists declare unanimously that it is the consequence of tobacco intoxication, citing as proof that – apart from too far advanced cases – all patients recover spontaneously once they have renounced the pleasure of smoking.*

A great deal of attention is devoted to the anomalies of refraction, especially by Couper.[289] *He claims maximum success is achieved by prescribing glasses aiming at perfect correction, which he manages to do by instilling atropine and then taking into consideration even the least degrees of astigmatism. These glasses patients are supposed to wear all day, even when looking at nearby objects; they are, as it were, to merge into one with their glasses. Couper uses this method for myopia up to ⅕ and claims it causes near-sightedness to make no or, at most, very little progress. He believes that the reason for this is that progressive myopia is caused by convergence rather than by accommodation.*
The refraction ophthalmoscope used by Couper is characterised by a very simple mechanism, which allows the examiner to place the mirror plate at an angle to the lens bearing disc so that he is not forced to look through the convection lens at an oblique angle.
My stay in London was cut short after a fortnight when my colleague Dr Karl Denk[290] *was called up to join his regiment, forcing me to return to the clinic. I only had time to spend two days with Donders*[291] *and Snellen*[292] *in Utrecht. Both are engrossed at present in the study of colour perception and colour blindness. Donders*[293] *is focused above all on the question of whether there is only red-green blindness or whether red blindness and green blindness should be kept separate as two distinct anomalies, a question of great import especially in the case of theories propounded by Young*[294]*-Helmholtz*[295] *and Hering.*[296]
On 15 October 1878 I was back in Vienna·
Vienna, October 1878. Signed:

Dr Ernst Fuchs,
assistant at the Eye Clinic
of Professor Hofrath v. Arlt
in Vienna.[297]

In addition to this official document private notes related to Fuchs's study trip have survived. During his stay in Paris Fuchs sent a detailed report to his teacher, Arlt, to acquaint him with the latest innovations in both clinical and operative aspects of their speciality. In spite of his relative youth, Fuchs emerges as remarkably self-confident:

Paris, 5 September 78.

Verehrter Herr Hofrath!

Having been in Paris now for almost one month I feel obliged to send you a brief report to let you know how I am spending my time. As all clinics keep the same hours (1–3 p.m.), it is difficult to visit more than one per day. Wecker is still in Biarritz – he is expected to return tomorrow or the day after tomorrow; I have therefore put off a visit to his clinic until he gets back. I first visited the clinic of Landolt, even though it is inferior to the other clinics in number of patients; Landolt himself is head and shoulders above the French ophthalmologists as for as expertise is concerned. I have seen quite a number of his cataract extractions. He uses a small, downward curved incision, roughly located in the scleral border; the lens is by no means easy to extract, firstly, because the incision is rather small; and, secondly, because the iris (no atropine is instilled) holds back the swelling lens equator. The iris is then repositioned, which is usually easy. In some cases it was found during evening rounds to have prolapsed and had to be cut off later. The great majority of cases, however, heal beautifully without coloboma; iritis and iridocyclitis are said to be no more common than otherwise, in spite of the strong strain on the iris.

On the whole this mode of operation closely resembles Wecker's, the only difference being that Wecker operates upwards. Landolt performs iridectomy with the narrow cataract knife and cuts off the prolapsed iris with pince-ciseaux instead of scissors.

Landolt has some rather nice things in the exhibition:[298] *a new, pretty straightforward ophthalmometer, a modification of Maxwell's disc for the determination of colour blindness, etc. Very appealing (and perhaps of use also at your clinic) is the fixation forceps he uses. Instead of teeth it is lined with caoutchouc, without any detriment to its grip. It helps to prevent any tearing of the conjunctiva. Meyer's clinic is distinguished by meticulous order, accurate sight tests and determination of the field of vision. The patient volume is not great. Meyer's treatment methods are similar to those in use by most German ophthalmologists. It is worth noting that, like Becker and many others, he uses thick Bowman*[299] *probes (No. 6 and thicker), claiming that these enable him to cure most tear sac blennorrheas within a fortnight. Like most French ophthalmologists he hardly bends his probes at all, which makes it difficult for him to work his way down.*

Instead of eserine he always resorts to pilocarpine. The advantages claimed for the latter are that it does not decompose, does not irritate the conjunctiva even after protracted use and does not cause oppressive headaches. Its efficacy is said to be on a par with that of eserine.

The genuinely French ophthalmologists have the greatest volume of patients, especially Galezowski, for whom no day passes without 20 new patients. Examination of the patients is extremely cursory and the therapy he administers to them in common with the other Frenchmen is highly idiosyncratic. For every catarrh leeches, atropine and poultices, as hot as they can be tolerated. Later a solution of silver nitrate, which is instilled. Mustard dough bandages and cupping glasses for every form of iritis, keratitis, chorioiditis, etc. His cataract operation mode resembles that of Landolt, but he is a poor surgeon. While the incision is still in progress, he presses down so hard with the fixation forceps that not infrequently the result is a prolapse of the vitreous body. I was also present when he whittled down the anterior bulbus segment because of staphyloma.
Panas is not in town at present. He is being covered for by a surgeon called Marchand[300] *who, on his own admission, has no expertise whatever in ophthalmology.*
Of the French oculists in the narrow sense of the term it is decidedly Abadie who leaves the best impression. Patients are painstakingly examined. His therapy is rather similar to yours. He also seems to be perfectly conversant with the literature in German. He is perhaps the most deserving candidate for the chair of ophthalmology as the Germans – Wecker, Meyer, Landolt – are ruled out a priori. However, the most promising candidate is Javal.[301] *To refute the charge that he cannot operate, he recently performed an iridectomy on a boy suffering from a stationary cataract. He then formally presented the boy to a meeting at the Institut de France. Badal*[302] *is also said to have a sporting chance. Of foreign oculists I have met here Prof. Becker from Heidelberg, Brettauer,*[303] *Hirschberg,*[304] *and Dufour.*[305] *Cohn*[306] *and Businelli*[307] *are also here, but I have not seen them. Let me assure you of my respect and gratitude.*

Ihr ergebenster
Fuchs.
Rue des Écoles 6.[308]

A brief account of his study trip features in Fuchs's autobiography, which was published in 1946 and has already been referred to repeatedly. In keeping with the private character of that autobiography, the account is less formal and conveys a more colourful and more personal insight into this formative episode in his training as an ophthalmologist:

In 1878 I was awarded the Haber-Linsberg travel grant[309] *in line with a decision taken by the Faculty to enable me to spend half a year abroad. One half of the grant, whose amount now escapes me, was paid in advance, the other half was to be paid to the recipient on return from his travels, on the obvious presupposition that the recipient would borrow the money he needed for the second half of his travels. I was given six months leave of absence and in the spring I went first to Paris, at that time hosting a World Exhibition. By a rare coincidence Dr. Wiethe*[310] *happened to be waiting at the station. I knew him well from Vienna. Slightly younger than me, he had accepted the position of assistant Landolt had offered him, having been a junior doctor in Vienna under Jäger.*[311] *However, he did not remain in Paris for long and when I saw him again in Vienna, he was seriously ill. Wiethe had not been waiting for me. Initially, I put up at a student hostel in the Rue des écoles in the Quartier Latin because it was cheap. Each of the students shared his room with his girl, and these girls, usually seamstresses and the like, regularly joined the students at the table d'hôte at mealtime. I could have lived with this, but what I could not live with was the terrible dirt in the hostel so I left after a few days. I found a nice mansard let by a widow in a nearby street. Houses in Paris often have a balcony that runs along the topmost storey, which is accessible through the glass doors of the mansards. These rooms have no windows, only doors. The balcony section belonging to each mansard was only marked off from its neighbouring spaces by a few flower pots, which were easy enough to negotiate so that in the evening a lively toing and froing developed on the balcony, presumably involving the swapping of the girls. When none moved in with me, the widow asked me, with all the signs of being non-plussed, why I chose to remain single.*

At one of the clinics I then made the acquaintance of Dr Oeller,[312] *who had also come to Paris to study. He was to become professor in Erlangen later. When the French heard that he was from Bavaria they were decidedly less obliging, since in 1870–71, during the war, the Bavarian regiments had made themselves particularly feared, while they extolled the fact that I was from Austria.*

There was no university eye clinic yet in Paris, only private clinics, all of them small, cramped and dirty. The most frequented clinic belonged to Wecker, a Frankfurt Jew, who still spoke his Frankfurt French. He has a large out-patient clinic and allowed the patients after a cataract operation to go home by omnibus. One day he urgently recommended an operation to a patient with an immature cataract in one eye, while the other was still good. When I asked him in German why he did not opt for waiting, he replied: "Well, in that case it would be one of my colleagues that gets the chance to operate on her."

On one occasion he performed a tenotomy on a boy,[313] *without anaesthetic and, of course, without cocaine, which was not yet known at the time. The boy was wailing most pitifully. It was midsummer, the windows, which gave on to the street, were open (the clinic was on the ground floor) and the boy's lamentations caused a growing crowd to gather, blocking the street. I asked Wecker whether I should close the window so that the wailing should become less audible. He replied: "On the contrary, the wailing is the best advertisement for me. People in the street will say, 'This is Dr Wecker performing one of his operations'. He was very proud of his title of nobility: he was indebted to Austria for his "de Wecker" in some way that is unknown to me.*[314] *He was an excellent surgeon, acquitting himself brilliantly even in the most difficult bulbus operations, even though binocular vision was denied to him. He was afflicted with marked exotropia. He had been operated on in his youth by v. Graefe for esotropia, with the result common at the time of a later onset of exotropia. Wecker was an inveterate bachelor, who earned an inordinate amount of money and lived in a nice palais. The bulk of his patients were people from countries far away, Spaniards, South Americans, Mexicans, etc. Landolt, who was still comparatively young, had, as has already been mentioned, the newly arrived Wiethe as assistant. Landolt was not a good surgeon; his forte was refraction, which was only rarely practised at that time, and muscle anomalies. He charged 20 francs for an astigmatism determination, which was a lot of money at the time.*

Meier,[315] *another Jew from Frankfurt, turned out to be a genial, highly cultivated gentleman, who speaks French like a Frenchman and has a highly lucrative practice among the high aristocracy. He was always very nice to me.*

Sichel,[316] *the son of the famous ophthalmologist Sichel,*[317] *is on his last legs. Another son of a famous father is young Desmarres,*[318] *who seeks to capitalise on the name of his father.*[319] *He adds the numbers of his operation logs to those of his father and uses those numbers, which exceed 100,000, to impress the patients of the polyclinic. The only genuine Frenchmen were Abadie, Perrin, and a few others, whose achievements as ophthalmologists are so insignificant that when a chair for ophthalmology was created in Paris, a Greek, Dr Panas, was entrusted with it, even though he was not even an ophthalmologist. He was a surgeon at Lariboisière Hospital, where he had shown great interest in eye diseases. Taking a German was of course out of the question. Panas learned the ropes extremely quickly; he proved a genial, highly cultivated and highly knowledgeable gentleman.*

Perhaps the most frequented ophthalmologist was Professor Galezowski, because he is cheap. He is a real charlatan. Treacher Collins[320] *told me the following story about him: "You know that at one stage I operated on the Shah's wife. She had been referred to me as reputedly suffering from cataract and other people had raised the prospect of an operation restoring good eyesight to her. However,*

she was suffering from advanced glaucoma and was already blind on one eye. The other eye was reduced to finger counting; even though the iridectomy was successful, the disappointment of the patient and her relatives was acute since more had been expected. It was impossible to explain the true state of things to her or to her companions and it is likely that the shortfall was imputed to me. The net result of this was that when the heir to the Persian throne was afflicted with an eye disease, it was not me who was called to Teheran but Nettleship, who was requested to repair thither along with Galezowski. Nettleship declined and suggested I join Galezowski. On the way there and also during our return journey Galezowski operated on a number of patients suffering from optic atrophy, which he misleadingly declared to be glaucoma simplex. Later, I myself saw two patients he had performed operations on. In Teheran we found that little was actually amiss with the heir apparent, other than perhaps a trachoma that had healed already, but Galezowski insisted (because of the fee) on performing an operation and it was only with a great deal of effort that I got him to agree that he would confine his operation to slitting open a lacrimal canal so that at least he did no harm."[321]
I paid several visits to Javal in his lab at the Sorbonne, with its rather sparse equipment; at the time a very young man, the Dane Tscherming [sic],[322] *was working there.*
These private clinics usually do not open until 11 or 12 o'clock. I therefore put the morning hours to good use by going to the Louvre or one of the other museums, and Sundays were earmarked for excursions with Oeller to the environs of Paris, which are especially charming in spring. In the afternoon there was often a visit to the World Exhibition. One of the sights there was a ballon captif[323] *construed by Godard,*[324] *in which Meier,*[325] *Landolt, I, and others ascended at a cost of 20 frs. It was already evening and as we were rising to ever greater heights, the sun reappeared behind Mont Valérian* [sic].[326]
In general, my stay in Paris was extremely rewarding, not as far as ophthalmology was concerned, where there was only little I found useful, but on account of my getting to know the city itself and its art treasures really well.
After a sojourn of three months I travelled via Rouen and Dieppe to Newhaven and then on to London, where I stayed at a boarding house. It is impossible to imagine a greater contrast than the one offered by Paris and London at that time. In London there was great deal to learn for an ophthalmologist already well versed in the trade. I was a frequent visitor to Thomas Hospital, where I met Nettleship, with whom I was soon on friendly terms, and to Moorfields, where Brayley,[327] *Gunn,*[328] *and several other highly competent men were at work. They had no time*

for beginners, which is the reason why so often Americans come from London to Vienna, where they find what they need: "spoon-feeding".[329]
However, the doctors at Moorfields were willing enough to discuss special cases with me and even asked me on one occasion to perform an enucleation to show them Arlt's method. Old Critchett is no longer active at the hospital, but he allowed me to witness a cataract operation at his private practice. It was then usual to perform operations at the patient's home and only people who could not afford this went to hospital, as was also the case in Vienna.
I met Hutkinson [sic],[330] *who was still an ophthalmologist at the time before wholly switching to dermatology later; he gave me his famous book on keratitis parenchymatosa*[331] *as a gift, which is now in the library of the 2nd Eye Clinic.*[332]
Bowman is still around but unfortunately does not practise any longer; it is a pity I decided not to visit him for fear of disturbing him.
In England it is usual to anaesthetise patients for bulbus operation with ether. Chloroform is not used.
I was told a story about Bowman at Moorfields Hospital, where he used to work: while a patient was being anaesthetised for the operation, Bowman used to stand there waiting, with his back to the fireplace, ready to go to the patient as soon as he was told that he or she was ready; on one occasion there was a sudden commotion among the assistants and one of them finally came up to Bowman, saying "Patient is dead", whereupon Bowman is reputed to have said, "Next patient".
Unfortunately, my stay in London lasted only three weeks instead of three months. In the meantime, Austria had occupied Bosnia and Herzegovina and my colleague at the clinic, Denk, if my memory serves me right, had been called up and I had to go back. I only had enough time to have a look around in the Netherlands and to visit Donders.[333]

"Amerikanerkurse"

After Fuchs's return from his study trip in October 1878, the first *Amerikanerkurs*, albeit still in German, was realised in November 1878 on the personal initiative of Lawrence Webster Fox (1853–1931).[334] (Fig. 23) Fox, who spent four years in Europe studying with eminent specialists, had come to Vienna from Berlin, where he organised theoretical and practical classes given to a group of ten American medical doctors by Mauthner,[335] who, as has already been mentioned, had trained under Jaeger, and by Fuchs. When, more than half a century later, Fox wrote a heartfelt obituary for Ernst Fuchs, he had no problem recalling the precise details of their first meeting:

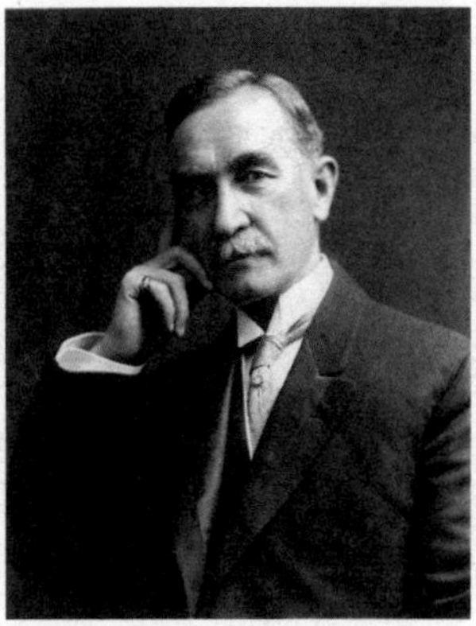

Fig. 23. Lawrence Webster Fox

It is with no little pride that I recall a certain Sunday morning in 1878, when the late Dr David H. Cooper[336] *of Denver and myself, anxious to see the great Arlt operate at his clinic in Vienna, first came across Fuchs in the hospital. He was quite tall and apparently rather spare in build. Prosperity had not yet marked him for her own. Sensing from our dress and mannerisms that we were Americans, he addressed us in English, and after the usual salutations inquired, in the characteristic kindly way which distinguished him throughout his life, as to what service he might render us. When we replied that we wished to see Professor Arlt operate, he told us that could be readily accomplished since he was Professor Arlt's first assistant. Suiting the action to the word, he escorted us into the operating room and we were afforded a choice view of the master at work.*[337]

A few months later, in May 1879, Fuchs achieved a pioneering feat that was to leave its mark for times to come on the curriculum of the Vienna Medical University. He, too, had no problems recalling it in detail almost fifty years later:

The incremental increase in medical specialisation all over the world was the reason why an ever greater number of foreign medical doctors were flocking to Vienna, where they found better opportunities for specialisation than elsewhere. This demand Viennese lecturers met by offering an ever increasing number of more and more specialised courses. My time as an assistant at the clinic in the second half of the '70s coincided with the beginnings of this development. It so happened at the time that several of my American students proposed a course on an especially difficult chapter of ophthalmology – difficult because it involved some maths – of a kind that had never before been taught; at the same time they voiced their apprehension that, in light of the complexity of the topic, they might not be able to follow the lectures in a language they were only insufficiently conversant with. I therefore offered to lecture in English to the best of my powers and held the first course in English at Vienna's Medical Faculty. Several years ago, I was, to my great joy, hosted in the United States by two of my former students.[338] *My first course in English had no [immediate] sequel because I left Vienna soon afterwards, having received a call for a professorship abroad. Nor do I know when and by whom the tradition of lecturing in English was continued. It has now become a fixture.*[339]

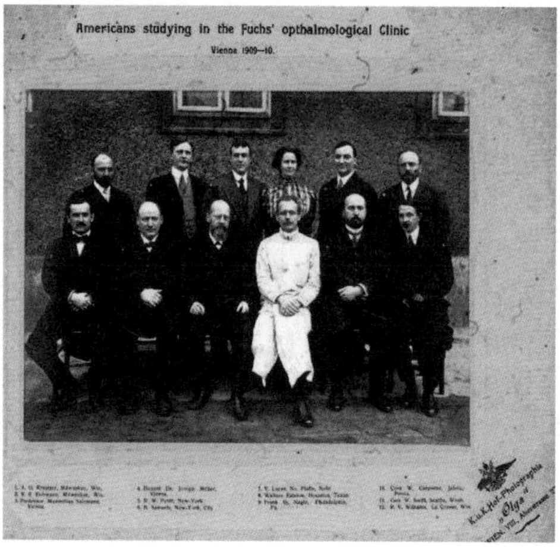

Fig. 24. "Amerikanerkurs" at Fuchs's Eye Clinic in 1909–1910

This was the beginning of a lifelong friendship between Ernst Fuchs and Lawrence Webster Fox, who reminisced about the beginnings as follows:

Shortly afterward Dr Coover and myself prevailed on Fuchs to give us, in English, a course of instruction in refraction and ophthalmology in general. It was necessary to make up a class of ten to satisfy the requirements, and in that class were Coover of Denver, Ryerson[340] *of Toronto, Charnley*[341] *of Shrewsbury, England, Linton Forbes of Belfast, Ireland, Knaggs*[342] *and Tom Dixon of Australia, Palmer*[343] *of Toronto, and myself, with two others whose names, for the time, escapes my memory. So instructive was the course and so delightful the instructor, that other English-speaking students rapidly embraced the opportunity to repeat the course, and Fuchs's popularity with the embryonal English-speaking ophthalmologists became assured from that moment.*[344]

The list drawn up by Fox goes to show that Ernst Fuchs's *Amerikanerkurse* were attended from the very first also by others than US-Americans. From the moment they took off in 1878 in German, they attracted postdoc students from all over the Anglophone world, as is shown here by the presence of two Canadians (Ryerson, Palmer), a Briton (Charnley), an Irishman (Forbes) and two Australians (Knaggs, Dixon). The commonly used term *Amerikanerkurse* probably arose because the "founding fathers" Coover and Fox as well as the majority of participants came from the United States and because the course was in English. First held in 1879, it was a premiere for the curriculum of the Medical University of Vienna.

The group of twenty-three Anglo-American doctors, who continued their postdoc studies under Fuchs in May 1879, were so taken by the content and by the way it was presented by Ernst Fuchs that only one month later they founded the Austro-American Medical Society.[345] The original mission statement of this association called for the organisation of additional courses lasting several weeks led by Fuchs. In the wake of Fuchs's spectacularly successful teaching experiment, courses in English began to be offered by other specialist clinics only a few years later. In 1904, the Austro-American Medical Society established its own office in the immediate vicinity of the hospital (Lazarettgasse 13 in the 9th district). Evidence of courses held in 1909 and 1910, taught by Fuchs's assistants Maximilian Salzmann[346] and Josef Meller,[347] has survived in the form of original photos with the names of all the participants. (Figs. 24, 25) Later the society extended its services to Asian medical doctors with an English-speaking background.[348]

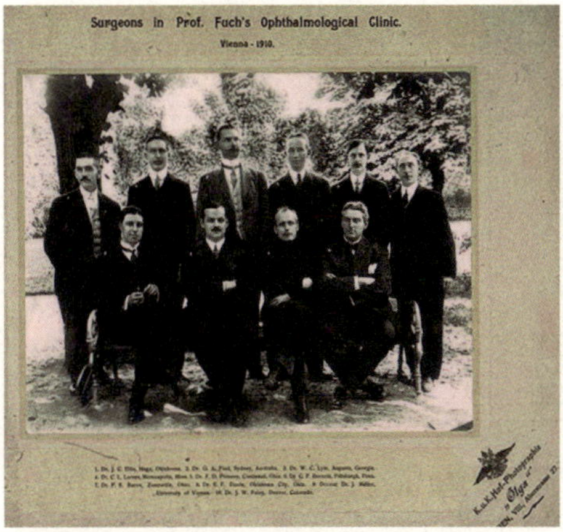

Fig. 25. Surgeons in Prof. Fuchs's Eye Clinic (1910)

During his assistantship under Arlt and before his "habilitation" in 1880, Fuchs held three so-called privatissima, normally a lecture for an invited audience, in this case really a series of private lessons. Fuchs's first private student was Adolph Barkan (1844–1935),[349] originally from Hungary, who had established himself in San Francisco in 1872 and taught at Stanford. Barkan was followed by Joseph Nelson (1840–1910).[350] Nelson had worked for a time in India but wished to return to his native Belfast. As he wanted to establish himself there as an eye specialist, but had not yet received any specialist training, he decided to spend the entire year of 1878–79 in Vienna. During this time, he worked under Fuchs at Arlt's clinic every day and paid his tutor a fee of 1,000 fl. Fuchs valued the intensive contact with Nelson very highly, not least because it helped him to perfect his own command of English to a degree that enabled him to hold the *Amerikanerkurse* mentioned above and to accept invitations to hold courses and deliver lectures in the English-speaking world later. After the end of Nelson's time in Vienna, Fuchs remained on friendly terms with him and paid him two visits in Belfast.[351]

Fuchs's most prominent ophthalmological private student was Carl Theodor Herzog in Bayern (1839–1909),[352] the brother of Empress Elisabeth von Österreich:

He had obtained his MD from Munich and came to Vienna to specialise as an ophthalmologist under Arlt. Arlt in turn handed me the Duke, and I instructed him in the use of the ophthalmoscope, in operations and diagnosis; he shared my workroom. He was an uncommonly nice and unassuming person of great diligence.[353]

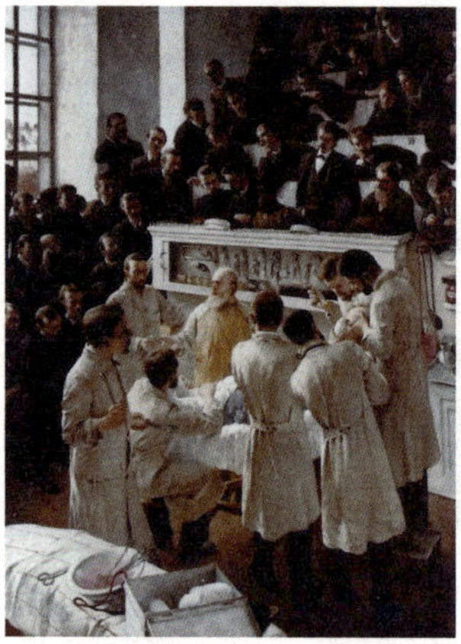

Fig. 26. Billroth in the Lecture Hall

The duke continued to hone his skills in 1882 at Eduard Jaeger von Jaxthal's Eye Department at the Allgemeines Krankenhaus.[354] His repeated stays in Vienna allowed him to make friends with Theodor Billroth. Adalbert Franz Seligmann (1862–1945),[355] the son of the Viennese medical historian Franz Romeo Seligmann (1808–1892),[356] included him in 1890 in his painting *Billroth im Hörsaal* [Billroth in the Lecture Hall].[357] (Fig. 26) Author of several ophthalmological papers, the duke founded his own eye clinic in Munich in 1895. As "Augenklinik Herzog Carl Theodor" it is still a going concern.[358]

Before Fuchs was given the green light for his "habilitation" by Arlt in the spring of 1880, he had to prove himself in years of hard work. In addition to research this involved a great deal of teaching at the clinic. During his assistantship, as Fuchs admitted later, he was inclined to take a rather dim view of his academic prospects and, alongside plans for setting up practice in one of the Monarchy's other major cities, he even contemplated emigration to America:

During my time as an assistant I had not given a great deal of thought to an academic career and rather than dwelling on considerations at the back of my mind, I had been doing my work for its own sake, because the questions I was dealing with were of interest to me. When Arlt in the end asked me to apply for a lecturership on the basis of my sarcoma paper, I did so without setting any great store by it. It seemed to me that my prospects of an academic career were more or less nil. I was toying with the idea of either establishing myself in Brünn after the end of my assistantship. As [...] *no eye specialist had set up practice there yet, I would have been sure to flourish – or I would emigrate to America. This idea appealed to me because several of my fellow students had done so with great success and because American participants in my course had described such a venture in glowing colours. One was not even required to sit the exams again in America; a diploma from Vienna was recognised anywhere. In order to give me a chance to at least have a brief look at America first, an Englishman in my course saw to it that I was offered the position of ship's doctor on a vessel bound for the West Indies, which would also have taken me to New Orleans. I had already been given the requisite leave when I was told that yellow fever had broken out in the West Indies, as so frequently happened at the time, and that quarantine regulations would prevent me from disembarking. I gave up the position, hoping to be offered another one in the near future. Then the call to Liège arrived completely out of the blue.*[359]

"Habilitation"

As Fuchs's time as assistant was coming to an end in late February 1880, Arlt, departing from established practice, applied for a third two-year extension of the assistantship towards the end of January 1880. [360] This enabled Fuchs to submit his application for "habilitation" in March 1880.[361] Fuchs specified the prospective *"Programme of Lectures"* as follows:

1. Normal and pathological anatomy of the human eye, in concert with the demonstration of preparations and practical exercises.
2. Theoretical and practical aspects of the ophthalmoscope, with demonstrations and exercises involving patients.[362]

In the assessment Arlt and Stellwag von Carion delivered as expert witnesses on 1 June 1880 to the Professorial Council of the Vienna Medical Faculty, they spelt out Fuchs's qualifications as follows:

What Prof. Arlt would like to stress in particular are his achievements in and his capacity for anatomical-microscopic anatomy. Fuchs has proved himself a worthy successor of his predecessors O. Becker and H. Sattler and has augmented in the most commendable way possible the collection of pathological eye preparations for clinical tuition initiated by those two.
It is his intention, according to the attached curriculum, to lecture initially on normal and pathological anatomy and on theoretical and practical aspects of the ophthalmoscope. The first topic in particular makes it highly desirable that a lecturer devote his attention to it since both the professor's and the assistants' commitments do not allow the time that would be required for it. All that remains for Prof. Arlt to do is to express the wish that someone who is so diligent and so gifted is not lost to teaching.[363]

The habilitation procedure passed through the following stages:

"Herr Dr Ernst Fuchs, assistant at the Eye Clinic of Herr Hofrath Professor v. Arlt, has submitted the attached application, dated 17 March this year, for his habilitation as private lecturer in ophthalmology, which was passed on for report

to Professors von Arlt und von Stellwag in the meeting of the Professorial College on 17 April.
This report was made on 12 June this year. Herr Dr Fuchs was admitted to the colloquium with 15 votes in favour, 1 against, and Herr Hofrath von Arlt was asked to take charge of it. The colloquium took place on 10 July 1880 and Herr Dr Fuchs was admitted to a trial lecture, with 16 votes in favour, 2 against. The topic chosen for the test lecture was "On Cyclitis". The lecture was delivered on 16 July this year in the presence of the undersigned, Herr Hofrath v. Arlt, and a numerous audience and was received with general satisfaction.
The Professorial College was notified of this result in the meeting on 23 October this year and on that occasion approved of the habilitation of Dr Ernst Fuchs as private lecturer in ophthalmology with 18 votes in favour, 2 against.
The undersigned respectfully herewith submits all the requisite documents to the Ministry, asking for confirmation of this habilitation.
Vienna, 25 October 1880.

Signed: E. Hofmann,[364]
Dekan[365]

Roughly a month later, on 20 November 1880, a character reference attesting Ernst Fuchs's integrity as a citizen was supplied to the Minister für Cultus und Unterricht by the Office of the Imperial Royal Lower Austrian Governor:

Medicinae Doctor Ernst Fuchs, the son of Imperial Royal Professor Adalbert Fuchs resident in Vienna, born in Vienna, 29 years old, Catholic, single, has been an assistant of Ophthalmology of the Imperial Royal Hospital since 1873, where he has been resident since 1876.
He lives in ordered circumstances, appears above reproach both as a moral subject and citizen and enjoys a good reputation everywhere.[366]

Having delivered his trial lecture[367] on 16 July 1880, Fuchs took part in the annual conference of the British Medical Association one month later in Cambridge, where he was the only non-British speaker and where, in all probability, he presented his first paper in English at a conference outside Austria.[368] His topic was an innovative therapeutic intervention involving cauterization of the cornea developed and propagated to a significant extent by himself at the Vienna University Eye Clinic under Arlt.[369]

The Ministry's confirmation of Ernst Fuchs's habilitation in Ophthalmology at Vienna University dates to 25 November 1880.[370] His habilitation thesis is a comprehensive study of the sarcoma of the uveal tract, which was to be published two years later as a three-hundred-page monograph.[371] (Fig. 27) The manner in which Fuchs deals with the topic is an early indication of what was to become his mastery of the description and the assessment of pathohistological changes in the eye. Altogether, Fuchs drew in his thesis on the statistics of 259 cases, 22 of which were marked as his own cases, which came with detailed case reports. What is noteworthy even at this early stage is that Fuchs already had his own collection of pathological section preparations of the eye at his disposal, a collection he had started putting together as soon as he joined Arlt's clinic.[372] The other case studies used by Fuchs were taken from international specialist publications accurately indexed to the 270 items in the alphabetically listed bibliography.

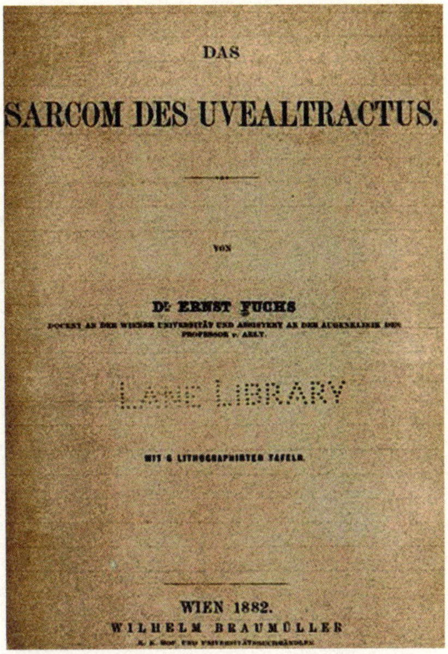
DAS

SARCOM DES UVEALTRACTUS.

VON

Dr. ERNST FUCHS

WIEN 1882.

WILHELM BRAUMÜLLER

Fig. 27. Ernst Fuchs's habilitation thesis

He discovered the diffuse form of the sarcoma, studied the necrosis of the ulcer and its symptoms, and identified its unusual form of sympathetic inflammation.[373]

Fuchs's exact work met with immediate recognition both in the Austrian and international specialist press. The Viennese ophthalmologist Leopold Königstein (1850–1924),[374] for instance, wound up his review of the monograph with the following conclusion:

FUCHS has acquitted himself to the fullest extent of the task he set out to accomplish – to draw as complete a picture of the uveal sarcoma as possible – and has managed both to end his assistantship in Vienna and commence his professorship in Liège in a perfectly congenial manner.[375]

Fuchs's first monograph impresses with its accuracy of observation and the resulting clear description of the specific pathological substrate. In addition, this work by an author who was only twenty-nine provides a foretaste of things to come. Fuchs was in a league entirely of his own when it came to distilling the characteristics typical of any given pathology from details stored in his phenomenally selective memory and synthesizing them into discrete entities. For this, he often had to make do with only a handful of individual cases he had observed over the course of several years. In the sarcoma monograph, painstaking observation enabled him to distinguish between fourteen different types of uveal sarcoma based on differences in their cellular structure.

What assures Fuchs of a lasting place not only in the history of ophthalmic oncology but of oncology in general is his discovery of a universal law. His research on the sarcoma of the uveal tract enabled him to formulate the "seed and soil" theory of the pathogenesis of metastases, which will always be associated with his name:

It is not to be doubted that with melanosarcoma the general infection of the organism happens via embolism. It is therefore crucial to determine whether the primary tumour provides favourable conditions for tumorous cells to be dislocated and swept along by the bloodstream. This will be facilitated all the more the more numerous the vessels of the tumour are, the wider their calibre is and the thinner is their wall. The smallness of the cells and the deficiency in the formation of the stroma, which make the tumour soft and friable, are additional contributory factors. Taken together, these qualities cause the different degrees of malignity of the various sarcoma types.[376]

In the Anglo-American world the discovery of the causal link between the primary site of a tumour and the organ or tissue it "seeds" with characteristic metastases is commonly attributed to English surgeon Stephen Paget (1855–1926),[377] the son of the renowned surgeon and pathologist Sir James Paget (1814–1899).[378] Stephen Paget postulated this law in 1889 in light of bone metastasis in cases of breast cancer.[379] Paget himself noted explicitly at the time that the priority for this discovery belongs to Ernst Fuchs, when he pointed out that *"the chief advocate of this theory of the relation between the embolus and the tissues which receive it is Fuchs.*[380]

Fuchs's habilitation thesis, which was published in 1882, caused interest in research on this rare tumour of the uvea to surge over the next decades. From among the many publications on sarcoma formation in the eye there is room here to mention only a few papers published in German. In the year of Fuchs's monograph, 1882, Berlin ophthalmo-historian Julius Hirschberg,[381] who was later to become a world celebrity, published his study on the prognosis for choroidal sarcoma.[382] This was followed by three doctoral theses that originated from the eye clinics of the universities of Halle and Königsberg.[383] In 1890 Arlt student Rosa Putjata-Kerschbaumer published a comprehensive pathological-anatomical monograph.[384] In the introduction to this volume, Hubert Sattler, whose collection had provided the preparations discussed by Putjata-Kerschbaumer, made explicit mention of Fuchs.[385] At the instigation of the Director of the Eye Clinic of Göttingen University, Theodor Leber,[386] another thesis took shape,[387] whose author refers to Fuchs's exemplary basic research in an introductory statement.[388] Similar citation is given in another paper coming out of Göttingen on the same group of disorders.[389] The Fuchs students Maximilian Salzmann (1862–1954)[390] and Oskar Kopetzky von Rechtperg (1873–1963) contributed a collection of case studies[391] and decades later Fuchs himself revisited his earlier observations on the formation of sarcoma of the uvea.[392] Fuchs's scientific achievement in the description of the exceedingly rare melanosarcoma is still being appreciated to this day in specialist oncological literature:

His paper about malignant sarcomas continues to have a huge impact after more than 100 years. He is thought [of] as the father of modern ophthalmology; the ophthalmologist who paved the way for future research on uveal melanoma.[393]

The Vienna University publishing house Wilhelm Braumüller, which had published Fuchs's sarcoma monograph in 1882, reacted in its own way to the fact that Fuchs was a rising star in the world of science. A full-page ad for Fuchs's habilitation thesis was included in Braumüller's later publications in addition to a portrait of the author, which was highly unusual at that time. (Fig. 28)

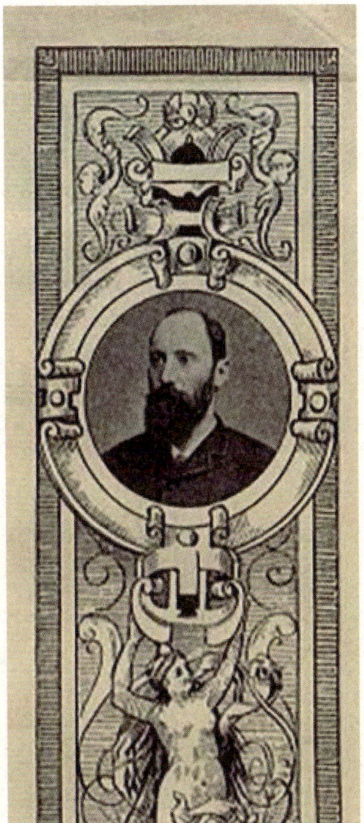

Fig. 28. Advertisement of the publishing house Braumueller with Ernst Fuchs's portrait

The summer semester of 1881–82 was Fuchs's first term as a private lecturer at Vienna University. He announced a free course in testing eye function to be held every Saturday and Sunday between 8 and 9 a.m. in the lecture hall of Arlt's clinic.[394] For the ensuing winter semester of 1881–82 Fuchs announced a course on the normal and pathological anatomy of the eye.[395]

When he sat down four decades after his habilitation to write his autobiography, he was no longer quite sure about his beginnings as a lecturer, being of the opinion that he had received the call from Liège immediately after his habilitation: *"I had not yet got round to making use of my venia legendi."*[396] Since he habilitated in the winter semester of 1880–81, it appears plausible, however, that he in fact held the course that was announced for the ensuing summer semester. His call to the Chair of Ophthalmology at the University of Liège[397] coincided with the beginning of the winter semester of 1881–82 so that the course announced for that term at Vienna University had to be cancelled.

Notes

51 This institution had been founded in 1735 for the training of engineer officers and had been raised to the status of an academy in 1769. For more details, see A. SCHMIDL, *Wien wie es ist. Ein Gemälde der Kaiserstadt und ihrer nächsten Umgebungen in Beziehung auf Topographie, Statistik und geselliges Leben, mit besonderer Berücksichtigung wissenschaftlicher Anstalten und Sammlungen nach authentischen Quellen vorgestellt.* Carl Gerold, Vienna 1833, pp. 110–113; Friedrich GATTI, *Geschichte der K. K. Ingenieur- und K. K. Genie-Akademie 1717–1869.* Wilhelm Braumüller, Vienna 1901.

52 Carl Graf VASQUEZ, *K. K. Polizey-Bezirk MARIAHILF bestehend a. d. Vorstädten Laimgrube, Mariahilf, Windmühle, Magdalenagr[und] & Gumpendorf nebst 14 Ansichten der vorzüglichsten Gebäude.*

53 Then Mariahilfer Hauptstraße No. 186, today Stiftgasse 2–2a in Vienna's 7th district, Neubau. Cf. Robert MESSNER, *Mariahilf im Vormärz. Historisch-topographische Darstellung der westlichen Vorstädte (südliche Hälfte) auf Grund der Katastralvermessung (= Topographie von Alt-Wien* VI. Teil*)*. Verband der Wissenschaftlichen Gesellschaften Österreichs. Vienna 1982, pp. 79–80.

54 Cf. *Hof- und Staats-Schematismus des österreichischen Kaiserthums.* II. Theil. K. K. Hof- und Staats-Aerarial-Druckerey Vienna 1822, p. 140; *Militär-Schematismus des österreichischen Kaiserthumes.* K. K. Hof-und Staats-Druckerey, Vienna 1837, p. 422.

55 *Hof- und Staatsschematismus des österreichischen Kaiserthumes.* II. Theil. K. K. Hof- und Staats-Aerarial-Druckerey, Vienna 1843, p. 114.

56 Then the corner of Windmühl Gasse/Kleine Kirchen Gasse/Hollerbeer Gasse, today Windmühlgasse 30 and 32/corner Barnabitengasse 2 in Vienna's 6th District, Mariahilf. Cf. MESSNER, *Mariahilf* (as in FN 53), p. 178.

57 ÖBL (as in FN 11); Lambert M. SURHONE, Miriam T. TIMPLEDON, Susan F. MARSEKEN (eds.), *Adalbert Nikolaus Fuchs. Wieden, Kritzendorf, Technische Universität Wien, Ernst Fuchs, Schottengymnasium.* ßetascript publishing und Verlag Dr Müller 2010.

58 Karl (Carl) Fuchs (1812–1. 8. 1881), Dr med. (Grad. 5 Aug. 1837), Dr chir. (doctorate 2 Aug. 1840) and Master's degree in obstetrics 1840. Cf. UA Wien, Medizinisches Hauptrigorosen-Protokoll 1821–1871. In compliance with the study regulations in force at the time he submitted the following doctoral thesis: Carolus FUCHS, *Dissertatio inauguralis medico-practica de Endocarditide quam consensu et auctoritate illustrissimi ac magnifici domini Praesidis et Directoris, perillustris ac spectabilis domini Decani, nec non clarissimorum et celeberrimorum D. D. Professorum, pro doctoris medicinae laurea summisque in medicina honoribus ac privilegiis rite et legitime obtinendis in antiquissima ac celeberrima Universitate Vindobonensi publicae eruditorum disquisitioni submittit.* Schmid 1837.

59 During the revolution in Vienna in 1848 he served as a first lieutenant in the National Guard in the suburb Mariahilf, which remained loyal to the Emperor. He was a member of the college of doctors of the Med. Fac. of Vienna Univ. Residence: Mariahilf, Josefigasse 80. Together with his brother Adalbert Nikolaus he took part in the 32nd Versamml. dt. Naturforscher and Ärzte in Vienna 1856. Nobilitated with the predicate "Edler von". Died in 1881 at the age of 69. Interment at the Kritzendorf cemetery. Cf. *Allgemeines Beamten-Adressbuch für die k. k. Haupt- und Residenz-Stadt Wien. Systematische Zusammenstellung sämmtlicher k. k. Hof- und Staats-Aemter, der*

städtischen Behörden, öffentlichen Anstalten, Vereine etc. und bei denselben angestellten Beamten, Functionäre und Diener, mit Angabe des Namens, der Diensteigenschaft und der Wohnung nebst alphabetischen Registern. Yr. 1. Friedrich Manz, Vienna 1853, p. 173; Paul SCHULZ, *Marginalien über die Wiener Revolution vom Jahre 1848 und ihre wichtigsten Folgen in der spätesten Zeit*. W. Gerhard, Leipzig 1856, p. 246; *Tageblatt der 32. Versammlung deutscher Naturforscher und Aerzte in Wien 1856*. Editions 1–8, p. 25; Joseph Alexander Frh. von HELFERT, *Österreichisches Jahrbuch*. Vol. 7. Verlag des Österreichischen Volksschriften-Vereins in Kommission bei Kubasta & Voigt, Vienna 1883, p. 342; In memoriam card (original in the Family archive).

60 *Genealogisches Handbuch des Adels*. Vol. 58. C. A. Starke, Limburg 1974, p. 383.

61 FUCHS, *Augenarzt* (as in FN 2), p. 16. The contact with Czaderski proved so long lived that in 1851, many years later, Adalbert Nikolaus Fuchs's first-born son was given the first name Ernst in Czaderski's honour. Ibid.

62 UA Wien, Med. Hauptrigorosen-Protokoll 1821–1871. Award of Dr med. on 6 Aug. 1839. No evidence has been found of an additional doctorate in surgery from Vienna Univ.

63 Letter from the Lower Austrian Provinc. Governm., No. 12994, dated Vienna, 28. Feb. 1846, to Dr A[da]lbert Fuchs, Mariahilf No. 27: *"According to the Imperial-Royal Morav. Siles. government in a letter dated 17th of this month, Z. 6949, His Royal Imperial Majesty has deigned to dispose of this chair otherwise."* Original in the Family archive.

64 UA Wien, *Verzeichnis d. a. d. Philosoph. Fak. d. Univ. Wien von 1774 bis zum 2. Juli 1873 promovierten Doktoren d. Philosophie*. Vienna 1954, p. IV.

65 FUCHS, *Augenarzt* (as in FN 2), p. 16.

66 Ibid., FN 2.

67 For more details, see: Carl Heinrich SCHULTZ, *Natürliches System des Pflanzenreichs nach seiner inneren Organisation, nebst einer vergleichenden Darstellung der wichtigsten aller früheren künstlichen und natürlichen Pflanzensysteme*. August Hirschwald, Berlin 1832.

68 Österreichisches Staatsarchiv/Allgemeines Verwaltungsarchiv Vienna [= ÖSTA/AVA Wien], 6 Technik Fuchs, Ministerium des Cultus und Unterrichtes No. 3159. Gracious Decree Issued by His Majesty Emperor Franz Joseph, dated 15 April 1850: *"I herewith give my consent to the institution of lectures on agronomy at the Polytechnic Institute in Vienna, and appoint Dr Adalbert Fuchs, hitherto Professor of Agronomy and General Natural History at Innsbruck University, Full Professor of Agronomy at the aforementioned Institute, on conditions as agreed."* For more details, see: *Die K. K. Technische Hochschule in Wien 1815–1915. Gedenkschrift herausgegeben vom Professorenkollegium redigiert von Hofrat Prof. Dr Josef Neuwirth*. Selbstverlag d. K. K. Technischen Hochschule in Wien in Kommission bei Gerold & Co. Vienna 1915, p. 230; Alfred LECHNER, *Geschichte der Technischen Hochschule in Wien (1815–1940)*. Vienna 1942, p. 72.

69 Cf. FN 3, Ahnenpaß Hofbauer, p. 14, and HOFBAUER, *Edelhof* (as in FN 7), pp. 32–33.

70 Josef Ludwig Ritter von Schreibers (1793–1874). Jurist and member of the k. k. Landwirthschaftsgesellsch. Translator of the manual compiled by Sir John SINCLAIR (1754–1832), *The Code of Agriculture; Including Observations on Gardens, Orchards, Woods and Plantations; With an Account of all the Recent Improvements in the Management*

of Arable and Grass Land. Sherwood, Neely & Jones, London 1817 = *Grundgesetze des Ackerbaues, nebst Bemerkungen über Gartenbau, Obstbaumzucht, Forst-Cultur und Holzpflanzung*, von Sir John Sinclair, Gründer der königl. Gesellschaft des Ackerbaues in Großbritannien. Mit 9 Kupfern. Auf Veranlassung der k. k. Landwirthschafts-Gesellschaft in Wien aus dem Englischen übersetzt von Joseph Ritter v. Schreibers, Mitgliede der Gesellschaft. Heubner, Vienna 1819. – Joseph Ludwig's elder brother, Karl Franz Ritter von Schreibers (1775–1852), was the director of the K. K. Hof-Naturalien-Cabinet [today's Naturhistorisches Museum] in Vienna. Cf. ÖBL (as in FN 11).

71 First documented address: Vorstadt Landstraße, Rennweg Gasse Konskriptionsnummer 540, from 1830, after the reordering of house numbers: Konskriptionsnummer 638, today Rennweg 14 in Vienna's 3rd district, Landstraße. Cf. Franz Heinrich BÖCKH (ed.), *Wiens lebende Schriftsteller, Künstler, und Dilettanten im Kunstfache. Dann Kunst- und Naturschätze und andere Sehenswürdigkeiten dieser Haupt- und Residenz-Stadt. Ein Handbuch für Einheimische und Fremde. Auf Kosten des Verfassers.* Gedruckt bey B. Ph. Bauer, Vienna 1821, pp. 459–461; Carl Graf VASQUEZ, *Kais. Königl. Polizey Bezirk Landstrasse bestehend aus den Vorstädten Landstrasse, Erdberg und Weissgerber nebst 14 Ansichten der vorzüglichsten Gebäude daselbst*; Walter ÖHLINGER (ed.), *Die Pläne der k. k. Haupt- und Residenzstadt Wien von Carl Graf Vasquez*. Edition Winkler-Hermaden, Schleinbach 2011, p. 17 (with reprints of the original lithographs in the holdings of the Wien Museum, Inv. No. 105.971/4).

72 HOFBAUER, *Edelhof* (as in FN 7), p. 47.

73 Anton BEHSEL, *Verzeichniß aller in der kaiserl. königl. Haupt- und Residenz-Stadt Wien mit ihren Vorstädten befindlichen Häuser, mit genauer Angabe der älteren, mittleren und neuesten Nummerirungen, der dermahligen Eigenthümer und Schilder, der Straßen und Plätze, der Grund-Obrigkeiten, dann der Polizey- und Pfarr-Bezirke*. Carl Gerold, Vienna 1829, p. 138.

74 MESSNER, *Mariahilf*, p. 85.

75 Roman-Cath. Parish Mariahilf (today, Barnabitengasse 14, 6th district). Tauf-Register (vols. unnumbered) fol. 159, Juni 1851. The Family archive features the following certificate of baptism issued on 5 May 1860, presumably on the occasion of Ernst's enrolment at the Schottengymnasium: *"This is to certify on the basis of the baptismal register kept at this parish that ERNST JOSEF is the legitimate son of H. Adalbert Nikolaus Fuchs, doctor of medicine and philosophy, k. k. Professor of Agriculture at the Polytechnisches Institut* – [himself] *the son of H. Adalbert Fuchs, ret. k. k. Professor at the Ingenieur Akademie, and Fr. Theresia Ferdinanda Cremes – and his wife, Fr. Isabella née Ritter v. Schreibers, resident in Mariahilf No. 80, born on 14 June 1851 and baptised on 23 June 1851 … in the presence of … the godfather, the honourable Josef Ritter v. Schreibers, Chairman of the k. k. pr. Fire Insurance Institute and gentleman farmer."*

76 A. E. KOMERS, A. (ed.), *Jahrbuch für österreichische Landwirthe*. I und II. Jahrgang. J. G. Calve'sche k. k. Universitäts-Buchhandlung, Prag 1863, p. 351.

77 FUCHS, *Augenarzt* (as in FN 2), p. 45.

78 *Reden, gehalten bei der feierlichen Inauguration des für das Studienjahr 1869/70 gewählten Rectors des k. k. polytechnischen Institutes, Dr Adalbert Fuchs am 12. October 1869*. Vienna 1870.

79 Wilhelm HERZIG, *Das Medicinische Wien. Wegweiser für Aerzte und Naturforscher, vorzugsweise für Fremde. Nach Originalquellen.* Braumüller & Seidel, Vienna 1844, pp. 138–139; Josef HÄUSLER, *Die Entwicklung der K. K. Landwirtschafts-Gesellschaft in Wien während ihres hundertjährigen Bestandes.* Österreichische Land- und Forstwirtschaftsgesellschaft, Vienna 1907, pp. 24 and 88.

80 *Amtlicher Bericht über die im Mai 1857 abgehaltene fünfzigjährige Jubelfeier der k. k. Landwirthschafts-Gesellschaft in Wien an ihre allgemeine Versammlung am 26. Jänner 1858 erstattet im Auftrage des General-Comité von dessen Schriftführer, dem beständigen Secretär der Gesellschaft, Prof. Dr Ad. Fuchs.* K. K. Hof- und Staatsdruckerei, Vienna 1858.

81 *Allgemeiner Bericht über die land- und forstwirthschaftliche Ausstellung zu Wien im Jahre 1866,* in: *Bericht über die von der k. k. Landwirthschafts-Gesellschaft veranstaltete land- und forstwirthschaftliche Ausstellung zu Wien im Jahre 1866.* Herausgegeben durch das Ausstellungs-Comité. Selbstverlag, Vienna 1867, pp. I–III.

82 *Jahrbuch für Landeskunde von Niederösterreich.* Vol. 56–58 (1991), pp. 221ff.; FUCHS, *Augenarzt* (as in FN 2), pp. 17–18; HOFBAUER, *Edelhof,* pp. 34–35.

83 Sigmund Conrad Freiherr von Eybesfeld (1821–1898). Studied at the Univ. of Graz and Vienna (Dr jur.). 1841 Entry into the Civil Service: 1852 Dir. of the District Commission of Leibnitz and Marburg, 1853 Governor's Councilor in Temesvár, 1854 in Milan. 1857 Hofrat, Deputy of the Ban of Croatia, 1861 Deputy Governor of Trieste, 1865 Deputy Governor of Venice, 1867 Country President of Carniola, 1871 Governor of Upper Austria, 1872–1880 Governor of Lower Austria, 1880–1885 Minister f. Cultus and Unterricht. Cf. ÖBL (as in FN 11).

84 ÖSTA/AVA Wien. 6 Technik Fuchs, K. K. Ministerium für Cultus und Unterricht No. 17565 of 5. Sept. 1884.

85 Cf. *Landwirthschaftliche Zeitschrift* 12 (1886), pp. 1–2, and the obituary notice in the Family archive.

86 The Bärenmühle was located in the Vienna suburb Wieden, No. 790, [then Wienstraße 1, today Rechte Wienzeile in Vienna's 4th district] on the as yet unfortified right-hand bank of the Wien river. Cf. *Neuester Plan von Wien und seinen Vorstädten.* Artaria & Comp., Vienna 1856; Robert MESSNER, *Wien vor dem Fall der Basteien. Häuserverzeichnis und Plan der Inneren Stadt vom Jahre 1857.* Österr. Bundesverlag, Vienna 1958, p. 182; Gustav Adolph SCHIMMER, "Notizen über das Kärnthnerthor, die alte verschwundene Kärnthnervorstadt und die Vorstadt Wieden", in: *Das alte Wien. Darstellung der alten Plätze und merkwürdigsten jetzt größtenteils verschwundenen Gebäude Wiens.* Mit einem Vorwort zur Neuauflage von Isabella Wasner-Peter. Reprint of issues 1–12 of the originals from the years 1854–1856, now in the Townhall's Wienbibliothek. Ed. Winkler-Hermaden, Schleinbach 2009, V. Heft, pp. 1–14. – The Bärenmühle was powered by a millstream, which was a side arm of the Wien river. It was the property of the Ritterorden v. Hl. Geist, the Order of the Knights of the Holy Spirit, which had also been operating a hospital at the same site since the early 13th century. In Fuchs's days the mill was still referred to as the *Heilige-Geist-Mühle.* Legend has it that at the time of the second Turkish siege of Vienna (1683), the miller was attacked by a bear at night. His assistant saved his life and the miller commemorated the event by attaching the effigy of a bear to the building. In 1705 the Bärenmühle

was replaced by a new building. There was a pub next door, "Zum Schwarzen Bären", which was also referred to by the name *Bärenmühle*, as was the multi-storey block of flats erected there later. The mill was operational until 1856, when the millstream was filled in. Between 1913 and 1937 a newly installed passageway was known as the *Bärenmühlgasse*. Today, the *Bärenmühldurchgang*, linking Rechte Wienzeile 1–1A and Operngasse 18–20, serves as the last reminder of the historical mill. Cf. CZEIKE (as in FN 13); Maria PACOLT, *Sagen aus Alt-Wien*. Alexa & Co, Vienna 1946, pp. 43–45; Joh. W. HOLCZABEK, Adalbert WINTER, *Sagen und geschichtliche Erzählungen der Stadt Wien. Nebst einer kurzen Geschichte der k. k. Reichs-, Haupt- und Residenz-Stadt Wien und der Vororte*. Nach besten Quellen bearbeitet. Reprint of the ed. of 1900. Geyer Edition Vienna 1978, pp. 24–25; *Richard GRONER, Wien wie es war. Ein Auskunftsbuch für Freunde des alten Wien*. 3rd ed., Hain, Vienna 1934, p. 30; Felix F. CZEIPEK, *Wien-Wieden. Historische Bezirksbilder*. Sutton, Erfurt 2004, pp. 10 and 16; Carola LEITNER, Kurt HAMTIL, *Wiens 4. Bezirk Wieden in alten Fotografien*. Carl Ueberreuter, Vienna 2007, pp. 91–92.

87 Address at the time: Am Glacis No. 28 [today Techn. Univ., Karlsplatz 13, 4st district]. Cf. Johann ZIEGLER, *Aussicht vom Glacis gegen St. Karolikirche, Belvedere und Fürstl. Schwarzenberg. Garten;* ZIEGLER, *Aussicht gegen die Vorstädte. Vieden und Vien*. Kolorierter Kupferstich. Artaria, Vienna 1780; Carl Graf VASQUEZ, *K. K. Polizey-Bezirk Wieden bestehend a. d. Vorstädten Wieden, Margarethen, Schaumburger-Grund, Hungelbrunn, Nikolsdorf, Reinprechtsdorf, Hundsthurm, Matzleinsdorf, Laimgrube and Lorenzergrund nebst 14 der vorzüglichsten Ansichten*. Vienna 1830; Leopold SCHMIDT, *Zwischen Bastei und Linienwall. Wiener Vorstädte und ihre Gäste*. Wiener Verlag 1947, pp. 44–52.

88 UA Wien, Nationale der Juridischen Fakultät. Wilhelm Fuchs 3. Sem. 1872, fol. 279.

89 Ibid., Promotionsprotokoll der Juridischen Fakultät No. 2403.

90 ÖSTA/AVA Wien, 4 Jus FUCHS. K. K. Ministerium für Cultus and Unterricht. No. 11662 from 1877, dated 12 July 1877: *"Bericht der rechts-und staatswissenschaftlichen Facultät an der Wiener k. k. Universität betreffend die Zulassung des Doct. Wilhelm Fuchs zur Privatdocentur für österreichisches materielles Privatrecht."* Cf. *Übersicht der akademischen Behörden, Professoren, Privatdocenten, Lehrer, Beamten etc. an der k. k. Universität zu Wien für das Studienjahr 1877/78*. K. K. Hof- und Staatsdruckerei, Vienna 1877, p. 15.

91 Cf. Family archive.

92 The last course Wilhelm Fuchs had announced was one dealing with the Austrian law of obligations in the summer term of 1893. Cf. *Öffentliche Vorlesungen an der k. k. Universität zu Wien im Sommer-Semester 1893*. Adolf Holzhausen, Vienna 1893, p. 7. – In the course catalogues, Wilhelm Fuchs's name is listed until the academic year of 1896–97 among those of the lecturers and professors of the Faculty of Law and Political Science of Vienna University who were unable in the term in question to deliver any lectures. Cf. *Übersicht der akademischen Behörden, Professoren, Privatdocenten, Lehrer, Beamten etc. an der k. k. Universität zu Wien für das Studienjahr 1896/97*. Adolf Holzhausen, *Vienna 1896*, p. 12; *Öffentliche Vorlesungen an der k. k. Universität zu Wien im Sommer-Semester 1897*, p. 10.

93 *Die feierliche Inauguration des Rectors der Wiener Universität für das Studienjahr 1897/98*. Selbstverlag d. k. k. Univ. Wien 1897, p. 9.

94 Cf. *Todten Protokoll der Pfarre St. Rochus 1897–98,* Tom. 28, Sterbe-Register N°. 167, fol. 30. Wilhelm Fuchs's last address was Reisnerstr. 20 (today in the 3rd district of Vienna, Landstrasse).

95 Wilhelm FUCHS, *Das Ehehinderniss des bestehenden Ehebandes nach österreichischem Rechte und seine Umgehung.* Alfred Hölder, Vienna 1879; FUCHS, *Die Rechtsvermuthung der ehelichen Vaterschaft nach römischem und neuerem Rechte mit besonderer Berücksichtigung des österreichischen Rechtes.* Alfred Hölder, Vienna 1880 (Habilitation thesis); FUCHS, *Rechtsfälle zum Allgemeinen Bürgerlichen Gesetzbuche. Für den akademischen Gebrauch bearbeitet.* Alfred Hölder, Vienna 1881; FUCHS, *Die sogenannten Siebenbürgischen Ehen und andere Arten der Wiederverehelichung geschiedener österreichischer Katholiken.* Manz, Vienna 1889, FUCHS, *Der Hausmeister und sein Recht. Eine juristische Studie aus dem Wiener Leben.* Manz, Vienna 1891; FUCHS, *Beiträge zur Lehre von der Religionsfreiheit in der Praxis.* Manz, Vienna 1894.

96 FUCHS, *Augenarzt* (as in FN 2), p. 21, FN 6.

97 Anton KÖHLER (ed.), *Curiositäten- und Memorabilien-Lexicon von Wien. Ein belehrendes und unterhaltendes Nachschlag- und Lesebuch in anekdotischer, artistischer, biographischer, geschichtlicher, legendarischer, pittoresker, romantischer und topographischer Beziehung.* Vol. 1. Realis, Vienna 1846, pp. 497–498; Gottfried HEINDL, *Wien. Brevier einer Stadt.* Paul Neff Verlag, Vienna/Berlin 1972, pp. 72–73; Walter HUMMELBERGER, Kurt PEBALL, *Die Befestigungen Wiens* [= Peter PÖTSCHER (ed.), *Wiener Geschichtsbücher* Vol. 14]. Paul Zsolnay Verlag, Vienna/Hamburg 1974.

98 Walter ÖHLINGER (ed.), *Rundpanorama von Wien. Ansicht der k. k. Haupt- und Residenz-Stadt Wien vor Beginn der Stadterweiterung und Demolierung der Basteien im Jahre 1858 von C. Zacijek.* Edition Winkler-Hermaden, Schleinbach 2010.

99 FUCHS, *Augenarzt* (as in FN 2), pp. 21–22.

100 Ibid., pp. 27–28.

101 Han(n)s Frh. von Chiari (1851–1916). Studied at Vienna Univ. (Dr med. 1875). 1875–1879 Assist. at the pathol.-anatom. Inst. under Carl v. Rokitansky (cf. FN 15) and R.'s successor Richard Heschl (1824–1881). 1878 Habilitation in Pathol. Anat. at Vienna Univ. 1881/82 Substitute teacher for the chair. 1882–1906 initially Associate Prof., from 1883 Full Professor and Dir. of the Pathol.-Anatom. Inst. of the German Univ. of Prague (1900/01 Rector). 1906–1916 in the same function at Strasbourg Univ. (1914/15 Rector). Cf. CZEIKE; EULNER (as in FN 13); FISCHER (as in FN 28); Obituaries: *Wiener klin. Wochenschr.* 29 (1916), pp. 688ff.; *Centralbl. Allg. Pathol. and pathol. Anat.* 27 (1916), pp. 289ff.; *Münch. med. Wochenschr.* (1916), pp. 1080ff.

102 Friedrich Schauta (1849–1919). Studied at the Univ. of Vienna, Würzburg and Innsbruck (Dr med. 1874, Vienna). Trainee surgeon at the 1st Surg. Univ. Clinic (Johann Dumreicher, 1815–1880), 1875/76 prov. assist., 1876–81 definit. assist. at the 2nd Obstet. Univ. Clinic. (Joseph Spaeth). 1881 Habilitation in Obstetrics and Gynaecol. at Vienna Univ. 1881/82 Substitute teacher for the Chair of Obstetrics, 1883 Assoc. Prof., 1884 Full Prof. at Innsbruck Univ., 1887 Full Prof. at the Germ. Univ. of Prague, from 1891 Full Prof. and Dir. of the 1st Geburtshilfl. Klinik at Vienna Univ. Contributed to the developm. of operat. techniques, e.g. the repair of uterine prolapse. Most important of all was his development of the expanded vaginal total exstirpation of the uterus in cases of collum carcinoma. Together with Rudolf Chrobak (cf. FN 688) he developed the blueprints for the new construction of the Women's Univ.

Clinics in Vienna's Allgem. Krankenhaus. Cf. CZEIKE; EISENBERG 2; EULNER (as in FN 13); FISCHER (as in FN 28); PAGEL (as in FN 13); ÖBL (as in FN 11); Isidor FISCHER, *Geschichte der Geburtshilfe in Wien*, pp. 397ff.; LESKY, *Wien. Med. Schule* (as in FN 12), cf. Ind.; Obituaries, in: *Monatsschr. f. Geburtsh. Gynäkol.* 49 (1919), pp. 151ff.; *Arch. Gynäkol.* 111 (1919), pp. XXI ff.; *Zentralbl. Gynäkol.* 43 (1919) pp. 129ff (Josef Halban); *Wiener klin. Wochenschr.* 32 (1919), pp. 98ff. (Ludwig Adler); *Med. Bl.* 41 (1919), pp. 29–30; *Feierl. Inauguration … Univ. Wien 1919/20* (1919), pp. 46–47.

103 Heinrich Friedjung (1851–1920). Originally from Moravia. Studied history at the Univ. of Prague, Vienna and Berlin and, from 1871 to 1873, at the Inst. f. österr. Geschichtsforschung in Vienna (Dr phil 1872, Vienna). Well-known historian, politician and publicist. Cf. ÖBL (as in FN 11).

104 Max Ritter von Gruber (1853–1927). Studied chemistry and medicine at the Univ. of Vienna, Munich and Leipzig (Dr med. 1876, Vienna). After three years as an assistant at the Chem. Inst. in Vienna, he moved to Munich, where he specialised under the renowned hygienist Max von Pettenkofer (1818–1901). 1882 Habil. in Hygiene at Vienna Univ. 1884 Assoc. Prof and Dir. of the Inst. of Hygiene and Bacteriol. at Graz Univ. From 1887 Dir. of the Hygien. Inst. at Vienna Univ. (1891 Full Prof). In 1896 together with Herbert Edward Durham (1866–1945) discovery of agglutination, which made him the founder of serol. 1902 Full Prof. of Hygiene and Dir. of the Hygiene Instit. of Munich Univ. Supporter of the Nazi racial ideology. Cf. GERABEK et al. (as in FN 13); ÖBL (as in FN 11); NDB (as in FN 15), cf. Ind.; LESKY, *Wien. Med. Schule* (as in FN 12), cf. Ind.

105 Cf. FUCHS, *Augenarzt* (as in FN 2), p. 28.

106 *"As I wanted to be at the top of the form, I had to work hard at home, especially for the Matura* [the school leaving exam], *for which I read the entire Iliad and the Odyssey in the company of Schauta* (Friedrich Schauta, cf. FN 102) *and Doblhoff* [Rudolf Frh. v. Doblhoff, 1849–1924, later a politician and industrialist]. *To prepare for the exam, which in those days comprised oral exams in all subjects apart from Natural History, I got up at 4 a.m. for several months."* Ibid., p. 29.

107 Cf. FN 11.

108 Hans CHIARI, *Eine Erinnerung an Prof. Sigismund Gschwandner*, in: Heinrich Ritter von WITTEK (ed.), *Festgabe zum 100jährigen Jubiläum des Schottengymnasiums gewidmet von ehemaligen Schottenschülern*. Wilhelm Braumüller, Vienna 1907, pp. 36–38.

109 Gymnasium zu den Schotten in Wien: Katalog der fünften Klasse vom Schuljahre 1864/65, Katalog der sechsten Klasse vom Schuljahre 1865/66, Katalog der siebenten Klasse vom Schuljahre 1867.

110 Ibid. Katalog der achten Klasse vom Schuljahre 1868. The grades in the individual subjects for the second term in the final year were as follows: *"Application satisfactory; Religious Instruction laudable; Latin excellent; Greek excellent; German laudable; Geography and History laudable; Mathematics excellent; Sciences excellent; Philosophical Propaedeutics excellent"*.

111 Cf. *"testimonio maturitatis Gymnasii Viennensis de dato 29. Julii 1868"* according to the protocol of the 1st Rigorosum at the Med. Fac. of Vienna Univ. of 18 February 1873. (The only extant copy in the Family archive); UA Wien, Medizinisches Rigorosenprotokoll: Vom October 1872/73.

112 Ernst FUCHS, "Auf Xenophons Spuren", in: WITTEK, *Schottengymnasium* (as in

FN 108), pp. 96–106, and FUCHS, *Augenarzt* (as in FN 2), pp. 149–150.

113 FUCHS, *Augenarzt* (as in FN 2), p. 32.

114 Ibid., p. 33.

115 UA Wien. Nationale der Medizinischen Fakultät, Wintersemester 1868/69. Erstinskription von Ernest Fuchs v. 2. 10. 1868.

117 Cf. FN 13.

116 *Öffentliche Vorlesungen an der k. k. Universität zu Vienna im Winter-Semester 1868/9.* K. K. Hof- und Staatsdruckerei, Vienna 1868, p. 10.

118 FUCHS, *Augenarzt* (as in FN 2), p. 33.

119 UA Wien. Nationale der Medizinischen Fakultät, Sommersemester 1869, Ernest Fuchs, Inskription für das 2. Studiensemester vom 9. 4. 1869.

120 Cf. FN 14.

121 LESKY, *Wien. Med. Schule* (as in FN 12), p. 259 and Gabriela SCHMIDT, "Zur Entwicklung der Fächer Klinische Chemie und Laboratoriumsdiagnostik in der Wiener Schule", in: *Berichte zur Wissenschaftsgesch.* 14 (1991), pp. 231–239.

122 Cf. ALBERT/EDWARDS (as in FN 38), pp. 128–129; Hans TUPPY, "Physiologie und Biochemie 1820–1930", in: Karl ACHAM (ed.), *Geschichte der österreichischen Humanwissenschaften.* Vol. 2: *Lebensraum und Organismus des Menschen.* Passagen Verlag, Vienna 2001, pp. 235–269 (for Brücke, see pp. 237–245); IBBO (as in FN 18).

123 Ernst BRÜCKE, "Anatomische Untersuchungen über die sogenannten leuchtenden Augen bei den Wirbelthieren", in: *Archiv für Anatomie, Physiologie und wissenschaftliche Medicin* [= *Müllers Archiv*] Yr. 1845, pp. 387–406.

124 Jeremy NORMAN (ed.), *Morton's Medical Bibliography. An Annotated Check-List of Texts Illustrating the History of Medicine* [= GARRISON/MORTON]. Fifth Edition, Scolar Press 1991, p. 917.

125 Hermann Ludwig Ferdinand von Helmholtz (1821–1894), like Brücke a student of the leading Berlin physiol. Johannes Müller (1801–1858). In the 2nd half of the 19th century, Helmholtz held a dominating position in German-speaking science as physiol., physicist, mathematician and philosopher: 1849 Prof. of Physiol. at Königsberg Univ., 1855–1858 Prof. of Anat. and Physiol. at Bonn Univ., then at Heidelberg Univ., 1871 Prof. of Physics in Berlin, 1888 Pres. of the newly founded Physikal.-Techn. Reichsanstalt in Berlin-Charlottenburg. Helmholtz' *Handbuch der physiologischen Optik* (1867) remained unsurpassed for decades. Cf. FISCHER (as in FN 28); HIRSCHBERG, *Geschichte der Augenheilkunde* (as in FN 18), vol. 15/1 [= Reprint vol. VI], § 1021, pp. 73–81; IBBO (as in FN 18); KRAFT (as in FN 40); PAGEL (as in FN 13); Leo KOENIGSBERGER, *Hermann von Helmholtz.* Reprint of the ed. of 1902/03. 3 vols., Thoemmes Press 2001; Paul HERTZ, Moritz SCHLICK (ed.), *Hermann von Helmholtz. Schriften zur Erkenntnistheorie.* Springer, Berlin 1921; Karl LINDNER, "Hermann Helmholtz, zum 50. Todestag", in: *Wiener med. Wochenschr.* 94 (1944), p. 433; David CAHAN (ed.), *Hermann von Helmholtz and the Foundations of Nineteenth-Century Science.* University of California Press, Berkeley/Los Angeles 1993; Lorenz KRÜGER (ed.), *Universalgenie Helmholtz. Rückblick nach 100 Jahren.* Akademie-Verlag, Berlin 1994; Gregor SCHIEMANN, *Wahrheitsgewissheitsverlust. Hermann von Helmholtz' Mechanismus im Aufbruch der Moderne. Eine Studie zum Übergang von klassischer zu moderner Naturphilosophie.* Wissenschaftliche Buchgesellschaft 1997; Michel MEULDERS, *Helmholtz. From*

Enlightenment to Neuroscience. Translated and edited by Laurence Garey. MIT Press 2010.

126 Hermann HELMHOLTZ, *Beschreibung eines Augen-Spiegels zur Untersuchung der Netzhaut am lebenden Auge*. A. Förstner, Berlin 1851. Cf. GARRISON/MORTON (as in FN 124), p. 917; HIRSCHBERG, *Geschichte der Augenheilkunde* (as in FN 18), vol. 15/1 [= Reprint vol. VI], § 1022, pp. 82–88; J. E. SCHMIDT, *Medical Discoveries Who and When. A dictionary of medical and related scientific discoveries in alphabetic order, giving in each case the name of the discoverer, his profession, nationality, and floruit, and the date of the discovery*. Charles Thomas, Springfield 1959, p. 334; LESKY, *Wien. Med. Schule* (as in FN 12), pp. 260–261.

127 Ernst BRÜCKE, "Über den Musculus Cramptonianus und den Spannmuskel der Chorioidea", in: *Müllers Archiv* Yr. 1846, pp. 370–382.

128 Ernst BRÜCKE, *Anatomische Beschreibung des menschlichen Augapfels*. G. Reimer, Berlin 1847.

129 Ernst BRÜCKE, *Vorlesungen über Physiologie*. Unter dessen Aufsicht nach stenographischen Aufzeichnungen herausgegeben. Vol. 2. Wilhelm Braumüller 1873, pp. 106–207.

130 Theodor von FRIMMEL, "Erinnerungen an Josef Hyrtl", in: Alois TROST (ed.), *Alt-Wiener Kalender für das Jahr 1919*. Kunstverlag Anton Scholl & Co., Vienna 1919, pp. 53–57; EULNER (as in FN 13), pp. 46–65; Karl Eduard ROTHSCHUH, "Hyrtl contra Brücke. Ein Gelehrtenstreit im 19. Jahrhundert und seine Hintergründe", in: Erna LESKY (ed.), *Wien und die Weltmedizin. 4. Symposium der Internationalen Akademie für Geschichte der Medizin veranstaltet im Institut für Geschichte der Medizin der Universität Wien 17.–19. September 1973*. Hermann Böhlaus Nachfolger, Vienna/Cologne/Graz 1974, pp. 159–169; Herbert HÖRZ, *Physiologie und Kultur in der zweiten Hälfte des 19. Jahrhunderts. Briefe an Hermann von Helmholtz*. Basilisken-Presse/Verlag Natur & Text 1994, pp. 188ff.

131 By constituting epistemology as the foundation from which to attempt to grasp natural phenomena, the Königsberg philosopher Immanuel Kant (1724–1804) exerted a powerful influence on the development of scientific thought and experimental research not only in the German-speaking world throughout the 19th century. This is true of Kant's *Kritik der reinen Vernunft* (1781; *Critique of Pure Reason*) and of the *Kritik der Urteilskraft* (1790; *Critique of Judgment*) and even more so of his seminal treatise *Metaphysische Anfangsgründe der Naturwissenschaft* (1786; Metaphysical Foundations of Natural Science). Cf. KRAFT (as in FN 40); Werner SAUER (as in FN 131), *Österreichische Philosophie zwischen Aufklärung und Restauration*. Beiträge zur Geschichte des Frühkantianismus in der Donaumonarchie [= Richard HALLER (ed.), *Studien zur österreichischen Philosophie* vol. II]. Königshausen und Neumann, Würzburg 1982; Georgi SCHISCHKOFF (ed.), *Philosophisches Wörterbuch*. Begründet von Heinrich Schmidt. 22nd ed. Alfred Kröner, Stuttgart 1991 (= *Kröners Taschenausgabe* vol. 13), pp. 368–371; Konstantin POLLOK, *Kants "Metaphysische Anfangsgründe der Naturwissenschaft". Ein kritischer Kommentar.* (= *Kant-Forschungen* 13). Meiner, Hamburg 2001.

132 As a spokesman of utilitarianism, John Stuart Mill (1806–1873) is one of the most prominent exponents of positivism. Fuchs is arguably referring to an epistemological work by Mill which was seminal for scientific thought: John Stuart MILL, *A System of*

Logic, Ratiocinative, and Inductive, Being a Connected View of the Principles of Evidence, and the Methods of Scientific Investigation. John W. Parker, London 1843. (German transl.: J. SCHIEL, *System der deduktiven und induktiven Logik. Eine Darlegung der Principien wissenschaftlicher Forschung, insbesondere der Naturforschung von John Stuart Mill.* Friedrich Vieweg & Sohn. Braunschweig 1849). Cf. J. SCHIEL, *Die Methode der inductiven Forschung als Methode der Naturforschung in gedrängter Darstellung hauptsächlich nach John Stuart Mill.* Friedrich Vieweg & Sohn, Braunschweig 1865; Georgi SCHISCHKOFF (as in FN 131), p. 484–485.

133 FUCHS, *Augenarzt* (as in FN 2), p. 35.

134 Ernst BRÜCKE, *Über Gravitation und Erhaltung der Kraft.* K. K. Hof- und Staatsdruckerei, Vienna 1857; Joseph HYRTL, *Die materialistische Weltanschauung unserer Zeit. Rede bei dem Antritte der Rectorswürde an der Wiener Universität am 1. October 1864.* Adolf Holzhausen, Vienna 1865. Cf. also: LESKY, *Wien. Med. Schule* (as in FN 12), pp. 259–260; SAUER (as in FN 131), pp. 325–326; Kurt BAYERTZ, Walter JAESCHKE, Myriam GERHARD (eds.), *Weltanschauung, Philosophie und Naturwissenschaft im 19. Jahrhundert.* Vol. 1: *Der Materialismusstreit.* Meiner, Hamburg 2007.

135 As a 25-year-old university professor in Bonn, Johannes Müller (1801–1858) had published a comparative treatise on the sense of sight of animals and human beings: Johannes MÜLLER, *Zur vergleichenden Physiologie des Gesichtssinnes des Menschen und der Thiere nebst einem Versuch über die Bewegungen der Augen und über den menschlichen Blick.* Leipzig 1826. Especially innovative is the introduction entitled *"Von dem Bedürfniß der Physiologie nach einer philosophischen Naturbetrachtung"* [Physiology's need for a philosophical approach to nature], a lecture he had given as early as 1824 as a public university lecturer in Bonn. (Ibid., pp. 1–36). Cf. Michael HAGNER, Bettina WAHRIG-SCHMIDT (eds.), *Johannes Müller und die Philosophie.* Akademie-Verlag, Berlin 1992.

136 Estelle du BOIS-REYMOND (ed.), *Jugendbriefe von Emil Du Bois-Reymond an Eduard Hallmann.* Berlin 1918, p. 108. Cited in Gunter MANN (ed.), *Naturwissen und Erkenntnis im 19. Jahrhundert: Emil Du Bois-Reymond.* Gerstenberg, Hildesheim 1981, p. 126. Cf. Hermann HELMHOLTZ, *Ueber die Erhaltung der Kraft. Eine physikalische Abhandlung, vorgetragen in der Sitzung der Physikalischen Gesellschaft zu Berlin am 23. Juli 1847.* G. Reimer, Berlin 1847; Sven DIERIG, *Wissenschaft in der Maschinenstadt. Emil Du Bois-Reymond und seine Laboratorien in Berlin.* Wallstein, Göttingen 2006.

137 Sigmund Exner v. Ewarten (1846–1926). Studied at the Univ. of Vienna and Heidelberg (Dr med. 1870, Vienna) as a student of Brücke (Vienna Univ.) and Helmholtz (Heidelberg Univ.). Habilitation in Physiolog. at Vienna Univ. 1871 (tit. Associate Prof. 1875), 1891–1917 Full Prof. at Vienna Univ. as Brücke's successor. Cf. CZEIKE; EISENBERG 2; EULNER; HIRSCH (as in FN 13); ÖBL (as in FN 11); *Feierl. Inauguration … Studienjahr 1926/27*, pp. 46ff. (A. Durig); LESKY, *Wien. Med. Schule* (as in FN 12), pp. 541–544.

138 Sigmund EXNER, *Ernst v. Brücke und die moderne Physiologie*, in: *Wiener klin. Wochenschr.* 3 (1890), pp. 807–812 (here: p. 811).

139 Cf. FN 15.

140 SCHISCHKOFF (as in FN 131), pp. 463–464.

[141] Gabriela SCHMIDT, "Rokitansky als Patho-Philosoph", in: *Sudhoffs Archiv* 89 (2005), pp. 170–195; Felicitas SEEBACHER, "'Freiheit der Naturforschung!' Carl Freiherr von Rokitansky und die Wiener Medizinische Schule. Wissenschaft und Politik im Konflikt" (ibid.).

[142] Ernst Fleischl v. Marxow (1846–1891). Studied at Vienna Univ. (Dr med. 1870). While still a student, prosector under the patholog. Rokitanksy (cf. FN 15). After a study visit to physiol. Carl Ludwig (1816–1895) in Leipzig from 1873 Brücke's assist. in Vienna. 1874 Habilitation in Physiol. at Vienna Univ.; 1880 Assoc. Prof.; focus of work: muscle-nerve physiol., physiol. optics. Cf. CZEIKE; EISENBERG 2; HIRSCH (as in FN 13); ÖBL (as in FN 11); PAGEL (as in FN 13); LESKY, *Wien. Med. Schule* (as in FN 12), pp. 538–540.

[143] Josef Paneth (1857–1890). Studied at the Univ. of Vienna and Heidelberg (Dr med. 1879, Vienna). First trainee surgeon at Vienna's 2nd Surg. Univ. Clinic under Theodor Billroth. Then histol. research at the Breslau Physiol. Institute and the Zoolog. Station in Villefranche-sur-Mer. 1886 Habilitation in Physiol. under Brücke in Vienna. Pioneering work in research on nerve physiology. 1888 Initial description of the coarsely granular granule cells of the Lieberkuhn crypts in the small intestine. Cf. CZEIKE (as in FN 13); FISCHER (as in FN 28); GERABEK et al. (as in FN 13); ÖBL (as in FN 11); LESKY, *Wien. Med. Schule* (as in FN 12), p. 542.

[144] Cf. FN 32.

[145] Heinrich Obersteiner (1847–1922). Studied at Vienna Univ. (Dr med. 1870). Introduction to experiment. work in Brücke's physiolog. laboratory, where he also acquired the experim. methodol. tools for his multifaceted research on the anatomy of the brain. From 1872 Dir. of the Sanatorium for the Mentally Ill founded by his father (together with Maximilian Leidesdorf (1816–1889)) in Oberdöbling. 1873 Habilitation in anat. and pathol. of the nervous system at Vienna Univ. (1880 Assoc. Prof., 1898 tit. Full Prof.). 1882 Foundation of a neurol. institute dedicated to research on the brain. Named after him – Obersteiner-Institut –, it quickly gained internat. reputation, attracting students from all over the world. Cf. CZEIKE; EISENBERG 2 (as in FN 13); FISCHER (as in FN 28); NDB (as in FN 15); ÖBL (as in FN 11); PAGEL (as in FN 13); LESKY, *Wien. Med. Schule* (as in FN 12), pp. 386–388; Obituaries, in: *Arbeiten aus dem Neurol. Inst.* 24 (1923), Issues 2/3; *Wiener klin. Wochenschr.* 35 (1922), p. 946; Appreciation: Erwin STRANSKY, "Erinnerungen an Heinrich Obersteiner", in: *Wiener klin. Wochenschr.* 69 (1957), pp. 537–538.

[146] Carl Wedl (1815–1891). Studied at Vienna Univ. (Dr med. 1841). Medical practitioner in Bad Ischl for a few years. At his teacher Rokitansky's request return to Vienna Univ. (1849 Habilitation in Histology, 1853 Assoc. Prof.). 1854–1883 Foundation of the first Univ. Institute of Histology in the German-speaking world; Dir. of the Institute (Full Prof. 1872). He aimed at grounding all clin. manifestations in the microscopic observation of tissue. His textbook, *Grundzüge d. pathol. Histologie*, published as early as 1854, reflected these intentions and established his close collaboration with the leading clinicians of the 2nd Vienna Medical School. 1883 Rector of Vienna Univ. Cf. CZEIKE; EISENBERG 2; EULNER; HIRSCH (as in FN 13); IBBO (as in FN 18); PAGEL (as in FN 13); LESKY, *Wien. Med. Schule* (as in FN 12), pp. 249–251; Viktor PATZELT, "Carl Wedl, der erste Vorstand einer deutschsprachigen Lehrkanzel für Histologie", in: *Anatomischer Anzeiger* [= Anat. Anz.] 100 (1953/54), pp. 147–156

(with bibliography); PATZELT., "Zum 100jährigen Bestand der Wiener Lehrkanzel für Histologie", in: *Wiener klin. Wochenschr.* 66 (1954), pp. 775–779.

147 FUCHS, *Augenarzt* (as in FN 2), pp. 36–37.

148 UA Wien. Nationale der Medizinischen Fakultät. Inskription von Ernest Fuchs für das 3. Studiensemester vom 5. 10. 1869 sowie Protokoll d. 1. Rigorosums an d. Med. Fak. d. Univ. Wien v. 18. Februar 1873 (Only extant copy in the Family archive).

149 Carl WEDL, *Grundzüge der pathologischen Histologie.* C. Gerold und Sohn, Vienna 1854.

150 Georg DHOM, *Geschichte der Histopathologie* (as in FN 40), pp. 208–213.

151 Then Währinger Gasse Nos. 201 and 202 in the Alsergrund suburb, today Währingerstraße 11–13/Corner Schwarzspanierstraße 17 in Vienna's 9th district). Cf. CZEIKE (as in FN 13); Anton ZIEGLER, Carl Graf VASQUEZ (eds.), *Polizey-Bezirk Alsergrund. Alsergrund, Breitenfeld, Michelbeurischergrund. Mit einem Grundrisse.* Vienna 1828; Robert MESSNER, *Der Alsergrund im Vormärz. Historisch-topographische Darstellung der nordwestlichen Vorstädte und Vororte Wien auf Grund der Katastralvermessung.* Notring d. wissenschaftl. Verbände Österr., Vienna 1970, p. 150.

152 Cf. FN 146 (Appreciation of Wedl by Patzelt).

153 Wilhelm HERZIG, *Das medicinische Wien. Wegweiser für Aerzte und Naturforscher, vorzugsweise für Fremde. Nach Originalquellen bearbeitet.* 3rd ed., Wilhelm Braumüller, Vienna 1863, pp. 55–56. Cf. Sigmund EXNER, "Das neue physiologische Institut in Wien. Eröffnungsrede, gehalten am 2. Mai 1904", in: *Wiener klin. Wochenschr.* 17 (1904), pp. 712–716.

154 Cf. the advertisement in the course catalogue: Praktische Histologie, fünfmal wöchentlich, von 9–3 Uhr, von dem k. k. a. ö. Professor Herrn Dr. Carl Wedl; im histologischen Laboratorium des physiologischen Institutes, im 2. Stock des Vorgebäudes der gewesenen k. k. Gewehrfabrik, Alsergrund, Währingergasse Nr. 1 (monatliches Honorar für Doctores 10 fl., für Candidaten der Medicin 5 fl.) [Practical Histology, five times weekly, from 9 a.m. to 3 p.m., k. k. a. ö. Professor Herr Dr Carl Wedl; at the histological laboratory of the Institute of Physiology, on the 2nd floor of the building in front of the former k. k. Gewehrfabrik, Alsergrund, Währingerg. Nr. 1 (monthly fee for doctors 10 fl., for students of medicin 5 fl.)], in: *Öffentliche Vorlesungen an der K. K. Universität zu Wien im Winter-Semester 1869/70.* K. K. Hof- und Staatsdruckerei, Vienna 1869, p. 11.

155 Payment of the fee of 5 fl. for this one-month course is noted on the *Nationale* under the date of 10 March 1870. Cf. UA Wien, Nationale der Medizinischen Fakultät, Wintersemester 1869. Inskription von Ernest Fuchs für das 3. Studiensemester.

156 Paul TOWER, "Carl Wedl. Histopathology of the Eye in the Nineteenth Century", in: *Archives of Ophthalmology* [= Arch. Ophthalmol.] 63 (1960), pp. 756–760.

157 Cf. FN 18.

158 *Die Deutsche Karl-Ferdinands-Universität in Prag unter der Regierung Seiner Majestät des Kaisers Franz Josef I.* Verlag der J. G. Calveschen K. u. K. Hof- und Universitätsbuchhandlung (Josef Koch), Prague 1869, pp. 346–354; Walter KOERTING, *Die Deutsche Universität in Prag. Die letzten 100 Jahre ihrer Medizinischen Fakultät* [= Schriftenr. d. Bayer. Landesakademie vol. 11]. Richard Pflaum Verlag, Munich 1968, pp. 229–230.

159 LESKY, *Wien. Med. Schule* (as in FN 12), pp. 220–226 and p. 478.

160 Ferdinand ARLT, *Meine Erlebnisse*. J. F. Bergmann. Wiesbaden 1887, p. 43.

161 Ibid.

162 Anton Elfinger (1821–1864). Studied at the Akademie d. bild. Künste under Leopold Kupelwieser (1796–1862); then medical studies at Vienna Univ. (Dr med. 1845). Junior doctor at Vienna's Allgem. Krankenhaus and prosector under the dermatol. Ferdinand R. v. Hebra (cf. FN 163), whose monumental atlas of skin diseases he skilfully illustrated together with Carl Heitzmann (cf. FN 167). The Med. Fac. of Vienna Univ. employed him between 1849 and 1858 as artist for div. spec. publ.; much sought-after draughtsman for such periodicals as *Wiener Allgem. Theaterzeitg.* and various polit. journals. Cf. CZEIKE (as in FN 13); Margarete POCH-KALOUS, *Cajetan. Das Leben des Wiener Mediziners und Karikaturisten Dr Anton Elfinger*. Wiener Bibliophilen-Gesellschaft, Vienna 1966; Isolde EMICH, "In memoriam Dr med. Anton Elfinger", in: *Materia therapeutica* 17 (1971), pp. 117–144; Karl PORTELE, "Dr med. Anton Elfinger, ein vergessener medizinischer Modelleur", in: *Annalen d. Naturhist. Museums Wien* 78 (1974), pp. 95–102; Manfred SKOPEC, "Anton Elfinger (1821–1864) – a forgotten medical illustrator", in: *International Journal of Dermatology [Internat. J. Dermotol.]* 22/4 (1983), pp. 256–259; Ingrid HACKSTOCK, *Die wissenschaftlichen Illustrationen der Wiener Medizinischen Schule vom Ende des 18. bis Mitte des 19. Jahrhunderts*. Phil. Diss., Vienna Univ. 1988; Karl HOLUBAR, Cathrin SCHMIDT, "Art in Dermatology versus Dermatology in Art. Anton Elfinger (1821–1864) and Carl Heitzmann (1836–1896): Hebra's forgotten Painter-Physicians", in: *Internat. J. Dermatol.* 33 (1994), pp. 385–387; Stella FATOVIĆ-FERENČIĆ, "Anton Elfinger (1821–1862 [sic]) in: Christoph LÖSER, Gerd PLEWIG (eds.), *Pantheon der Dermatologie*. Springer, Heidelberg 2008, pp. 256–259.

163 Ferdinand Ritter v. Hebra (1816–1880). Originally from Brünn (today Brno/Czech Republic). Studied at Vienna Univ. (Dr med. 1841). 1843 Junior doctor at a ward for chest diseases in Vienna's Allgem. Krankenhaus under Joseph Škoda (cf. FN 16). Conjoined with that ward was one for patients with chron. skin rashes. Meticulous observation and self-experiments allowed Hebra in 1844 to show that scabies, a then common skin disease, was caused by mites, and he developed a local therapy. Following in the footsteps of Rokitanksy and Škoda (cf. FN 15 and 16), Hebra recast for dermatology the doctrine of efflorescence in 1845 on the basis of pathol. morphology (Second Vienna Medical School). 1844 Habilitation at Vienna Univ. 1845 Dir. of a Dept. of Skin Diseases created for him at the Allgem. Krankenhaus (1848 Head physician), 1849 Assoc. Prof. and Dir. of the newly established first Dermatolog. University Clinic in the German-speaking world; 1869 Full Prof. ad pers.; 1856–1876 Publication of his monumental *Atlas d. Hautkrankheiten*, whose illustrations by Anton Elfinger (cf. FN 162) and Carl Heitzmann (cf. FN 167) are as instructive as they are satisfying from an artistic point of view. Hebra's activities made Vienna the centre of Dermatol. both in teaching and research. 1876 Publication of his seminal textbook (tog. with his son-in-law Moriz Kaposi, 1837–1902). Cf. CZEIKE; EISENBERG 2; EULNER (as in FN 13); FISCHER (as in FN 28); NDB (as in FN 15); PAGEL (as in FN 13); LESKY, *Wien. Med. Schule* (as in FN 12), pp. 153–160; Obituaries: *Vierteljahresschr. f. Dermatol.* 7 (1880), pp. 1 ff.; *Archiv f. Dermatol.* 12 (1880); *Almanach d. Akad. d. Wissensch.* 31 (1881), pp. 194 ff.; *Wiener med. Wochenschr.* 31 (1881), Nr. 4; *Feierl. Inaug. … Studienjahr*

1880/81, pp. 9ff. Appreciations: Leopold ARZT, "Ferdinand von Hebra und die Dermatologie unserer Zeit", in: *Wiener med. Wochenschr.* 76 (1926), cols. 1316ff.; Josef TAPPEINER, "Ferdinand von Hebra und die Wiener Dermatologenschule. Hebra und die Gesellschaft der Ärzte", in: Ibid. 116 (1956), Special issue Oct. 1956; Karl HOLUBAR, "Ferdinand von Hebra und das Allgemeine Krankenhaus in Wien", in: Ibid. 132 (1982), cols. 423ff.; Gabriela SCHMIDT-WYKLICKY, "Ferdinand Karl Franz Ritter von Hebra (1816–1880)", in: Christoph LÖSER, Gerd PLEWIG (eds.), *Pantheon der Dermatologie*. Springer, Heidelberg 2008, pp. 417–432.

164 *Horizontaler Durchschnitt des menschlichen Auges nach Präparaten des Professors Dr. Arlt gezeichnet von Dr. Elfinger. 1862.* Wilhelm Braumüller, Vienna 1875.

165 Carl (Karl) Stellwag von Carion (1823–1904). Studied at Vienna Univ. (Dr med. 1847). 1853–1856 Publication of his monumental, three-volume *Die Ophthalmologie vom naturwissenschaftlichen Standpunct aus betrachtet.* 1854 Habilitation in Ophthalmology at Vienna Univ.; 1857 Prof. at the med.-surg. Josephs-Akademie in Vienna until its dissolution in 1873. *Lehrbuch der praktischen Ophthalmologie* (1861), Italian, Engl. and Hungar. translations. 1874 Creation of a Second Eye Clinic at the Allgem. Krankenhaus with an ad personam chair; 1884–1894 Dir. of the 1st Univ. Eye Clinic in Vienna as the successor of Arlt. Infrequent or incomplete blinking as a symptom of morbus Basedow is referred to even today as Stellwag's sign in med. terminology. Cf. CZEIKE; EISENBERG 2 (as in FN 13); Dieter HEID *Personalbibliographien der Professoren und Dozenten der Ophthalmologie an der Medizinischen Fakultät der Universität Wien, im Zeitraum von 1812 bis 1884.* Med. Diss., Univ. Erlangen-Nürnberg 1972, pp. 92–99; HIRSCH; PAGEL (as in FN 13); ÖBL (as in FN 11); HIRSCHBERG, *Geschichte der Augenheilkunde* (as in FN 18), vol. 15/2 (Reprint vol. VI), § 1247–1251, pp. 407–429); Salomon KIRCHENBERGER, *Lebensbilder hervorragender österreichisch-ungarischer Militär- und Marineärzte* [= Militärärztliche Publikationen No. 150]. Šafář Vienna/ Leipzig 1913, pp. 198–202; IBBO (as in FN 18); LESKY, *Wien. Med. Schule* (as in FN 12), pp. 226–229; Helmut WYKLICKY, *Das Josephinum. Biographie eines Hauses. Die medicinisch-chirurgische Josephs-Akademie seit 1785. Das Institut für Geschichte der Medizin seit 1920.* Christian Brandstätter, Vienna 1985, pp. 116–117; Gabriela SCHMIDT-WYKLICKY, Helmut GRÖGER, "Carl Stellwag von Carion. Vorstand der I. Universitäts-Augenklink in Wien 1884 bis 1894", in: *Spektrum Augenheilk.* 26 (2012), pp. 303–308. See Ch. 4.

166 Carl WEDL, *Atlas der pathologischen Histologie des Auges.* Unter Mitwirkung des Herrn Prof. Dr C. Stellwag von Carion herausgegeben. Erste bis Vierte Lieferung. Georg Wigand, Leipzig 1861.

167 Carl (Karl) Heitzmann (1836–1896). Originally from Croatia. Studied medicine at the Univ. of Pest and Vienna (Dr med. 1859). Assist. at the 2nd Surg. Univ. Clinic under Franz Schuh and the dermatol. Ferdinand R. v. Hebra (cf. FN 163). After the death of Anton Elfinger (cf. FN 162), completion of the illustrations of Hebra's epoch-making *Atlas d. Hautkrankheiten* (1856–1876). Illustrator of works by the following professors of the Second Vienna Med. School: Ludwig Türck (1810–1868, *Kehlkopfkrankheiten* 1866); Moriz Heider (1816–1866, *Pathologie d. Zähne* 1868/69 tog. with Carl Wedl); Otto Becker (cf. FN 178, *Topograph. Anat. d. Auges* 1874–1878). Together with his younger brother Julius Heitzmann (1847–1922) author of the *Atlas d. deskript and topograph. Anatomie* (1870–1875) and the *Kompendium d. Chir. Med.* Experimenter

under Salomon Stricker (cf. FN 610). Prosector at the Wiedner Krankenhaus. 1873 Habilitation in Pathol. Anatomy at Vienna Univ.; 1874 Emigration to New York, establishment of a highly frequented private teaching institute for microscopy. 1883 Publication of an overview of his own research on the microscop. anat. of healthy and diseased animals. Cf. CZEIKE; EISENBERG 2; HIRSCH; PAGEL (as in FN 13); LESKY, *Wien. Med. Schule* (as in FN 12), pp. 564–566; Carl HEITZMANN, "20 Jahre wissenschaftliche Thätigkeit in Amerika", in: *Wiener klin. Wochenschr.* 8 (1895), pp. 561ff.; Karl HOLUBAR, Klaus WOLFF, "The Genesis of American Investigative Dermatology from its Roots in Europe", in: *J. Invest. Dermatol.* 92 (1989), Suppl. Nr. 4, pp. 14ff.; Ingrid HACKSTOCK, "Carl Heitzmann (1836–1896): physician and illustrator", in: *Intern. J. Dermatol.* 37 (1998), pp. 235–240; Karl HOLUBAR, Stella FATOVIĆ-FERENČIĆ, Gerd PLEWIG, *Looking at Eyes and Faces. Ophthalmologic watercolours drawn largely by physician-artists Vienna late 18th and 19th centuries.* Austrian Academy of Sciences Press, Vienna 2006; Stella FATOVIĆ-FERENČIĆ, "Carl Heitzmann (1836–1896)", in: LÖSER/PLEWIG, *Pantheon der Dermatologie* (as in FN 162), pp. 433–437.

168 Karl STELLWAG von CARION, *Abhandlungen aus dem Gebiete der praktischen Augenheilkunde. Ergänzungen zum Lehrbuche.* Unter Mitwirkung der Herrn Prof. Dr C. Wedl und Dr E. Hampel. Wilhelm Braumüller, Vienna 1882.

169 Emil Bock (1857–1916). Originally from Galicia. Studied at Vienna Univ. (Dr med. 1881). 1882–1887 Assist. under Stellwag, 1886 Habilitation at Vienna Univ. 1890 Head physician at the newly established Eye Department at the Landeskrankenhaus Laibach (today Ljubljana/Slovenia). Cf. FISCHER (as in FN 28); HEID (as in FN 165), pp. 106–115; HIRSCHBERG, *Geschichte der Augenheilkunde* (as in FN 18), Reprint vol. VI (15/2, § 1258, pp. 445–447; IBBO (as in FN 18).

170 Carl WEDL, Emil BOCK, *Pathologische Anatomie des Auges.* Systematisch bearbeitet. Mit einem Atlas von XXXIII Tafeln. K. K. Hof- und Staatsdruckerei. In Commission bei Carl Gerold's Sohn, Vienna 1886.

171 Carl WEDL, Emil BOCK, *Atlas zur pathologischen Anatomie des Auges.* XXXIII Tafeln in Lichtdruck ausgeführt in der k. k. Hof- und Staatsdruckerei. In Commission bei Carl Gerold's Sohn, Vienna 1886.

172 Ibid., p. III.

173 Cf. Jonas S. FRIEDENWALD, "The contributions of Professor Ernst Fuchs to ophthalmic pathology", in: *Am. J. Ophthalmol.* 14 (1931), pp. 138–140; Jens Martin ROHRBACH, "Ophthalmopathology between yesterday and tomorrow", in: *Klin. Monatsbl. Augenheilk.* 221/2 (2004), pp. 87–91.

174 FUCHS, *Augenarzt* (as in FN 2), p. 41.

175 Cf. UA Wien. Nationale der Medizinischen Fakultät, Sommersemester 1872, Inskription von Ernest Fuchs für das 8. Studiensemester.

176 Maximilian Ritter von Vintschgau zu Altenburg und Hohenhaus (1832–1913). Originally from the Tyrol. Studied at Vienna Univ. (Dr med. 1856). Assist. under Brücke, who kindled his interest in research topics related to the physiology of the senses. 1857 Establishment of the Institute of Physiol. at what was then the Austrian University of Padova (Full Prof. 1860). 1867 Call to Prague Univ. to ensure that physiol. was taught also in German alongside the physiol. Jan Evangelista Purkinyě (1787–1869), who lectured in Czech. From 1870 first Dir. of the Institute of Physiol.

at the Med. Fac. of Innsbruck Univ., building the institute from scratch; 1874/75 and 1881/82 Rector of Innsbruck Univ. Cf. PAGEL (as in FN 13); Cf. also: Carl v. Rokitansky's expert opinion on appointing Maximilian v. Vintschgau as Professor of Physiology at Prague University, in: Erna LESKY, "Purkyněs Weg. Wissenschaft, Bildung und Nation", in: *Sitzungsber. d. ÖAW.* Phil.-hist. Kl., vol. 265, 5. Abhandl. [= Veröffentlichungen d. Kommission für Geschichte d. Erziehung and d. Unterrichtes Issue 12]. Hermann Böhlaus Nachf., Vienna/Cologne/Graz 1970, Appendix pp. 62–64; Luisa BIZZOTTO, Giorgio RIALDI, "L'attività didattica e scientifica del fisiologo Maximilian Vintschgau (1832–1902) all'Università di Padova", in: *Acta medicae historiae pataviana* [*Acta Med. Hist. Patav.*] 22 (1975), pp. 9–20; Karl SABLIK, "Hering, Vintschgau und das Problem der Nachfolge Purkinjes", in: *Archiv für Geschichte der Medizin [= Sudhoffs Archiv*] 73 (1989), pp. 78–87; Heinz HUBER, *Geschichte der Medizinischen Fakultät Innsbruck und der medizinisch-chirurgischen Studienanstalt (1673–1938).* Unter Mitarbeit von Verena Plankl. Böhlau, Vienna/Cologne/Weimar 2010, pp. 189–191.

177 Ferdinand SCHEMINZKY, Th. WENSE, "Die Geschichte des Physiologischen Institutes der Universität zu Innsbruck", in: *Forschungen und Forscher der Tiroler Ärzteschule (1948–1950).* Vol. 2. Oberösterr. Landesverlag, Wels 1950, pp. 145–150; Helmut WYKLICKY, "Von der Begründung der III. Medizinischen Fakultät in Innsbruck im Jahre 1869", in: *Wiener med. Wochenschr.* 119 (1969), col. 535; Franz HUTER (ed.), *Hundert Jahre Medizinische Fakultät Innsbruck 1869 bis 1969. II. Teil. Geschichte der Lehrkanzeln, Institute und Kliniken*, in: *Veröffentlichungen der Universität Innsbruck* 17 [= Forschungen zur Innsbrucker Universitätsgeschichte vol. VII/2]. Innsbruck 1969; pp. 217–219; *Die Medizinische Fakultät der Leopold-Franzens-Universität Innsbruck* [= Veröffentlichungen der Universität Innsbruck 190]. Universität Innsbruck 1992; HUBER, *Med. Fakultät Innsbruck* (as in FN 176), p. 283. (To be used with caution on account of faulty dates.)

178 Otto Becker (1828–1890). Originally from Ratzeburg/Germany. 1847 Studied theology and philology at Erlangen Univ.; 1848–1851 Studied mathematics and science at the Univ. of Berlin; 1854–1859 Studied medicine at Vienna Univ. 1861 Junior doctor at the Eye Department of Vienna's Allgem. Krankenhaus under Eduard Jaeger v. Jaxtthal. 1862–1867 Arlt's assist. at the 1st Univ. Eye Clinic in Vienna (1863 Habilitation). 1868–1890 Full Prof. and Dir. of the Univ. Eye Clinic Heidelberg, which he had rebuilt from scratch. Cf. EULNER (as in FN 13); HEID (as in FN 165), pp. 36–44; HIRSCH, vol. 1; HIRSCHBERG, *Geschichte der Augenheilkunde* (as in FN 18), vol. 15/2 [= Reprint vol. 6], § 1188–90, pp. 266–274; IBBO (as in FN 18); PAGEL (as in FN 13).

179 Otto BECKER, *Die Universitäts-Augenklinik Heidelberg. Zwanzig Jahre klinischer Tätigkeit.* J. F. Bergmann, Wiesbaden 1888; Adelheid BOECKER-REINARTZ, *Die Augenkliniken der Universitäten des deutschen Sprachgebietes (1769–1914).* Med. Diss., Univ. Cologne 1990, p. 55 and 76; Hans-Joachim KÜCHLE, *Augen-Kliniken deutschsprachiger Hochschulen und ihre Lehrstuhlinhaber im 19. und 20. Jahrhundert.* Biermann, Cologne 2005, pp. 125–126.

180 FUCHS, *Augenarzt* (as in FN 2), p. 41.

181 Michael Josef Dietl (1847–1887). Originally from Königsberg/Eger/Bohemia (today Kynšperk nad Ohří/Czech Republic). Studied medicine at the Univ. of Prague

and Innsbruck (Dr med. 1872, Dr chir. 1873). Assist. of the physiol. Vintschgau. Habilitation in Histology; 1876 Habilitation in Gen. and Experim. Pathology at Innsbruck Univ.; first Chair of Gen. and Experim. Pathology at Innsbruck Univ. (1878 unsalaried Assoc. Prof.). Left the Univ. in 1884 to become a spa physician in Marienbad/Bohemia (today Mariánské Lázně/Czech Republic). It took until 1887 for the Innsbruck Univ. Institute of Physiol. to become an autonomous entity under Moritz Loewit (1851–1918); (1887 Assoc. Prof., 1890 Full Prof.). Cf. Theodor WENSE, "Die Lehrkanzel für allgemeine und experimentelle Pathologie in Innsbruck und ihr Vorstand Prof. Dr Gustav Bayer", in: *Forschungen und Forscher der Tiroler Ärzteschule (1948–1950)*. Vol. 2. Oberösterr. Landesverlag, Wels 1950, pp. 199–211; EULNER (as in FN 13), p. 649; Peter GOLLER, *Die Matrikel der Universität Innsbruck*. Hrsg. im Auftrage d. Akad. Senats. Abt. Med. Fak. Vol. 1: 1869–1900. Universitätsverlag Wagner, Innsbruck 1995, p. 83; HUBER, *Medizinische Fakultät Innsbruck* (as in FN 176), p. 191.

182 Archiv d. Innsbruck Univ. [= UA Innsbruck]. Akten d. Med. Fak. No. 249 from 1872/73.

183 Ibid. Ernst Fuchs's letter of application: *"The Deanery of the Medical Faculty of Innsbruck University. Ernst Fuchs, MD student, herewith applies for the vacant post of assistant for physiology."* His father Adalbert Nikolaus Fuchs complemented the application of his son with the following handwritten declaration of consent: *"The above application of his son Ernst has the consent of Dr Fuchs, o. ö. Professor at the Imperial Royal Technical University."* This consent was required for legal reasons because according to legal provisions in force in Austria at the time citizens did not come of age until they reached their twenty-fourth year. Cf. Joseph UNGER, *System des österreichischen allgemeinen Privatrechts*. Vol.1. Breitkopf und Härtel, Leipzig 1856, p. 284.

184 Anton Tinzl, b. 1846. Cf. GOLLER, *Matrikel* (as in FN 181), p. 87.

185 UA Innsbruck, Akten d. Med. Fak. No 249 from 1872/73. Vintschgau's assessment dated 16 March 1873.

186 Ibid. Decree of 16 April 1873, Z. 4759. This procedure was necessary because, with Fuchs, a student rather than a fully graduated medical doctor had been appointed as assistant. Tenure could therefore only be temporary. – The Ministerium für Cultus und Unterricht was in charge of religious – not, as one might be led to believe, of cultural – affairs, and education.

187 UA Innsbruck, Akten d. Med. Fak. No. 280 from 1872/73. HUBER, *Med. Fakultät Innsbruck* (as in FN 176), pp. 283–284, unfortunately gives several wrong dates.

188 *Personalstand und Ordnung der öffentlichen Vorlesungen an der K. K. Leopold-Franzens-Universität zu Innsbruck im Sommer-Semester 1873*. Wagner'sche Universitäts-Buchdruckerei, Innsbruck 1873, p. 6.

189 UA Innsbruck, Akten der Med. Fak. No. 249 from 1872/73: *"Herrn Ernst Fuchs, Student of Medicine at the Imperial Royal University of Vienna. – The Professorial Council of the Medical Faculty of the Imperial Royal Univ. of Innsbruck has appointed you at the request of Prof. Dr v. Vintschgau in accordance with the resolution passed on 22 March of this year as temp. assistant at the Department of Physiology at this Imperial Royal University for the duration of two years. This post comes with an annual salary of 600 fl.*
You are herewith notified accordingly, with the caveat that in case you decide to resign from this post before the time as specified above you will notify your superior six weeks in advance;

you are expected to arrive in Innsbruck in early April. Innsbruck, 23 March 1873. On behalf of the Professorial Council of the Medical Faculty: Tschurtschenthaler"

190 UA Innsbruck, Schreiben d. k. k. Statthalters in Tirol and Vorarlberg a. d. Landeshauptkasse No. 7527 v. 26. April 1873 [copy] and Akten d. Med. Fak. No. 317 from 1872/73.

191 GOLLER, *Matrikel* (as in FN 181), p. 91.

192 UA Innsbruck, Nationale der Medizinischen Fakultät, Sommersemester 1874. Inskription von Ernest Fuchs mit "Verzeichniß der Vorlesungen, welche der Studirende zu hören beabsichtigt" [List of lectures the student is planning to attend].

193 Anton Alois Tschurtschenthaler (1815–1900, 1885 Edler v. Helmheim). Studied at the Univ. of Padova and Vienna (Dr med. 1841, Dr chir. 1842, Mag. obstetr. 1843); from 1845 Med.-clin. assist. and junior doctor at Innsbruck's Allgem. Krankenhaus. 1846–1847 and 1851–1853 Subst. lecturer for the Chair of Theoret. Med. 1856–1869 Full Prof. and Dir. of the Pharmacolog.-Pharmacognost. Collection 1846–1850. Initially assist. at the Department of Pract. Med., 1855/56 subst. lecturer for this professorship. 1855–1857 Extracurricular lectures on Spec. Med. Pathol. and Therapy. 1857–1859 Pract. demonstrations in pharmacognosy. 1859–1869 Extracurricular pediatr. lectures. 1859/60 Lectures on physiol. and general pathol. 1869–1886 First Full Professor of Gen. Pathol., Pharmacol. and Pharmacognosy and 1869–1896 First Full Prof. of Pediatrics at the newly built Med. Fac. of Innsbruck Univ. 1872/73 and 1878/79 Dean of the Med. Fac. 1884/85 Rector of Innsbruck Univ. Cf. EULNER (as in FN 13); ÖBL (as in FN 11); Adolf JARISCH, "Zur Geschichte des Pharmakologischen Instituts der Universität Innsbruck", in: *Forschungen und Forscher d. Tiroler Ärzteschule* (1948–1950). Vol. 2. Oberösterr. Landesverlag, Wels 1950, pp. 179–182. HUBER, *Med. Fakultät Innsbruck* (as in FN 176), pp. 117–118.; W. EPPACHER, "Die Tschurtschenthaler, ein uraltes Tiroler Geschlecht", in: *Amtsblatt d. Landeshauptstadt Innsbruck* 23/No. 9, September 1960, pp. 1–2; Med. Innsbruck Univ./Division für Biochem. Pharmakologie/Aus der Institutsgeschichte: http://www.i–med.ac.at/ibp/institutsgeschichte.html [last accesssed 6 July 2020].

194 Karl Wilhelm von Heine (1838–1877). Originally from Cannstatt/Germany. Studied at the Univ. of Tübingen and Würzburg (Dr med. 1861, Tübingen). Study trips to Paris, London, Glasgow and Dublin. 1865 Habilitation in Surgery at Heidelberg Univ. (Assoc. Prof. 1868). 1869–1873 Full Prof. of Surgery at the reopened Univ. of Innsbruck; 1873–1877 in the same function at Prague Univ.; successful establishment of Prague's newly founded 2nd Surg. Univ. Clinic. Cf. EULNER; HIRSCH (as in FN 13); NDB (as in FN 15); PAGEL (as in FN 13); HUBER, *Med. Fakultät Innsbruck* (as in FN 176), p. 256.

195 "Wissenschaftliche Institute und Sammlungen. a) Bei der medicinischen Facultät: Physiologisches Institut", in: *Öffentliche Vorlesungen an der K. K. Leopold-Franzens-Universität zu Innsbruck im Winter-Semester 1873/74*. Wagner'sche Univ.-Buchdruckerei, Innsbruck 1873, p. 13.

196 "Wissenschaftliche Institute und Sammlungen. a) Bei der medicinischen Facultät: Physiologisches Institut", in: *Personalstand und Ordnung d. öffentl. Vorlesungen a. d. K. K. Leopold-Franzens-Universität zu Innsbruck im Sommer-Semester 1874*. Wagner'sche Univ.-Buchdruckerei, Innsbruck 1874, p. 21. Cf. HUBER, *Med. Fakultät Innsbruck* (as in FN 176), p. 283. – No evidence has been found to date of Ernst Fuchs's presence

at Innsbruck Univ. in the relevant documents held at the ÖSTA/AVA Wien. The reason could be that temporary assistants were not registered as such. Cf. AVA 5 Assis[tenten] Innsbr. Mediz[in] 1848–1909.

197 FUCHS, *Augenarzt* (as in FN 2), p. 42.

198 UA Wien. Nationale der Medizinischen Fakultät. Inskription von Ernest Fuchs für das 7. Studiensemester.

199 FUCHS, *Augenarzt* (as in FN 2), p. 41.

200 Ludwig Mauthner (1840–1894). Originally from Prague. Dr med. Vienna Univ. 1861. Study trip to London, Utrecht (Donders), Paris and Berlin (A. Graefe); 1864 Habilitation in ophthalmolog. at Vienna Univ. Assist. at the Eye Department of Eduard Jaeger v. Jaxtthal at Vienna's Allgem. Krankenhaus. 1869–1877 Full Prof. of Ophthalmology at reopened Innsbruck Univ. Return to Vienna, where he operated a highly frequented practice, gave free rein to his didactic skills and carried out important research work in neuro-ophthalmology. 1890 Head physician at Vienna's Allgem. Poliklinik. 1894 Call to succeed Stellwag as Full Professor at Vienna's 1st Univ. eye clinic. Died one day after his appointment. Mauthner represented the physical-optical orientation within the Vienna School of Ophthalmol. His monographs on Ophthalmoscopy (1868) and on diseases of the eye (1872–1876) gained internat. recognition. Cf. *Austrian Ophthalmologists*, pp. 15–16.; CZEIKE; EISENBERG 2; EULNER (as in FN 13), p. 559 and 561; HIRSCH (as in FN 13); HIRSCHBERG, *Geschichte der Augenheilkunde* (as in FN 18), vol. 15/2 [= Reprint vol. 6], § 1242–44, pp. 398–408; IBBO (as in FN 18); ÖBL (as in FN 11); PAGEL (as in FN 13); Franz DAXECKER, *125 Jahre Universitäts-Augenklinik in Innsbruck 1869–1994.* Ihre Vorstände [= Veröffentl. d. Innsbruck Univ. 201/Forschungen zur Innsbrucker Universitätsgeschichte XVIII]. Wagner, Innsbruck 1994, pp. 11–17; DAXECKER, "Das Schicksal des Prof. Ludwig Mauthner (1840–1894). The Fateful Life of Prof. Ludwig Mauthner (1840–1894)", in: *Klin. Monatsbl. Augenheilk.* 225 (2008), pp. 173–174; Erich DEIMER, *Chronik der Allgemeinen Poliklinik in Wien im Spiegel der Medizin- und Sozialgeschichte.* Göschl, Vienna 1989, pp. 158–160; HEID (as in FN 165), pp. 129–138; HUBER, *Med. Fakultät Innsbruck* (as in FN 176), pp. 278–280; KÜCHLE (as in FN 179), pp. 401–402; LESKY, *Wien. Med. Schule* (as in FN 12), pp. 479–482; James E. LEBENSOHN, "The Eye and Sleep", in: *Archive of Ophthalmology* [*Arch. Ophthalmol.*] 25 (1941), pp. 401–411; Ernst August SEYFARTH, Steven J. ZOTTOLI, "Ludwig Mauthner (1840–1894): neuroanatomist and noted ophthalmologist in Fin-de-Siècle Vienna", in: *Brain, Behavior and Evolution [Brain Behav. Evol.]* 37 (1991), pp. 252–259; Helmut GRÖGER, Gabriela SCHMIDT-WYKLICKY, "Ludwig Mauthner, berufen zum Vorstand der I. Universitäts-Augenklinik in Wien 1894", in: *Spektrum Augenheilk.* 26 (2012), pp. 319–320. For the competition between Mauthner and Fuchs when the position of Eduard Jaeger von Jaxtthal in Vienna's 2nd Univ. Eye Clinic fell vacant after the latter's death in 1884, see Ch. 4.

201 Ferdinand Plenk (b. 1846), studied at the Univ. of Vienna and Innsbruck; assist. of Mauthner (Habilitation 1876); 1877 included in the shortlist of candidates to succeed Mauthner in Innsbruck. From 1883 head physician in Brno. Cf. Ferdinand PLENK, "Bericht über die k. k. Augenklinik der Universität zu Innsbruck für das Studienjahr 1871/72", in: *Berichte d. naturwissenschaftl.-med. Vereins in Innsbruck*, Folge 3 (1873), pp. 223–230; Peter GOLLER, *Osttiroler Studenten an der Philosophischen Fakultät*

der Universität Innsbruck in der zweiten Hälfte des 19. Jahrhunderts (1848–1904), in: *Osttiroler Heimatblätter* [= Heimatkundliche Beilage des *Osttiroler Bote*] 70 (2002), No. 11 [n. p.].

202 FUCHS, *Augenarzt* (as in FN 2), p. 42.

203 UA Innsbruck, Akten d. Med. Fak. No. 284 from 1873/74. The original of Ernst Fuchs's letter of application and the two attachments mentioned in it are no longer part of this file. What the file does comprise is a letter from the then Dean Tschurtschenthaler to the Professorial Council of the Med. Fac. of Innsbruck Univ. of 25 April 1873, and evidence of Fuchs's application being forwarded to the Ministerium für Cultus and Unterricht in Vienna on 3 May, signed by all the professors of the Faculty.

204 UA Innsbruck, Letter No. 6527 from Minister Stremayr to the Med. Professorial Council in Innsbruck dated 24 May 1873.

205 UA Wien, Rigorosenprotokoll d. Med. Fak.: October 1872/73.

206 UA Wien, Med. Dekanat, No. 118 from 1873/74. Fuchs's request was acceded to by the Ministerium für Cultus and Unterricht in a letter to the deaneries of the Med. Fac. in Vienna and Innsbruck dated 25 November 1873 (No. 15.731.)

207 FUCHS, *Augenarzt* (as in FN 2), p. 44. Here Fuchs's memory seems to have played a trick on him. The grade he achieved for his 3rd *Rigorosum* on 28 January 1874 was "Sufficient". Graduation date: 18 February 1874. Cf. UA Wien, Rigorosenprotokoll der Medizinischen Fakultät vom October 1872/73 sowie Promotionsprotokoll für das Doktorat der Medizin, Kod. M 33.5 (1874–1890). Prot. Nr. 48, Promotion von Ernst Fuchs zum Dr med. am 18. 2. 1874.

208 This is a reference to Vienna's Allgem. Krankenhaus with its univ. clinics.

209 As the disciple of Rokitansky and Škoda, Arlt, as has already been mentioned, had grounded ophthalmology in Vienna in the achievements of pathol. anatomy. He discovered the causes of myopia, a feat that was made possible by his connection to his Prague teacher, Johann Nepomuk Fischer. Fischer's wife, whose pronounced near-sightedness was generally known, had left her eyes to Arlt for the purpose of dissection. This allowed Arlt to show in 1854 that the cause of myopia was an elongation of the visual axis. Cf. Ferdinand ARLT, "Myopischer Bau des Bulbus. Vortrag von Professor Arlt im Prager Medicinischen Doctorencollegium", in: *Dr Altschuls Monatsschrift*, June issue. Prague 1854; Ferdinand ARLT, *Ueber die Ursachen und die Entstehung der Kurzsichtigkeit*. Wilhelm Baumüller, Vienna 1876; Ernst FUCHS, "Die Augen der Frau Fischer. Aus der Geschichte der Wiener Augenheilkunde", in: *Neues Wiener Tagblatt* No. 322, 23 November 1930, p. 6; Karl David LINDNER, "Zur Geschichte der Kurzsichtigkeit von Kepler bis Arlt", in: *Klin. Monatsbl. Augenheilk.* 107 (1941), pp. 320–328; FUCHS, *Augenarzt* (as in FN 2), p. 61, and LESKY, *Wien. Med. Schule* (as in FN 12), p. 223. For Arlt's ophthalmol. merits and his influence on Fuchs, cf. Alexander JOKL, "Ferdinand Arlt and Ernst Fuchs. Two Representatives of the Vienna School of Ophthalmology", in: *Suid-Afrikaanse Tydskrip vir Geneeskunde/South African Med. Journal*, 15 Maart 1958, pp. 301–303, and *Internat. Rec. Med.* 170 (1957), pp. 702–707. Cf. also.: Erna LESKY, "Aus dem Nachlaß Ferdinand von Arlts im Wiener medizinhistorischen Institut", in: *Klin. Monatsbl. Augenheilk.* 139 (1961), pp. 847–856.

210 FUCHS, *Augenarzt* (as in FN 2), p. 44.

211 Cf. UA Wien, Med. Deanery, No. 133 from 1874/75 comprising the decree of the

Ministerium f. Cultus and Unterr. No. 16770 of 29 November 1874 to the Deanery of the Med. Fac. of the University of Vienna. In his memoir, which was written from memory and published in 1946 Fuchs himself noted (erroneously): "*Operationszögling an der Billrothschen Klinik 1. 3. 1874–1. 3. 1876*" [Trainee surgeon at Billroth's clinic 1 March 1874 – 1 March 1976]. Cf. FUCHS, *Augenarzt* (as in FN 2), p. 52. He added: *"As a surgeon I received a stipend of 30 fl. and felt I was very rich after my previous pocket money of 3 fl a month."*

212 See Ch. 1 and FUCHS, *Augenarzt* (as in FN 2), pp. 52–54.

213 Cf. FN 176.

214 Cf. FN 27.

215 FUCHS, *Augenarzt* (as in FN 2), pp. 55–56.

216 As noted by Fuchs's youngest student, Karl David Lindner, at the *Trauersitzung zum Andenken an weil. Prof. Dr Ernst Fuchs* on 28 November 1930 at the Gesellsch. der Ärzte in Vienna: "Offizielles Protokoll der Gesellschaft der Aerzte in Wien", in: *Wiener klin. Wochenschr.* (1930), pp. 1517–20.

217 The website of the City of Vienna only features the following general remarks: *"In c. 1870 skiing arrived from Norway in the Alpine regions, where it was modified significantly (Austria had a decisive influence on the technical development) … In 1891, the 'Erster Wiener Skiverein' was founded."* Accessible online at: https://www.geschichtewiki.Vienna.gv.at/Skisport (last 21 Aug. 2018).

218 Andreas MÜLLER, Charles N. J. McGHEE, "Professor Ernst Fuchs (1851–1930). A Defining Career in Ophthalmology", in: *Arch. Ophthalmol.* 121/6 (2003), pp. 888–891.

219 FUCHS, *Augenarzt* (as in FN 2), p. 57.

220 Hubert Sattler (1844–1918). Son of the Salzburg landscape painter of the same name, grandson of the renowned portrait and landscape painter Johann Michael Sattler (1786–1847, "Sattler Panorama" of the City of Salzburg). 1869 Dr med., Dr chir. at Vienna Univ. 1869/70 Aspir. under Arlt, 1870–1872 Trainee surgeon under Billroth. 1872–1876 Assist. under Arlt. 1873 Study trip to Prague, Breslau (today Wrocław/Poland), Berlin, Utrecht, London and Paris. 1876 Habilitation in Ophthalmology at Vienna Univ. 1877 Full Prof. at the Univ. Eye Clinic Gießen; 1879–1886 Erlangen; 1886–1891 Prague and 1891–1920 Leipzig. Outstanding surgeon. Initiated at Arlt's Clinic the turn towards the histol. examination of the eye, which was perfected to mastery after his departure by Fuchs. Cf. EULNER (as in FN 13); HEID (as in FN 165), pp. 67–76; HIRSCH (as in FN 13); IBBO (as in FN 18); KÜCHLE (as in FN 179), p. 73, pp. 172–173 and 247, ÖBL (as in FN 11); PAGEL (as in FN 13); HIRSCHBERG, *Geschichte der Augenheilkunde* (as in FN 18), vol. 15/2 [= Reprint vol. VI], § 1156–57, pp. 197–198.

221 Cf. UA Wien, Med. Dekanat, No. 327 from 1875/76. Letter from Arlt to the Professorial Council of the Med. Fac. of Vienna Univ. dated 11. February 1876.

222 FUCHS, *Augenarzt* (as in FN 2), p. 54.

223 Otto Bergmeister (1845–1918). Originally from the Tyrol. Studied at Vienna Univ. (Dr med. et chir. 1870). 1872–1874 Assist. under Arlt. 1874 Habilitation at Vienna Univ. 1892 Full Prof. 1893 Head physician at the Eye Department of the Krankenanstalt Rudolfstiftung in Vienna. Cf. EISENBERG 2 (as in FN 13); HEID (as in FN 165), pp. 63–66; HIRSCH; PAGEL (as in FN 13); HIRSCHBERG, *Geschichte*

der Augenheilkunde (as in FN 18), vol. 15/2 [= Reprint vol. VI], § 1235, p. 378.

224 Friedrich Kerschbaumer (1847–1906). Studied at Vienna Univ. (Dr med. univ.1873). Trainee surgeon under Billroth, then assistant under Arlt. 1877 Married Russian-born Raissa (Rosa) Putjata (1851–1923), whom he had met during one of his courses at the clinic. Establishment of a medical practice in their private apartment in Salzburg, which soon burgeoned into a private eye clinic. Cf. Sabine VEITS-FALK, *Rosa Kerschbaumer-Putjata (1851–1923). Erste Ärztin Österreichs und Pionierin der Augenheilkunde. Ein außergewöhnliches Frauenleben in Salzburg* [= Schriftenreihe des Archivs der Stadt *Salzburg* 23] Salzburg 2008.

225 FUCHS, *Augenarzt* (as in FN 2), p. 54.

226 Cf. UA Wien. Med. Deanery, No. 376 from 1875/76 comprising the decree of the governor Erlass Z. 5089 dated 1 March 1876 about the transfer of the salary for newly appointed assistant Fuchs.

227 FUCHS, *Augenarzt* (as in FN 2), p. 57.

228 Ibid.

229 Lint (French/German charpie, German also Scharpie, from the Latin verb carpere, to pick). Picking apart cotton or canvas strips yielded fibres that were used in wound dressing up until the early twentieth century. Cf. Walter GUTTMANN, *Medizinische Terminologie. Ableitung und Erklärung der gebräuchlichsten Fachausdrücke aller Zweige der Medizin und ihrer Hilfswissenschaften.* 6th and 7th revised and augm. editions. Urban & Schwarzenberg, Berlin 1913, col. 209.

230 FUCHS, *Augenarzt* (as in FN 2), p. 58.

231 Ernst FUCHS, "Herpes iris conjunctivae. Beobachtet an der Klinik des Professor von Arlt," in: *Klin. Monatsbl. Augenheilk.* 14 (1876), pp. 333–351.

232 See Ch. 7.

233 Ernst FUCHS, "Ueber Keratitis traumatica. Vorläufige Mitteilung", in: *Centralblatt für die medicinischen Wissenschaften* [Centralbl. med. Wissensch.] 14 (1876), pp. 113–114.; FUCHS, "Ueber die traumatische Keratitis", in: *Archiv für pathol. Anat. and Physiol. and für klin. Med.* [Virchows Archiv] 66 (1876), pp. 401–445.

234 Ernst FUCHS, "Beitrag zur Kenntnis des Froschblutes und der Froschlymphe", in: *Virchows Archiv* 71 (1877), pp. 78–107.

235 Albert ESSER, *Geschichte der Deutschen Ophthalmologischen Gesellschaft. Zur ersten Säkularfeier im Auftrage der Gesellschaft geschrieben.* J. F. Bergmann, Munich 1957.

236 Albrecht v. Graefe (1828–1870), son of the renowned surgeon Carl Ferdinand v. Graefe (1787–1840). Studied at Berlin Univ. (Dr med. 1847), 1848–1850 Ophthalmol. special training in Prague, Paris, Vienna, London and Utrecht. In 1851, Graefe was one of the first ophthalmologists to actually put the ophthalmoscope constructed by Helmholtz to practical use. 1852 Habilitation at Berlin Univ., 1854 Establishment of the eponymous *Graefe's Archiv für Augenheilkunde* (from 1855 jointly edited with Arlt and Donders), 1866 Full Prof. in Berlin. Graefe distinguished himself, among other things, through the propagation of iridectomy in cases of glaucoma. His method of cataract operation with its modified, peripheral lens extraction yielded markedly improved results compared with flap extraction of the lens. Cf. EULNER (as in FN 13), pp. 325–333; GARRISON/MORTON (as in FN 124); HIRSCH (as in FN 13); HIRSCHBERG, *Geschichte der Augenheilkunde* (as in FN 18), vol. 15/1 [= Reprint vol. VI], § 1050–88, pp. 208–314; IBBO (as in FN 18); KÜCHLE (as in FN 179),

pp. 43–56, PAGEL (as in FN 13); Julius HIRSCHBERG (ed.), *Professor A. v. Graefe's klinische Vorträge über Augenheilkunde;* A. Hirschwald, Berlin 1872; Hubert SATTLER (ed.), *Albrecht von Graefe's grundlegende Arbeiten über den Heilwert der Iridectomie bei Glaukom*, in: Karl SUDHOFF (ed.), *Klassiker der Medizin*. vol. 11. J. A. Barth, Leipzig 1911; Charles SNYDER, *Our Ophthalmic Heritage*. Little, Brown & Comp., Boston 1967, pp. 13–17; Blida HEYNOLD von GRAEFE, *Albrecht von Graefe. Mensch und Umwelt.* Stapp, Berlin 1969 (Reprint 1991); George GORIN (as in FN 38), pp. 132–139; ALBERT/EDWARDS; ALBERT/HENKIND (as in FN 38), pp. 361–369; BOECKER-REINERTZ (as in FN 179), pp. 37–42; Hans REMKY, "Albrecht von Graefe – Facets of his work", in: *Graefes Archive of Clinical and Experimental Ophthalmology* [*Graefes Arch.* Clin. Exper. Ophthalmol.] 233 (1995), pp. 537–548.

237 Wilhelm v. ZEHENDER (ed.), *Die Ophthalmologische Gesellschaft während der ersten fünfundzwanzig Jahre ihres Bestehens von 1863 bis 1888* [= Ausserordentl. Beilagenheft z. d. Klin. Monatsbl. Augenheilk. Yr. XXVI]. Ferdinand Enke, Stuttgart 1888, p. 94.

238 Ernst FUCHS, "Otto Becker †", in: *Wiener klin. Wochenschr.* 3 (1890), p. 159.

239 Some of Becker's tissue sections, marked Heidelberg, their place of origin, have survived. They were a gift from the former 1st Univ. Eye Clinic in Vienna to the former Institute for the History of Medicine of Vienna University (today: Sammlungen d. Med. Univ. Wien). Becker was co-editor of the performance report of Vienna's Eye Clinic for 1863–1865 and was responsible for the posthumous publication of the memoirs of his teacher, Arlt. Cf. Max TETZER, Lucian RYDEL, Otto BECKER, *Bericht über die Augenklinik der Wiener Universität. 1863–1865.* Unter Mitwirkung des Prof. Dr Ferdinand Arlt. Wilhelm Braumüller, Vienna 1867; ARLT, *Meine Erlebnisse.* – In the days when Fuchs was still a student and, later, an assistant under Arlt, Becker, even though he was Chair in Heidelberg, insisted on having his illustrated books on ophthalmology published by the Viennese publishing firm of Wilhelm Braumüller. For this, he relied on the proven collaboration with the brothers Carl and Julius Heitzmann (cf. FN 167) as draughtsmen. Furthermore, Becker used Braumüller for a first attempt to photograph drawings of eye preparations and published them in the form of three series of loose sheets: Otto BECKER (ed.), *Atlas der pathologischen Topographie des Auges.* Gezeichnet von Carl Heitzmann. I. Lieferung. Mit 9 Tafeln und 7 Holzschnitten. Wilhelm Braumüller, Vienna 1874; II. Lieferung. Mit 9 Tafeln. Gezeichnet von Carl und Julius Heitzmann, Robert Sattler und Friedrich Veith. Wilhelm Braumüller, Vienna 1875; III. Lieferung. Mit 12 Tafeln. Gezeichnet von Julius Heitzmann, Hubert Sattler und Friedrich Veith. Wilhelm Braumüller, Vienna 1878; BECKER, *Photographische Abbildungen von Durchschnitten gesunder und kranker Augen.* Gezeichnet von Friedrich Veith, photographirt von J. Schulze in Heidelberg. Wilhelm Braumüller, Vienna. I. Serie 1875, II. und III. Serie 1876.

240 UA Wien, Med. Dekanat, No. 183 of 16 March 1878.

241 Ibid.

242 Cf. UA Wien, Med. Deanery, No. 278 from 1877/78 comprising the governor's decree No. 9392 of 12 April 1878 to the Deanery of the Med. Fac. concerning the continued payment of the salary.

243 Fuchs kept accurate records of course attendance in copybooks expressly dedicated to this purpose. These have unfortunately not come down to us, but in a footnote in his father's autobiography Adalbert Fuchs supplies the following impressive figures:

"Between 10 September 1877 and 25 April 1881 my father held thirty courses in German on the use of the ophthalmoscope and he himself supplied a statistic of the participants. Of these, 765 were from North America, 325 from Great Britain, 220 from Germany, 119 from Scandinavia, 61 from Austria, 23 from Russia, 19 from Switzerland, 7 from South America, 174 from other countries." FUCHS, *Augenarzt* (as in FN 2), p. 59, FN 25.

244 Albert Neisser (1855–1916). Born in what was then Germ.-Silesian Schweidnitz (today Świdnica/Poland). Studied at the Univ. of Breslau and Erlangen (Dr med. 1877, Breslau). Then assistant at the Univ. Skin Clinic in Breslau for 2 years. 1880 Habilitation in Dermatol. at Leipzig Univ.; 1882–1916 Dir. of the Univ. Skin Clinic in Breslau (1882 Assoc. Prof., 1907 Full Prof. ad personam, 1912 Full Prof.). 1889 Cofounder of the Dt. Dermatol. Gesellschaft. 1892 Inauguration of the newly built clinic, to whose planning he made a substantive contribution. 1902 Founder of the Dt. Gesellsch. zur Bekämpfung d. Geschlechtskrankheiten [German Society for Control of Sexually Transmitted Diseases]. Chief areas of work and research: STD, skin infections, bacteriol. and social hygiene. 1879 Identification of the pathogen causing gonorrhea, invention of the first practicable colouring technique for the detection of lepra bacteria. Joint research with August Paul von Wassermann (1866–1925) on the serolog. test for syphilis (1906 Wassermann reaction). 1892 Start of human experiments (infection of adults with the syphilis pathogen without their knowledge and consent and of minors without the knowledge or consent of their legal guardians) – 1900 Trial and conviction for breach of duty. Cf. GERABEK et al. (as in FN 13); NDB (as in FN 15); PAGEL (as in FN 13); Sigrid SCHMITZ, *Albert Neisser Leben und Werk auf Grund neuer, unveröffentlichter Quellen.* Triltsch Verlag, Düsseldorf 1968 [= Düsseldorfer Arbeiten z. Geschichte d. Medizin vol. 29, at the same time med. diss., Univ. Düsseldorf 1967]; Obituary, in: *Dermatol. Wochenschr.* 131 (1955), pp. 214–216; Feliks WASIK, Albrecht SCHOLZ, Günther SEBASTIAN, "Erinnerungen an Albert Neisser", in: *Der Hautarzt.* 31 (1980), p. 328–333.

245 Adolf von Strümpell (1853–1925). Born in the Baltics, then part of the Russian Impire (today Latvia). Studied at the Univ. of Dorpat and Leipzig (Dr med. 1875). 1876 Assistant at the Leipzig Med. Univ. Clinic under Carl Reinhold August Wunderlich (1815–1877) and Ernst Leberecht Wagner (1829–1888). 1878 Habilitation in Intern. Med. 1883 Assoc. Prof. and Dir. of the Med. Univ. Clinic Leipzig. 1886 Full Prof. at Erlangen Univ., 1903 at Breslau Univ., 1909/10 at the 3rd Med. Univ. Clinic in Vienna, 1910–1925 at the Med. Univ. Clinic in Leipzig. 1915 Rector of Leipzig Univ. Focused predominantly on neurological topics in the context of internal medicine. Discovered several new pathologies eponymously named after him. His textbook of special pathology and therapy became a work of reference, appearing in 30 editions and translations into many languages between 1884 and 1930. Cf. EULNER (as in FN 13); FISCHER (as in FN 28); GERABEK et al. (as in FN 13); FUCHS, *Augenarzt* (as in FN 2), p. 59.

246 Adolf STRÜMPELL, *Aus dem Leben eines deutschen Klinikers. Erinnerungen und Beobachtungen.* Vogel, Leipzig 1925, pp. 102–103. Fuchs was in close contact with Strümpell in 1909/10, when the latter was Dir. of the 3rd Med. Univ. Clinic in Vienna for two years. Cf. FUCHS, *Augenarzt* (as in FN 2), p. 59.

247 Cf. UA Wien, Med. Dekanat, Z. 13 aus 1877/78, dated 3 Jan. 1878.

248 Ibid.

[249] Cf. UA Wien, Med. Deanery, No. 196 from 1877/78 (Award Decree), comprising a decree of the Academic Senate of Vienna Univ. No. 405 of 26 February 1878.

[250] Ernst FUCHS, "Chorioiditis bei Glaukom", in: Frans Cornelis DONDERS, Wilhelm HESS, Wilhelm ZEHENDER (eds.), *Bericht über die elfte Versammlung der Ophthalmologischen Gesellschaft Heidelberg 1878*. Universitäts-Buchdruckerei von Adler's Erben. Rostock 1878, p. 65. Cf. also: ZEHENDER, *Ophthalmol. Gesellschaft*, p. 73.

[251] Louis-Antoine Ranvier (1835–1922). Studied at the Univ. of Lyon and Paris (Graduation 1865): Directeur adjoint at the histol. laboratory of the Collège de France, from 1875 Titular Professor of the Chair of General Anatomy in Paris, which had been created especially for him. Cf. GERABEK et al.; HIRSCH; PAGEL (as in FN 13).

[252] Ludwig Wecker/Louis de Wecker (1832–1906). Originally from Frankfurt. Studied medicine at Würzburg Univ. (Dr med. 1855). Specialised in ophthalmol. in Berlin, Vienna and Paris. 1862 Establishment of a prosperous private clinic in Paris. Invented a great number of specialist instruments and modifications to ophthalomolog. surgery; Professeur libre d'ophtalmologie. Cf. GORIN (as in FN 38), pp. 189–190, HIRSCH (as in FN 13); HIRSCHBERG, *Geschichte der Augenheilkunde* (as in FN 18), vol. 15/II [= Reprint vol. VI], § 1263–1266, pp. 471–497; IBBO (as in FN 18); PAGEL (as in FN 13); Gabriela SCHMIDT-WYKLICKY, "Die Beziehungen des Graefe-Schülers Louis de Wecker (1832–1906) zur Wiener Ophthalmologischen Schule und zur österreichisch-ungarischen Monarchie", in: *Mitteilungen der Julius-Hirschberg-Gesellschaft zur Geschichte der Augenheilkunde* vol. 14–2012 (2016), pp. 219–235.

[253] Edmund/Edmont Landolt (1846–1926). Originally from Aarau/Switzerland, studied medicine at the Univ. of Heidelberg, Zurich, Vienna, Berlin and Utrecht (Dr med. 1860, Berlin). In Zurich assistant at the Surg. Univ. Clinic, then at the Univ. Eye Clinic under Johann Friedrich Horner (1831–1886). 1874 Established himself in Paris (highly frequented eye clinic). Cf. GORIN (as in FN 38), p. 191; HIRSCH (as in FN 13); HIRSCHBERG, *Geschichte der Augenheilkunde* (as in FN 18), vol. 15/II [= Reprint vol. VI], § 1273, p. 512; IBBO (as in FN 18); PAGEL (as in FN 13).

[254] Eduard/Edouard Meyer (1838–1902). Originally from Dessau. Ophthalmol. specialisation under Graefe in Berlin. 1863 Established himself in Paris. Soon considered to be a leading practitioner of ophthalmol. Cf. GORIN (as in FN 38), p. 190; HIRSCH (as in FN 13); HIRSCHBERG, *Geschichte der Augenheilkunde* (as in FN 18), vol. 15/II [= Reprint vol. VI], pp. 1267–68, pp. 497–503; IBBO (as in FN 18).

[255] Charles Abadie (1842–1932). Originally from Paris. Studied at Paris Univ. (Graduation 1868). Ophthalmol. specialisation in Vienna and Berlin (Graefe). Return to Paris. Joined Wecker's clinic. Establishment of a grand private eye clinic on the Boulevard St. Germain. Glaucoma specialist, supporter of iridectomy. Cf. GORIN (as in FN 38), p. 195; HIRSCHBERG, *Geschichte der Augenheilkunde* (as in FN 18), vol. 15/II [= Reprint vol. VI], § 1300, p. 575; IBBO (as in FN 18); PAGEL (as in FN 13).

[256] Arthur Sichel (life data not retrievable), student of Graefe. Son of the outstanding ophthalmol. Julius/Jules Sichel (1802–1868) from Frankfurt, founder of the first eye hospital in Paris. Cf. HIRSCHBERG (as in FN 18), vol. 14/3 [= Reprint vol. III], § 595, p. 232 and vol. 15/I [= Reprint vol. VI], § 1053, p. 216 (FN).

[257] Xaver/Xavier Galezowski (1832–1907). Originally from Poland. Studied medicine in St. Petersburg (Graduation 1858). Establishment of a highly successful private clinic in Paris. Distinguished himself by improving many existing instruments and operation methods and inventing new ones. Cf. GORIN (as in FN 38), p. 191; HIRSCH (as in FN 13); HIRSCHBERG, *Geschichte der Augenheilkunde* (as in FN 18), vol. 15/II [= Reprint vol. VI], § 1269–71, pp. 503–509; IBBO (as in FN 18).

[258] Photinos Panas (1832–1903). Originally from Greece. Studied medicine in Paris (Graduation 1860). Eye surgeon at various hospitals in Paris: Hôpital Lariboisière (from 1872) and Hôtel Dieu (from 1879). From 1873 lecturer in Ophthalmol. at the Paris Med. Fac. (1879 tit. Full Prof.). Author of a popular textbook and a great number of specialist publications. Significant contributions to the progress of ophthalmol. in France. Cf. GORIN (as in FN 38), p. 192; HIRSCH (as in FN 13); HIRSCHBERG, *Geschichte der Augenheilkunde* (as in FN 18), vol. 15/II [= Reprint vol. VI], § 1274, pp. 514–523; IBBO (as in FN 18); PAGEL (as in FN 13).

[259] Maurice Constantin Perrin (1826–1889). Studied at Paris Univ. (Graduation 1851). Career as a military doctor and lecturer, winding up as Prof. and Dir. of the Hôpital d'instruction des armées du Val-de-Grâce in Paris. Cf. GORIN (as in FN 38), pp. 193–194; HIRSCH (as in FN 13); HIRSCHBERG, *Geschichte der Augenheilkunde* (as in FN 18), vol. 15/II [= Reprint vol. VI], § 1293, pp. 563–565; IBBO (as in FN 18); PAGEL (as in FN 13).

[260] The miotic effect of extracts from the Calabar bean was first described by Sir Thomas Richard Fraser (1841–1919) at Edinburgh Univ. in 1862. More accurate examinations of its effects on the pupil and on accommodation were carried out in 1863 by Douglas Argyll Robertson (1837–1909) and Graefe. Graefe used these extracts also as an efficacious miotic during iridectomy. Obtained from Calabar beans, eserine had been described as a pure alkaloid in 1865, after physostigmine, which is identical with it, had been isolated from it as a first product in the preceding year. One of Graefe's students, Adolf Weber (1829–1915), is credited with having pioneered the study of the effects of these substances on intraocul. pressure. Cf. Adolf WEBER, "Ueber Calabar und seine therapeutische Verwendung", in: *Graefes Archiv* 22 (1876), pp. 215–232; WEBER, "Die Ursachen des Glaukoms", in: *Graefes Archiv* 23 (1877), pp. 1–91; ALBERT/EDWARDS, p. 220; GORIN (as in FN 38), pp. 151–152.
At Arlt's clinic, silver nitrate cautery was used before the discovery of eserine to cause the pupil to contract. Ernst Fuchs reminisced about this in a conversation in 1925 with his Berlin fellow ophthalmol. Carl Hamburger (1870–1944), who delivered a paper on "Das Erweichungsprinzip bei der Glaukombehandlung" to the Ophthalmological Conference in Heidelberg in that year. Cf. Carl HAMBUR GER, "Glaukomprobleme", in: *Klin. Monatsbl. Augenheilk.* 78 (1927), pp. 189–205 (p. 201, FN 1).

[261] In 1877, roughly conjointly with eserine, Weber studied another substance, pilocarpine, which also reduced intraocular pressure and had fewer side effects. Cf. Adolf WEBER, "Ueber die Wirkung des Pilocarpinum muriaticum", in: *Centralbl. med. Wissensch.* 14 (1876), pp. 769–772; W. ENGELMAYR; G. K. KRIEGLSTEIN, *Pilokarpin. Ein Jahrhundert in der Glaukomtherapie*. Kaden, Heidelberg 1980, pp. 16–17.

[262] These experiences caused Fuchs in September 1878 to publish his own observations: Ernst FUCHS, "Ueber die Verwendung des Pilocarpins in Augenkrankheiten", in: *Wiener med. Wochenschr.* 28 (1878), cols. 997–999 and 1013–17. This paper is a report

on 18 patients suffering from eye diseases such as iridocyclitis acuta, iridochorioiditis chronica, opacitates corporis vitrei, ablatio retinae, neuroretinitis haemorrhagica and keratitis parenchymatosa, who were being treated at Arlt's clinic with subcut. injections of pilocarpinum muriaticum. Fuchs justfied the form of application he had chosen as follows: *"The miotic effect of pilocarp. mur., which is achieved when it is instilled as a solution into the conjunctival sac, was not used, seeing that we have a much more efficacious and safer miotic in eserine."* (Ibid., col. 997). – Especially in those acute indications where a quick intervention had taken place, often combined with a significant secretion of fluids, Fuchs had succeeded in restoring the acuity of vision. He summed up his own results as follows: *"I therefore believe that in addition to those cases where p[ilocarpinum] is used because of its resorbent properties, it should be used on a trial basis more frequently where we are aiming to put an end to an existing acute inflammation with its concomitant pain by relieving the strain on the vessels."* (Ibid., col. 1017).

263 Carl Friedrich Richard Förster (1825–1902). Studied at the Univ. of Breslau, Heidelberg and Berlin (Dr med. 1849). 1857 Habilitation in Ophthalmology at Breslau Univ. and founder of the Univ. Eye Clinic (Head 1857–1899, Assoc. Prof. 1863, Full Prof. 1873). Inventor of the photometer (1857) and the perimeter (1868). Cf. BOECKER-REINARTZ (as in FN 179), p. 69; EULNER (as in FN 13), p. 556; GORIN (as in FN 38), p. 155; HIRSCH (as in FN 13); HIRSCHBERG, *Geschichte der Augenheilkunde* (as in FN 18), vol. 15/II [= Reprint vol. VI], § 1138–1141, pp. 159–170; IBBO (as in FN 18); KÜCHLE (as in FN 179), pp. 163–164, PAGEL (as in FN 13).

264 William Nicati (1850–1931). Swiss ophthalmol., later active in Marseille. Cf. IBBO (as in FN 18).

265 James Clerk Maxwell (1831–1879). Originally from Edinburgh. Fellow of Trinity College, Cambridge, from 1856 Prof. of Natural Philosophy in Aberdeen (main areas of interest: electricity, magnetism). 1860 King's College, London (main areas of study: colour theory and colour blindness). 1860 Invention of a colorimeter, in c. 1865 Conception of the electromagnet. theory of light. 1871 Cavendish Professor of Physics, Cambridge. Cf. ALBERT/EDWARDS (as in FN 38), p. 144; IBBO (as in FN 18); Lewis CAMPELL, William GARNETT, *The Life of James Clerk Maxwell. With a Selection of His Correspondence and Occasional Writings and a Sketch of His Contribution to Science*. London, Macmillan 1882.

266 Richard Liebreich (1830–1917). Originally from Königsberg/Prussia (today Kaliningrad, a Russian exclave between Poland and Lithuania). Studied at the Univ. of Königsberg, Berlin and Halle (Dr med. 1853). Special. in ophthalmol. under Donders in Utrecht; introduced to experim. work by Ernst Wilhelm v. Brücke in Berlin. 1854–1862 Assist. under Graefe in Berlin (1854–1862). Special. in ophthalmoscopy (modification of Helmholtz's ophthalmoscope, first atlas in the world of ophthalmoscopy in German and French 1863). 1862 Established himself in Paris. Owing to the Franco-Prussian war move to London in 1870. From 1878 Dir. of the Eye Dept. at St. Thomas Hospital. Returned to Paris. After the winding down of his private practice trained as an artist at the École des Beaux-Arts. Cf. HIRSCH (as in FN 13); HIRSCHBERG, *Geschichte der Augenheilkunde* (as in FN 18), vol. 15/2 [= Reprint vol. VI], § 1094–1095, pp. 10–16; IBBO (as in FN 18); PAGEL (as in FN 13).

267 Christian Georg Theodor Ruete (1810–1867). Studied at Göttingen Univ. (Dr med. 1833). Special. in ophthalmol. and habilitation under Carl Himly (1772–1837) at Göttingen Univ.; 1852–1867 Full Prof. of Ophthalmology at Leipzig Univ. and 1853–1861 Dir. of the Leipzig Med. Policlinic. Only one year after the invention of the ophthalmoscope by Helmholtz in 1852 Ruete inaugurated inverted-image ophthalmoscopy. Arlt learnt this method from Ruete, but preferred Liebreich's ophthalmoscope later. Cf. HIRSCH (as in FN 13); HIRSCHBERG, *Geschichte der Augenheilkunde* (as in FN 18), vol. 14/2 [= Reprint vol. III], § 483, pp. 17–25; IBBO (as in FN 18); PAGEL (as in FN 13).

268 Crètes, an optician who made instruments for renowned ophthalmol. in Paris, e.g. for Wecker. Registered at 66, rue de Rennes. Cf. *Centralbl. prakt. Ophthalmolog.* 7 (1883), p. 586.

269 Edward Treacher COLLINS, *The History and Traditions of the Moorfields Eye Hospital. One Hundred Years of Ophthalmic Discovery and Development.* H. K. Lewis and Co., London 1929.

270 Cf. ALBERT/HENKIND, pp. 89–104; GORIN (as in FN 38), pp. 170ff.; HIRSCHBERG, *Geschichte der Augenheilkunde* (as in FN 18), vol. 14/4 [= Reprint vol. IV], § 633, pp. 97ff.; G. Barry CARRUTHERS, Leslie A. CARRUTHERS, *A History of Britain's Hospitals and the Background to the Medical, Nursing and Allied Professions.* Book Guild Publishing, Sussex 2005, p. 189.

271 George Critchett (1817–1882). Renowned surgeon at the Royal London Ophthalmic Hospital (Moorfields). Developed, among other techniques, a subconjunct. strabismus operation (iridodesis) and a new enucleation procedure. Cf. GORIN (as in FN 38), p. 170; HIRSCH (as in FN 13); HIRSCHBERG , *Geschichte der Augenheilkunde* (as in FN 18), vol. 14/4 [= Reprint vol. IV], § 642–648, pp 168–197; IBBO (as in FN 18); PAGEL (as in FN 13).

272 John Fremlyn Streatfield (1828–1886). Assistant surgeon at Moorfields Hospital, then eye surgeon at University College Hospital and Professor of Eye Surgery at Univ. College London. Cofounder of the British Ophthalmol. Society. Cf. HIRSCH (as in FN 13); HIRSCHBERG, *Geschichte der Augenheilkunde* (as in FN 18), vol. 14/4 [= Reprint vol. IV], § 650, pp. 226–228; IBBO (as in FN 18).

273 Thomas Wharton Jones (1808–1891). Studied in Edinburgh and Paris, Prof. of Physiol. at Charing Cross Hospital and the Royal Institution, Prof. of Ophthalmolog. at Univ. College Hospital. Cf. HIRSCHBERG, *Geschichte der Augenheilkunde* (as in FN 18), vol. 14/4 [= Reprint vol. IV], § 671, pp. 299–303; IBBO (as in FN 18).

274 John Couper (1835–1918). Studied at Glasgow Univ. Specialisation in London. Eye surgeon at several London hospitals. Cf. IBBO *(as in FN 18).*

275 Sir Jonathan Hutchinson (1828–1913). Eye surgeon at Royal London Ophthalmic Hospital Moorfields (1868–1883). One of the most highly respected ophthalmologists of his time. Leading position in the Ophthalmol. Soc. of the United Kingdom. Initial description of the symptom triad – sensorineural deafness, interstitial keratitis and malformed teeth (Hutchinson incisors and mulberry molars) in presumptive cases of syphilis – Hutchinson's triad: *Clinical Memoir on Certain Diseases of the Eye and the Ear Consequent on Inherited Syphilis* (John Churchill, London 1863). Cf. GARRISON/MORTON (as in FN 124); GORIN (as in FN 38), pp. 171–172; HIRSCH (as in FN 13); HIRSCHBERG, *Geschichte der Augenheilkunde* (as in FN 18), vol. 14/4

[= Reprint vol. IV], § 651, pp. 234–238; IBBO (as in FN 18); P AGEL (as in FN 13); Maurice-P. RAVAULT, *Syndromes en Ophtalmologie* (Guide-Dictionnaire). Doin-Deren, Paris 1970, pp. 185–186; Rickman GODLEE, "Sir Jonathan Hutchinson, F. R. S. (1828–1913)", in: *Brit. J. Ophthalmol.* June 1925/9, pp. 257–281 [= British Masters of Ophthalmology Series 15]; Almut BÖER, "Sir Jonathan Hutchinson (1828–1913)", in: LÖSER/PLEWIG (eds.), *Pantheon der Dermatologie* (as in FN 162), pp. 471–488.

276 Edward Nettleship (1845–1913). Initially vet. surgeon, then studied human medicine at King's College and London Hospital. Specialisation in infantile eye diseases. Eye surgeon at South London Ophthalmic Hospital (later Royal Eye Hospital for Sick Children), under Hutchinson at Royal London Ophthalmic Hospital Moorfields (1882–1898) and at St. Thomas Hospital (1875–1895). Cofounder of the Brit. Ophthalmol. Soc. 1880. Cf. GORIN (as in FN 38), p. 172; HIRSCHBERG, *Geschichte der Augenheilkunde* (as in FN 18), vol. 14/4 [= Reprint vol. IV], § 652, pp. 239–245; IBBO (as in FN 18); Sarah ROTHBÜHR, Thorsten ZUBERBIER, "Edward Nettleship (1845–1913)", LÖSER/PLEWIG (eds.), *Pantheon der Dermatologie* (as in FN 162), pp. 738–741.

277 James Edward Adams (1845–1890). Ophthalmol. at Moorfields Hospital. 1883 Construction of an ophthalmoscope with indir. light source, which, like the otoscope, was attached to a headband to free up both hands of the examiner. Cf. Obituary in: *Brit. Med. J.* February 1, 1890, pp. 271–272; ALBERT/EDWARDS, p. 196; GORIN (as in FN 38), p. 179.

278 John Soelberg Wells (1834–1879). Studied at Edinburgh Univ. (1856), ophthalmol. specialisation under Graefe in Berlin. 1860 Joined Moorfields Hospital; Prof. at King's College (1865). Brought scientific and clin. innovations in ophthalmology from Berlin, Vienna and Utrecht to London. Cf. GORIN (as in FN 38), p. 172; HIRSCHBERG, *Geschichte der Augenheilkunde* (as in FN 18), vol. 14/4 [= Reprint vol. IV], § 651, pp. 238–239; IBBO (as in FN 18).

279 Charles Higgins (1846–1920). Eye surgeon at Guy's Hospital. Cf. IBBO (as in FN 18).

280 Arthur R. Dunnage (life data not retrievable). Surgeon at Central London Ophthalmic Hospital (1873–1879). Cf. Charles DICKENS (Jr.), *Dickens's Dictionary of London 1879. An Unconventional Handbook*. Macmillan & Co., London 1879, p. 85 (Entry: Doctors).

281 Warren Tay (1844–1927). Like Nettleship student and assistant under Hutchinson. After the retirement of Sir William Bowman (1816–1892, cf. FN 299) and Critchett 1877 at Moorfields Hospital, Tay and Adams took over. 1875 Description of chorioiditis guttata together with Hutchinson and, in 1881, of the changes to the eyes consequent on infantile amaurotic family idiocy. The Tay-Sachs syndrome is named after him and neurologist Bernard Sachs (1858–1944). Cf. FISCHER (as in FN 28); GARRISON/MORTON (as in FN 124); GORIN (as in FN 38), p. 173; H. V. NEMA, *Ophthalmic Syndromes*. Butterworth, London 1973, pp. 250–251; RAVAULT (as in FN 275), p. 189 and pp. 346–347; IBBO *(as in FN 18).*

282 Pierre Desiré Lebrun (1836–1900). Studied at Löwen University (Leuven/Louvain in Flanders/Belgium). Ophthalmol. training in Paris under Sichel, Charles M. Edouard Chassaignac (1805–1879) and Louis-Auguste Desmarres (1810–1882) and in London

under Bowman and Critchett. Established himself in Brussels. Initial description of leucosarcoma of the iris and of a new type of incision for the removal of cataracts without iridectomy. 1885 Director of the Institut ophtalmologique du Brabant. Cf. IBBO (as in FN 18); Daniel Van DUYSE, *Coup d'œil sur l'histoire de l'ophtalmologie en Belgique au XIXe siècle.* Ad. Host, Gand 1912, p. 49; P. LEBRUN, "Tumeur sarcomateuse de l'iris. Extirpation du globe. Guerison", in: *Annales d'Oculistique* 1869, p. 208; P. LEBRUN, "New Mode of Operating for Cataract by Median-Sphero-Cylindrical Flap", in: Henry P. MENESES, George CRITCHETT (eds.), *Report of the Fourth International Ophthalmological Congress Held in London, August, 1872.* vol. 4, Savill, Edwards 1873, p. 205.

283 The reference is to Albrecht von Graefe.

284 This relic of humoral pathol. medicine was still in use in Arlt's clinic. Cf. HIRSCHBERG, *Geschichte der Augenheilkunde* (as in FN 18), Reg.; FUCHS, *Augenarzt* (as in FN 2), pp. 48–49.

285 Cf. FN 275 (Hutchinson Triad).

286 Poor eyesight. Functional deficiency in one or, more rarely, both eyes.

287 Ferdinand ARLT, "Ueber Retinitis nyctalopica", in: Max TETZER, Lucian RYDEL, Otto BECKER (eds.), *Bericht über die Augenklinik der Wiener Universität 1863–1865. Unter Mitwirkung des Prof. Dr Ferdinand Arlt.* Wilhelm Braumüller, Vienna 1867, pp. 123–132. Cf. Hermann Cohn's summary, in: *Klin. Monatsbl. Augenheilk.* 6 (1868), pp. 21–23.

288 Theodor Leber (1840–1917). Studied at Heidelberg Univ. (Dr med. 1862). Ophthalmol. specialisation above all in Berlin under Graefe (Assistant 1867–1870). During Graefe's last illness (†1870) he substituted for him. 1871 Assoc. Prof. at Göttingen Univ. (1873–1890 Full Prof.). 1890–1910 Full Prof. at Heidelberg Univ. Cf. BOECKER/REINARTZ (as in FN 179); EULNER (as in FN 13); FISCHER (as in FN 28); HIRSCHBERG, *Geschichte der Augenheilkunde* (as in FN 18), vol. 15/2 [= Reprint vol. VI], § 1107, pp. 52–60; IBBO (as in FN 18); KÜCHLE (as in FN 179); PAGEL (as in FN 13).

289 Cf. FN 274.

290 Karl Denk (1850–1927). Specialist training under Arlt, then priv. eye clinic in Linz. Father of Wolfgang Denk [(1882–1970), 1931–1953 Full Prof. of Surgery, Dir. of the 2nd Surg. Univ. Clinic in Vienna]. Denk's call-up to military service referred to by Fuchs had to do with mobilisation in the context of the Russo-Turkish War 1877/78. When the path was cleared for Bosnia and Herzegovina to be put under Austrian administration by the Reichenbach Agreement (15.1./18.3.1877), the war between a Russian-backed alliance and the Ottoman Empire broke out, in which the Slavic alliance sought to expel the Turks from the Balkans.

291 Frans Cornelis Donders. Cf. FN 38. His opus magnum is a comprehensive monograph published in English in 1864: F. C. DONDERS, *On the Anomalies of Accommodation and Refraction of the Eye. With a Preliminary Essay on Physiological Dioptrics.* Translated from the Author's Manuscript by William Daniel Moore. The New Sydenham Society, London 1864. A German translation by Otto Becker followed two years later: F. C. DONDERS, *Die Anomalien der Refraction und Accomodation des Auges.* Deutsche Originalausgabe unter Mitwirkung des Verfassers herausgegeben von Dr Otto Becker. Braumüller, Vienna 1866. – A friendship comparable in closeness to the one between

Arlt and Donders was to develop later between Fuchs and Donders, who was the driving force behind Fuchs's call to Liège (see Ch. 3). The cordiality of their relationship is in evidence in Fuchs's obituary for Donders: Ernst FUCHS, "Franz Cornelius Donders †", in: *Wiener klin. Wochenschr.* 2 (1889), pp. 271–272.

292 Herman Snellen (1834–1908). Studied under Donders. 1862 Successor of Donders at the Nederlandsch Gasthuis voor ooglijders in Utrecht. Introduction of a practicable measurement of the acuity of vision by means of square capitals ("Optotypes"): Herman SNELLEN, *Letterproeven, tot bepaling der gezichtsscherpte.* P. W. Van de Weijer, Utrecht 1862. 1877 Full Prof. of Ophthalmolog. at Utrecht Univ. Cf. Obituary, in: *Wiener klin. Wochenschr.* 21 (1908), p. 157 (Ernst Fuchs). Cf. ALBERT/EDWARDS (as in FN 38); GARRISON/MORTON (as in FN 124); GORIN (as in FN 38), pp. 215–216; HIRSCH (as in FN 13); HIRSCHBERG, *Geschichte der Augenheilkunde* (as in FN 18), vol. 14/7 [= Reprint vol. V], § 839, pp. 117–118; IBBO (as in FN 18).

293 Frans Cornelis DONDERS, "Ueber Farbensysteme", in: *Graefes Archiv* 27/Abth. 1 (1881) pp. 155–223 and DONDERS, "Noch einmal die Farbensysteme", in: Ibid. 30/ Abth. 1 (1884), pp. 15–90.

294 Thomas Young (1773–1829). Studied medicine at the Univ. of London, Edinburgh and Göttingen (Graduation 1796). In 1793, when he was only 20, he showed that the accommodation of the eye is effected by changes in the form of the lens – in recognition of this achievement he was awarded a fellowship by the Royal Society, London. Exponent of the wave theory of light vs. the corpuscle theory of Isaac Newton (1643–1727). 1800 Established himself in London; scientific studies. 1800–1804 Prof. of Physics at the Royal College, London. 1801 Initial description of astigmatism. Initially he supported the view that colour vision depended on structures of the retina that correspond to the spectral colours of red, green and violet. 1822 Member of the Am. Acad. of Arts and Sciences. 1807 Development of the first kymograph, a pioneering device for the recording of sound. Significant contributions to deciphering Egyptian hieroglyphs. Cf. IBBO (as in FN 18); KRAFT (as in FN 40); Thomas YOUNG: "The Bakerian Lecture: On the Theory of Light and Colours", in: *Philosophical Transactions of the Royal Society of London* [= Phil. Transact. Royal Soc. London] 92 (1802) pp. 12–48.

295 The Young-Helmholtz theory rests on the assumption that the three components of the spectral colours (red, green, violet) are localised in the cones of the retina. Cf. GARRISON/MORTON (as in FN 124); "Hermann von HELMHOLTZ, 'Ueber die Theorie der zusammengesetzten Farben'", in: *Arch. Anat. Physiol. wiss. Med.* Yr. 1852, pp. 461–482 and *Annalen der Physik und Chemie* [Ann. Phys. Chem.] 87 (1852), pp. 45–66; Ernst Wilhelm von BRÜCKE, "Ueber einige Consequenzen der Young-Helmholtz'schen Theorie." 1. Abhandlung, in: *Sitzungsber. d. k. k. Akad. d. Wissensch. Math.-Naturwiss. Cl. Abt. 3,* vol. 80. Gerold, Vienna 1880, pp. 18–72; Paul D. SHERMAN, *Colour Vision in the Nineteenth Century: The Young-Helmholtz-Maxwell Theory.* Institute of Physics Publishing 1981.

296 Carl Ewald Hering (1834–1918). Studied at Leipzig Univ. (Dr med. 1858). 1862 Post-doc in Physiol. at Leipzig Univ. under the sensual physiolog. Ernst Heinrich Weber (1795–1878). 1865 Prof. in Physiol. as the successor of Carl Ludwig (1816–1895) at the med.-surg. Josephs-Akademie (Josephinum) in Vienna. 1870–1895 Successor of Purkinyě at Prague Univ. 1895 Prof. of Physiol. at Leipzig as the successor of

Carl Ludwig (1816–1895). Main areas of interest: physiol. optics, "opponent colour theory". 1868 with Josef Breuer (1842–1925) discovery of the mechanism for the self-regulation of breathing by the nervus vagus. Cf. EULNER (as in FN 13); GARRISON/MORTON (as in FN 124); LESKY, *Wien. Med. Schule* (as in FN 12), pp. 530ff.; WYKLICKY, *Josephinum* (as in FN 165), p. 118; Karl SABLIK, "Hering, Vintschgau und das Problem der Nachfolge Purkinjes", in: *Sudhoffs Archiv* 73 (1989), pp. 78–87.

297 Cf. UA Wien, Med. Dekanat, No 73 from 1878/79, travel report by Ernst Fuchs from October 1878.

298 The reference is to the Paris World Exhibition from 1 May–31 October 1878 on the Champ du Mars. Cf. W. H. UHLAND, *Illustrirter Katalog der Pariser Weltausstellung von 1878*. Brockhaus, Leipzig 1880.

299 Sir William Bowman (1816–1892). Trained at Birmingham General Hospital and at King's College, London. Study trips to Leiden, Amsterdam, Bonn, Heidelberg, Munich, Vienna and Berlin. Then Chair of Physiol., gen. and pathol. anatomy at King's College. From 1843 at the Royal Ophthalmic Hospital Moorfields. Initial description of the anterior elastic lamina of the cornea (Lamina limitans anterior), which still bears his name today. Examination and description of the ciliary muscle almost at the same time as Ernst Wilhelm v. Brücke. For the probing of the lacrimal pathways construction of the probes mentioned by Fuchs. Cf. ALBERT/EDWARDS, pp. 82–87 and Index; ALBERT/HENKIND (as in FN 38), pp. 300–316; Daniel M. ALBERT, Edward W. D. NORTON, Reva HURTES, *Source Book of Ophthalmology*. Blackwell Science 1995, pp. 44–45; GARRISON/MORTON (as in FN 124); GORIN (as in FN 38), pp. 142–144; HIRSCH, *Geschichte der Augenheilkunde*, p. 367; HIRSCHBERG, *Geschichte der Augenheilkunde* (as in FN 18), vol. 14/4 [= Reprint vol. IV], § 647–649, pp. 197–225 and Index; IBBO (as in FN 18); PAGEL (as in FN 13).

300 A. Marchand (1841–1899). Initially apprenticed to a shop keeper, then pharmacist. Studied medicine in Tours. From 1866 in Paris. From 1872 active in var. surg. positions at several hospitals. Cf. PAGEL (as in FN 13).

301 Louis Émile Javal (1839–1907). Originally from Paris, initially trained as a mining engineer. Deeply impressed by a consultation of Albrecht v. Graefe, he decided to study medicine and to specialise in ophthalmology. 1878 Dir. of the ophthalmol. laboratory at the École des Hautes Études in Paris, 1885 Received into the Académie de Médecine. Charismatic teacher and researcher, especially in the field of physiol. optics (Main works: *Mémoires d'Ophtalmometrie* 1886, *Manuel du Strabisme* 1896). Prior to this, excellent translation of Helmholtz's *Physiologische Optik*. Inventive instrument builder (e.g. ophthalmometer). Owing to chron. glaucoma bilateral age-related blindness. Coped with this blow by, among other things, writing a popular guidebook: Émile JAVAL, *Entre Aveugles. Conseils à l'usage des personnes, qui viennent de perdre la vue*. Masson et Cie., Paris 1903. Cf. HIRSCH (as in FN 13); HIRSCHBERG, *Geschichte der Augenheilkunde* (as in FN 18), vol. 15/2 [= Reprint vol. VI], § 1280–1282, pp. 535–547; ÖBL (as in FN 18); PAGEL (as in FN 13).

302 Jules Badal (1840–1929). Studied medicine at the École impériale du Service de santé militaire (Graduation 1864). Specialisation in ophthalmol. under Maurice Perrin (cf. FN 259) and Marc Antoine Louis Félix Giraud-Teulon (1816–1887). 1875 Invention of a perimeter. 1876 Invention of an optometer, whose use, along with gen. ophthalmol. and cataract operation, he taught at the École pratique de Faculté de médicine in Paris.

1878 tit. Prof. of Theoret. Ophthalmolog. at Bordeaux Univ.; 1882–1910 tit. Prof. and Dir. of the newly established eye clinic at this Univ. Main area of interest: physiol. optics. Cf. HIRSCHBERG, *Geschichte der Augenheilkunde* (as in FN 18), vol. 14/4 [= Reprint vol. IV], § 622; IBBO (as in FN 18).

303 Josef Brettauer (1835–1905). Originally from Ancona, studied at the Univ. of Prague and Vienna (Dr med. 1859). Ophthalmol. specialisation under Arlt in Vienna. Further special. in Berlin, Utrecht and Paris. Eye specialist in Trieste (1871–1904 Head physician at the municip. hospital. On behalf of Carl Koller (at the time junior doctor at Vienna's Allgem. Krankenhaus, Cf. FN 591) announcement of Koller's discovery of local anaesthesia of the eye by instilling a watery solution of cocaine at the Dt. Ophthalmologenkongress in Heidelberg 1884. Major collection of paintings and engravings with a bearing on the med. profession and of med. coins and medals (c. 7,000 items); bequest to Vienna Univ. (since 1931 in the Bundessammlung für Medaillen, Münzen und Geldzeichen at Vienna's Kunsthist. Museum). Cf. CZEIKE (as in FN 13); ÖBL (as in FN 11); Eduard HOLZMAIR, *Medicina in nummis. Katalog der Sammlung Dr Josef Brettauer*. Vienna 1937. Unchanged reprint Vienna 1989 [= Veröffentl. d. Numismat. Komm. d. ÖAW 22].

304 Julius Hirschberg (1843–1925). Originally from Potsdam. Studied at Berlin Univ. (Dr med. 1866). Ophthalmol. special. in Berlin under Graefe. 1870 Private lecturer in surg. and ophthalmolog. (1879 Assoc. Prof.). Studied further maths and physics, collaborator in the lab of Hermann von Helmholtz (cf. FN 125). Extensive study trips and visits to eye clinics in Prague, Vienna, Heidelberg, Düsseldorf, Paris, Marseille, London, Dublin, Glasgow, Edinburgh, Barcelona, Madrid, Sevilla, Rome, Naples, Palermo, Athens, Stockholm, St. Petersburg, Moscow, Alexandria, Cairo, Mumbai, Kolkata, Tokyo, Kyoto, San Francisco, and New York. Founder of the *Centralblatt für praktische Augenheilkunde* (1877). Author of *Geschichte der Augenheilkunde* (1899–1918, last part of the 2nd ed. of the *Handbuch der gesamten Augenheilkunde* initiated by Graefe and Theodor Saemisch (1833–1900), an indispensable work of reference even today. After World War I he sold his private library to his student Jujiro Komoto (1859–1938, cf. FN 1565), who also studied under Fuchs (now the Komoto Library at Tokyo's Univ. Lib.) Cf. ALBERT/NORTON/HURTES (as in FN 299), pp. 157–158.; GORIN (as in FN 38), pp. 149–151 and Ind.; HIRSCH (as in FN 13); HIRSCHBERG, *Geschichte der Augenheilkunde* (as in FN 18), vol. 15/2 [= Reprint, vol. VI], § 1109, pp. 60–68; IBBO (as in FN 18); PAGEL (as in FN 13); *Katalog der Büchersammlung von J. Hirschberg*. Berlin 1901.– At the 84th Versammlung d. Dt. Ophthalmol. Gesellsch. in Aachen in 1986, foundation in his honour of the Julius-Hirschberg-Gesellschaft, a German-speaking association for research on the history of ophthalmology at the Institut f. Geschichte d. Medizin d. Univ. Wien, where it was headquartered at the time. Now headquartered at the Sammlungen d. Univ. Wien; address unchanged: 1090 Vienna, Währingerstraße 25. Cf. www.jhg-online.org [last accessed: 9 Aug. 2022].

305 Marc Dufour (1843–1910). Studied at Zurich Univ. (Dr med. 1865). Ophthalmol. specialist training at Zurich Univ. (Horner), Paris (Liebreich) (Paris) and Berlin (v. Graefe). While studying under Graefe, call in 1869 to head the Asile des Aveugles in Lausanne. 1870 Prof. at Lausanne Univ.; member of the jury that awarded Fuchs the first prize in 1884 for his monograph *Die Ursachen und die Verhütung der Blindheit*

(cf. Ch. 3). Cf. HIRSCHBERG, *Geschichte der Augenheilkunde* (as in FN 18), vol. 14/7 [= Reprint vol. V], § 782, pp. 34–37; IBBO (as in FN 18).

306 Hermann Ludwig Cohn (1838–1906). Studied chemistry and physics at the Univ. of Heidelberg and Breslau (Dr phil 1860), studied medicine at the Univ. of Breslau, Heidelberg and Berlin (Dr med. 1863). Ophthalmol. specialist training under Richard Förster (cf. FN 263) in Breslau and under v. Graefe (Berlin), de Wecker (Paris) and v. Arlt (Vienna). 1868 Habilitation at Breslau Univ. (1874 Assoc. Prof.). Area of special interest: eye hygiene. Operated a priv. eye clinic, providing free treatment to indigent patients. Member of the jury that awarded Fuchs in 1884 the first prize in the competition organ. by the Society for the Prevention of Blindness (see Ch. 3). Cf. HIRSCH (as in FN 13); HIRSCHBERG, *Geschichte der Augenheilkunde* (as in FN 18), vol. 15/2 [= Reprint, vol. VI], § 1142, pp. 170–174; IBBO (as in FN 18); PAGEL (as in FN 13).

307 Francesco Businelli (1828–1908). Studied medicine at Padova Univ. (Graduation 1853). Trainee surgeon at the 2nd Surg. Univ. Clinic in Vienna under Franz Schuh (1804–1865) and private assist. at the Eye Dept. under Eduard Jaeger v. Jaxtthal; 1857–1859 Assist. at Arlt's clinic; 1861 Prof. in Sassari/Sardinia, 1862–1872 Prof. at Modena Univ.; 1873–1899 Full Prof. and Dir. of the Eye Clinic of Rome Univ. Cf. HIRSCH (as in FN 13); HIRSCHBERG, *Geschichte der Augenheilkunde* (as in FN 18), vol. 14/5 [= Reprint vol. IV], § 734, pp. 82–84; IBBO (as in FN 18); PAGEL (as in FN 13).

308 Sammlungen d. Med. Univ. Wien; Handschriftenarchiv No. 2107/1. Initial publication: Erna LESKY, "Aus dem Nachlaß Ferdinand von Arlts im Wiener medizinhistorischen Institut", in: *Klin. Monatsbl. Augenheilk.* 139 (1961), pp. 847–856 (here: pp. 852–853)

309 Named after industrialist Louis Freiherr Haber v. Linsberg (1804–1892). Cf. ÖBL (as in FN 11).

310 Johann Theodor Wiethe (1851–1894) was Ernst Fuchs's junior by one day.

311 The reference is to Eduard Jaeger von Jaxtthal.

312 Johann Nepomuk Oeller (1850–1932). Studied at Munich Univ. (Dr med. 1877). 1879 Habilitation in Ophthalmolog., until 1900 assist. under August v. Rothmund (1830–1906). 1900–1920 Full Prof. and Dir. of the Univ. Eye Clinic at Erlangen Univ.; impassioned draughtsman and talented painter. Monumental main work: *Atlas der Ophthalmoskopie* (J. F. Bergmann, Wiesbaden 1896–1899), published simultaneously in German and Engl., transl. by Herman(n) Knapp (1832–1911, cf. FN 1352) in New York, and OELLER., *Atlas seltener ophthalmoskopischer Befunde. Zugleich Ergänzungstafeln zu dem Atlas der Ophthalmoskopie. Atlas of Rare Ophthalmoscopic Conditions and Supplementary Plates to the Atlas of Ophthalmoscopy. The Text translated into English by Thos. Snowball.* [Thomas Snowball (1873–1940)]. J. F. Bergmann, Wiesbaden 1900/12. Cf. EULNER (as in FN 13); HIRSCH (as in FN 13); HIRSCHBERG, *Geschichte der Augenheilkunde* (as in FN 18), vol. 15/1 [= Reprint vol. VI], § 1029, p. 124; IBBO (as in FN 18); PAGEL (as in FN 13).

313 Surgical division of a tendon to correct strabismus.

314 Ludwig/Louis (de) Wecker. Cf. FN 252. 1870 Given an Austrian hereditary knighthood. Publication of his monograph on pathologies of the ocular fundus in combination with the French translation of Eduard Jaeger v. Jaxtthal's *Ophthalmologischer Handatlas* (First public. in German in 1869) with a dedication to Eduard Jaeger's father, Friedrich

Jaeger v. Jaxtthal: L. de WECKER, E. de JAEGER, *Traité des maladies du fond de l'œil et atlas d'ophtalmoscopie.* Adrien Delahaye/Imprim. Impériale et Royale, Paris/Vienne 1870. Cf. ÖSTA/AVA Wien, Ministerium d. Inneren, Faszikel 43 Ritterstand, No. 245 from 1870: Wecker Ludwig, Medicinae Dr in Paris, um Erhebung i. d. Ritterstand auf Grundlage d. Ordens d. eisernen Krone 3ter Klasse; Gabriela SCHMIDT-WYKLICKY, "Die Beziehungen des Graefe-Schülers Louis de Wecker (1832–1906) zur Wiener Ophthalmologischen Schule und zur österreichisch-ungarischen Monarchie", in: *Mitteil. d. Julius-Hirschberg-Gesellschaft zur Geschichte d. Ophthalmologie* vol. 14/2012 (2016), pp. 219–235.

315 A reference to Edouard Meyer (cf. FN 254).

316 Arthur Sichel, cf. FN 256 and HIRSCHBERG, *Geschichte der Augenheilkunde* (as in FN 18), vol. 14/3 [= Reprint vol. III], § 595, p. 232.

317 Julius Sichel, ibid.

318 Alphonse Desmarres (1840–1913) was supposed to undergo training in Berlin, but never attended Graefe's clinic. Cf. HIRSCHBERG, *Geschichte der Augenheilkunde* (as in FN 18) vol. 14/3 [= Reprint vol. III], § 594, p. 232.

319 Louis Auguste Desmarres (1810–1882). Studied medicine at Paris Univ.; private training in ophthalmol. under Sichel the elder, who made him his private secretary. 1841 Establishment of a private ophthalmol. hospital that attracted many students, including Albrecht v. Graefe. Highly skilled surgeon, developed a great number of new techniques and instruments, e.g. an eyelid retractor, a strongly curved eyelid clamp with a long handle still in use today. Cf. ALBERT/NORTON/HURTES (as in FN 299), p. 82; GORIN (as in FN 38), pp. 84–85.; HIRSCH (as in FN 13); HIRSCHBERG, *Geschichte der Augenheilkunde* (as in FN 18) vol. 14/3 [= Reprint vol. III], § 591–594, pp. 205–232; IBBO (as in FN 18).

320 Edward Treacher Collins (1862–1937). Studied at Middlesex Hospital Univ. College London. House surgeon at Moorfields Eye Hospital; pathol. and curator of the hospital's museum. Special field: histopathol. of the eye. Lecturer and Dir. of the Eye Department of Charing Cross Hospital, London. Lectured also at the Royal College of Surgeons. Meritorious organiser of worldwide ophthalmol. conferences for the Internat. Fed. of Ophthalmol. Soc., in whose foundation he had been involved. Close friend of Ernst Fuchs. Cf. ALBERT/NORTON/HURTES (as in FN 299), pp. 65–66; FISCHER (as in FN 28); GORIN (as in FN 38), p. 174 and 178; IBBO (as in FN 18).

321 Edward TREACHER COLLINS, *In the Kingdom of the Shah.* T. F. Unwin, London 1896. Cf. J. G. RAVIN, "In the Kingdom of the Shah: Treacher Collins' Persian adventure", in: *Surv. Ophthalmol.* 43 (1999), pp. 361–367.

322 Reference to the Danish ophthalmol. Marius Hans Erik Tscherning (1854–1939). 1910–1925 Prof. and Dir. of the Eye Department of the Rigshospitalet in Copenhagen. Cf. M. NORN, O. A. JENSEN, "Marius Tscherning (1854–1939): his life and work in optical physiology", in: *Acta Ophthalmologica Scandinavica [= Acta Ophthalmol. Scand.*] 82 (2004), pp. 501–508.

323 Pierre Eugène Godard (1827–1890) and his brother Louis. 1846/47 Pioneers in the construction of hot-air balloons.

324 Captive balloon.

325 Eduard/Edouard Meyer (cf. FN 254).

326 Reference to the Mont Valérien. A 162 metre high hill in the Île de France 12 km from

Paris, since 1840 site of a fortress. During France's occupation by the Nazis execution site for resistance fighters. Today, US soldiers' cemetery and the site of the Mémorial de la France Combattante as the key French national site of remembrance (inauguration 1960). Cf. *Le Mont Valérien – Haut lieu de la mémoire nationale.* www.mont-valerien.fr/ (last accessed: 6 Sept. 2022).

327 Reference to William Arthur Brailey (1845–1915). Studied at Cambridge and at Guy's Hospital in London (M.D. 1874). 1880 Cofounder of the Ophthalmol. Soc. of the United Kingdom. 1882 Resident surgeon at Guy's Hospital. 1885/86 Hunterian Prof. at the Royal College of Surgeons. Cf. FISCHER (as in FN 28); IBBO (as in FN 18); Obituary: "William Arthur Brailey, M. A., M. D. Cantab., Consulting Ophthalmic Surgeon, Guy's Hospital", in: *Brit. Med. J.* 1 (1915), p. 701.

328 Robert Marcus Gunn (1850–1909). Originally from Scotland, with a Scandinavian family background. Studied medicine at Edinburgh Univ.; December 1874–June 1875 study visit to the two Viennese Univ. Eye Clinics and to Eduard Jaeger v. Jaxtthal's Eye Dept. at the Allgem. Krankenhaus. Preferred Jaeger as teacher over Arlt and Stellwag. Impressed by the systemat. tuition in the form of spec. courses in ophthalmol., Gunn practised this didactic method from 1876 as a surgeon at Royal London Ophthalmic Hospital Moorfields. Eye surgeon at the National Hospital for the Paralysed and Epileptic, at the Hospital for Sick Children and at University College Hospital. 1896–1899 Vice Pres., 1907–1909 Pres. of the Ophthalmol. Soc. of the United Kingdom. Research on the anat., physiol. and pathol. changes of the nervus opticus, the retina and the cornea. He has given his name, among other things, to the crossing sign in arteriolar sclerosis. Cf. GORIN (as in FN 38), pp. 172–173; HIRSCHBERG, Geschichte der Augenheilkunde (as in FN 18), vol. 14/5 [= Reprint vol. IV], § 653, pp. 245–246; IBBO (as in FN 18); Obituaries: The Lancet, Dec. 11, 1909, pp. 1786–87; Brit. Med. J. 2 (1909), pp.1719–21; Am. J. Ophthalmol. 27 (1910), p. 49. Appreciation: Gill ROPER-HALL, "Historical Vignette: Robert Marcus Gunn (1850–1909): Scottish Ophthalmologist, Skilled Observer, and Gifted Teacher", in: American Orthoptic Journal [Am. Orthoptic J.] 65/1 (2015), pp. 121–127.

329 Henry HUN, *A Guide to American Medical Students in Europe*. William Wood & Comp., New York 1883.

330 Reference to Sir Jonathan Hutchinson (cf. FN 275). Correct version of the name in Ernst Fuchs's original typescript. The typo seems to have occurred in Adalbert Fuchs's editing of the memoir of his father. Cf. Family archive and FUCHS, *Augenarzt* (as in FN 2), p. 65.

331 Jonathan HUTCHINSON, *Clinical Memoir on Certain Diseases of the Eye and the Ear Consequent on Inherited Syphilis.* John Churchill, London 1863. Cf. his earlier monograph: HUTCHINSON, "*On the different forms of inflammation of the eye consequent to inherited syphilis", in: Ophthalmic Hospital Reports*, London 1 (1858), pp. 191–203 and pp. 226–244; ibid. 2 (1859), pp. 54–105; ibid. 3 (1860), pp. 258–283 and the later description of his findings: HUTCHINSON, *"New facts and opinions as to inherited syphilis", in: London Hospital Reports* II (1865), pp. 145–204.

332 Cf. *Wissenschaftlicher Katalog der Bibliothek der zweiten Augenklinik.* Abteilung 1: *Allg. ophthalm. Literatur – Lehrbücher, Atlanten.* Bound manuscript. Private collection.

333 FUCHS, *Augenarzt* (as in FN 2), pp. 62–66.

334 Lawrence Webster Fox (1853–1931). Originally from Pennsylvania. Studied at

Jefferson Med. College in Philadelphia (M. D. 1878). Ophthalmolog. specialist training in Berlin, Vienna and London. 1882–1885 ophthalmol. assist. at his alma mater. 1883–1893 Eye surgeon at Germantown Hospital. 1893 Prof. at the Medico-Chirurgical College in Philadelphia, 1922 Prof. at the Graduate School of Medicine of Pennsylvania Univ. – In his later years, his work took him to the western United States to treat the Blackfeet Indians. In recognition of his role in eliminating trachoma, an eye disease prevalent among native Americans, he was adopted into the Blackfeet tribe. Cf. FISCHER (as in FN 28); IBBO (as in FN 18); Daniel M. ALBERT, Harold G. SCHEIE, *A History of Ophthalmology at the University of Pennsylvania*. Charles C. Thomas, Springfield 1965, p. 345.

335 Cf. FN 200.

336 Reference to David H. Coover. 1911–1917 Prof. of Ophthalmolog. of the Univ. of Colorado Med. School in Denver. Cf. "Directory, Officers and Graduates, 1877–1921", in: *Univ. of Colorado Bulletin* 21 (1921), p. 20.

337 Lawrence Webster FOX, "Obituary Ernst Fuchs", in: *Am. J. Ophthalmol.* 14/3 (1931), pp. 166–167.

338 Reference to Ernst Fuchs's trip to America in 1921/22. One of the people Fuchs refers to here was the initiator of the *Amerikanerkurse*, Lawrence Webster Fox (cf. FN 334 and Ch. 11).

339 Ernst FUCHS, "Wien, das Mekka der amerikanischen Ärzte", in: *Österreich 2* (1928), p. 109 and FUCHS, *Augenarzt* (as in FN 2), pp. 331–341 (here pp. 337–338.).

340 John Sterling Ryerson (1855–1925). Originally from Toronto. Studied at Trinity Med. School, Toronto (M. D. 1876). Postgrad. ophthalmol. specialisation: study trip to Europe – Edinburgh, London, Paris, Vienna and Heidelberg. 1880 Establishment of a private practice in Toronto. Full Prof. of Eye, Ear and Throat Diseases at Trinity Med. School and Eye surgeon at the Andrew Mercer Ear and Eye Infirmary of Toronto Gen. Hosp.; 1895 Founder of the St. John Ambulance Assoc. in Ontario and in 1896 of the Canad. Red Cross. Main areas of interest: colour vision; colour vision testing; the application of radium in ophthalmol.; introduction of the local anaesthesia of the eye with cocaine in Toronto. Cf. Website of the Dept. of Ophthalmol. and Vision Sciences of the Univ. of Toronto: John Sterling Ryerson (1855–1925), accessible online: https://www.utovs.com/history/early–history/ryerson_ansel_sterlin_15E.html (last accessed: 6 Sept. 2022).

341 William Charnley (1845–1911). Studied at Univ. College London (M.D. 1875). Postgrad. ophthalmol. specialis. in Paris and Vienna (Ernst Fuchs). 1878 Member of the Royal College of Surgeons in London. Surgeon at the London Ophthal. Hospital and at other hospitals. Cf. *The Eagle: A Magazine Supported by Members of St. John's College*, vol. 22 (1901), p. 256.

342 Samuel Thomas Knaggs (1842–1921). Originally from Ireland. 1848 Emigrated with his family to Australia, settled in Sydney. Studied at the Univ. of Dublin and Aberdeen (M. D. 1873). Study trip to Paris and Vienna; initially general practitioner in Newcastle/New South Wales, then specialis. as surgeon in Europe (and as eye surgeon in Vienna under Fuchs). 1883–1893 Prof. of Clin. Surg. at Sydney Univ.; active in the area of public health. Cf. Obituary, in: *Med. J. of Australia*, 16 Apr. 1921, pp. 320–321; Entry in the National Library of Australia, accessible online: https://www.nla.gov.au/nla.party–577734 (last 22 Aug. 2018) and in the *Australian Dictionary*

of Biography, accessible online: https://www.adb.anandedandau/biography/knaggs-samuel-thomas-3965 (last accessed: 9 July 2020).

343 R. Johnston Palmer. Originally from Detroit. Later surgeon in Toronto. Cf. Clarence Monroe BURTON, *The City of Detroit*. vol. 5. S. J. Clarke Publ. Comp. 1922, p. 766.

344 Cf. FN 337.

345 Cf. Franz LACKNER, *Hunderte amerikanische Jungärzte jährlich zur Fortbildung in Wien. Zur Geschichte der Wiener "American Medical Association/Society"*. Internetpubl. accessible via the Gesellschaft d. Ärzte in Wien: info@billrothhaus.at (last accessed: 9 July 2020).

346 Cf. FN 45

347 Cf. FN 46.

348 Cf. *100 Jahre Wiener Medizinische Akademie. Universimed, Vienna 1996*, p. 31. – A folder from ca. 1910 with the registration forms of the course participants and their different specialities has been preserved, alongside a volume of photographs of Fuchs and, later on, his assistants surrounded by a great number of students.

349 Adolph Barkan (1845–1935). Originally from Hungary (Bárkány Adolf). Studied at Vienna Univ. (Dr med. 1866). Ophthalmol. specialist training in Vienna (Univ. Eye Clinic unter Arlt) and other ophthalmol. hotspots in Europe. 1868 Emigration to the USA, where after a year in Baltimore he established himself in San Francisco. 1872–1883 Prof. of Ophthalmol. and Otol. at the Med. College of the Pacific. 1884–1891 in the same function at Cooper Med. College. 1892–1908 Prof. of Ophthalmol., Laryngol. and Otol. Ibid. 1895–1912 Eye and Ear Surgeon at Lane Hospital. 1909–1911 Professor of Structure and Disease of Eye, Ear, and Larynx at Stanford University, School of Medicine. Prof. emer. 1912–1935. Member of the Stanford College of Directors. Signif. contribution to the creation of a substantive med. and medico-hist. library at Stanford Univ. (Lane Med. Library). Cf. Obituaries: *J. Am. Med. Assoc.* 105 (1935), p. 1538; *Calif. West. Med.* 43 (1935), p. 307; *Am. J. Ophthalmol.* 18 (1935), p. 1156 (Lawrence T. Post); Am. J. Ophthalmol. 19/3 (1936), pp. 260–262 (Edward Jackson); *Brit. Med. J.* 20 (1936), pp. 188–189; Appreciation: J. Fraser MUIRHEAD, *Adolph Barkan (1845–1935), European Ophthalmologist in San Francisco*, in: *JAMA Ophthalmol.* 132/3 (2014), pp. 346–349.

350 Joseph Nelson (1840–1910). 1858 Queen's Univ. in Belfast (M. D. 1863). 1860 Interrupted his studies to take part in the rebellion of the unification movement led by Giuseppe Garibaldi (1807–1882) in southern Italy. After his graduation emigration to India, where he remained for 14 years as a surgeon at a tea plantation. 1877 Return to Ireland, ophthalmol. specialisation in Dublin. Learnt German. 1878 One-year study visit to the Univ. Eye Clinic as assistant under Arlt and Fuchs. 1880 Head Surgeon at the newly created Eye, Ear and Throat Department of the Royal (Victoria) Hospital and the Hospital for Sick Children in Belfast. Pres. of the Ulster Med. Soc. 1898/99. Cf. Obituary, in: *Brit. Med. J.* 2 (1910), pp. 823–824; Appreciation: *Dictionary of Ulster Biography*, accessible online: www.newulsterbiography.co.uk (entry: NELSON, Garibaldi (last accessed: 6 Sept. 2022).

351 FUCHS, *Augenarzt* (as in FN 2), p. 59.

352 Carl Theodor Herzog in Bayern (1839–1909). Son of Maximilian Joseph Herzog in Bayern (1808–1888) and Ludovika Wilhelmine Herzogin v. Bayern (1808–1892), a daughter of the Bavarian King Maximilian I. Joseph (1756–1825). Studied at the

Ludwig-Maximilians-Univ. München first philosophy, law and economics, then medicine (Dr med. 1880). Ophthalmol. specialis. under Jaeger and Arlt in Vienna and under Horner in Zürich. Practised as an eye specialist for a decade and a half in Munich, Tegernsee and Merano, before setting up his own private eye clinic (1895). Cf. Oskar EVERSBUSCH, "Zum 70. Geburtstag von Dr. med. Carl, Herzog in Bayern", in: *Münchner medizinische Wochenschrift* [Münch. med. Wochenschr.] 56 (1909), pp. 1648–49; Richard SEXAU, *Fürst und Arzt. Dr med. Herzog Carl Theodor in Bayern. Schicksal zwischen Wittelsbach und Habsburg*. Styria, Graz/Vienna/Cologne 1963, pp. 271ff.; Uwe CLASEN, "Carl Theodor, Herzog in Bayern und Augenarzt (1839–1909)", in: Julius Hirschberg Gesellschaft (Deutschsprachige Vereinigung für Geschichte der Augenheilkunde) – Société francophone d'histoire de l'ophtalmologie: *33 Beiträge zur Geschichte der Augenheilkunde – Contributions à l'Histoire de l'Ophtalmologie*. Facultas, Vienna 1991, pp. 211–220.

353 FUCHS, *Augenarzt* (as in FN 2), pp. 59–60.

354 Letter from Herzog Carl Theodor to Eduard Jaeger v. Jaxtthal dated 8 Dec. 1882. Cf. Helmut WYKLICKY, *Zur Geschichte der Augenheilkunde. Ophthalmology in Vienna. 100 Jahre II. Universitäts-Augenklinik in Wien.* Christian Brandstätter, Vienna 1984, p. 51.

355 Adalbert Franz Seligmann (1862–1945). Studied at the Academy of Fine Arts (Vienna 1880–1884, Munich 1884–1887). History painter, art critic and essayist. 1897 Prof. at the Academy in Vienna, 1926–1932 at the Wr. Kunstschule f. Frauen und Mädchen (later Frauenakad.) he had founded himself, 1911 Lecturer in Fashion History and Art History at the Akad. f. Musik und darstellende Kunst in Vienna. Cf. ÖBL (as in FN 11).

356 Franz Romeo Seligmann (1808–1892). Originally from what was then Austrian Nikolsburg/Moravia (today Mikulov/Czech Republic). Studied medicine and orient. languages (notably Persian) at Vienna Univ. (Dr med. 1830). Junior doctor at Vienna's Allgem. Krankenhaus; cholera specialist and epidemiologist. Belonged to the circle around the Austrian national poet Franz Grillparzer (1791–1872) and Ottilie v. Goethe. 1869 Full Prof. at the newly founded department of History of Medicine at Vienna Univ. Cf. GERABEK et al. (as in FN 13); ÖBL (as in FN 11); WURZBACH (as in FN 15).

357 Adalbert SELIGMANN, "Der Billroth'sche Hörsaal im Allgemeinen Krankenhause in Wien", in: *Wiener med. Wochenschr.* 77 (1927), p. 368. Cf. Robert BUCHBERGER, "Der Billrothsche Hörsaal im Wiener Allgemeinen Krankenhaus. Gemälde von Adalbert F. Seligmann", in: *Wiener klin. Wochenschr.* 78 (1966), pp. 853–856; Helmut WYKLICKY, "Theodor Billroth (1829–1894)", in: *Kunst des Heilens. Aus der Geschichte der Medizin und Pharmazie*. Katalog d. Niederösterr. Landesausstellung in d. Kartause Gaming v. 4. Mai bis 27. Oktober 1991. Katalog d. Niederösterr. Landesmuseums. N.F. 276. – Vienna: Amt d. Niederösterr. Landesregierung, Kulturabteilung 1991, Objekt-Nr. 17.04, p. 651 (caption).

358 Max OPPEL (ed.), *Festschrift zum 100-jährigen Bestehen der Augenklinik Herzog Carl Theodor in München 1995*. Selbstverlag, Munich 1995; Gregor WOLLENSAK, Holger VOGTEN, "Herzog Carl Theodor in Bayern – ein adliger Ophthalmologe", in: Frank KROGMANN (ed.), *Mitteilungen der Julius-Hirschberg-Gesellschaft zur Geschichte der Augenheilkunde*, vol. 7 – 2005. Königshausen & Neumann, Würzburg

2010, pp. 217–237.

359 FUCHS, *Augenarzt* (as in FN 2), p. 67.

360 UA Wien, Med. Dekanat No. 199 from 1879/80 and No. 300 from 1879/80: "*Herr Hofrath Professor von Arlt beantragt die Verlängerung der Dienstzeit für den Assistenten Herrn Dr Ernst Fuchs auf ein fünftes und sechstes Jahr.*" [Herr Hofrath Professor von Arlt requests the prolongation of the employment of assistant Herr Dr Ernst Fuchs for a fifth and sixth year].

361 UA Wien. Med. Dekanat. from 1879/80 and ÖSTA/AVA Wien. K. K. Ministerium für Cultus und Unterricht 4 Med. Fuchs Ernst No. 17. 336, dated 25 Oct. 1880, and 4 Medicin /: Docenten:/ Fuchs No. 18708, dated 20 Nov. 1880.

362 Ibid.

363 UA Wien, Med. Dekanat No. 109 from 1880/81 and ÖSTA/AVA Wien 4 Medicin Docenten Fuchs, K. K. Ministerium für Cultus und Unterricht No. 17.336 from 1880.

364 Eduard Ritter von Hofmann (1837–1897). Studied at Prague (Dr med. 1861). Assist. at the Department of Staatsarzneikunde (i. e. Forensic Pathology, lectures in Czech). 1865 Habilitation in *Staatsarzneikunde* at Prague Univ.; 1869–1875 Full Prof. of *Staatsarzneikunde* at Innsbruck Univ.; 1875–1897 Full Prof. of Forensic Pathology at Vienna Univ.; in keeping with the maxims of the Second Vienna Medical School, he grounded forensic pathology on histol. examinations and experim. works on a scientific basis. Creation of a comprehensive Museum of Forensic Pathology. 1878 Publication of his seminal textbook, supplemented later by an instructive atlas. Cf. CZEIKE; EISENBERG 2; EULNER; HIRSCH (as in FN 13); NDB (as in FN 15); ÖBL (as in FN 11); PAGEL (as in FN 13); LESKY, *Wien. Med. Schule* (as in FN 12), pp. 606–611. Obituaries: *Wiener klin. Wochenschr.* 10 (1897), pp. 797ff.; *Prag. med. Wochenschr.* 22 (1897), pp. 453ff.; *Wiener med. Bl.* 20 (1897), p. 584.

365 ÖSTA/AVA Wien, as in FN 361, No. 285.

366 ÖSTA/AVA Wien, 4 Medicin /: Docenten:/ Fuchs No. 18708, dated 20 November 1880.

367 Cf. FN 365.

368 *Daily Journal of the British Medical Association: Forty-Eighth Annual Meeting*, Cambridge 1880. Friday August 13th, Section H. – Ophthalmology, p. 13. Ernst Fuchs's personal programme with his own annotations and markings. Private collection.

369 "Forty-Eighth Annual Meeting of the British Medical Association", in: *Brit. Med. J.* II (1880), p. 780ff. See Ch. 10.

370 ÖSTA /AVA (as in FN 361).

371 Ernst FUCHS, *Das Sarcom des Uvealtractus*. Wilhelm Braumüller, Vienna 1882.

372 See Ch. 7.

373 Cf. MÜLLER, McGHEE (as in FN 218).

374 Leopold Königstein (1850–1924). Originally from Moravia. Like Fuchs, his junior by one year, engaged on experiment. work in Brücke's lab.; student of Arlt and Eduard Jaeger. 1881 Habilitation in Ophthalmology at Vienna Univ.; 1900 tit. Assoc. Prof., assistant at the Eye Department Vienna's Allgem. Poliklinik under Jakob Hock. Cf. EISENBERG 2 (as in FN 13); FISCHER (as in FN 28); HIRSCHBERG, *Geschichte der* Augenheilkunde (as in FN 18); IBBO (as in FN 18); ÖBL (as in FN 11); Obituary, in:

Die feierliche Inauguration des Rektors der Universität Wien für das Studienjahr1924/25. Vienna Univ. 1924, pp. 22–23. (Moriz Sachs). For the question of priority reg. Königstein vs. Koller and the discovery of cocaine as the first anaesthetic for the eye: cf. LESKY, *Wien. Med. Schule* (as in FN 12), p. 489 and FN 586.

375 Leopold KÖNIGSTEIN, "Das Sarkom des Uvealtraktus. Von Dr Ernst Fuchs, Professor der Ophthalmologie in Lüttich", in: *Wiener med. Presse* 22 (1881), cols. 1612–14.

376 FUCHS, *Sarcom des Uvealtractus* (as in FN 371), p. 200.

377 Stephen PAGET ((1855–1926). Born in London the son of eminent surgeon and pathologist Sir James Paget (1814–1899, cf. below). Studied at St. Bartholmew's College. Fellow of the Royal College of Surgeons (F.R.C.S.). Having originally contemplated a career as a surgeon, he was forced to give up the idea for health reasons and concentrated on experimental basic research. Cf. Obituaries: *Nature* 117 (1926), p. 831; Appreciation: George POSTE, Linda PARUCH, "Stephen Paget, M.D., F.R.C.S. (1855–1926). A retrospective", in: *Cancer and Metastasis Reviews* 8 (1989), pp. 1–97.

378 Sir James Paget (1814–1899). After five years of surgical training from 1834 a two-year residence at St. Bartholomew Hospital in London and surg. qualification. Then museum curator and demonstrator of pathol. anat. at this hospital. 1843 Lecturer in physiol. 1847–1871 Surgeon at St. Bartholomew's, successful teaching activities. 1876 Initial descript. of osteitis deformans. Cf. Shirley ROBERTS, *Sir James Paget – the Rise of Clinical Surgery.* Royal Society of Medicine Services Ltd., London 1989.

379 Stephen PAGET, "The Distribution of Secondary Growths in Cancer of the Breast", in: *The Lancet* 67/1 (1889), pp. 571–573. Cf. Domenico RIBATTI, G. MANGIALARDI, A. VACCA, "Stephen Paget and the 'Seed and soil' theory of metastatic dissemination", in: *Clin. Exp. Med.* 6 (2006), pp 145–149; Adriano PIRIS, Manfred MIHM, "Mechanisms of Metastasis: Seed and Soil. Cancer Metastasis and the Lymphovascular System: Basis of Rational Therapy", in: Stanley P. L. LEONG (ed.), *Cancer Treatment and Research.* Springer, New York 2007, p. 119: *"Stephen Paget published in 1889 in* The Lancet *a paper by the title 'The distribution of secondary growths in cancer of the breast' inspired by the work of Fuchs 'Das Sarkom des Uvealtraktus' in 1882 published in* Graefe's Archiv für Ophthalmologie.[1] *Although Fuchs has written previously about the metastatic embolus and its relationship to the recipient tissue, it is Paget who spread the concept of the 'Seed and soil' that continues to be regarded as a major contribution to the area of cancer metastasis. The 'seeds' refer to certain tumor cells with metastatic capability, and the 'soil' is any organ or tissue providing a proper environment for growth of the seeds. Paget suggested that the spread of metastatic cells was organ specific and not merely anatomic."* Cf: Sadhan MAJUMDER (ed.), *Stem Cells and Cancer.* Springer, New York 2009, p. 171; Kenneth G. MANTON, Igor AKUSHEVICH, Julia KRAVCHENKO, *Cancer Mortality and Morbidity Patterns in the U. S. Population. An Interdisciplinary Approach.* Springer, New York 2009, p. 4.

[1] It is to be regretted that both in the Anglo-Saxon and the German specialist literature the same bibliographical mistake is being perpetuated in that Fuchs's monograph is treated as if it had been an original contribution to *Graefes Archiv.* The damage is completed by citing an illusory volume and sometimes even an illusory page: "vol. XII/2, p. 233".

380 Ibid. (Stephen Paget).

381 Cf. FN 304.

382 Julius HIRSCHBERG, "Zur Prognose der Aderhautsarcome", in: *Virchows Archiv* 90/Abth. I (1882), pp. 1–23.

383 W. SAUER, *Beitrag zur Casuistik der Irissarkome*. Med. Diss. Univ. Halle 1883; H. MASCHKE, *Ein Beitrag zur Lehre der Aderhautsarcome*. Med. Diss. Univ. Königsberg 1884; W. MARTIN, *Zur Prognostik der Uvealsarcome*. Med. Diss. Univ. Halle 1885.

384 Rosa PUTJATA-KERSCHBAUMER, *Das Sarkom des Auges*. J. F. Bergmann, Wiesbaden 1890.

385 Sattler began his introduction by saying: *"In the years that have passed since the publication of E. Fuchs's comprehensive monograph on the sarcoma of the uveal tract a great deal has happened. An overwhelming number of individual observations have been made, many valuable new perspectives have been opened up at the pathological-anatomical level, and our oncological views have changed and expanded in several directions. It may certainly be said therefore that the time has come to subject the topic again to an extensive examination and treatment.* Ibid., n.p.

386 Cf. FN 288.

387 Gustav FREUDENTHAL, "Ueber das Sarcom des Uvealtractus", in: *Graefes Archiv* 37/Abth. I (1891), pp. 137–184.

388 *"In his excellent monograph on the sarcoma of the uveal tract Fuchs explicitly emphasises the importance of further statistical reports on the successful operative treatment of this disease."* Ibid., p. 137.

389 S. WEINBAUM, "Beitrag zur Kenntniss der Sarkomerkrankung der Augenhäute", in: *Graefes Archiv* 37/Abth. I (1891), pp. 185–202.

390 Cf. FN 45.

391 Maximilian SALZMANN, "Fall von Sarkom der Iris und des Ciliarkörpers", in: *Wiener klin. Wochenschr.* 6 (1893), pp. 166–167. (Officielles Protokoll d. k. k. Gesellschaft d. Aerzte in Wien, Sitzung v. 24. Februar 1893) and SALZMANN, "Studien über das Myxosarkom des Sehnerven", in: *Graefes Archiv* 39/Abtheil. IV (1893), pp. 94–130; Oskar KOPETZKY von RECHTPERG, "Ringförmiges Sarkom der Iris und des Ciliarkörpers", in: *Graefes Archiv* 52 (1901), pp. 330–335.

392 Ernst FUCHS, "Über Sarcom der Aderhaut nebst Bemerkungen über Nekrose der Uvea", in: *Graefes Archiv* 77/III. Abth., (1910), pp. 304–392; FUCHS, "Smallest Sarcoma of the Choroid", in: *Transact. Am. Ophthalmol. Soc.* 12/Part III, pp. 787–789 [47th Annual Meeting, New London/Conn. July 11–12, 1911. Exhibition of Specimens, Discussion, pp. 789–790]; FUCHS, "Nachtrag zur Arbeit 'Ueber Sarkom der Aderhaut' im LXXVII. Bd. dieses Archivs", in: *Graefes Archiv* 81 (1912), pp. 556–562.

393 Maria ZOZOLOUL, Gregory TSOUCALAS, Marianna KARAMANOU, Konstantinos LAIOS, Ilias GEORGALAS, Athanasios DOUZENIS, George ANDROUTSOS, "The distinguished Austrian ophthalmologist Ernst Fuchs (1851–1930) and the 'sarcom des uvealtractus'", in: *Journal of the Balkan Union of Oncology* 23 (2018), pp. 1563–1568. – That Ernst Fuchs's "habilitation" thesis is a standard work not only of ophthalmic oncology but also of the modern international book trade is attested by two recent reprints and the freely accessible digitisation by Google.

394 *Öffentliche Vorlesungen an der K. K. Universität zu Wien im Sommer-Semester 1881.* Kaiserlich-Königliche Hof- und Staatsdruckerei, Vienna 1881, p. 23.

[395] *Öffentliche Vorlesungen an der K. K. Universität zu Wien im Winter-Semester 1881/82.* Kaiserlich-Königliche Hof- und Staatsdruckerei, Vienna 1881, p. 26.

[396] FUCHS, *Augenarzt* (as in FN 2), p. 67.

[397] See the next chapter.

3. Professor at the University of Lüttich/Liège 1881–1885

There are three authentic sources for the four years Fuchs spent in Lüttich/Liège in his first fully autonomous academic position. These are the relevant passages from his two autobiographies and the letters to his former teacher Arlt, in which he reported in detail on what went on in Liège.[398] Only a brief excerpt from the first of these letters has been published to date by medical historian Erna Lesky in 1961;[399] the others have never been published in full. These different sources make it possible to form some idea of Fuchs's life in the period in question with regard to both his scientific and his private concerns.

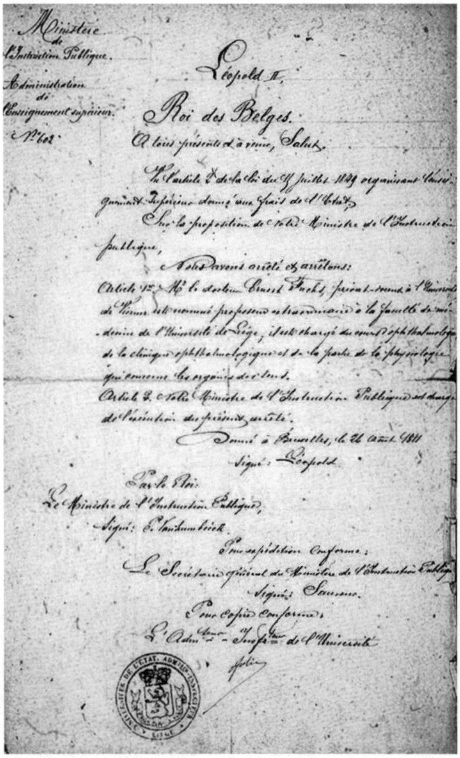
Ministère de l'Instruction Publique.
Administration de l'Enseignement supérieur.
N° 602
Léopold II,
Roi des Belges.
A tous présents et à venir, Salut.
Vu l'article 2 de la loi du 15 juillet 1849 organisant l'enseignement supérieur donné aux frais de l'État;
Sur la proposition de Notre Ministre de l'Instruction publique,
Nous avons arrêté et arrêtons:
Article 1er. Mr le docteur Ernest Fuchs, privat-docent à l'Université de Vienne est nommé professeur extraordinaire à la faculté de médecine de l'Université de Liège; il est chargé du cours d'ophthalmologie, de la clinique ophthalmologique et de la partie de la physiologie qui concerne les organes des sens.
Article 2. Notre Ministre de l'Instruction Publique est chargé de l'exécution du présent arrêté.
Donné à Bruxelles, le 26 Août 1881
Signé: Léopold
Par le Roi:
Le Ministre de l'Instruction Publique,
Signé: E. Van Humbeeck.
Pour expédition conforme:
Le Secrétaire général du Ministère de l'Instruction Publique
Signé: Sauveur.
Pour copie conforme,
L'Administrateur-Inspecteur de l'Université

Fig. 29. Certificate of Ernst Fuchs's appointment as Associate Professor at the University of Liège on 26 August 1881

On the technicalities of his call to Liège Fuchs had this to say:

One day in the spring of 1881 an old gentleman attended a course lecture. He subsequently joined us for a visit to the ward and I thought he was a medical doctor. He then asked to see me and I invited him to my room. He introduced himself as Transenster[400] [sic], *a mining engineer and Rector of Liège University, an integral part of which is the école des mines. He had come to Vienna with the express purpose of seeing me and had very nearly fallen victim to a train accident on the way. The proposal had been submitted for me to occupy the newly created Chair of Ophthalmology and he had wanted to see first what kind of a person I was, how I lecture, etc. I owe the call above all to Winiwarter,*[401] *the Professor of Surgery in Liège, and to Donders, who had been asked to recommend a candidate since no one suitable was to be found in Belgium. He had recommended me.*
We soon came to terms. My salary as an Associate Professor was higher than the regular initial salary of a Full Professor in Vienna. My parents gave their wholehearted consent. What remained to be done now was for me to improve my French in a hurry and I made use of the vacations to spend some time in Evian, on the French side of Lac Leman, and then went on to Paris for further language studies. Towards the end of September I travelled to Lüttich.[402]

By a decree of 26 August 1881 issued by the Belgian King, Leopold II, Ernst Fuchs was appointed Associate Professor of Ophthalmology at Liège University.[403] (Fig. 29) Two weeks after his arrival Fuchs sent the following report to Arlt in Vienna:

Lüttich, 12/10 81.

Verehrter Herr Hofrath!
Allow me to share my news from my new home. From Heidelberg I went to Paris, where I remained until the end of October.[404] *My most frequent visits were to the clinics of Landolt and Wecker. The latter surpasses himself in the invention of new operations, which have the indisputable value of demonstrating what the human eye will tolerate. To treat retinal detachment he burns a hole into the sclera with a pointed galvanocauter to obtain the mouth of a fistula that does not close up again immediately. I watched him perform this operation on a man who had only one eye left. In cases of optic atrophy, where one eye is wholly blind and the other has some sight left, Wecker stretches the optic nerve of the blind eye to allow him to intervene – through the chiasma – on the optic nerve of the other eye. In cases of cyclitis, choroiditis [and] glaucoma Wecker's student Abadie performs a denudation de l'œil, i.e. he exposes from outside the sclera as far as the optic nerve and severs all the ciliary vessels to reduce the blood flow to the eye. None of these operations invites imitation. In late September I travelled from Paris directly to Liège, where I was received most cordially by all. At the hospital I found two rooms with 15 beds altogether, an ensemble that represents the entire eye clinic. Even these rooms had stood empty over the last few years owing to the fact that my predecessor Borlé [e]*[405] *did not concern himself with the clinic at all. Ophthalmoscope room, lecture hall, etc. were all non-existent. What instruments there were at the clinic were truly antediluvian,*[406] *with no more than historical value at most; the clinic presumably never had such things as optotypes. I have now managed to obtain three rooms with 34–36 beds altogether. I will also be able to install a waiting room, a lecture hall and a refraction and ophthalmoscope room. Furthermore, I will be given a new clinic in about three years' time; the construction of a new, pavilion-style hospital is about to begin. I have an assistant, who draws an annual salary of 2500 frc., and a chef de clinique, a medical student in his final year, with an annual salary of 600 frc. Only the latter has an apartment in the hospital.*
The greatest problem to be overcome are the patients. As the clinic remained closed for almost an entire year, people have forgotten about the eye clinic. It will therefore take some time for a substantial patient volume to develop. Nursing is

in the hands of nuns who are hopeless; there is an incessant stream of complaints from all concerned.
Lüttich is pleasantly located, quite populous (130,000 inhabitants) and there are densely inhabited industrial towns nearby. I therefore do not doubt that there is considerable potential for the future, and I hope that the 34 beds will soon prove inadequate.
I often recall with a sense of intense gratitude the instructive years I spent at your clinic, to which I now owe this position.

Ihr ergebener und dankschuldiger Schüler
Fuchs
1 Rue des Anges.[407]

No other writer has described the atmosphere of Liège, an ancient city of culture and a burgeoning industrial metropolis, as graphically as Austrian writer Stefan Zweig (1881–1942), who paid the city a visit two decades after Fuchs's sojourn there, in August 1914, only a few weeks after the outbreak of World War I. The temptation to include this authentic testimony in full has proved too great to resist:

It reminds one a little bit of Salzburg, this Walloon city, with its citadel on the commanding hill and the river dividing the unruly residential areas into unequal halves. What it shares with Salzburg are the many churches, which in this instance do not strain upwards into a clear sky in the delicate, sinuous forms of the Italian baroque, but rise, heavy and massive, to northern clouds, always a little veiled by the coal haze emanating from its many factories. An episcopal see like Salzburg and at a thousand years old its contemporary – Walter Scott[408] *has left a masterful description of the days of its glory in one of his novels – Liège has lost many of its ancient traits to luxury: broad avenues, unattractive and noisy, have, with their lights and posters, cut swathes through ancient quarters, and the solemn cathedrals stand there forlorn amid the tumult. Everywhere one senses that bane of small cities, their inclination to let external growth overthrow inner charm, the provincial hankering after boulevards of the sort sported by Brussels or Paris, the useless striving for a cosmopolitan allure oblivious of congenital dimensions. There is, with the exception of Nuremberg, hardly another city for whose beauty industrialisation and its rapidly acquired wealth constitute such a threat as for this Walloon bishop's see, which has transformed itself over the last fifty years into a capital of material gain.*

You only need to board one of the small steamers for a trip up or downstream on the Maas to become keenly aware of the change that has befallen the city. As long as you are within sight of the city bridges, all is quiet, you hear the sound of bells from the many churches and, judging from the peaceful facades of houses and villas, you might think you were in a small town. But the moment the river's banks turn green, you can hear the thumping of the ironworks. Wherever you look, the red shafts of factory chimneys have been planted in the lovely landscape, and coal haze shrouds the sky. Behind this, ash grey pyramids tower like mountains; blast furnaces and coal pits abound, there is a ceaseless string of barges laden with black coal, and trains thunder along on their way to or from the city. You may think you have reached unspoilt nature at last, but the black wall of pits still keeps spreading outwards. The activities of a thousand enterprises, visible or subterranean, are unfathomable. From the vantage point of the citadel at night you can see the red beacons of the blast furnaces in the distance, the perpetual flames of labour that continue to burn when the light in the windows has long gone out.
A city of music for centuries, from Orlando di Lasso[409] *to César Franck,*[410] *Liège has now become a city of labour, a vigorous, flourishing industrial workshop. Ever since the unification of the Provinces it has been another of Belgium's large cities, but it is still a capital in spirit, the centre of the Walloon race. The University has become a focal point of French intellectual life, increasingly so in direct proportion to the pace at which the discord between Flemings and Walloons, reflecting the relationship between France and Germany, has been gathering momentum in political life. Everything here is directed towards Paris, and where Antwerp is the centre towards which the Flemish element gravitates, and Brussels sits on the fence, keeping the two nations in a state of equilibrium, Liège, rarely called Lüttich by the locals, is an unrepentant stronghold of Frenchness, despite sitting so close to Germany. The professors, first of all Maurice Wilmotte,*[411] *admonish the younger generation to be mindful of French culture and lay down the intellectual groundwork for a merger with the* [French] *Republic, a move the Walloon party subscribes to quite openly. By virtue of their temperament and language the population are closer to their western than their eastern neighbours and the strong push of the German army against Liège was an incursion into enemy territory in fact, if not in politics.*[412]

Fuchs's first home was a flat near the Botanical Gardens at 1, rue des Anges. After his marriage in 1882, which will be dealt with in more detail below, he moved to a small house with a garden at 13, rue Fusch, behind the Botanical Gardens.[413]

He was helped to find his feet in Liège by his friend Alexander von Winiwarter, who had succeeded Carl Gussenbauer as Professor of Surgery at Liège University. This allowed him to concentrate straightaway on sizing up the work that was waiting for him at his post:

In Lüttich I was especially cordially welcomed by Winiwarter and his young wife, and by van Aubel [sic],[414] *Professor of Thérapeutique Générale, and his wife. The two women found a charming four-room bachelor's flat in an annex located in a small garden. …*
Things went less easily at the clinic. As no chair of ophthalmology has previously been in existence,[415] *there is no clinic as such; Winiwarter was supposed to touch on eye diseases in his lectures and had a ward with 8–10 beds, which he gave up for my benefit straightaway. This, however, was too little and I had no lecture hall, no workroom. To fill the position of assistant, Winiwarter parted company with his chef de clinique (a position that roughly corresponds to that of aspirant), the terribly simple-minded Dr X., and I was also assigned a servant. I went to Brussels to acquaint the minister with my needs and was told that my colleagues at the hospital would not hesitate to cede other hospital rooms to me. This was of course not the case but at least I managed to secure funding from the ministry so that I will be able to carry out my plans.*
The clinics are located in an age-old monastery building called Hôpital de Bavière, because an archbishop of Liège, who reputedly founded the monastery, had been a Bavarian prince.[416] *The building has a huge loft of the type one often finds in such old structures and I could install several quite large wards there, a lecture hall, an ophthalmoscope room and two small workrooms. It was, however, only in the nature of things that below the roof it was cold in winter and hot in summer. The worst thing was that there was only one very long wooden staircase; when fire broke out in it on one occasion, all of us would have been burnt to death if it had not been very quickly extinguished. My successor Nuel,*[417] *by the way, had to make do with the loft for years until a new clinical hospital was built.*[418]
For a time, things hung so much in the balance that I was about to resign from my position as it seemed impossible to me to make a success of it.
Another difficulty concerned the volume of patients. There was this charitable foundation, the Institut ophtalmique, that had been around for a very long time. Its head was an old eye specialist, Dr Jamain,[419] *who was an excellent surgeon. Patients had become used to going there and the existence of a new eye clinic at the University Hospital remained virtually unknown for quite some time. This meant in my first years I had only slightly more than a thousand new patients annually,*

and each new case had to be exploited as a teaching resource. The number of students was usually between 30 and 40 so that one could really get to know each one and they received good tuition.
The arrangement for tuition in ophthalmology was comparable to that in the other specialties in that twice a week an hour was devoted to theory and the other days to the clinic – to the demonstration of cases. So, before the clinic was established, I confined myself to two theoretical lectures a week, which I delivered in one of the University's lecture halls at some distance from the hospital.
As the government was loath to appoint a professor for a minor field of study such as ophthalmology (for other such minor fields there were lecteurs), the Professor of Physiology, Fredericq,[420] *hit upon the idea of adding to my teaching commitment a course in the physiology of the senses, a course I was supposed to hold twice a week during two terms. I didn't mind having to lecture on physiological optics, even though I had to get the hang of it as I went along. It interested me. What presented difficulties of a different order was the physiology of hearing, as I could not read music and indeed knew next to nothing about music as such. I got round this difficulty by treating the physiology of the eye at such lengths that the second semester ended without my ever reaching acoustics. As it was up to me to examine the students in this specialty, it was easy for me to confine myself to physiological optics. Nor did it irk Fredericq to have got rid of the physiology of the senses, in which he had little interest. I continued the lectures on physiological optics for four years.*
When I arrived in Liège, I was surprised to find Professor Schwann[421] *among my active colleagues. As the first proponent of the doctrine that the animal organism is made up of cells,*[422] *his name features on the very first pages of all textbooks of histology. I had been of the opinion that he belonged to a past century.*
He had made a name for himself as a young lecturer in Berlin with a monograph, the one on the cellular structure of the body of animals,[423] *and a second one on fermentation*[424] *and had received a call to Liège many years ago. Once there, he had not distinguished himself any further through scientific achievements. He became a cleric*[425] *and, to all intents and purposes, an exceedingly kind old gentleman and famous wine connoisseur. We were colleagues only for one semester. During the Easter vacation he paid a visit to his native Düren near Düsseldorf, where he suffered a stroke. In Liège he had no longer spoken German really well, without having acquired perfect command of French in exchange. After his stroke he was afflicted with aphasia in the sense that he only retained his command of German. He died in Düren not long afterwards.* […]
Another great friend was van Beneden,[426] *an outstanding anatomist and a very witty gentleman, with whom I used to dine every day while I was still single.* […]

From among other colleagues to whom I became attached I would like to mention the anatomist S[w]aen,[427] *the internist Masius,*[428] *and the pathological anatomist Vanlair.*[429] *My closest contact was of course Winiwarter's family, where I often went for dinner. I was soon assigned a new, excellent assistant, Leplat,*[430] *who has retained his affection for me to this day.*[431]

His gift for languages and his medical professionalism made sure that Fuchs was soon in complete control of his tasks as a teacher:

In Lüttich I had to deliver two lectures a week on theoretical aspects of ophthalmology. As the lectures had to be held in French, I elaborated lecture notes for this purpose, which, rather than reading them out, I then delivered ex tempore. These lecture notes later formed the basis, the skeleton, as it were, of my textbook. … On the days reserved to the clinic in Lüttich I demonstrated to the students such cases as turned up. I stuck to this method of demonstration later on in Vienna.[432]

Fuchs's next letter to Arlt is dated eleven months after his first description of the situation in Liège and offers a vivid insight into the work he was pursuing there, in spite of the difficulties he had mentioned earlier.

Lüttich, 27. Nov. 1881.
Rue des Anges

Sehr geehrter Herr Hofrat!
I beg your permission to ask a favour of you. Recently the view has been gaining more and more adherents that sympathetic inflammation proceeds along the optic nerve. I would like to mount a few arguments against this, especially in view of the most recent paper on this subject (by Knies,[433] *Festgabe für Horner),*[434] *which in my view will prove irrefutably that first and foremost the pathologies always occur in the areas supplied by the ciliary nerves. Nor do I approve of the strict separation of sympathetic irritation and sympathetic inflammation, as postulated by Leber*[435] *and Knies. The latter postulate that symp. irritation proceeds via the ciliary nerves, symp. inflammation via the optic nerve, which makes the two complexes of symptoms utterly different. By contrast, I would like to take up the cudgels for the old doctrine, which interprets the prodromal symptoms of symp. ophthalmia as merely those manifestations of irritation to be observed in any organ before the outbreak of the actual inflammation.*[436] *– I would like to ask your permission to use for this short paper, which I want to publish in French, several of the case histories I made notes on while I was still at your clinic – unless,*

of course, [you] *are planning to make use of them yourself. I am unable to retrieve the notes on one particular patient, the brush maker Rieger, who was put up in Room 58c in March 1880. He remained in the clinic for a very long time before being discharged, ostensibly fully cured. Shortly before my departure I had his case history copied for you, because* [you] *thought it might be of use to you in Heidelberg. If this* [case history] *is still among your papers I would ask you to kindly let me have it so that I can copy it. I will then send it back by return of post.*

I am reasonably content here. The only thing that needs to be improved is the volume of patients. As the eye clinic of the University Hospital was totally neglected over the last few years, standing in fact entirely empty for most of the time, [the] *caravan of eye patients has turned towards the two free out-patient clinics that still exist here. They are under the direction respectively of Dr Romiée*[437] *and Dr Jamin.*[438]

Among the patients I have performed operations on here there is one whose case is not without interest. A miner, he had come down with a type of glaucoma I want to call gl. fulminans. The patient reported he had lost all perception of light simultaneously with the onset of acute pain. At his admission to the hospital a few days after the glaucoma attack it was impossible to establish with any certainty whether any sensitivity to light was still left. I first performed an iridectomy on the other eye, which displayed prodromal symptoms of gl[aucoma], in order to forestall an acute attack, and 6 days later I iridectomised the inflamed eye to put an end to what were still considerable pains. These disappeared shortly after the operation. The day before yesterday the patient could discern hand movements and today, 10 days after the iridectomy, he was able to count fingers at a distance of 4 m; however, his field of vision is still severely restricted.

I also performed a sclerotomy on a trial basis, even though I am by no means partial to this operation. A roughly 55-year-old man presented with bilateral glaucoma simplex. At no stage was there any indication of elevated intraocular pressure. Visual acuity is the same in both eyes (5 6/24). I performed a sclerotomy on the left eye (according to Wecker's method) and will soon perform an iridectomy on the right eye. As both eyes are affected to the same degree, this case may be ideal for a comparison between the two methods of operation. The sclerotomy went without a hitch and without the least incarceration of the iris.

I commit my request for the case history to your kind discretion.

Ihr ergebenster und dankbarer Schüler

E. Fuchs.[439]

A letter to Arlt dating from three months later illustrates especially clearly the exchange of scientific ideas that went on between the two men and the competition for Arlt's succession that was already gathering momentum in Vienna:

Lüttich 20. Februar 1882

Verehrter Herr Professor!
It had been my firm resolve for days to write to you and today I wanted to use the leisure offered by Sunday to do so, when I received your letter. – If I remember correctly, you will be celebrating your 70th birthday sometime at the end of this month.[440] *I know there is no need for me to assure you how fervently I wish that you may be preserved to us for a long time to come in your full physical and mental health. I share with all your students the hope that you will not turn your back on your clinic any time soon. It is a depressing thought for all of us that the clinic may end up in the hands of Stellwag, who, apart from a host of other concerns, cannot pretend to be a good teacher capable of firing up students.*
I have read roughly the first half of the book Stellwag has just published.[441] *I am not quite sure what purpose it is meant to serve. Is it really, as the title claims, meant as a supplement to his textbook? In that case, most chapters are much too long-winded and not at all clearly structured. If, on the other hand, it is meant to be a series of original papers, then I for one do not see what the entire chapter devoted to the development* [of the eye] *is supposed to do. It is no more than a compilation of already well-known facts that Stellwag can only have extracted from various works, since he is at present hardly concerned with microscopy and least of all with embryology.*
I have noticed that, in the chapter on keratitis, Stellwag finds fault with the view that ker[atitis] interstit[itialis or parench[ymatosa] is very often hereditary-syphilitic in origin. He cites a compilation done by his assistant, Hampl,[442] *according to which only four cases out of 110 are said to be have been linked to syphilis (p. 49). However, it becomes apparent later on how little this compilation is to be trusted. On p. 57 the reader learns that these 110 cases are in fact a farrago of widely different types of keratitides. Furthermore, the diagnoses of k[eratitis] parench [ymatosa] do not always appear to have been correctly made since they include two patients older than fifty!*
The more cases of k [eratitis] parench [ymatosa] I see – they are relatively common here – the more I am convinced that the great majority of them has to be linked to syph[ilis]. Admittedly, it is often difficult to diagnose hereditary syph. and especially to distinguish it from scrofulosis, which it resembles in so many respects. This Hampl seems to have omitted.

In the chapter on diseases of the retina Stellwag has failed to distinguish his herpes from herpes zoster and even from herpes Horneri. His argument concerning affection of the nerves in conj[unctivitis] lymph[atica] is based on a single case,[443] *the one studied by Iwanoff.*[444] *– That in cases of conj. lymph., round cells, making their way from the corneal parenchyma to below the epithelium to form nodules there, should do so by following nerves does not surprise me. The lymphatic spaces surrounding nerves are the only physiologically preformed pathways leading across the corneal lamellae and finally through Bowman's membrane. I have been able to form an adequate picture of the important role of these pathways through the study of glaucomatous corneal clouding.*[445] *This behaviour does not justify talk about a specific pathology of the nerves, just as no one will diagnose an inflammation of a muscle if pus from an abscess spreads between the epimysia on its way down.*

As for cysticercus, this can only refer to one of the following two cases: a young girl had in her right (?) eye a cyst. ubretin. located far forward on the outside, which you extracted with resounding success. It should be possible to find this girl in the log of Room No. 58 a b, I believe in the autumn of 1878, on no account after 1. Dec., but maybe much earlier, perhaps in the spring of 1878 or earlier still. – Another young girl (a housemaid from Reitergasse?) had come to the clinic in the winter of 79/80 only once and was probably not recorded in the outpatient log as she arrived when the clinic was already closed. She presented with a clearly circumscribed, blueish-white retinal detachment at the posterior pole of one eye roughly the size of 4–5 disc diameters and an intensely white spot, which seemed to correspond to the head of a cyst[icercus]. Unfortunately, she did not keep her promise to come back the following day, but I learnt later that Dr Hock[446] *had presented her to the Doctorencollegium (or the Ärzteverein).*[447]

As for my essay on sympathetic ophthalmia, I have strong misgivings that you expect more from it than it can deliver. It is basically only two case histories, the brush maker Rieger and one Baumann, plus a couple of notes. I have expanded the first case history with anatomical findings on the enucleated eye. I have cut the eye, which I have taken with me, in half, but did not want to destroy it by searching for the foreign body. I'd rather cut it up into sections with the microtome, which will deliver the foreign body in any case. I have delayed the procedure until the arrival of the new microtome I ordered from Heidelberg and will now settle down to it very soon. A few weeks ago, I asked Dr Herz[448] *to write to the brush maker. I would like to know whether he has been lastingly cured. However, I have not yet heard from him.*

I believe it would be a mistake for me to attempt a major work on sympath[etic] ophthalmia, since I have no new, decisive material at my disposal and would therefore be reduced to rehearsing well-known arguments that have already been

discussed many times. What I will do later, undeterred as I am by the failure of others, is to try and get to grips with this matter through experiments. Perhaps dogs will facilitate the breakthrough that those all too indolent rabbits have denied me. Only now have I finally reached the stage, after countless difficulties, where I can establish my definitive clinic, having had to make do until now with two small, provisional hospital rooms. I will have at my disposal 3 hospital rooms with a total of 32 beds, a lecture hall, an ophthalmoscope and a refraction room and 2 workrooms; all this is of course on the smallest possible scale. As the hospital does not have any labs I had to resort to a trick to establish the two workrooms. I claimed that these two rooms were dedicated to the examination of patients. All this will take another 2–3 weeks to be completed so I won't be able to start working properly until then.
On the whole I would be quite content with my situation if it wasn't for this pervasive sense of loneliness. My colleagues, the other professors, are all married, and I do not have a great deal of contact with them. Nor do I have many other acquaintances. – All this means that I am lacking scientific stimulation; there is nobody with whom I can discuss an interesting case or scientific questions concerning ophthalmology.
I gather from your letter that there is a shortage of workers at your clinic. Herz, who is now the only one in charge of the assistants' workload, is no doubt full of good will, but he may not have the requisite talent. I am very sorry and have charged myself with ingratitude many times that I left at a time when I had finally acquired the knowledge that would have made me a really useful assistant. It is unfortunate that the prospects for young ophthalmologists are so bad that I was forced to take the leap when an opportunity offered.
I fear I am abusing your patience with this long letter. I am planning to go to Vienna at Easter and am tremendously looking forward to seeing you again in full health, as I hope.

Mit den herzlichsten Grüßen
hr dankbar ergebener
Fuchs.[449]

The spring of 1882 was entirely given over to a redefinition of Ernst Fuchs's personal circumstances: he married his fiancée Julia-Rosina (Julie) Mayr.[450] (Fig. 30) The civil ceremony took place on 21 May 1882 in Liège. [451] The church wedding took place on 22 June 1882 at the parish church of St. Rochus and Sebastian on Landstraße in Vienna (Fig. 31). His wife's family lived in the Viennese suburb Landstraße in a house named "Zum Einsiedler" (today Landstraßer Hauptstraße 75, 1030 Vienna), which had been acquired by Julie's grandparents.[452]

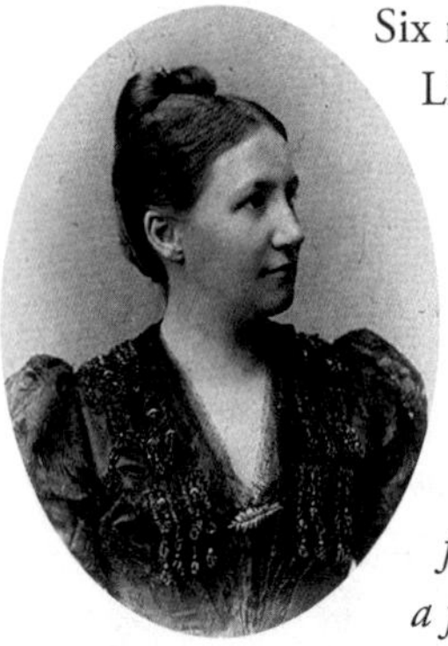

Fig. 30. Julia Rosina Fuchs

Six months later Fuchs resumed his correspondence with Arlt from Liège:

Lütich, 24 Sept 1882.

Hochverehrter Herr Hofrath!

Not having been in touch for so long I'm ashamed of myself as I write again at last. First of all I would like to thank you for being present at my wedding. My honeymoon consisted in my taking four weeks for the return journey, stopping off here and there for a few days. In early September I made a round trip with my wife in Belgium itself. This meant that to my great regret I was unable to go to Heidelberg.[453] *Since my return the clinic has been fully in operation and I have resumed my work, which was interrupted for so long by my getting married.*

I have little to report as far as the clinic is concerned. Iodoform, which is now in fashion, I have found of significant use in only a few cases of suppurating progressive corneal ulcer. I sprinkled it as a very fine powder on the cornea, especially on the ulcer itself, and then bandaged the eye. I am convinced that the shrinkage of the ulcer and its healing were effected much sooner than would have been the case with bandages alone or together with cataplasms.[454]

12 days ago, I performed a blepharoplastic according to Meyer's method.[455] *The patient, a woman, having suffered burns from petroleum, had such extensive scars that an operation with a pedicle flap would hardly have been viable. The ectropion concerned the right upper lid, where all the skin had been lost so that the ciliary row had become fused with the eyebrows. In keeping with Meyer's instructions, the piece of skin taken from one of the patient's upper arms was considerably larger than what had been lost; it measured 5 ½ by 8 cent[imeters]. The graft has healed very well apart from isolated spots at the edges; should it shrink ever so much, it will presumably still be large enough, for at present it is much too large; the upper lid protrudes over the lower one on to the cheek. I had refrained during the operation from temporarily attaching the eyelids to each other (as is otherwise common practice); instead, I had pulled down the edge of the upper lid and attached it to the cheek by means of a thread loop (and a glass bead) to be able to graft the large piece of skin comfortably on to the wound.*

My attempts to induce sympathetic ophthalmia in dogs and rabbits have not led to any results so far. I have operated on quite a number of animals, always by implanting a foreign body (iron wire or a piece of a sewing needle) into the interior of the eye in the region of the ciliary body. When after some time (with dogs this happens rather quickly) iridocyclitis and the discolouration of the eye subsides,

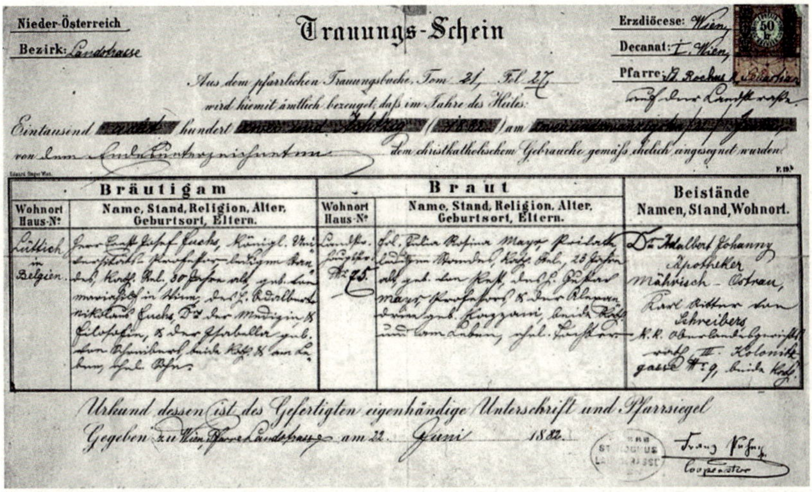
Nieder-Österreich
Bezirk: Landstrasse

Trauungs-Schein

Erzdiöcese: Wien
Decanat: I. Wien
Pfarre: St. Rochus [illegible]

Aus dem pfarrlichen Trauungsbuche, Tom 21, Fol. 27
wird hiemit ämtlich bezeuget, daß im Jahre des Heiles:
Eintausend [redacted] hundert [redacted] ([redacted]) am [redacted]
von [illegible] dem christkatholischem Gebrauche gemäß ehelich eingesegnet wurden:

Bräutigam		Braut		Beistände
Wohnort Haus-Nº	Name, Stand, Religion, Alter, Geburtsort, Eltern.	Wohnort Haus-Nº	Name, Stand, Religion, Alter, Geburtsort, Eltern.	Namen, Stand, Wohnort.
Lüttich in Belgien	[illegible] Ernst Josef Fuchs, [illegible]	Landstr. [illegible] Nº 25	Frl. Julia Rosina Mayr, [illegible]	Dr. Adalbert Johanny Apotheker Mährisch-Ostrau, Karl Ritter von Schreibers [illegible] Kolonitzgasse Nº 9, [illegible]

Urkund dessen ist des Gefertigten eigenhändige Unterschrift und Pfarrsiegel
Gegeben zu Wien, Pfarre Landstrasse am 22. Juni 1882.
[illegible]
Cooperator

Fig. 31.
Ernst Fuchs's and Julia Rosina Mayr's Catholic marriage certificate of 22 June 1882

I perform the same operation again in the same manner, because I believe it is crucial to maintain an acute state of irritation for as long as possible. That I have failed to achieve a sympathetic inflammation so far I find easily understandable. Even among human beings who suffer from traumatic iridocyclitis only a certain insignificant percentage develop a sympathetic inflammation. I therefore believe that the animal experiments must be quite numerous and must be performed continuously in order to yield a result.
Some dogs are offered a considerable daily dose of brandy to slake their thirst and I want to inject some of them with nicotine. This experiment is to be continued over some time until it is time to examine the optic nerves. Perhaps evidence will be found of the same chronically inflammatory processes that alcoholism triggers e.g. in the liver and in other organs.
At present I am busy with the microscopic study of the eyes I brought with me from Vienna. I can leave this to my servant, whom I have taught to operate the microtome, so that I am making good progress.
Dr Nelson,[456] *who spent a great deal of time in '78 and '79 at your clinic and worked hard there, is planning to return to Vienna in the near future. He will ask you for a testimony on that occasion and has asked me to remind you of him. You will no doubt recall him when you see him. I can confirm that he was an assiduous visitor at your clinic and that he benefited very much.*
Kindly bear with my endless effusions.
Mit ehrerbietigen Grüßen Ihr dankbar ergebener

E. Fuchs.[457]

Fuchs's next letter to Arlt dates from January 10, 1883. This time the topics include histological examinations in the context of the pathogenesis of glaucoma, a focus of attention for Fuchs at the time, and a new method of embedding the sections he collected:

Verehrter Herr Hofrath!
The book in question has been returned to me in good order. – As for my case (Dimm), while the ciliary body is hypertrophic, it is not inflamed; the inflammation is only observable in the choroid proper, mainly in the form of a general, moderate cellular infiltration of the kind usually found to accompany a distinct iridocyclitis. The iris is absolutely normal – there are no symptoms of inflammation, edema or atrophy.
At the hyaloidea there are drusy or crumbly bulges; the vitreous body itself is normal. I have come across eyes with glauc[oma] simplex or relatively little advanced glauc[oma] infl[ammatorium acutum]. Among my bulbi I have only been able to find a single glaucomatous eye with the optic nerve still attached – all the others have already been processed. I will mail this bulbus to you tomorrow and beg you to make whatever use of it you see fit. It comes from your own private practice. You gave it to me in May 1877, saying that it used to belong to a 55-year-old Greek (or Turk?) and that the diagnosis was being kept in the balance between glaucoma and tumour chor[ioideae]. I noted on the enucleated bulbus at the time: Moderately deep chamber, very wide pupil, with some protrusive synechiae. Lens transparent. – You will find a second preparation in the box that I take the liberty of sending you. It is a sarcoma of the chor[ioidea], embedded in gelatin according to the method of Priestley-Smith. These preparations keep as long as those in alcohol and are very handy for use in classes as they have the advantage of being kept safe from the clumsy hands of the students and can be handed out without fear. I have prepared a number of bulbus halves in this way for use in my classes and am sending this one as a sample, in case you have not yet seen this mode of preparation. As for Brailey's[458] *hypothesis (dilation of the ciliary arteries, espec[ially] the circ[ulus] art[eriosus] ir[idis] major), I must say that I have not found any confirmation in the eyes I have examined so far.*
If there is anything I can do for you, I am at your service.
Mit den besten Grüssen Ihr
dankbar ergebener

E. Fuchs[459]

The next letter in Fuchs's correspondence with Arlt that has come down to us was written five months later:

Lüttich 17. Juni 1883.

Hochverehrter Herr Professor!

As I told you in a letter this winter, I went to Italy with my wife, where we spent two months relaxing at the Lago maggiore. I have now been back for almost six weeks and have resumed my lectures on diseases of the eye and physiological optics with redoubled energy, in order to make up at least in part for what was left undone. This is also the reason why I did not write to you any earlier. I gather, partly from the papers, partly from what relatives of mine tell me in their letters, how much distress and frustration you have had to endure recently, giving a bitter taste to what is effectively the last year in your career as a teacher. Unfortunately, the principle at work here is Nemo propheta in patria, and your word, which carries the greatest weight everywhere outside Austria, is nil and void against the machinations of a coterie[460] *in Austria itself.*

My work was interrupted by my illness and this has also affected the great number of experiments on sympathetic ophthalmia. While I have been unable to provoke the onset of it, I have at least a collection of acutely inflamed eyes now that enables me to study the optic nerve and the ciliary nerves along their entire extension. I will, however, be unable to finish this in time for the Heidelberg Conference, all the more since I won't be here during August.

My clinic has of course suffered due to my long absence so that the patient volume is still not what I want it to be. This leaves me with nothing to report on. In case you have not tried iodoform yourself in the meantime, allow me to point out its excellent efficacy for corneal ulcers, provided they are not yet too far advanced.

I am planning to go to Heidelberg in the summer and hope very much that we will meet there. I am looking forward to this all the more since I cannot tell when I will be able to go to Vienna.

Mit den herzlichsten Grüßen

Ihr dankbar ergebener
E. Fuchs[461]

The illness Fuchs mentions in this letter was a case of sepsis caused by an unguis incarnatus on his right foot. He was physically so weak that his mother came to Liège for a time to attend to him. His wife could not do that because she had come down with typhus, which was raging in Liège at the time as a regular epidemic.[462]

The next letter to Arlt that has come down to us dates from half a year later:

Lüttich 13. Dec. 1883.

Hochverehrter Herr Professor!

I have enquired about the book you have asked for at our library; unfortunately, we don't have it nor is it available from the library of the Royal Academie de Médecine in Brussels, whose catalogue I have been able to consult in our library. The librarian has already written to Ghent to find out whether their University Library has a copy. The answer will take 2–3 days. Failing that, I will turn to Amsterdam. I will send you the volume by registered mail as soon as I have got hold of it. If you want me to have it translated here, please tell me. Obtaining a second-hand copy is impossible because there are no major antiquarian bookshops either here or in Brussels that stock scientific literature.

I have been doing a great deal of anatomical work since my return from Heidelberg but have not yet got around to publishing anything. You will find the results of an examination of two glaucomatous eyes on an attached sheet, albeit in a highly condensed form. Should you need more details, they are at your disposal.

I was very sorry not to have met you in Heidelberg, all the more since I had counted on it. There was no one who did not react to your absence with regret. I had spent the summer with my wife partly in Vorarlberg, partly in Switzerland and did not go to Vienna. We are both well now; my wife is expecting a baby this coming February or March.[463]

This summer I had a very severe case of keratitis parenchymatosa at the clinic. The opacity had a strong tinge of yellow and a central deep ulcer was developing on both corneas. It was this fact about the first eye that made me hesitate in the diagnosis. However, when the disease took the same course in the second eye and finally, when the patient's sister presented at the clinic with a bilateral keratitis parenchymatosa (which had already run its course), all doubts were dispelled. – Recently I performed the extraction of an iron splinter with Hirschberg's magnet. The operation was very easy to do and was crowned with success: the severe iridocyclitis subsided almost immediately so that now not even any synechiae are left.

I would ask you to be patient for a few days with regard to the book you need.

Ihr dankbar ergebener

E. Fuchs[464]

Attached to this letter was the case history of a patient, Dimm, whom Fuchs had already mentioned in his letter of January 10, 1883. Fuchs seems to have taken this case history with him from the Vienna University Eye Clinic:

[…] *A highly instructive photograph of such sections is provided by Priestley Smith,*[465] *Ophthalmic Hosp. Reports (the volume number has unfortunately slipped from my memory).*[466] *The enlargement of the ciliary body is not due to any swelling (edema or inflammation), because its texture is entirely normal (at least 1½ years passed between the glaucoma attack and death). Nor was there any evidence of significant hypermetropia, with both eyes measuring 24 mill[imeters]. The ciliary processes extended close to the posterior area of the iris without actually touching it, let alone pushing it forward. When opening the eyes, I unfortunately omitted to pay attention to the interstice between the ciliary processes and the lens wall. When I examined the eyes this year, the lenses had dropped out.*
In the choroidea a slightly inflammatory infiltration distributed fairly evenly across the entire membrane; no distinct foci, no obliterated vessels. The delicate capillaries at the anterior edge of the choriocapillaris described by Sattler[467] *consistently fully developed. Pigment epithelium normal. A very remarkable change observable on several nerves of the choroidea: enormous bulges in specific places of the nervous fibres, filled with a finely dotted matter in which neither cross cylinders nor pith were distinguishable any longer. I detected these changes only on lesser nerve cords and only in the r[ight] eye. Retina normal, no traces of retinitis (Mauthner).*[468] *At the papilla, the lamina crib[rosa] bulges very slightly backwards, but the level of the papilla surface is normal. A slight atrophy at the optic nerve trunk, to the extent it is still attached to the bulbi.*
This atrophy is most strongly in evidence in the nerve bundles immediately below the pial sheath[469] *and in those adjacent to the central vessel. In addition, many other bundles display a slight atrophy at their margins. The connective-tissue septa are somewhat bloated. The atrophy decreases from front to back.*
Lens, incipient cataract, equat[orial] diameter 8.22, sagittal diameter 4.72 m[m]. Measurement is not totally reliable because it was made at the cross-section of the lens and there is no telling whether the latter was placed exactly in the middle of the lens.[470]

One year later, Fuchs published this patient's case history, together with a comprehensive discussion of the pathogenesis of glaucoma.[471]

Working conditions at his eye clinic in Liège consistently failed to come up to Fuchs's expectations. In spite of his repeated lobbying of the competent university authorities, the establishment of a congenial working environment at the clinic eluded him. Even though Fuchs intervened repeatedly both in faculty meetings and with the ministry in Brussels, he failed to bring about the changes he was asking for.[472]

It was with these unsatisfactory working conditions in mind that Fuchs wrote to Arlt in early 1884 the following letter:

Lüttich 19. Jänner 1884

Verehrter Herr Hofrath!
Eight days ago I learnt from the papers that there is talk in Prague of proposing me to succeed Hasner.[473 474] *Unfortunately I do not know for sure whether this has actually happened by now as I have had no direct news from Prague. The prospect of taking up the post of a professor of ophthalmology in that city fills me with the greatest joy. It is a great honour – almost too great an honour – to teach at the same clinic that you yourself led for such a long time. I hope I will not be disappointed. If the Professorial College really put me forward as a candidate, the Minister will no doubt turn to you to enquire about my qualifications. May I entertain the hope that you will pass a favourable judgement? I am convinced that a great deal, if not everything, depends on that. This is why I have taken the liberty of writing to you and of asking you for a favourable assessment, if you believe me worthy of the position in question. You may rest assured that I will do anything to prove myself worthy of my teacher and mentor.*
Ihr dankbar ergebener

E. Fuchs[475]

A search for the relevant files of the Medical Faculty of Prague University[476] in Vienna failed to retrieve Arlt's letter of recommendation, but three weeks after the letter reprinted above Fuchs thanked his teacher for acceding to his request:

Lüttich 3. Feb. 1884.

Hochverehrter Herr Hofrath!
Many thanks for your exceedingly generous letter. The Prague Faculty has not yet made any decision about filling the vacant position and the news item in the Med. Wochenschrift *was just another canard.*[477]

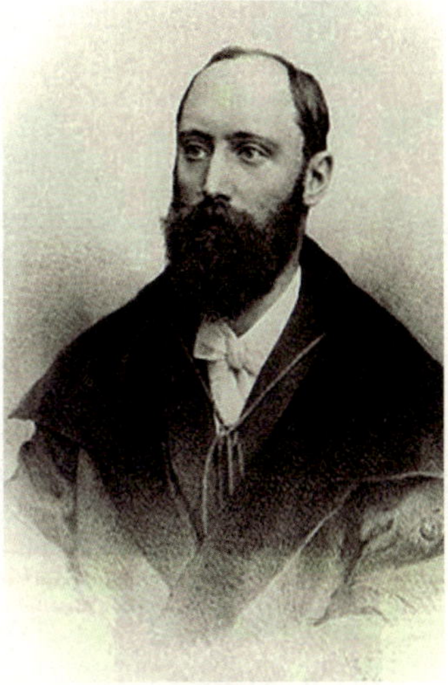

Fig. 32.
Ernst Fuchs as Full Professor at the University of Liège in 1885

I would like to share with you the preparation of gelatin specimens. Priestley Smith presented this novel method in Ophthalmic Review in March 1883;[478] *I have seen such preparations in Torino made by Reymond.*[479] *If the specimen was preserved in alcohol, it is soaked in fresh water for a day and is then refined in glycerine of 10%, 25% and 50%. In each of these solutions, it remains for a day or longer. Preparations preserved in Mueller's solution*[480] *must first be rid of their yellow colour before being put into glycerine. Discolouration is achieved by putting them in a 5% solution of chloral hydrate, which is renewed every second or third day. From the 50% solution of glycerine the preparation is transferred to gelatin. For the gelatin 1 part colourless glue (in Vienna, if I am not mistaken, this is referred to as Kölner Leim* [Cologne glue]*; it is used in gilding) is dissolved in 6 parts of hot water. Once this has dissolved completely, 6 parts of glycerine and some phenol solution are added. The hot solution is filtered and becomes solid as it cools.*
To embed the preparation the gelatin is liquefied by applying heat and is poured into a glass box. The preparation, which is taken from the 50% glycerine solution, is embedded in it and is kept on the floor of the box with a needle until it is fixated there by the gelatin as that substance solidifies again. If the specimen is a half eye, it is first placed so that the concavity faces upward; the gelatin then seeps into all the hollow spaces; it is then turned around so that the cut surface comes to rest on the bottom of the box. Care must be taken in the process to prevent any air bubbles from being caught in the eye.
Priestley claims that such specimens are perfectly suitable for microscopic examination even years later. All that is needed for this purpose is to liquefy the gelatin again by warming it. The same method is used if embedding has not gone according to plan.

Mit ehrerbietigen Grüßen
Ihr dankbar ergebener
E. Fuchs[481]

In the autumn of 1884 Fuchs was appointed Full Professor at Liège University.[482] In keeping with the University's academic traditions, the occasion was marked by his students and colleagues commissioning a portrait lithograph, which was executed by the well-known lithographer Florimond van Loo (1823–1901) in February 1885.[483] (Fig. 32)

The scientific exchange between Fuchs and Arlt continued unabated. In the autumn of 1884 Fuchs sent his teacher this report:

Lüttich 9. October 1884.

Verehrter Herr Hofrath!
I have just received your book on glaucoma.[484] *Let me thank you most cordially and let me express my sincere admiration. Despite your age Ernst Fuchs as Full*[485] *you still best the younger generation in alacrity and energy. The pleasure I draw from this is all the greater the more I feel devoted to you in respect and gratitude. Unfortunately, I was denied the pleasure of seeing you this year in Heidelberg. I made use of the vacations by travelling to England and frequenting the eye clinics there for some time. Nettleship, Priestley Smith, and Brailey are excellent men from whom one can learn a great deal. From England I made a detour to Ireland, which meant it was too late to go to Heidelberg. I subsequently learnt from Professor Swanzy,*[486] *who paid me a visit here on his return* [to Ireland], *that you were in Heidelberg and in good health.*
I am at present engaged in work on the optic nerve (pathol[ological] anatomy),[487] *whose completion will take some time.*
My wife and my little daughter are both well. The former has asked me to convey her cordial greetings to you.

Mit ehrerbietigen Grüssen
Ihr aufrichtig ergebener
E. Fuchs[488]

Fuchs's last letter in this series dates to early February 1885:

Lüttich 6/2 85.

Verehrter Herr Hofrath!
I am happy that what I have done meets with your approval; this is the most rewarding recognition I could wish for. – If I may, I would like to propound in greater detail my views on the point you have touched on. You mention that in the description of glaucomatous eyes I have stated that sometimes there are manifestations of an inflammation of the papilla at the beginning of the glaucomatous process. I have only ever observed this in cases of inflammatory glaucoma and with some regularity when an iridectomy was performed after the first attack. An examination with the ophthalmoscope, once the clarification of the media is far enough advanced, often does not yet reveal an excavation;

instead, it reveals slightly inflamed changes at the head of the optic nerve. If I am not mistaken, I discussed this at one time with Sattler,[489] *who had made similar observations. I have, however, never seen this as a genuine disease of the optic nerve but have treated it as being in the same league as the inflammatory oedema of the conjunctiva, the iris and the ciliary body in acute glaucoma attacks and I have never been in any doubt that the excavation is the result of an increase in pressure. Especially in cases of chronic simple glaucoma, where Jäger*[490] *and his adherents insist on the presence of a primary disease of the optic nerve, I have never seen this moderate inflammation of the optic disc and am quite convinced it simply does not occur.*
If, as you say in your letter, you feel motivated to do work on other topics, I can assure you that the entire ophthalmic world would be deeply beholden to you. The recognition that your work on myopia[491] *alone has met with is conveyed best by the fact that nowadays the majority of ophthalmologists is already eyeing convergence as the root cause of myopia. This turnaround in received wisdom is arguably owed first and foremost to your work.*
I spent the last week in Paris, where I took part in the Conference of the Ophth[almological] Society. It went on for four days and was remarkable for its lack of scientific content. In part utterly nonsensical views were put forward, such as that astigmatism is the main cause of senile cataract, or long exploded treatments were duly rehashed, such as partial tenotomy (Graefe) or the aspiration of soft cataracts, which was practised in England for so long before it was given up. The reception the Parisian ophthalmologists gave their guests was charming and most hospitable. I have not seen anything new by way of operating technique. I myself delivered a brief paper on the anatomy of the optic nerve.[492]
My award-winning monograph[493] *on the prevention of blindness is now available in print and I will send you a copy within the next few days (thanks to the good offices of my father).*
My family are all well. My wife asks me to remember her to you.

Mit ehrerbietigen Grüßen
Ihr aufrichtig ergebener
E. Fuchs[494]

In Liège Fuchs paid special attention to the description of the conus inferior:[495]

Lüttich has at last seen me finish my work on the conus downward. I was the first to draw attention to the categorical difference between the common conus outward, which is usually not congenital but acquired, and the congenital conus downward

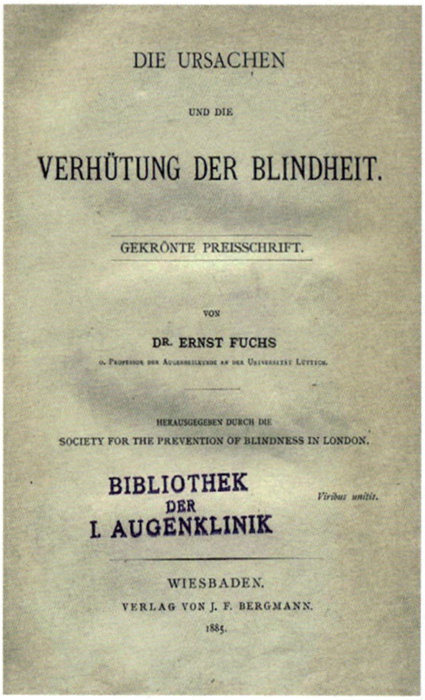
DIE URSACHEN
UND DIE
VERHÜTUNG DER BLINDHEIT.
GEKRÖNTE PREISSCHRIFT.
VON
DR. ERNST FUCHS
o. Professor der Augenheilkunde an der Universität Lüttich.
HERAUSGEGEBEN DURCH DIE
SOCIETY FOR THE PREVENTION OF BLINDNESS IN LONDON.
Viribus unitis.
BIBLIOTHEK DER I. AUGENKLINIK
WIESBADEN.
VERLAG VON J. F. BERGMANN.
1885.

Fig. 33. Ernst Fuchs's prize essay of 1885

and to demonstrate that only the latter often goes hand in hand with a downward tilt of the papilla, pseudoneuritis, higher astigmatism and often deficient acuity of vision. All intermediary stages of the development of optic nerve colobomas were present as well.
This work has met with general approval, and it may well be that even today the conus downward is referred to as Fuchs coloboma[496] *in England.*[497]

Other publications mentioned by Fuchs include his work on the normal anatomy of the eyeball,[498] anomalies of refraction and accommodation,[499] the peripheral atrophy of the optic nerve,[500] lid closure[501] and the normal anatomy of the iris.[502] His former student Daniel Van Duyse (1852–1924)[503] has left detailed notes on the chronology and the content of Fuchs's main areas of work in Liège.[504]

International Recognition for Fuchs's Essay on the Prevention of Blindness (1884)

The crowning achievement of Fuchs's years in Liège was the prize essay on the causes and the prevention of blindness, which he mentioned in the letter to Arlt quoted above. (Fig. 33) This topic had been chosen towards the end of November 1882 for a competition organised by the newly founded Society for the Prevention of Blindness, and the Improvement of the Physique of the Blind at the instigation of its founder, honorary secretary and treasurer, Mathias Roth (1818–1891).[505] The winner of the competition, which was open to essays in German, English, French or Italian, was to be awarded a prize of 2,000 Swiss francs/£80. It was arranged for the award to be presented at the 5th International Congress of Hygiene and Demography in The Hague two years later. The programme for the prize essay was formulated as follows:

1. Causes of Blindness. – a. Influence of heredity, diseases of parents, consanguineous marriages, &c. b. Eye diseases of infancy, various inflammations. c. School period, progressive myopia, &c. d. General diseases, diatheses, various fevers, poisoning, &c. e. Influence of occupations, accidents and injuries, sympathetic ophthalmia. f. Social and climatic influences; infectious eye diseases; unwholesome, overcrowded, ill-lighted dwelling places, &c. g. Defective or total absence of treatment of eye affections.

2. The most appropriate preventive measures are to be stated for each of these groups. a) Legislative measures. b) Hygienic and professional measures. c) Pedagogic measures. d) Medical and philanthropic measures.[506]

After two originally nominated members had withdrawn and had been replaced, the international jury comprised twelve experts from six nations:

Germany:	Professor of Ophthalmology Rudolf BERLIN (1833–1897), Stuttgart[507]
	Professor of Ophthalmology Hermann Ludwig COHN, Breslau[508]
England:	Secretary and Treasurer of the Society for the Prevention of Blindness Mathias ROTH[509]
	Professor of Ophthalmology John Fremlyn STREATFIELD (1828–1886), London[510]
France:	Ophthalmologist Henri COURSSERANT, Paris
	Ophthalmologist Jean-Marie-Théodore FIEUZAL (1836–1888), Paris[511]
	Professor of Hygiene Alexandre-Elzéar LAYET (1840–1916), Bordeaux
Italy:	Professor of Ophthalmology Carlo REYMOND, Torino[512]
	Italy's first Professor of Hygiene, Giuseppe SORMANI (1844–1923), Pavia[513]
Netherlands:	Professor of Ophthalmology Herman SNELLEN, Utrecht[514]
Switzerland:	Professor of Ophthalmology Marc DUFOUR, Lausanne[515]
	Lecturer in Ophthalmology and Secretary Georg/Georges HALTENHOFF, (1843–1915),[516] Lecherer in Ophthalmology (Geneva), Secretary.

Each of the submitted essays featured a motto which was also inscribed on an envelope, alongside the author's name, title and address. These envelopes remained sealed until the submission deadline had expired and the jury had passed the relevant resolution.[517]

By March 31, 1884 seven manuscripts had been submitted – four in German, two in English and one in French. Ernst Fuchs had chosen the motto "Viribus Unitis" [518] for his essay, summing up in a nutshell his conviction that combating the causes of blindness required a multi-faceted attack carried out by a multitude of actors. The jury's decision in favour of Fuchs's essay was unanimous.[519]

The jury's verdict as read out by Haltenhoff in his capacity of secretary reads in translation as follows:

This 545-page manuscript treatise in two volumes, entitled "Die Ursachen und die Verhütung der Blindheit" is an original work of great merit and provides better and more complete answers than its competitors to the wide range of questions raised by this programme. Combining the clinician's personal experience with fail-proof familiarity with the specialist literature on the subject, the author has covered all aspects with a competence, accuracy, sweep and high-mindedness that have captivated all the members of the jury. Having the spirit and the practical, philanthropic purpose of the competition always at the back of his mind and predicating his work on a definition of blindness based on the condition of the social and economic dependency of the blind, the author of the treatise "Viribus unitis" has managed to do justice both to completeness and to science, while at the same time avoiding superfluous statistical data and considerations of pathology and therapy that lie more or less outside the scope of the subject. His work presents a well-coordinated whole, where each chapter may also be profitably consulted on its own. By far the most space is devoted to prophylactic measures designed to reduce the number of the incurably blind. The jury considers it their duty to express the desire that this remarkable treatise be published soon and, if at all possible, translated into other languages, be it at the behest of the English Society for the Prevention of Blindness or on the basis of some other arrangement.[520]

The assessment passed on the treatise Fuchs had submitted underscores its undisputed scientific credentials, the author's comprehensive knowledge of the specialist literature and the wide-ranging perspectives opened up in dealing with the given questions. It was especially praiseworthy in the eyes of the jury that Fuchs had taken practical aspects and the philanthropic orientation of the competition as much into account as a wealth of practical advice on how to avoid irreversible blindness. Here the socio-medical aspects of the competition came into play, reinforced by the presence of the two hygienists in the jury, Layet and Sormani. Fuchs had, for example, given ample space to social hygiene in his discussion of what kind of lighting in schools and at workplaces was considered desirable from an ophthalmologically prophylactic point of view. This is why the prize was awarded to Fuchs and why the jury recommended its early publication in several languages to ensure an international readership.[521]

Two other names stand out among the competitors in the field:[522] the German neuro-ophthalmologist Hermann Wilbrand (1851–1935)[523] and the English innovative eye surgeon Philip Henry Mules (1843–1905).[524]

With his brilliant treatise Fuchs had shown himself fully in line with the ophthalmological tradition of the Vienna Medical School. In 1800, Georg Joseph Beer,[525] founder of the First University Eye Clinic in the world (1812) in Vienna's Allgemeines Krankenhaus, had published at his own initiative a popular treatise on eye care with advice on how to shield the eyes from damage.[526] Beer's grand-disciple Arlt had published a similar monograph in 1846.[527]

In Vienna, Fuchs's treatise was the subject of at least one lengthy, though unbylined, review,[528] which even found space for a quotation of Europe's blindness statistics, which Fuchs himself had put together, and the burden this placed on Europe's economy. In R. E. Dudgeon's translation this reads as follow:

In Europe there is on an average one blind to every 1,000 of population, which will give for all Europe 311,000 blind persons. If we take the daily cost of these per head at only 10d., this implies a yearly cost of above £4,520,000. If we take for granted that one quarter of the blind need no pecuniary assistance, either because they are in easy circumstances or because they can earn their own living, there still remain £3,400,000. If we allow that one-third of all the blind, that is 103,666 persons, would earn 1s. 8d. per diem if they could see, that would make – reckoning 300 working days – £2,480,000. This added to the cost of maintenance, involves an annual loss of £5,880,000 for the states of Europe. On the part of the State, hitherto nothing has been done for the prevention of blindness […].[529]

Breslau ophthalmologist Hermann Cohn,[530] a recognized expert in the field of ophthalmological school hygiene[531] and a member of the jury, called Ernst Fuchs's seminal treatise from a German perspective a *"work of art rich in ideas"*.[532] The work has arguably been appreciated most extensively in the Anglo-American world, which did a great deal towards spreading Fuchs's fame in international specialist circles.[533]

Professor Fuchs's book … appears to us to be a work of exceptional practical value. It connects in a manner hardly to be met with elsewhere the most important results of ophthalmic science with wide questions of philanthropy and social economy. We hope and believe that it will be productive of widespread good, and thus fulfil the aims of its author and of the Society who were the means of calling it into existence.[534]

The French medical press covered the translation of Fuchs's essay in 1885 extensively in a series of announcements and brief reviews.[535]

Liège University was at that stage already beginning to resign itself to Fuchs's departure for Prague. The university's rector filed the following report to the Minister of Interior Affairs and Education on July 6, 1885:

Liège University is at present under threat from a double calamity. The University of Prague wants to carry off Professors Van Beneden and Fuchs.
The Faculty of Medicine has been debating the considerable loss the departure of these two distinguished colleagues would entail. I have the honour of presenting to you a record of the entreaties the Faculty has put forward to the two to persuade them not to accept the advantageous offers they have received.
You have already been preoccupied, Monsieur le Ministre, with steps to ensure that M. Van Beneden will not leave. There is nothing I can add to the representations I have already had the honour of submitting to you.
M. Fuchs, like M. Van Beneden, is a leading exponent of the science he teaches. In spite of still being quite young, his reputation already spans the whole of Europe. The courses he gives are truly remarkable. I would like to add that ophthalmology at a scientific level has been neglected rather badly in Belgium and that the departure of M. Fuchs would leave a void that would oblige us to seek for help from abroad to fill. All that M. Fuchs demands are the material means that would both enable his students to work and him to train specialists. It would, as is well known, be necessary to increase funding for his courses. At a different level, I will continue to plead for a replacement for Hôpital de Bavière and a reconstruction of the buildings housing the clinics.[536]

The entire staff of the Medical Faculty of Liège University closed ranks behind intense efforts to persuade Fuchs not to leave.[537] This went so far as an official petition addressed to Fuchs. In a specially convened meeting of the Faculty on June 11, 1885, the Secretary of the Medical Faculty, Léon Frédéricq, submitted to the Professorial College Fuchs's detailed answer to this petition:

M. Fuchs would like to thank his colleagues for the flattering petition with which they have chosen to honour him and would like to inform them of the state of play concerning the calls he has received from Vienna and Prague. He rates as very low the probability of an appointment to Vienna [University]*; that he has been singled out among the candidates is in his view no more than a honorific gesture that was felt to be his due.*
As for his appointment to [the University of] *Prague, it is not assured either, as the minister has not yet ratified the Faculty's choice. The chair in Prague offers the advantage of a solid material [basis] whereas in Liège the facilities for teaching and the hospital rooms leave a great deal to be desired in every respect. M. Fuchs deplores this state of affairs, which is not conducive to the academic progress of his students, since they are denied the possibility of availing themselves of his laboratory to work there. However, if the University of Liège does not compare favourably with German universities as far as facilities are concerned, it is superior to them by virtue of the cordial relationships between the different members of the Faculty. M. Fuchs doubts whether he will find in Prague as many excellent friends as in Liège, and he assures his colleagues that these considerations will weigh more heavily for his decision than any pecuniary advantages that might be offered to him.*[538]

However, the minister, who had been asked by the Medical Faculty of Liège to support the proposals submitted by Fuchs to improve the situation at the Eye Clinic and the training of the students and medical doctors, failed to rise to the occasion. This finally led Fuchs, who was still without news from Prague, to accept the call the Vienna Medical Faculty had issued in the summer of 1885 and to return to his native Vienna.[539]

According to academic traditions still adhered to at the time, Fuchs organised a formal farewell dinner for his Faculty colleagues. Even decades later, his memories of his first academic position that had given him full autonomy were coloured by nostalgia:

I left Liège with a heavy heart. I had been very happy there: what a beautiful city, what beautiful surroundings, what excellent friends – and time galore for scientific work.[540]

On the occasion of his return to Vienna Fuchs had a portrait photograph made and sent as a memento to several of his former colleagues in Liège. For the chemist Lucien Louis de Koninck (1844–1921) Fuchs added a handwritten, telling dedication:

M. Fuchs, professeur d'ophtalmologie à Liège, où le gouvernement n'a pas su le retenir et d'où il a été appelé à Vienne.[541]

Fuchs's acceptance of the chair in Vienna did not, however, spell the end for his contact with Belgian ophthalmologists. In 1892,[542] 1897,[543] and 1906[544] his former clinical assistant Lucien Leplat,[545] of whom Fuchs thought very highly, was in charge of the French translation of his epoch-making textbook. Even years later Fuchs was still being honoured for what he had achieved in his four years in Liège: in 1901, he was received into the Académie royale de médecine de Belgique as a foreign corresponding member.[546] In 1905, he was awarded honorary membership in the Maatschappij tot Onderstand der Blinden/Société Protectrice des Aveugles in Antwerp/Anvers[547] and in 1907 the Société belge d'ophtalmologie followed suit. His former student Daniel Van Duyse, founder and General Secretary of this society and Professor of Ophthalmology at Gand/Ghent, testified in his comprehensive history of ophthalmology in Belgium in the nineteenth century to Ernst Fuchs's extraordinary capacity by succinctly calling him an "*ophtalmologiste de réputation mondiale*".[548]

Notes

[398] Sammlungen d. Med. Wien. Univ.; Handschriftenarchiv No. 2107.

[399] Erna LESKY, "Aus dem Nachlaß Ferdinand von Arlts im Wiener medizinhistorischen Institut", in: *Klin. Monatsbl. Augenheilk.* 139 (1961), pp. 847–856.

[400] Louis Trasenster (1816–1887). Rector of Liège Univ. until 1886. Cf. Léon-E. HALKIN, *Trasenster contre Kurth*, in: Marcel FLORKIN, Léon-E. HALKIN (ed.), *Chronique de l'Université de Liège*. Université, Liège 1967, pp. 319–333.

[401] Cf. FN 33.

[402] Cf. FUCHS, *Augenarzt* (as in FN 2), pp. 67–68.

[403] At the beginning of the academic year of 1881/1882 Rector Trasenster reported (originally in French) that *"by a decision taken on that same day* [i. e. 26 August 1881], *Dr Ernest Fuchs, private lecturer at the University of Vienna, has been appointed Associate Professor at the Faculty of Medicine. He will be in charge of a course of ophthalmology, of the eye clinic and of the physiology of the senses."* In: *Ouverture solennelle des cours, 17 octobre 1881. Des cours et rapport de M. le recteur Trasenster*. Liège 1881, p. 48. Original of the Certificate of Appointment in the Family archive.

[404] Recte: September, as Fuchs himself indicates in this letter a few lines later.

[405] Reference to Joseph-Augustin Borlée (1817–1907). Taught ophthalmology in addition to other surgical specialties between 1848 and 1881; author of the treatise *Précis clinique et pratique de pathologie chirurgicale spéciale y compris les maladies des yeux.* H. Manceaux, Bruxelles 1872. Cf. IBBO (as in FN 18).

[406] antediluvian = literally, dating from before the biblical Great Flood.

[407] Sammlungen d. Med. Univ. Wien; Handschriftenarchiv No. 2107.

[408] Sir Walter Scott (1771–1832). The novel by Sir Walter Scott Stefan Zweig alludes to is *Quentin Durward* (London–Edinburgh 1823).

[409] Orlando di Lasso, also known as Roland/Orlande de Lassus (1532–1594). Composer of German descent.

[410] César Auguste Jean Guillaume Hubert Franck (1822–1890), French composer of German-Belgian descent.

[411] Maurice Wilmotte (1861–1942), Belgian romanist and medievalist.

[412] Kurt BECK (ed.), *Stefan Zweig auf Reisen*. 2nd edition., S. Fischer Taschenbuch Verlag, Frankfurt a. Main 2004, pp. 173–175 [Stefan Zweig, *Journeys*, tr. Will Stone, Pushkin Press, London 2019 (2010) does not include the author's impressions of Liège, T/N]. Cf. K. BÆDEKER, *Belgien und Holland nebst dem Großherzogtum Luxemburg. Handbuch für Reisende*. Verlag v. Karl Bædeker, Leipzig 1900, pp. 23–33; *Souvenir de Liège*, n. p., n. d.; *Ville de Liége. Notice sur les curiosités à visiter. Nomenclature complète des Voies de Communication*. J. Claesen, Bruxelles 1905*; Exposition Universelle Liége 1905*; *Au Pays de Liége*. Ed. Mathieu Thone; *Souvenir de l'Exposition*. Ed. Nels, Bruxelles n. y.; Meyers Lexikon. 7th ed., vol. 7. Bibliograph. Inst. Leipzig 1927, cols. 1373–1375.

[413] *Plan de la Ville de Liége. Guide-Notice*. J. Claesen, Bruxelles, n. d.

[414] Reference to Jean-Charles van Aubel (1832–1904). Cf. Philipp Christiaan MOLHUYSEN, Petrus Johannes BLOK, *Nieuw Nederlandsch Biografisch Woordenboek* [= *NNBW*] IX, cols. 33–34, accessible online: http://resources.huygens.knaw.nl/retroboeken/nnbw/ (last accessed: 6 Sept. 2022).

[415] After Borlée (cf FN 405) had been pensioned off in February 1881, the entire surg. clinic was merged under Winiwarter, and the governm. decided to create an autonom.

Dept. of Ophthalmology. The Rector of Liège Univ., Louis Trasenster, asked Arlt ro recommend a suitable candidate, as none could be found in Belgium. Other applicants were Georges Claeys (1851–1922) from Ghent, Charles Jamain (b. 1837) from Liège, Constant Loiseau (1838–1890) from Leuven, H. Romiée (b. 1847) from Liège and Daniel van Duyse (1852–1924) from Ghent. Cf. Marcel FLORKIN, "Apports viennois à la Faculté de médecine de Liège", in: FLORKIN/HALKIN (as in FN 400), pp. 217–230, identical with Marcel FLORKIN, "Les Années de Professorat de Karl Gussenbauer, d'Alexander von Winiwarter et d'Ernst Fuchs à la faculté de médecine de Liège", in: Erna LESKY (ed.), *Wien und die Weltmedizin.* Hermann Böhlaus Nachfolger. Vienna/Cologne/Graz 1974, pp. 196–203; HIRSCHBERG , *Geschichte der Augenheilkunde* (as in FN 18), vol. 14/7 [= Reprint vol. V], § 806, p. 81.

416 Named after Ernst of Bavaria, b. 1554, son of Duke Albrecht V, who – in keeping with polit. usage at the time – was appointed to the bishopric of Freising at the age of 11 and to the bishopric of Hildesheim at age 21. In 1581 he was presented with the principality of Liège and in 1583 he became Prince Archbishop of Cologne. In 1585 he was appointed Bishop of Münster (without ordination). His scientific interests, especially in astronomy, inspired the wish to found a university in Liège, a plan that foundered on the resist. put up by Leuven Univ. The duke had acquired a large plot of land in Liège in 1584, which he left to a lay brotherhood called Compagnie de Miséricorde Chrétienne to atone for his lifestyle. The brotherhood built a hospital on the grounds; inauguration in 1606. In memory of Prince Bishop Ernst (d. 1612), the hosp. was called Hôpital de Bavière. Initially the care of the patients was left to the brotherhood. In 1626, the Congrégation des Sœurs Augustines de Bavière was founded, housed in the hospital as a religious community, and patient care was committed to the sisters. When Ernst Fuchs settled in Liège in 1881, the old buildings were still in use. Cf. Marcel FLORKIN, "Les origines de l'Hôpital de Bavière", in: FLORKIN/HALKIN (as in FN 400), pp. 9–22.

1817 Foundation of Liège Univ. at the initiative of King Wilhelm I. Cf. HIRSCHBERG, *Geschichte d. Augenheilkunde* (as in FN 18), vol. 14/VII [= Reprint vol. V], § 786, p. 42; Alphonse LE ROY, *Liber Memorialis. L'Université de Liége depuis sa fondation. Ouvrage rédigé et publié en vertu d'une décision du Conseil Académique, à l'occasion du premier jubilé semi-séculaire de l'Université (3 Novembre 1867).* Carmanne, Liége 1869; Lüttich (Belgium). *Université de Liége*, in: R. KUKULA, K. TRÜBNER (eds.), *Minerva.* Jahrbuch der gelehrten Welt. Yr. 2. 1892–1893. Karl J. Trübner, Strassburg 1893, pp. 399–403; *Liège et son Université.* Ed. Georges Thone, Liège 1929; Marcel FLORKIN, "Le 150e anniversaire de l'Université de Liège et l'histoire de sa Faculté de médecine", in: *Médecine et Hygiène* [Méd. et Hyg.] 25 (1967), pp. 537–538.

417 Jean-Pierre Nuel (1847–1920). Originally from the Grand-Duchy of Luxembourg. Dr med. Ghent (Gand) 1870. Ophthalmol. specialist training in Bonn, Vienna and Utrecht (Donders). 1877–1880 Professor of Ophthalmol. at the Cathol. Univ. of Löwen/Louvain. 1880–1885 Prof. of Physiol. at Ghent/Gand. Fuchs's successor as Professor of Ophthalmology and Physiol. of the Senses at Liège (1885–1919). Cf. VAN DUYSE, *L'Histoire d'Ophtalmologie en Belgique* (as in FN 282), pp. 156–166; IBBO (as in FN 18).

418 The new Univers. Hospital was not built until 1895. Cf. Marcel FLORKIN, "L'enseignement clinique au Vieux-Bavière et au Nouveau-Bavière", in: Marcel FLORKIN,

Léon-E. HALKIN (eds.), *Chronique de l'Université de Liège*. Université, Liège (as in FN 400), pp. 407–431. (For archival material related to the Departm. of Ophthalmolog. and the enforced resignation of Borlée, cf. p. 423).

419 Charles Jamain (b.1837). Originally from France. Studied medicine at Liège. Ophthalmolog. specialis. 1863–1864 under Desmarres and (de) Wecker in Paris. 1865 Established himself in Liège, 1866–1868 médecin-adjoint with the Dir. of the Institut ophtalmique, Nicolas-Joseph Ansiaux (1802–1882). 1868–1900 Ansiaux's successor. Cf. HIRSCHBERG, *Geschichte d. Augenheilkunde* (as in FN 18), vol. 14/VII [= Reprint vol. V], § 791, p. 54; van DUYSE, *L'Histoire d'Ophtalmologie en Belgique* (as in FN 282), pp. 53–54 and 200.

420 Léon Frédéricq (1851–1935). Originally from Ghent (Gand). 1879 Prof. of Physiol. at Liège as the successor of Theodor Schwann (cf. FN 40. From 1883 collaboration with Nuel on a series of treatises entitled *Élements de physiologie humaine à l'usage des étudiants en médecine*, which went through several editions. Cf. FISCHER (as in FN 28); IBBO (as in FN 18); PAGEL (as in FN 13).

421 Cf. FN 40.

422 Theodor SCHWANN, *Mikroskopische Untersuchungen über die Uebereinstimmung in der Struktur und dem Wachsthum der Thiere und Pflanzen*. Sander, Berlin 1839.

423 Cf. GARRISON/MORTON (as in FN 124); Marcel FLORKIN, *Naissance et déviation de la théorie cellulaire dans l'œuvre de Théodore Schwann*. Hermann, Paris 1960. Henry HARRIS, *The Birth of the Cell*. Yale University Press, New Haven/London 1999, pp. 98ff.

424 In 1836 Schwann had succeed in isolating pepsin – his coinage – from animal tissue as the first digestive enzyme. In 1837 he showed that the mechanism of fermentation is caused by yeast. Cf. GARRISON/MORTON (as in FN 124); Theodor SCHWANN, "Ueber das Wesen des Verdauungsprocesses", in: *Arch. Anat. Physiol. wiss. Med.* 1836, pp. 90–138; SCHWANN, "Vorläufige Mittheilung betreffend Versuche über die Weingährung und Fäulniss", in: *Annalen der Physik und Chemie [= Ann. Phys. Chem.]* 41 (1837), pp. 184–193.

425 Marcel FLORKIN, *La personnalité de Théodore Schwann*, in: Marcel FLORKIN, Léon-E. HALKIN (eds.), *Chronique de l'Université de Liège* (as in FN 400), pp. 147–167 and HALKIN, *Le passage de Théodore Schwann de la Faculté de médecine de Louvain à celle de Liège*, in: ibid., pp. 169–179.

426 Édouard Joseph Louis-Marie van Beneden (1846–1910). Originally from Leuven/ Louvain. First Prof. of Zoology in Leiden, 1874 Successor of Theodor Schwann as Prof. of Zoology in Liège. Pioneer in embryol. and genetics, two specialties first emerging at that time. 1883 Initial descript. of meiosis. Cf. HIRSCH; PAGEL (as in FN 13); Obituaries: *Naturwiss. Rundschau* 25 (1910), pp. 362–363; *Nature* 83 (1910), p. 344; Appreciation: Carl RABL, *Édouard van Beneden und der gegenwärtige Stand der wichtigsten von ihm behandelten Probleme*. F. Cohen, Bonn 1915.

427 Reference to Auguste Swaen (1847–1929), Prof. of Anat. and Histol. at Liège Univ., which he also served in the capacity of rector. Cf. Obituaries: *JAMA* 92/25 (1929), pp. 2118–2119.

428 Jean-Baptiste Nicolas Voltaire Masius (1836–1912). Disciple of Schwann and Claude Bernard (1813–1878), the founder of experiment. physiol. in Paris. 1867 Prof. of Descript. Anat. at Liège. Animal experiments. Examination of the medulla together

with Constant Vanlair (cf. FN 429). With the surgeon Winiwarter he played a leading role in the reform committee of Liège Univ., which pushed through Fuchs's call to the newly created ophthal. clinic. Cf. HIRSCH (as in FN 13); Constant VANLAIR, "Notice sur Voltaire Masius", in: *Annuaire de l'Académie royale des Sciences, des Lettres et des Beaux-Arts de Belgique* (1914), pp. 79–116.

429 Constant-François Vanlair (1839–1914). 1868 Assoc. Prof. of Pathol. Anat. and Forensic Pathology at Liège (1872 Full Prof.), where he lectured from 1872 also on the spec. pathol. of internal diseases; from 1873 he also lectured at the Clinic of Geriatric Diseases. Cf. HIRSCH; PAGEL (as in FN 13); Pierre NOLF, "Notice sur Constant Vanlair", in: *Annuaire Académie royale des Sciences, des Lettres et des Beaux-Arts de Belgique* 89 (1923), pp. 125–150.

430 Lucien Leplat (1859–1946). Studied at Liège (graduation in 1882). Joined Borlée's eye clinic while still a student and remained there under Fuchs and Nuel. Together with Camille Lacompte (1843–1930), Leplat took charge of all three French editions of Fuchs's *Textbook* (1892, 1897, 1906). Cf. IBBO (as in FN 18); Lucien LEPLAT, "Ernest FUCHS (1882)", in: Léon HALKIN, Paul HARSIN (eds.), *LIBER MEMORIALIS. L'Université de Liége de 1867 à 1935. Notices biographiques.* Tome III. Faculté de Médecine. Rectorat de l'Université, Liége 1936, pp. 122–124.

431 FUCHS, *Augenarzt* (as in FN 2), pp. 67–70.

432 Ibid., pp. 88–89.

433 Max Knies (1851–1917). Originally from Kassel. Studied at Heidelberg (Dr med. 1874). Ophthalmol. specialist training in Heidelberg (Kühne, Becker), Bonn (Saemisch) and Zürich (Horner, habilitation). 1888 Assoc. Prof. in Freiburg. Recognised authority on glaucoma. Cf. FISCHER (as in FN 28); HIRSCHBERG, *Geschichte der Augenheilkunde* (as in FN 18), vol. 15/2 [= Reprint vol. VI], § 1187, pp. 264–265; IBBO (as in FN 18).

434 Max KNIES, "Über sympathische Augenerkrankung", in: *Beiträge zur Ophthalmologie als Festgabe Friedrich Horner zur Feier des fünfundzwanzigsten Jubiläums seiner academischen Lehrthätigkeit gewidmet von Marc Dufour in Lausanne, Otto Haab und Max Knies in Zürich, Julius Michel in Würzburg, Wilhelm Schoen in Leipzig, und O. F. Wadsworth in Boston, USA.* J. F. Bergmann, Wiesbaden 1881, pp. 53–97.

435 Cf. FN 288.

436 See Ch. 7.

437 H. Romiée. Originally from Liège. 1872 Established himself in Liège as an eye specialist. Eye surgeon at Liège Hospital and the Hospices Civiles in Verviers. Cf. Van DUYSE, *Histoire d'Ophtalmologie en Belgique* (as in FN 282), p. 213.

438 Reference to Charles Jamain. Cf. FN 419.

439 Sammlungen d. Med. Univ. Wien; Handschriftenarchiv No. 2107.

440 For the record: Arlt was born on 18 April 1812.

441 Karl STELLWAG von CARION, *Abhandlungen aus dem Gebiete der praktischen Ophthalmologie. Ergänzungen zum Lehrbuche.* Unter Mitwirkung von K. Wedl und E. Hampel. W. Braumüller, Vienna 1882. Cf. FN 168.

442 A reference to Erasmus Hampel, who is attested as assistant at Stellwag's clinic (Rooms 57a, b) at the Allgem. Krankenhaus only for the winter semester of 1880/81.

443 Alexander IWANOFF, "Ueber Conjunctivitis und Keratitis phlyctaenularis", in: *Klin. Monatsbl. Augenheilk.* 7 (1869), pp. 462–470.

[444] Alexander Iwanoff (1836–1880). Studied in Moscow, Montpellier and St. Petersburg (Graduation 1867). While still an undergraduate, ophthalmol. specialist training in Heidelberg (Knapp), Wiesbaden (Pagenstecher) and Vienna (v. Arlt). After two more years he spent on study trips 1869 Prof. of Ophthalmology in Kiev. Cf. HIRSCH (as in FN 13); HIRSCHBERG, *Geschichte der Augenheilkunde* (as in FN 18), vol. 14/7 [= Reprint vol. III], § 917, pp. 247–250; IBBO (as in FN 18).

[445] Ernst FUCHS, "Ueber glaukomatöse Hornhauttrübung", in: *Bericht über die Dreizehnte Versammlung der Ophthalmologischen Gesellschaft. Heidelberg 1881*. Redigirt durch F. C. Donders, W. Hess and W. Zehender. Universitäts-Buchdruckerei von Adler's Erben. Rostock 1881, pp. 73–79 (discussion pp. 79–80); FUCHS, "Ueber die Trübung der Hornhaut bei Glaucom", in: *Graefes Archiv* 27/III (1881), pp. 66–92.

[446] Jakob Hock (1831–1890). Studied at Vienna Univ. (Dr med. 1861). Student of Eduard Jaeger v. Jaxtthal. 1872 Habilitation at Vienna Univ. One of the founder members and Head Physician of the Eye Dept. at the Wr. Allgem. Poliklink. 1882 Foundation of a priv. eye clinic. Eye surgeon at the Rothschildspital and at the Blindeninstitut at the Hohe Warte. Cf. HEID (as in FN 165), pp. 139–145; HIRSCH (as in FN 13); HIRSCHBERG, *Geschichte der Augenheilkunde* (as in FN 18), vol. 15/2 [= Reprint, vol. VI], § 1246, p. 406; IBBO (as in FN 18); PAGEL (as in FN 13); ÖBL (as in FN 11); DEIMER, *Poliklinik* (as in FN 200), pp. 157–158.

[447] Jakob HOCK, "Fall von Cysticercus cellulosae unter der Bindehaut des Augapfels", in: *Mittheil. d. aerztl. Vereins in Vienna* 3 (1874), pp. 89–95. Cf. the references in: *Vierteljahresschr. prakt. Heilk.* 32/3 (1875), p. 107.

[448] Ludwig Herz (b. 1855). 1881–1883 Assist. under Arlt, 1883–1888 Assist. under Stellwag, died prematurely. EISENBERG 2 (as in FN 13); HIRSCHBERG, *Geschichte der Augenheilkunde* (as in FN 18), vol. 15/2 [= Reprint, vol. VI], § 1246, p. 376.

[449] Sammlungen d. Med. Univ. Wien; Handschriftenarchiv No. 2107.

[450] Julia-Rosina Mayr (or Mayer, 28 March 1859–12 June 1919). Daughter of Gustav May(e)r, Prof. at the Industrialschule in Pest, and Alexandrine Pazzani. Cf. Certificate of Birth and Baptism, Parish Pest–St. Joseph 1520/1860 of 1 December 1860. Certified translation from Latin; Ahnenpaß Wilhelm Hofbauer (as in p. 11 Family archive).

[451] Cf. *Extrait des Registres de l'Etat-Civil de la Commune de Liège pour l'année 1882, reposant au Greffe du Tribunal civil de première instance, séant à Liège*. Original in the Family archive.

[452] Cf. Trauungs-Schein. Aus dem pfarrlichen Trauungsbuche Tom. 21, fol. 27, Pfarre Landstraße vom 22. Juni 1882 (copy in Family archive) and Trauungs-Protokoll 1882–1885, Tom. 21, fol. 27.

[453] Reference to Fuchs's participation in the annual Conference of the Dt. Ophthalmol. Gesellsch.

[454] Cataplasm = poultice, "a soft, usu. heated mass of material applied to the skin to alleviate pain, inflammation, or irritation, to act as an emollient, or to stimulate the circulation locally." (Shorter Oxford Dictionary, vol. 2, p. 2306). Cataplasms were commonly applied in an age where medical thinking still revolved around humoral-pathological ideas of the sort Fuchs had encountered early on in his career. They are still applied today, if in a modified form. Cf. "Cataplasma", in: *Universal-Lexicon der practischen Medicin und Chirurgie von Andral, Bégin, Blandin, Bouillaud, Bonvier, Cruveilhier, Cullerier, Devergie, Dugès, Dupuytren, Foville, Guibourt, Jolly, Lallemand,*

Londe, Magendie, Ratier, Rayer, Roche und Sanson. Frei bearbeitet [...] von einem Verein deutscher Aerzte. Dritter Band. Blepharoptosis – Cinae. H. Franke'sche Verlags-Expedition, Leipzig 1837, pp. 464–469; "Kataplasma", in: Irmgard FREY, Lenore LÜBKE-SCHMID, Walter WENZL, *Krankenpflegehilfe.* Alle Fächer für Ausbildung und Praxis. 11., völlig neue bearbeitete Aufl., Georg Thieme Verlag, Stuttgart 2002, pp. 443–444.

455 The reference is to Eduard/Edouard Meyer, cf. FN 254.

456 Cf. FN 350.

457 Sammlungen d. Med. Univ. Wien; Handschriftenarchiv No. 2107.

458 Cf. FN 327.

459 Sammlungen d. Med. Univ. Wien; Handschriftenarchiv No. 2107.

460 Coterie = a small group of people with shared interests or tastes, especially one that is exclusive of other people. It can no longer be established with any certainty what clique Fuchs is referring to here. They were obviously so well known that no names were needed.

461 Sammlungen d. Med. Univ. Wien; Handschriftenarchiv No. 2107.

462 Cf. FUCHS, *Augenarzt* (as in FN 2), pp. 73–74.

463 The Fuchses' first child, Rosa, was born on 17 February 1884. Cf. Family archive.

464 Sammlungen d. Med. Univ. Wien; Handschriftenarchiv Nr. 2107.

465 Joseph Priestley Smith (1845–1933). Training at Queen's Hospital of his native Birmingham and at Moorfields Hospital, London. 1874–1916 Eye surgeon at Queen's Hospital, 1895–1900 Lecturer in Birmingham, 1900–1916 Prof. in Birmingham. Worldwide recognition as an expert on glaucoma. Construction of a perimeter and a tonometer. 1881 Founder of the *Ophthalmic Review*. Cf. IBBO (as in FN 18); Obituaries: *Lancet I* (1933), p. 1039; *BMJ* 1933/1, p. 850 and 898; *Brit. J. Ophthalmol.* 17 (1933), p. 442.

466 A note has been added in pencil in the left margin of the page: *"X. part I. p. 25"*. It refers to (Joseph) Priestley SMITH, "Glaucoma", in: *Royal Ophthalmic Hospital Reports* [= *Ophth. Rev.*], vol. X (1882), pp. 25–32.

467 Hubert Sattler, cf. FN 220.

468 Ludwig Mauthner, cf. FN 200. Whether or not this cryptic remark implies criticism of Mauthner, it is presumably a reference to the latter's monograph *Die Lehre vom Glaukom*. Bergmann, Wiesbaden 1882.

469 Cf. Reinhard OTTO, "Über das Vorkommen Fuchs'scher peripherer Atrophie des Sehnerven", in: *Untersuchungen über Sehnervenveränderungen bei Arteriosclerose.* Springer. Berlin 1893, pp. 123–128.

470 Sammlungen der Med. Univ. Wien; Handschriftenarchiv No. 2107.

471 Ernst FUCHS, "Anatomische Miscellen: III. Glaucoma inflammatorium", in: *Graefes Archiv* 30/Abth. III (1884), pp. 123–138.

472 Interesting and instructive though it would be to study Fuchs's petitions in the original, the relevant files, according to a letter from the archivist of Liège Univ., Mme Marie-Élisabeth Henneau, to the author in February 2005, have not been preserved in the Archive of Liège University.

473 Joseph Hasner Ritter v. Artha (1819–1892). Originally from Prague where he also studied (Dr med. 1842). 1843 Assist. at the Eye Clinic of Prague Univ. under Johann Nepomuk Fischer (1777–1847). 1848 Habilitation in Ophthalmolog. 1852 Assoc.

Prof. 1853–1855 Dean of the Professorial College of the Med. Fac. 1856–1883 Full Prof. and Dir. of the Eye Clinic at Prague Univ. as successor of Ferdinand Arlt, when the latter had received a call to Vienna's Univ. Eye Clinic. Cf. HIRSCH; EULNER (as in FN 13); ÖBL (as in FN 11); PAGEL (as in FN 13); WURZBACH (as in FN 15).

474 Fuchs is obviously referring to two new items published in the *Wiener med. Wochenschr.* No. 1 of 5 January 1884 (a) and No. 2 of 12 January 1884 (b):

a) *Having had his clinic reduced by one half* [owing to the division in 1882 of the old Charles University Prague into the Deutsche Univ. Prag, which existed until 1945, and the Czech Univ. of Prague, A/N], *Herr Professor v. Hasner has recently handed in his resignation. The Professorial College of Prague Univ. has, with great regret, taken note of the resignation of this outstanding professor and has filed a report to the Ministry of Education. The German medical faculty in Prague suffers a great loss through the resignation of two excellent teachers, v. Hasner and, presumably, Toldt* [Carl Toldt (1840–1920) as in FN 599. Cf. *Wiener med. Wochenschr.* 34 (1884), cols. 22–23.

b) *We have received news from Prague that the medical Professorial College has agreed to propose Herr Prof. Fuchs, Lüttich, primo loco as the successor of Hasner. In addition to Prof. Fuchs's name those of Prof Sattler, Erlangen, and of the lecturers Bergmeister and Reuss have been put forward to the Ministry. Lecturer Dr Schenk* [recte: Adolf Schenkl, b.1841, Dr med. 1865, Dr chir. et Mag. obstetr. 1866 Prague Univ., 1870–1874 Assist. under Hasner, 1875 Habilitation, 1886 unsalaried tit. Assoc. Prof. Cf. ÖSTA/AVA Wien, 5 Prag Med Schenkl, Fasz. 1123 U2 Prof. Qu–Z], *has been charged with substituting for the Chair of Ophthalmology.* Cf. *Wiener med. Wochenschr.* 34 (1884), col. 54.

475 Sammlungen d. Med. Univ. Wien; Handschriftenarchiv No. 2107.

476 ÖSTA/AVA Wien, 5 G Prag Medicin Ophthalmologie Faszikel 1160. According to a letter from the archivist to the author (Nov. 2004), a number of files concerning the period of 1853–1883 have been transferred to Prague Univ. This may well account for the lacunae we will encounter further down this road.

477 The vacancy at the Eye Clinic of the Germ. Univ. of Prague was filled in 1886, all of three years later, with Arlt's former student Hubert Sattler (cf. FN 220), after Fuchs had been appointed Full Prof. at the 2nd Univ. Eye Clinic in Vienna. Initially, the Deanery of the Med. Fac. of the Dt. Univ. Prag had submitted on June 8, 1884 to the Ministerium f. Cultus und Unterricht in Vienna the following proposal: primo loco Otto Becker (cf. FN 178), secundo loco Ernst Fuchs, tertio loco Hubert Sattler. The reason why the Prague eye clinic had remained vacant for so long was stated as follows: *This proposal was not immediately acted upon because in consequence of the death of Professor Dr Jaeger Ritter von Jaxtthal in July 1884 the Second Department and the Clinic of Ophthalmology at Vienna University also fell vacant. The Professorial College of this University having also included Fuchs and Sattler in its* terna, *it was not considered feasible to prioritise Prague's German medical faculty over filling the vacancy at the University Eye Clinic in Vienna.* The Minister für Cultus und Unterricht, Paul Gautsch Frh. v. Frankenthurn (1851–1918), had given precedence to Sattler, primarily because, unlike Becker, he was an Austrian subject. The Emperor gave his consent to Sattler's appointment on 2 March 1886. Cf. ÖSTA/AVA Wien, 5 Prag Medizin Sattler. Vortrag d. Ministers Gautsch an Kaiser Franz Joseph I. v. 26. Februar 1886.

478 (Joseph) Priestley SMITH, "Modes of Preserving and Drawing Ophthalmic Specimens", in: *Ophthalmic Review* II (1883), pp. 69–76.

479 Carlo Reymond (1833–1911). Originally from Albertville/France. Studied in Torino, ophthalmol. specialist training under Desmarres and Sichel in Paris. 1876 Prof. in Torino. Pioneer of antisept. methods of operations in Italy. Member of the jury that awarded the first prize of the Society for the Prevention of Blindness in 1884 to Ernst Fuchs's *The Causes and the Prevention of Blindness*. (For more details, see the next section in this chapter). Cf. HIRSCHBERG, *Geschichte der Augenheilkunde* (as in FN 18), Vol 14/5-7 [= Reprint vol. IV (1977)], pp. 70–72.

480 Named after the Würzburg pathol. anatomist Heinrich Müller (1820–1864), who made a name for himself by discovering a great number of pathol. changes in the eye. Ingredients: potassium bichromate-sodium sulphate = bichromate potash 2.5 g, sodium sulphate 1.00 g, acqu. destil. 100,0 ccm. This was the recipe he provided in 1855 for a solution to make tissue sufficiently hard for microscop.-histol. examination. Cf. HIRSCHBERG, *Geschichte der Augenheilkunde* (as in FN 18), vol. 15/2 [= Reprint vol. VI], § 1181–83, pp. 243–255; Georg STEHLI, *Das Mikrotom und die Mikrotomtechnik. Eine Einführung in die Praxis der Mikrotomie*. Franckh'sche Verlagshandlung 1913, p. 28; Georg SCHMORL, *Die pathologisch-histologischen Untersuchungsmethoden*. 16th rev. ed., ed. by P. Geipel, F. C. Vogel, Berlin 1934, p. 35.

481 Sammlungen d. Med. Univ. Wien; Handschriftenarchiv No. 2107.

482 According to the records at Liège University, Fuchs's promotion became effective by royal decree of 13 September 1884. Cf. *Ouverture solennelle des cours 20 octobre 1884*. Discours et rapport du recteur Trasenster. Liège 1884, p. 42. Writing from memory, Fuchs later dated his promotion to the spring of 1884. Cf. FUCHS, *Augenarzt* (as in FN 2), p. 75.

483 Cf. WYKLICKY, *Geschichte der Augenheilkunde* (as in FN 354), p. 57.

484 Ferdinand ARLT, *Zur Lehre vom Glaucom*. Wilhelm Braumüller, Vienna 1884.

485 Arlt had turned 73 that year.

486 Sir Henry Rosborough Swanzy (1844–1913). Studied at Univ. Dublin, Vienna and Berlin. Ophthalmol. training as assist. under Albrecht v. Graefe in Berlin. 1866 Army surgeon during the Prussian-Austrian War. After his return to his native Ireland, leading position at the National Eye and Ear Infirmary in Dublin. 1897–1899 Chairman of the Ophthalmic Society of the United Kingdom, 1906–1908 Chairman of the Royal Society of Surgeons of Ireland. Cf. HIRSCHBERG, *Geschichte der Augenheilkunde* (as in FN 18) (Reprint vol. IV (1977), Vol. 3, Section 10, § 709, pp. 438–440.

487 Ernst FUCHS, "Die periphere Atrophie des Sehnerven", in: *Graefes Archiv* 31/Abth. I (1885), pp. 177–200.

488 Sammlungen d. Med. Univ. Wien; Handschriftenarchiv No 2107.

489 Hubert Sattler, cf. FN 220.

490 Reference to Eduard Jaeger v. Jaxtthal.

491 Ferdinand ARLT, *Über die Ursachen und die Entstehung der Kurzsichtigkeit*. Wilhelm Braumüller, Vienna 1876.

492 Ernst FUCHS, "Étude microscopique sur le nerf optique", in: *Arch. d'Ophtal.* 1885, p. 173. The paper was delivered to the Société Française d'Ophtalmologie in 1885.

493 For more details, cf. the section below.

494 Sammlungen d. Med. Univ. Wien; Handschriftenarchiv, No. 2107.

495 Ernst FUCHS, "Beitrag zu den angeborenen Anomalien des Sehnerven", in: *Graefes Archiv* 28/Abth. I (1882), pp. 139–169.

496 Cf. ALBERT/EDWARDS (as in FN 38), p. 88; Adolf Ritter von SZILY, "Der Conus nach unten", in: *Centralbl. prakt. Ophthalmolog.* 7 (1883), pp. 353ff; Ernst KRAUPA, "Beiträge zur Morphologie des Augenhintergrundes II", in: *Graefes Archiv* 105 (1921), pp. 865–879; Adalbert FUCHS, Erich PRESSBURGER, "Myopia inversa", in: *Arch. Ophthalmol.* 37 (1947), pp. 722–739; Malcolm V. GRAHAM, Graham J. WAKEFIELD, "Bitemporal visual field defects associated with anomalies of the optic discs", in: *Brit. J. Ophthalmol.* 57 (1973), pp. 307–314.

497 FUCHS, *Augenarzt* (as in FN 2), p. 76. See Ch. 7.

498 Ernst FUCHS, "Beiträge zur normalen Anatomie des Augapfels", in: *Graefes Archiv* 30/ Abth. IV (1884), pp. 1–60.

499 Ernst FUCHS, "Beiträge zu den Anomalien der Refraction und Accomodation. (Zur Entstehung der Myopie/Myopie bei Cataracta senilis incipiens/Sympathische Accomodationslähmung)", in: *Klin. Monatsbl. f. Ophthalmolog.* 22 (1884), pp. 14–24.

500 FUCHS, *Die periphere Atrophie des Sehnerven*, as in FN 487.

501 Ernst FUCHS, "Zur Physiologie und Pathologie des Lidschlusses", in: *Graefes Archiv* 31/Abth. II (1885), pp. 97–120.

502 Ernst FUCHS, "Zur Anatomie der Iris", in: *Klin. Monatsbl. Augenheilk.* 23 (1885), pp. 467–478; FUCHS, "Beiträge zur normalen Anatomie der menschlichen Iris", in: *Graefes Archiv* 31/Abth. III (1885), pp. 39–86.

503 Prof. of Ophthalmol. at the Univ. of Gand/Ghent 1905–1922. Cf. Obituary, in: *Brit. J. Ophthalmol.* Year 192, p. 42.

504 Duyse's list does not provide any details of Fuchs's actual publications. Some of the topics he mentions were dealt with in Fuchs's German publications. See Ch. 13 (Catalogue of Published Works): 1881 *"Phénomène entoptique; le cautère, à diriger contre les affections cornéennes; Le trouble cornéen dans la glaucome dépend d'un œdème; La conjunctivite gonorrhétique; 1882: Contribution à l'étude des anomalies du nerf optique; L'anatomie pathologique du sarcome du tractus uvéal; 1883: L'irido-dialyse sans hémorrhagie; 1884: Contributions à l'anatomie pathologique de l'œil; Glaucome inflammatoire; Iris syphilitique; Myopie dans la cataracte sénile débutante; Contribution à la genèse de la myopie; Paralyse sympathique de l'accommodation; 1885: Contribution à l'anatomie normale de l'iris humain; Contribution à la physiologie et à la pathologie de la fermeture des paupières; Kyste libre dans la chambre antérieure; Trouble visuel par anisométropie; Forme particulière d'asthénopie musculaire."* Cf. van DUYSE, *L'Histoire de l'ophtalmologie en Belgique* (as in FN 282), pp. 148–155.

505 Mathias Roth (1818–1891). Originally from Hungary. 1839 Dr med. Univ. of Pavia. In Hungary orientation towards homeopathy, practised also as an orthopaedist. Advocate for the use and continued development of physical treatment methods. Took an active part in the 1848 revolution under the leadership of Hungarian nationalist Lajos Kossuth (1802–1894) to bring about Hungary's secession from the Habsburg Monarchy. Fled to London in 1849. Active at the Hahnemann Hospital, member of the Hahnemann Med. Soc. Publications on homeopathic topics, movement therapy, social hygiene measures (prevention of blindness, improvement of the lot of the blind). 1880 Foundation of the Society for the Prevention of Blindness, headquartered at 48, Wimpole Street, London (address of Roth's practice). This put him in touch with

internationally renowned homeopath Robert Ellis Dudgeon (d. 1904), the translator of Fuchs's prize essay into English. Cf. https://www.sueyounghistories.com/2008-10-08-mathias-roth-1818-e28093-1891 (last accessed: 6 Sept. 2022); Robert Ellis DUDGEON, Obituary: "*The memory of Dr Robert E. Dudgeon we honor and we regard him as the greatest homeopathic physician that has lived*", in: *Medical Century* [= Med. Cent.] 12 (1904), p. 352.

[506] Cf. "Genf. Preisaufgabe über die Verhütung der Blindheit", in: *Klin. Monatsbl. f. Augenheilk.* 21 (1883), pp. 25–27, and Ernst FUCHS, *Die Ursachen und die Verhütung der Blindheit.* Gekrönte Preisschrift. Herausgegeben durch die Society of the Prevention of Blindness in London. Bergmann, Wiesbaden 1885, pp. 237–238.

[507] Rudolf Berlin (1833–1897). Studied medicine in Göttingen, Würzburg and Erlangen. Ophthalmolog. specialist training under Albrecht v. Graefe in Berlin, then assist. under Alexander Pagenstecher (1828–1879) in Wiesbaden and at the Surg. Clinic in Tübingen. 1861 Establishment of his own eye clinic in Stuttgart. 1870 Habilitation in physiol. optics at the Univ. of Techn. in Stuttgart. 1875 Prof. of Comparative Ophthalmology at Stuttgart's Veterinary University. 1882 Foundation of the *Zeitschr. f. vergleich. Ophthalmolog.* 1887 Coinage of the term dyslexia. 1889–1897 Full Prof. at Rostock Univ. (1895 Dean of the Med. Fac., 1897 Rector). Cf. EULNER; PAGEL (as in FN 13).

[508] Cf. FN 306.

[509] Cf. FN 505.

[510] Cf. FN 272.

[511] Jean-MarieThéodore Fieuzal (1836–1888). Studied medicine in Paris. Ophthalm. specialisation. Director of the Hospice national des Quinze-Vingts, which he made the leading ophthalmol. centre for France's poor, having equipped it with a laboratory. 1883 Foundation of the *Bulletin de la Clinique nationale ophtalmologique*. In the year before his death he inaugurated the *Annales du laboratoire de l'Hospice*. French translator of Fuchs's prize essay: Ernst FUCHS, *Causes et prévention de la cécité.* (Mémoire couronné). Traduction par le Docteur Fieuzal. G. Steinheil, Paris 1885. Cf. PAGEL (as in FN 13).

[512] Cf. FN 479.

[513] Giuseppe Sormani (1844–1923). 1879–1919 Chair of Hygiene. Founder of an experim. lab at Pavia Univ. as Italy's first Full Professor of this specialty. Experim. studies on the pathogen causing tuberculosis; prophylactic measures against infectious diseases and against epidemics (tuberculosis, cholera, typhus) and tetanus. Pres. of the Reale Società Italiana d'Igiene. Cf. FISCHER (as in FN 28); www.treccani.it/enciclopedia/giuseppe-sormani (last accessed: 6 Sept. 2022).

[514] Cf. FN 292.

[515] Cf. FN 305.

[516] Georg/Georges Haltenhoff (1843–1915). Studied in Würzburg and Zürich (Dr med.). Ophthalmol. specialist training under Horner (Zürich), Graefe (Berlin) and Liebreich (Paris). Founded a self-financed polyclinic for indigent eye patients in Geneva in the mid-1870s, which he led himself for more than 2 decades, then Director of the Eye Department of the Municipal Polyclinic; from 1910 Director of a small autonomous eye clinic. 1874 Habilitation in Geneva, 1891 Assoc. Prof., 1903 Full Prof. and founder of the Univ. Eye Clinic Genève. Special interest in eye hygiene.

1891 Founder of the Societé des Messieurs de la Croix-Rouge and, in 1902, of the Association suisse-romande pour le bien des aveugles. Cf. *IN MEMORIAM Dr Georges Haltenhoff, Professeur d'Ophtalmologie à l'Université de Genève.* 8 juin 1843–25 avril 1915. Lausanne, Imprim. Hoirs Borgeaud 1915. (With contributions by J. Reverdin, Weber, E. Götz, Rehfous, G. Porte, C. Picot, A. Bernoud, Gourfein-Welt and P.-G. Piccard).

517 Cf. "Genf. Preisaufgabe über die Verhütung der Blindheit", in: *Klin. Monatsbl. f. Ophthalmolog.* 21 (1883), pp. 25–27.

518 VIRIBUS UNITIS [= With united forces] was the motto of Austria's Emperor, Franz Joseph I. (1830–1916). It is just conceivable that Fuchs chose the motto as a public, if encoded, avowal of his loyalty to Austria-Hungary to recommend himself for a professorship in Vienna.

519 Cf. FUCHS, *Die Ursachen und die Verhütung der Blindheit*, as in FN 506, p. 238. *Annales d'oculistique* 92 (1884), p. 142; FUCHS, *Augenarzt* (as in FN 2), p. 78, FN 30; Cinquième Congrès International d'Hygiène et de Démographie à La Haye (du 21 au 27 août 1884). Comptes Rendus et Mémoires publiés par le Secrétaire Général avec le concours de MM. les Decrétaires des Sections. Tome 1. Imprimerie Sud-Hollandaise, La Haye 1884, p. 174.

520 Cf. FUCHS, *Die Ursachen und die Verhütung der Blindheit*, as in FN 506, p. 238. Part of the jury's verdict, which is marked by its sincere appreciation of Fuchs's achievement, in German translation in LESKY, *Wien. Med. Schule* (as in FN 12), p. 492.

521 The treatise was published in 1885 in German, English, French, and Russian, and in 1890 in Italian: Ernst FUCHS, *Die Ursachen und die Verhütung der Blindheit.* Gekrönte Preisschrift. Herausgegeben durch die Society of the Prevention of Blindness in London. Bergmann, Wiesbaden 1885; FUCHS, *The Causes and the Prevention of Blindness.* Translated by R. E. Dudgeon, with a Few Notes by M. Roth. Baillière, Tindall & Cox, London 1885; FUCHS, *Causes et prévention de la cécité.* (Mémoire couronné). Traduction par le Docteur Fieuzal. G. Steinheil, Paris 1885; FUCHS, *O prichinakh i preduprezhdenii sliepoti.* Perevod s niemetskavo. E. I. Fyodoroff, Kiev 1885; FUCHS, *Intorno alle cause della cecità ed al modo di prevenirla.* VIRIBUS UNITIS. Saggio che ottenne il Premio di L. 2000 dalla Società inglese di Prevenzione della Cecità. Tradotto e pubblicato a cura della medesima società italiana. Tipografia Bonducciana – A. Meozzi, Firenze 1890.

522 Cf. James E. LEBENSOHN, "Professor Ernst Fuchs (June 14, 1851–November 21, 1930)", in: *Americ. J. Ophthalmol.* 34 (1951), pp. 772–774.

523 Hermann Wilbrand (1851–1935). Studied at Gießen and Strasbourg (Dr med. 1875). Ophthalmol. specialist training in Strasbourg under Ludwig Laqueur (1819–1909) and in Breslau under Carl Friedrich Richard Förster (cf. FN 263). 1879 Established himself as an eye specialist in Hamburg. 1905 Dir. of the Eye Department at Hamburg's Municip. Hospital. 1919–1923 Full Prof. at Hamburg Univ.; main area of interest: neuro-ophthalmology. Together with Alfred Saenger (1860–1921) publication of the monumental work *Die Neurologie des Auges*, Munich/Wiesbaden 1899–1927. Cf. EULNER (as in FN 13); GORIN (as in FN 38), p. 158; IBBO (as in FN 18); PAGEL (as in FN 13).

[524] Philip Henry Mules (1843–1905). Surgeon at the Royal Eye Hospital in Manchester; eye surgeon at Wrexham Infirmary in Gresford/Denbighshire. Cf. FISCHER (as in FN 28); IBBO (as in FN 18); "Obituary Philip Henry Mules", in: *Brit. Med. J.* Sept. 9, (1905), p. 610.

[525] Georg Joseph BEER (1763–1821). Originally from Vienna. Initially destined for a theol. career, he used his artistic skills to become an anat. draughtsman and demonstrator under the anat. and ophthalmol. Joseph Barth (1745–1818), who refused to give him lessons in ophthalmology; studied at Vienna Univ. (Dr med. 1786). Established his own practice in his private apartment, with two rooms set aside for the free stationary treatment of indigent patients. 1802 Habilitation at Vienna Univ. 1806 Transformation of his practice into a state-funded out-patient clinic, appointment as eye specialist to minister to the city's poor. Tried for many years to bring about the emancipation of ophthalmology from general surgery and the creation of a Chair of Ophthalmology and a clinic at Vienna Univ. 1812 Creation in Vienna of the first eye clinic in the world attached to a university under his own direction as Assoc. Prof. at Vienna's Allgem. Krankenhaus. 1818 Full Prof. and elevation of ophthalm. to the status of an obligatory subject in tuition and testing. Trailblazing teacher of the new specialty, who attracted students from all over Europe and the USA. Main work: *Lehre von den Augenkrankheiten* (2 vols. 1813, 1817). Founding father of ophthalmol. on a clinical-empirical basis still heavily influenced by contemporary natural philosophical thinking. Advocate of intracapsul. cataract extraction and iridectomy for the formation of an artificial pupil. Cf. UA Wien, Akten d. Med. Fak. Personalakt Georg Josef Beer, Box 78; HIRSCHBERG, *Geschichte der Augenheilkunde* (as in FN 18), vol. 14/1, Engelmann, Leipzig 1911, pp. 325–342 and 491–499; IBBO (as in FN 18); ÖBL (as in FN 11); WURZBACH (as in FN 15); Georg PREYSS, *Rede zum Andenken Georg Josef Beer's, gehalten bei Gelegenheit der siebenten Jahresfeier der wissenschaftlichen Thätigkeit des Doctoren-Collegiums der Wiener medicinischen Facultät.* Ditmarsch, Vienna 1857; HEID (as in FN 165), pp. 13–17; Wolfgang MÜNCHOW, "Geschichte der Augenheilkunde", in: Karl VELHAGEN, *Der Augenarzt.* vol. IX, Thieme, Leipzig 1983, pp. 347–366; Gabriela SCHMIDT-WYKLICKY, Helmut GRÖGER, "Georg Josef Beer (1763–1821). Leben und Werk des Begründers der ältesten Universitäts-Augenklinik", in: *Spektrum Augenheilk.* 26 (2012), pp. 266–272.

[526] Georg Joseph BEER, *Pflege gesunder und geschwächter Augen, nebst einer Vorschrift, wie man sich bei plötzlichen Zufällen an den Augen, welche nicht eine eigentliche medicinisch-chirurgische Kenntniß fordern, selbst helfen kann.* Weidmannsche Buchhandlung, und zu haben bey dem Verfasser. Vienna/Leipzig 1800.

[527] Ferdinand ARLT, *Die Pflege der Augen im gesunden und kranken Zustande, nebst einem Anhange über Augengläser, allgemein fasslich dargestellt.* Prague 1846. Cf. Gabriela SCHMIDT-WYKLICKY, "Ansätze zur Prävention und Behandlung von Augenkrankheiten im Rahmen der Wiener Schule des 19. Jahrhunderts: Von der Volksaufklärung bis zur wissenschaftlichen Publizistik", in: *Mitteil. d. Julius-Hirschberg-Gesellsch. zur Geschichte d. Ophthalmologie* (in print).

[528] The title of the monograph, however, was misquoted as "Die Ursachen und die Verhinderung [sic!] der Blindheit" […], in: *Wiener med. Presse* 26 (1885), cols. 1031–1033.

[529] Ibid., col. 1033.

[530] Cf. FN 306.

[531] Hermann COHN, *Die Hygiene des Auges in den Schulen*. Urban & Schwarzenberg, Vienna/Leipzig 1883; COHN, *Lehrbuch der Hygiene des Auges*. Urban & Schwarzenberg, Vienna/Leipzig 1892.

[532] Hermann COHN, "Die Ursachen und die Verhütung der Blindheit. Gekrönte Preisschrift. Von Dr Ernst Fuchs, O. Prof. d. Ophthalmolog. a. d. Univ. Lüttich. – Herausgegeben von der Society for the Prevention of Blindness. – Motto: Viribus unitis. Wiesbaden. Verlag von J. F. Bergmann. 1885 Preis 2 M. 40 Pf.", in: *Deutsche medizinische Wochenschrift* [*Dt. med. Wochenschr.*] 11 (1885), pp. 240–241 and 258–259.

[533] (Ed.), Ernst Fuchs (Liège), "The Causes and Prevention of Blindness", in: *Ophthal. Rev.* 4 (1885), pp. 79–86, 93–105, 129–139, 157–168 and 207–212.

[534] Ibid., p. 212.

[535] Cf. e.g.: *Revue générale d'ophtalmologie* vols. 3–4 (1885), p. 401; *Revue d'hygiene et de la médecine preventive* vol. 8 (1885), p. 65.

[536] For the report in French, cf. Archives de l'Université de Liège. Fonds du Secrétariat central, Nr. 143. Registre de correspondance du recteur, 6 juillet 1885.

[537] It should, however, be borne in mind that Fuchs had failed to secure the support of the Faculty for his plea for additional funding and equipment for his clinic only shortly before.

[538] For the French original, cf. FLORKIN, *Apports viennois à la Faculté de médecine de Liège*, in: FLORKIN/HALKIN *Chronique de l'Université de Liège* (as in FN 415), pp. 226–228.

[539] Cf. the next chapter.

[540] FUCHS, *Augenarzt* (as in FN 2), p. 81.

[541] *"M. Fuchs, Professor of Ophthalmology in Liège, where the government did not find the means to retain him and whence he was recalled to Vienna."* Collection of the ophthalmol. and anat. Georges Leplat (1890–1985), whose father, Lucien Leplat, was Fuchs's assistant in Liège. Cf. FLORKIN, *Apports viennois à la Faculté de médecine de Liège*, as in FN 415, p. 227.

[542] Ernst FUCHS, *Manuel d'Ophtalmologie*. Traduit sur la deuxième édition allemande par le Docteur C. Lacompte et le Docteur L. Leplat. Georges Carré, Paris 1892.

[543] Ernst FUCHS, *Manuel d'ophtalmologie*. 2. éd. française, traduite sur la 5. éd. allemande par G. Lacomte et L. Leplat. G. Carré & C. Naud, Paris 1897.

[544] Ernst FUCHS, *Manuel d'Ophtalmologie*. Troisième édition française traduite sur la dixième édition allemande par le Dr L. Leplat et le Dr C. Lacompte. Steinheil, Paris 1906.

[545] Cf. FN 430.

[546] Letter of the Permanent Secretary of the Académie royale de médecine de Belgique, psychiatrist Ernest Masoin (1844–1915), to Ernst Fuchs, dated Bruxelles, le 25 mai 1901. Original in the Family archive.

[547] Letter of the Chairman of the Maatschappij tot Onderstand der Blinden in Antwerp, Herman Mulder, and the Vice Chairman, N. van der Ouderaa, to Ernst Fuchs, dated Antwerpen, den II November 1905. Original in the Family archive.

[548] Daniel Van DUYSE, *L'histoire de l'ophtalmologie en Belgique* (as in FN 282), p. 148.

4. The Foundation of the Second University Eye Clinic in Vienna (1883) and the Appointment of Ernst Fuchs (1885)

A World Premiere: the Foundation of a University Eye Clinic (1812)

The world's first eye clinic attached to a university was founded in Vienna in 1812. It was domiciled at the Allgemeines Krankenhaus.[549] Its first head, Georg Joseph Beer (1763–1821),[550] (Fig. 34) established clinical ophthalmology as an integral part of the university. Handing on his impressive practical skills and his expertise to his son-in-law, Friedrich Jaeger von Jaxtthal (1784–1871), who in turn handed them on to his own son, Beer's grandson Eduard Jaeger von Jaxtthal (1818–1884), he became the founding father of a highly respected dynasty of Viennese ophthalmologists. Their exceptional talents gave a distinctive shape to academic ophthalmology in Vienna for the first three generations after the foundation of the clinic and ensured it of an international pioneering role.

In 1818 the Vienna University Eye Clinic was raised to the rank of a tenured professorship. Ophthalmology was now an obligatory subject taught and examined in the degree course of Vienna's Medical University.[551] For the first time, ophthalmology was raised to the same status as internal medicine and surgery. In this historical context, ophthalmology in the form it assumed in Vienna has the permanent distinction of having been the first specialty to be separated off from university-taught surgery[552] at the beginning of the nineteenth century.

Friedrich Jaeger von Jaxtthal (1784–1871)

Beer's student and son-in-law Friedrich Jaeger von Jaxtthal[553] failed to succeed him as director of Vienna's Eye Clinic, even though he had deputised for Beer between 1819 and 1822 during the latter's last illness and after his death.[554] Instead, Friedrich Jaeger served as director of the eye clinic at the Josephinum between 1826 and 1848, a school for military surgeons founded in 1785 by Joseph II in the immediate vicinity of the Allgemeines Krankenhaus, whose foundation by Joseph predated the Josephinum by one year.

In addition to a call to Pest Jaeger rejected two calls to Bonn. Through his student Julius Sichel (1802–1868) he made a significant contribution to the consolidation of ophthalmology in France. Other students of his played an equally significant or indeed even foundational part in establishing the health care system of Turkey. From 1841 Jaeger was hoping to be appointed Oberster Feldarzt [Surgeon General of the k. k. Army] *and Director of the Josephinian Academy. Such hopes proved vain.*[555]

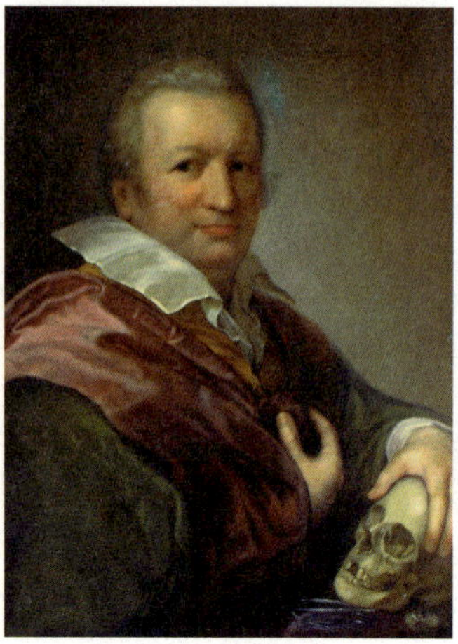

Fig. 34 Georg Joseph Beer (1763–1821)

These setbacks notwithstanding, Friedrich Jaeger was a much sought-after general practitioner in addition to being a highly respected eye specialist. His prominent patients included, admittedly only by chance, Franz Grillparzer (1791–1872). Austria's national poet gratefully mentions Friedrich Jaeger in his autobiography. Jaeger had cured him of a troublesome illness while the two were in Rome in 1844.[556] Friedrich Jaeger was accompanying Austria's State Chancellor Fürst Metternich, whose medical advisor and close friend he was for many years.[557]

What is less well known is the fact that Friedrich Jaeger was the first to put forward a proposal in 1849 for the establishment of a Second Eye Clinic at Vienna's Allgemeines Krankenhaus: after the Josephinum had been abolished for the second time and merged with the University following the revolutionary events of 1848. Jaeger, already 64 at the time, submitted a proposal in April 1849 to the Ministry of the Interior aimed at the establishment of a second university clinic or clinical ward.[558] The Ministry of the Interior passed on Jaeger's proposal, together with a thoroughly positive assessment, to the Ministerium für Cultus und Unterricht, headed since 1849 by Leopold Graf von Thun und Hohenstein (1811–1888).[559] The new clinic was to be assigned the hospital rooms 59 and 60, and, based on Friedrich Jaeger's excellent reputation, his appointment as director was strongly recommended.[560] However, the Minister rejected the proposal. He could not – or would not – see the need for such a foundation. The decision was formulated with great caution, almost as if it was only provisional:

I must herewith inform the [Ministry] that the difficulties linked to the establishment of a Second Eye Clinic and the significant expenses caused by it have, in view of the non-existent need for a Second Eye Clinic, led me to the decision to desist from appointing Professor Friedrich Jaeger to the University and from the establishment of that clinic for the time being. [561]

Friedrich Jaeger's expertise, talent and didactic skills had gained him a Europe wide reputation, which attracted students of the calibre of Julius Sichel, Louis de Wecker and Albrecht von Graefe. In a building belonging to the Schottenstift monastery in Vienna's inner city – then Schotten Hof, Schotten Gasse 136,[562] today Freyung 6, 1010 Vienna – he operated his own private clinic, where he also taught his son Eduard.

The likeable Swabian belongs [...] *to that group of researchers who preferred making their original ideas live on in their students rather than in any publications of their own.*[563]

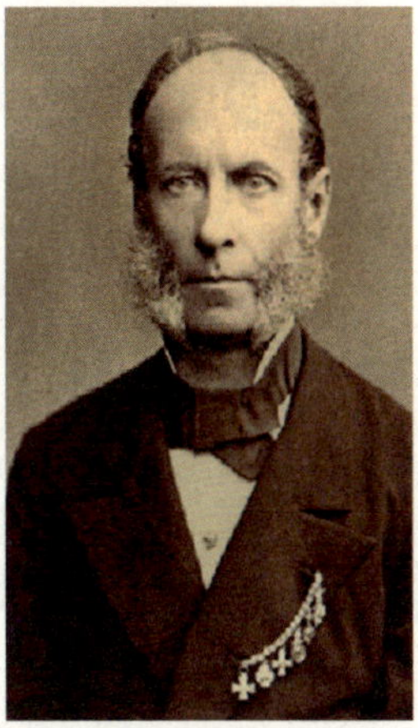

Fig. 35 Eduard Jaeger von Jaxtthal (1818–1884)

Eduard Jaeger von Jaxtthal (1818–1883)

Friedrich Jaeger's son Eduard[564] (Fig. 35) received his training at the Josephinum under the aegis of his father. On the basis of his 1844 doctoral thesis on cataract operations[565] he was appointed Associate Professor at Vienna University in 1856 and director of an eye department at the Allgemeines Krankenhaus in 1857. Beer's successor,[566] Anton Edler von Rosas (1791–1855),[567] who was director of the clinic between 1821 and 1855, held an initially unsalaried ad personam position and was assigned rooms 57a and 57b immediately adjacent to the Eye Clinic. When Rosas' successor, Ferdinand Ritter von Arlt,[568] left Prague University in 1856 to be appointed Director of Vienna's University Eye Clinic, Minister Thun-Hohenstein rolled out his plan to assign to Arlt's clinic only the two original rooms with no more than ten beds apiece. During the appointment negotiations Arlt objected to this and demanded he be assigned fifty beds altogether and an increase in his salary. Thun-Hohenstein conceded the latter but limited the number of beds to 30.[569] At the Prague University Eye Clinic Arlt had had at his disposal twice the number of beds.[570] The beds that were freed up in this way at the Allgemeines Krankenhaus were now assigned to the salaried position of a senior ophthalmologist, which was filled by Eduard Jaeger in 1857.[571]

Eduard Jaeger had to his credit outstanding achievements in the pathological anatomy of the eye and especially as a pioneer in the diagnostics of diseases of the ocular fundus,[572] involving the further development of the Helmholtz ophthalmoscope to render the fundus oculi in an upright image. Over the following twenty-five years he fought for academic recognition. As early as 1863 Eduard Jaeger put forward the proposal – as his father had done fourteen years earlier – of establishing a second University Eye Clinic at the Allgemeines Krankenhaus, which would have brought with it his appointment as Chair of Ophthalmology and as Director of this clinic. The clinic was to have become part of the University of Vienna – it was, in the bureaucratic parlance of the time, to have been 'systemised'.[573] The fate of his proposal at the time was sealed by the negative expert opinion submitted by Arlt, who in 1856 had still supported the appointment of Eduard Jaeger and Carl Stellwag von Carion[574] to associate professorships.[575]

The Foundation of the Second University Eye Clinic in 1883

In the spring of 1883, when Arlt's impending retirement from the First University Eye Clinic made finding a successor imperative, the Medical Faculty of the University of Vienna Wien finally acknowledged in its dealings with the Ministerium für Cultus und Unterricht the necessity of creating a second University Clinic of Ophthalmology. Eduard Jaeger now hoped to see the dream of a lifetime realised: his name was unanimously put at the top of the shortlist of candidates, with Ludwig Mauthner (9 votes for, 6 against) in second, and Hubert Sattler (8 votes for, 6 against) in third place.[576] The Professorial Council of the Medical University therefore proposed to appoint Carl Stellwag von Carion as Director of the First University Eye Clinic at the beginning of the winter semester of 1883/84. This involved the abolition of Stellwag's non-'systemised' clinic, 'systemising' Jaeger's existing department as the Second University Eye Clinic and appointing Jaeger as its chair. Stellwag had succeeded in 1874 where a quarter of a century earlier, in 1849, Friedrich Jaeger, and eleven years earlier, in 1863, the latter's son Eduard had failed: after the definitive abolition of the Josephinum, Stellwag was given a foothold inside the university provided by the creation of a second Eye Clinic at the Allgemeines Krankenhaus, comprising forty-eight beds in Rooms No. 57a and 57b. This enabled Stellwag to continue to teach. This Second Eye Clinic was not 'systemised' so that it was never referred to as the Second University Eye Clinic; instead, it was referred to in the bureaucratic Mandarin of the Ministries of the Interior and of Cultus und Unterricht as the "zweite oculistische Klinik".[577]

Jaeger's department, located in the first courtyard of the Allgemeines Krankenhauses directly above the main entrance in Alserstraße 4, comprised several hospital rooms with a total of 81 beds.[578] It had its own lecture hall, four small isolation rooms, a reception room for out-patients adjacent to the lecture hall and several smaller rooms suitable for use as ophthalmoscope and work rooms. Of the facilities that used to be part of Jaeger's department, the two larger hospital rooms with 45 to 50 beds, immediately adjacent to the lecture hall with an audience capacity of roughly 100, the lecture hall itself, the darkroom and the out-patient room were assigned to the new clinic. The remaining hospital rooms that were not needed for teaching purposes continued to be used for eye patients by the Allgemeines Krankenhaus.[579]

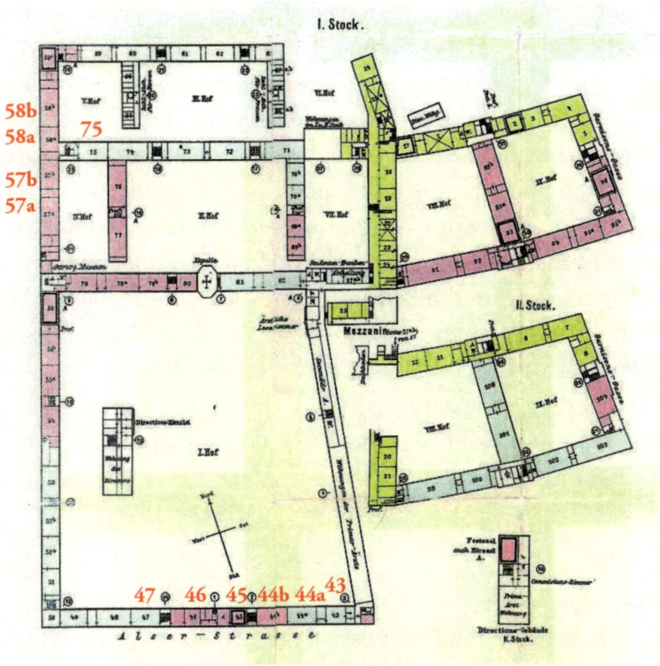

Fig. 36
Building Plan of Vienna's Allgemeines Krankenhaus according to J. F. Wagner 1886

Fuchs, at this stage still active in Liège, only knew about these developments from hearsay and is therefore understandably vague in his 1946 autobiography:

When the Josephinum was dissolved, Stellwag was assigned several rooms above the Skin Clinic [...] *After Arlt's departure Stellwag took over his clinic, and Stellwag's rooms were returned to the Department of Skin Diseases.*[580]

In addition to the regulation of Jaeger's salary, the following negotiations[581] introduced several other changes: Stellwag had had at the disposal of his clinic the two hospital rooms 57a and 57b with 48 beds, located on the first floor of the fourth courtyard of the Allgemeines Krankenhaus, and hospital room 75 with 25 beds, located between courtyards IV and V. When he assumed control of the First University Eye Clinic, Stellwag, like Arlt before him, was assigned hospital rooms 58a and 58b on the first floor of courtyard V with 30 beds. The two hospital rooms 57a and 57b were added to fall back on when the need arose, and hospital room 75 was returned to the hospital management.[582] (Fig. 36)

When in the autumn of 1883 Eduard Jaeger finally transformed his former department into the newly founded Second University Eye Clinic[583] – with hospital rooms 44 and 46 serving as the clinical rooms and room 45 having been adapted to serve as lecture hall and out-patient clinic[584] – he was already 65 and terminally ill. Credited with pioneering achievements in the study of the pathologically altered ocular fundus,[585] with the adaptation of the dioptric apparatus[586] and with having inaugurated the use of optotypes for the assessment of the acuity of vision,[587] his combined duties as director of the newly founded clinic and active clinical teacher were a burden he found increasingly hard to shoulder. On July 5, 1884 Eduard Jaeger passed away, having driven himself relentlessly for two semesters to realise his lifelong dream.[588] It was therefore necessary for the University after less than a year to enter into a new round of negotiations to fill the vacancy at the top of the Second University Eye Clinic.

Deputising for Jaeger (1884–1885)

After Jaeger's death August Leopold Ritter von Reuss (1841–1924)[589] deputised for him. He describes the first phase of the Second University Eye Clinic as follows:

When Hofrath v. Arlt resigned at the end of the summer semester 1883, the spatial arrangements in the Eye Clinic were reshuffled in that the rooms previously assigned to the two clinics were fused to form the First Eye Clinic, and what used to be known as the Department for Eye Patients was redesignated as the 2nd Eye Clinic. Two hospital rooms remained an integral part of the k.k. Allgemeines Krankenhaus as a Department for Eye Patients.

So the Second Eye Clinic has at its disposal two rooms with 21 beds for men and 19 for women and another two rooms with 22 beds for men and 14 for women in the Ward; furthermore, it has 5 isolation rooms with one bed each. While these are part of the women's room, they can be used for men or women, depending on need. The clinic therefore has 81 beds altogether. In addition, it comprises a lecture hall; a room for the treatment of out-patients and a waiting room for the latter; a small room for ophthalmoscopic examinations and another small room for microscopic work. Since the clinic lacks a room dedicated to sight tests, these have to be carried out in one of the clinical rooms.

Since early 1885, the medical staff has comprised, in addition to the professor, who is also Head Physician at the k. k. Allgemeines Krankenhaus, two assistants, two junior doctors 2nd class, who are assigned to the Department by the hospital director, a varying number of aspirants, and several volunteers, usually students, who devote their spare time to the clinic out of interest in the specialty.

The out-patient clinic is used by between 160 and 200 patients every day; on the evidence of its logs, 7,000 to 8,000 new patients a year seek treatment.[590]

Carl Koller and the Discovery of Cocaine as a Local Anaesthetic

Reuss's brief "interregnum" was distinguished by an event that sets it apart not only in the history of ophthalmology but in medical history in general. In the autumn of 1884, junior doctor at the Second University Eye Clinic's ward Carl Koller (1857–1944)[591] announced his discovery of local anaesthesia of the eye by applying an aqueous solution of cocaine.[592] Reuss immediately realised the beneficial implications for painless operations, provided ample scope for the new technique at his clinic and extolled Koller's merits in public.[593] Fuchs, incidentally, issued a warning in 1902 about the unthinking, uncritical and disproportionate use of cocaine in ophthalmology.[594]

Filling the Vacancy at the Top of the Second University Eye Clinic 1884/85

The search for a successor to Eduard Jaeger as Chair and Director of the Second University Eye Clinic cast a harsh light on a factional dispute that had been brewing for a long time and had acquired all the attributes of a bitter feud within Viennese ophthalmology, with representatives of the physical-optical school (Jaeger) on one side and those of pathological-anatomical persuasion (Arlt) on the other. The prize they were competing for was predominance in their specialty. It is noteworthy in this context that after Arlt's resignation in 1883 his position at the First University Eye Clinic was filled in 1884 not by one of his own students but by Stellwag von Carion.[595]

According to academic tradition, it was usual in such cases for the Professorial College of the Medical Faculty to agree on a shortlist that ranked the candidates according to qualification in the eyes of the College. To this end, a committee was formed on 25 October 1884, comprising surgeon Theodor Billroth,[596] pathological anatomist Hans Kundrat (1845–1893,)[597] internal clinician Hermann Nothnagel (1841–1905),[598] anatomist Carl Toldt (1840–1920)[599] and ophthalmologist Stellwag, the committee's chairman. The five candidates, whose respective merits were to be ranked, were Fuchs (Lüttich), Mauthner[600] (Vienna), Reuss (Vienna), Sattler[601] (Erlangen) and Schnabel[602] (Innsbruck). Stellwag as chairman did not take part in the ranking. As the committee proved unable to agree on a ranked shortlist of three candidates, it presented a majority and a minority shortlist.[603]

On December 2, 1884, the Dean of the Medical Faculty of Vienna University, August Emil Vogl (1833–1909),[604] was informed of the vote the Professorial College had submitted to the Ministerium für Cultus und Unterricht from their meeting on November 29, 1884:[605] in its shortlist approved by the majority, the committee had ranked three candidates as follows: primo loco: Fuchs; secundo loco: Sattler; and tertio loco: Mauthner. The Professorial College had rejected this proposal, with 11 against, 10 in favour. Nothnagel had then submitted his minority shortlist, with primo loco, Mauthner, secundo loco, Sattler, and tertio loco, Fuchs; in this version of the shortlist, Mauthner had therefore switched places with Fuchs. This proposal was accepted by the Faculty plenum with 11 in favour, 10 against.[606] Nothnagel may have given precedence to Mauthner, because the two shared a predilection for neurological topics.[607] It may also be that Nothnagel sided with Mauthner because of the latter's Jewish descent. A Protestant from Brandenburg, Nothnagel pointedly promoted assistants of Jewish descent and instigated the foundation of an association for the prevention of antisemitism, which was already beginning to rear its ugly head in Vienna at the time.[608]

The two shortlists mentioned above were supplemented by a third, which had been compiled by surgeon Eduard Albert (1841–1900),[609] experimental pathologist Salomon Stricker (1834–1898),[610] psychiatrist Theodor Meynert (1833–1892)[611] and two unnamed professors,[612] which had Mauthner in first place, Schnabel in second and Reuss in third. For this triad no majority could be found in the Faculty and it was therefore not put to the vote. In effect, Mauthner was present in all three shortlists, Fuchs and Sattler in two, Reuss and Schnabel in one.

Reuss went out of his way to make the committee see his scientific merits.[613] He listed in detail his commitment to the ophthalmological care he had provided to children of school age and the papers that had resulted from his focus on medical-social issues.

Only four days later – on December 6, 1884 – the *Wiener Medizinische Wochenschrift* published a diatribe in favour of the appointment of Ludwig Mauthner, dated "Wien, 3. Dezember 1884". Its polemical thrust, whose rancour is, to say the least, unusual by the standard of the time, was mainly directed against Fuchs:

Filling the Vacancy at the Eye Clinic
Last Saturday the question of filling the vacancy at the top of the Clinic of Ophthalmology caused by the death of Prof. v. Jäger was discussed by the medical Professorial College, a matter that stirred up a lot of dust. As is well known, a committee was appointed to provide a report, which elected Prof. Stellwag as a professor of the specialty in question as its chairman. Prof. Stellwag delivered a comprehensive report, in which he discussed the work of the five candidates, Professors Fuchs (Lüttich) and Mauthner (Vienna), Lecturer Reuss (Vienna), and Professors Sattler (Erlangen) and Schnabel (Innsbruck). The chairman did not file a motion; he did not want to express any preferences, any downgradings, any recommendations. The members of the committee, however, did not share this view; they declared themselves obliged to present to the College a shortlist of three candidates. As they failed to agree on the candidates and on any ranking, this resulted in a majority and a minority shortlist. The majority was in favour of the following order: Fuchs, Sattler, Mauthner. This proposal was kept under wraps until the plenary session. The surprise was all the greater when it was revealed that Prof. Fuchs had been ranked primo and Prof. Mauthner tertio loco. What might have been the reason for the singular decision of the majority? It is difficult to understand what could possibly have led to the young, albeit talented Professor from Lüttich to be preferred to all the other candidates. Little more than a year ago, when v. Jäger was appointed, Fuchs was not mentioned, let alone nominated, even by his own teacher, v. Arlt, and since then no special works, no outstanding achievements of his have come to public notice that would justify assigning him a place in the first row, unless one is prepared to consider his popular award-winning monograph[614] *as such a work.*

It is even more difficult to understand why the committee should have thought it necessary to downgrade Prof. Mauthner, who had been nominated a few years ago with a great majority alongside P[rof]. v. Jäger.

Prof. Mauthner is recognised as an outstanding exponent of his specialty both at home and abroad and has been as successful in his practical as in his scientific activities. There is no reason whatever to give precedence over him to another, albeit talented candidate, who has neither proved himself in practice over so many years nor is on a par with him in scientific achievements – no matter whether that candidate resides here or abroad.

It is a matter of fact that the majority of the entire College acknowledged these facts. The Professorial College decided in favour of a shortlist that ranked Prof. Mauthner primo loco; Prof. Sattler secundo, as before; and Prof. Fuchs tertio loco, a ranking that best depicts the candidates' entitlement according to achievement and seniority. It was Prof. Nothnagel who caused the committee's majority vote to be overturned by stating the objective reasons that spoke in favour of the minority vote. He declared that the ranking proposed [by the majority] was totally incompatible with its significance; by drawing attention to Mauthner's well founded reputation as a practising eye specialist, outstanding surgeon, excellent teacher and broadly recognised author of specialist publications, he managed to persuade the majority of the College. The minority vote was duly accepted and Mauthner was nominated primo loco, an outcome that has not failed to gain full acceptance in all medical circles.

Prof. Stellwag himself saw no reason to oppose this change. The fact that the greatest part of his report dealt with Prof. Mauthner proves that he would have been compelled to put Prof. Mauthner into first place, had he chosen to put forward a ranking. The Ministry of Education, which will decide this matter, will no doubt do so according to merit and entitlement.[615]

The Dean of the Medical Faculty passed on the shortlists to anatomist Carl Langer (1819–1887)[616] on the same day he had received them, December 2, 1884; they landed on Langer's desk on December 5. It was up to Langer in his capacity of advisor on medical matters to the Ministerium für Cultus und Unterricht to decide which shortlist was to be presented to the minister. To put himself in a better position to make an informed decision, Langer consulted a detailed memorandum that Prof. von Arlt had submitted to the competent minister on December 8, 1884. This memorandum casts a harsh – one might even say, shocking – light on the personal aspects behind the rivalries simmering within academic ophthalmology in Vienna in the late nineteenth century:

Pro memoria.
The shortlist designed to fill the vacancy left by the death of Prof. Ed[uard] von Jaeger put before the Professorial College of the Medical Faculty by the committee /: Prof. Stellwag, Billroth, Nothnagel, Kundrat and Toldt:/, which ranked the Professors Fuchs, Sattler, and Mauthner in this order, lost out with 10 votes in favour, 11 against to a minority shortlist presented by Prof. Nothnagel, which

reversed that order. This outcome may have been due to the fact that Prof. Kundrat was unable to take part in the vote.

If I take the liberty, even though I am no longer a member of the College, of drawing the attention of Your Excellency to several noteworthy facts, which are either represented not at all or only insufficiently in the Faculty's expert opinion, I am motivated to do so by a sense of respect for an institution which I myself presided over for twenty-seven years, as I believe, to the full satisfaction of the Ministry and whose reputation at home and abroad I would like to see assured for the future.

As for the nomination of Mauthner primo loco, it was justified mainly by reference to the candidate's eminent talent, even though Prof. Nothnagel does not know the other two candidates in person. I do not query that talent in the least, especially as regards oral delivery and written style but from a clinical teacher I would demand two additional qualities, which I would rank even higher: a love of truth in scientific matters and integrity of character. As I find M. lacking in both these qualities, I could not bring myself to include [him] in my shortlist, when I resigned from my position last year and a successor to the vacant second chair had to be nominated. I proposed at the time that in the case that Jaeger declined the appointment, citing health reasons, the position was to be offered to Sattler. My shortlist did not include any other names.

To justify my verdict on M. I must go back a little.

When the newly created position in Innsbruck had to be filled, I proposed Dr. Ritter v. Reuss, then assistant emeritus, who now deputises for Jaeger, to the satisfaction of all concerned, as I hear; however, under the aegis of Dr. Haser [sic],[617] *the position was given to Dr. Mauthner. As early as 1872 Mauthner submitted a request to the Ministry to relieve him of his post in Innsbruck and to award him an annual subsidy of 800 fl. to enable him to operate a clinic of his own devising in Vienna, which would have to be a model institution, as there was no eye clinic in Vienna that satisfied modern requirements and because he himself finally wanted to attain a "decent existence" again. In his eyes, life in Innsbruck was below human dignity! No honest person would, in trying to reach their aim, resort to casting aspersions against their colleagues or to peddling accusations against them, even if these did not happen to have been their own teachers. He is indebted* […] *for his training first to me, then to Prof. v. Jaeger as the latter's junior doctor or assistant. The Ministry, having sounded out the opinion of the Professorial College, rejected his request.*[618]

Mauthner's negative verdict cited above by Arlt on the academic institutions in Vienna where ophthalmology was taught – the University Eye Clinic under Arlt and the Eye Clinic at the Medical-Surgical Military Academy (Josephinum), then headed by Stellwag – is echoed in another pertinent, as yet unpublished document penned by Arlt. Faced with Mauthner's massive criticism regarding the poor quality of ophthalmological training, Arlt had submitted a detailed reply in an undated letter to the Ministerium für Cultus und Unterricht, which predates the above memorandum by more than a decade. The events described in it allow us to date it beyond doubt to the early summer semester of 1873. In it, Arlt seeks to refute Mauthner's criticism of him point by point. It is reprinted here to illustrate the multifaceted personal reasons that underpinned Arlt's objections to Mauthner. Tellingly, Arlt entitled the memorandum he submitted to the Ministry "Apologia against Mauthner".

Hohes Ministerium für Cultus und Unterricht!
In his proposal to set up an eye clinic Professor Mauthner has commented so contemptuously on the institutions already in existence in Vienna for the teaching of ophthalmology that as Director of the University Eye Clinic I believe it is my duty to draw the Ministry's attention to some facts that contradict Mauthner's claims.

Tuition at Vienna's University Eye Clinic is designed first and foremost as an obligatory subject for regular students. It is therefore elementary in nature and aims to teach students to observe accurately and to enable them to acquire the ophthalmological expertise any general practitioner needs. One semester – setting aside more was impossible in view of the other subjects – is enough for the stated purpose. It goes without saying that it is not enough to train eye specialists.

To offer those who want to train as ophthalmologists the opportunity to do so the Government itself has created the preconditions by employing two clinical assistants instead of the former one and by granting extra subsidies for the purchase from time to time of expensive teaching aids in addition to the clinic's annual endowment. While the professor is striving to do justice to the task set for him by the state without losing sight of his commitment to research and stimulation, the assistants are not only active in his support, but teach courses in their own right – docendo discimus – and are instructed to take care that all specific disciplines are represented, such as operating; ophthalmological examination; determination of refraction anomalies; and pathological-anatomical and microscopic examinations.

Assistants are no novices. As a rule, they have been interns or aspirants alongside former assistants for two to three years. From among the aspirants, of whom there are never fewer than 5 or 6, because this provides them with the best opportunity for further training, the most talented and diligent are chosen as assistants.

This well-ordered institution, which comprises all the different branches, is not designed to fascinate, to dazzle with lectures on any one topic, such as refraction anomalies or ophthalmoscopy: it constantly aims to offer to all who want to learn an opportunity for a comprehensive training. It is the result of many years' hard work and became possible only after space for patients was significantly enlarged. Now that Graefe's death[619] *has deprived Berlin of a comparable institution, it may well be that only London has anything analogous to offer.*

This is arguably the reason why there has been such an inrush of medical doctors from abroad over the last few years. The attached list[620] *of medical doctors from abroad who took part in tuition at the University Clinic during the winter semester of 1872/3 – not as one-off visitors, but as attendees for the entire semester, some of whom are still here at the beginning of this term – may be taken as proof of the operational efficiency of the clinic. As many of these gentlemen, especially those whose names have been underlined, have come to Vienna exclusively or at least mainly because of the Eye Clinic, it may be presumed that other countries and the public at large hold views on Vienna's ophthalmogical institutions that differ from those Professor Mauthner does not hesitate to peddle to the authorities. Calumniare audacter …*[621]

If Professor Mauthner claims that the training of capable ophthalmologists in Vienna is deficient, one is led to believe he himself does not in his own eyes belong to that group. Mauthner received his training in Vienna, apart from a 4–5-month study trip (Berlin, Utrecht). Or are we to be led to the conclusion that, in addition to him, there are other young men, as gifted and hard-working as he is, who also manage to reach high positions in practice and in science – in spite of the poor quality of Vienna's teaching institutions?[622]

Having listed in detail the reasons that in his eyes disqualified Mauthner as a candidate to succeed v. Jaeger as Director of the Second University Eye Clinic, Arlt was now faced with the task of recommending either Sattler or Fuchs for the position, both former students of his. Both had been assistants at his clinic before they received calls as full professors from abroad. Arlt acquitted himself of the delicate task of doing justice to both his former students as follows:

If I put Doctor Ernst Fuchs, who was my assistant for four years after Sattler's departure and whom I must give credit for being equally well qualified, secundo loco, this is due to the simple reason that Sattler is the elder. Describing the achievements and the capacity of Prof. Fuchs is in my view superfluous since a detailed assessment has presumably already been compiled by the Prague Medical Faculty.[623]

What prevented von Arlt from recommending Reuss was the fact that in his view he was not on a par with Sattler and Fuchs in pathological anatomy and microscopy. Arlt readily conceded, however, that Reuss, *"given his talent and widely known diligence"*, could be counted upon *"to remedy any deficiencies"*[624] in due time.

Taking into account the small majority in the vote of the Professorial College, the competent ministerial advisor Carl Langer reached the following decision roughly five months later, on December 31, 1884, for whose formulation he resorted to verbatim quotes from the original assessments and from Stellwag's presentation:

If the majority does not in itself carry a great deal of weight because of its smallness, it loses all claim to significance owing to the fact that Prof. Kundrat, who had voted in the committee for the first shortlist, with Fuchs primo loco, was not present at the plenum of the College, so that one can say that it was his absence that gave the second shortlist its headstart by one vote. [...] *Had he been present and had he voted along the same lines as in the committee, the vote in the plenum would have resulted in a hung decision.*

Therefore I cannot hail the result of this vote as being in any way significant for the decision; objective considerations need to be taken into account, based on the excellent expert opinion delivered by Prof. Stellwag and on the memorandum subsequently submitted by Prof. Arlt.

In a specialty as far reaching as ophthalmology, which takes as its domain several distinct fields of research, resting as it does not only on patholog[ical-] anatomical, but also on physical foundations, it stands to reason that eye specialists, while sharing the same command of the totality of the curriculum, differ in that they tend to favour now this direction, now that in their research and in their work. This is why one of the schools attaches greater weight to the pathological-anatomical direction, the other to the physical direction. It may be said that the school of Arlt has tended to favour the former, the school of Jaeger the latter.

This is of decisive importance for the assessment of the candidates. I therefore believe that I am doing the right thing when I only take into consideration the three candidates named in the first two shortlists, namely Fuchs, Mauthner and Sattler.

Fuchs is the youngest among the five candidates whom Stellwag profiled in his expert opinion. He is definitely not without merit. His monograph on the sarcoma of the eye has met with general recognition. Having said that, he does not on the whole surpass either Mauthner or Sattler, which is why I put him into the second rank.

Mauthner and Sattler are above the rest.

The majority of Mauthner's scientific achievements are in the difficult field of the optics of the eye. In several smaller treatises as well as in major works Mauthner treats this thoroughly complex subject in a manner of presentation that has been singled out for praise by the chairman, Prof. Stellwag. Mauthner has publications on a wide range of topics to his credit without therefore disregarding the clinical aspects. His qualification for a professorship is beyond doubt, all the more so since, as is well known, he is possessed of an eminent rhetorical talent. What has been widely remarked upon is his lack of interest in the cultivation of pathological anatomy, whose significance for ophthalmology he rates as low. [...] *According to Stellwag, "Sattler is capable of presenting extremely complex and tricky matters clearly and intelligibly". There is therefore no doubt that Sattler, too, is a suitable candidate.*

Mauthner is the product of the school of Jaeger, Sattler is the product of Arlt's school. Both are highly experienced practitioners and hard-working teachers with excellent reputations. For Mauthner this is the case especially in Vienna, while Sattler has two calls to German universities – Giessen and Erlangen – and Arlt's testimony in his favour.

Personally, I would rank the two ex aequo, but in keeping with Prof. Stellwag's presentation I have to admit that all three, Fuchs, Mauthner and Sattler, must be credited with having undergone sound practical training and all three would no doubt acquit themselves honourably of the task of teaching and of responsibly heading a major eye clinic.[625]

At this point, one last look at Arlt's role in the appointment procedure is needed. The outward equidistance he kept to Fuchs and Sattler does not seem to have reflected his real preference, which may in fact have been in favour of Sattler. An examination of his papers has revealed that Arlt tried to get Empress Elisabeth of Austria's brother, Herzog Carl Theodor in Bayern, a student both of Arlt and of Fuchs, as we have heard already,[626] to intervene with the Emperor in favour of Sattler's call to Vienna.[627] The evidence consists in two letters from the Duke to Arlt dating to the time of the protracted procedure in 1885, which he refers to. The first letter is kept in fairly general terms and mentions no names:

München 3 1 85

Verehrtester Herr Hofrath!
Having had an opportunity during my stay in Ofen to report the substance of our conversation at the highest level and having found both interest and the readiness to take care of the matter as desired, I would like to inform you with these lines of this result so that you may take the necessary steps and strike the iron while it is hot.

Mit herzlichen Grüßen
Ihr ergebener
Herzog Carl.[628]

Despatched three months later, the second letter is more explicit:

Meran den 15 IV. 85

Verehrtester Herr Hofrath!
Permit me after this long time to remind you of a matter that was of concern to both of us during my last stay in Vienna: filling the vacancy of the chair of ophthalmology in Vienna. I think if Herr Hofrath would be kind enough to ask for an audience with the Emperor, this might well decide the matter in Sattler's favour. When I spoke about this matter with the Emperor in Ofen, I mentioned Sattler's name, adding that you would be asking for an audience.
Hoping that this matter will find the desired resolution

Ihr ergebener,
Herzog Carl.[629]

The Duke's diction suggests that he himself was at least as interested as Arlt to see Sattler installed in Vienna as Jaeger's successor. From what can be established in retrospect, Arlt did not take up the Duke's suggestion of seeking to obtain an audience to involve Francis Joseph in the matter.[630]

The Minister für Cultus und Unterricht, Sigmund Freiherr Conrad von Eybesfeld, allowed another six and a half months to pass after Langer's assessment of December 1884 before passing on his decision, which he formulated and justified in an extremely interesting manner, to the Emperor. Citing verbatim the differences between the Jaeger and Arlt schools along the lines indicated by Langer, the minister, who, as we have seen, had not received any clear recommendation from his advisor, had reached a completely unexpected conclusion:

Having duly weighed all relevant facts and taken into equitable consideration the needs of medical tuition at Vienna's University, I take the liberty, in harmony with the proposal made by the Chairman of the Committee, Professor Stellwag, of humbly proposing that the Professor of Ophthalmology at Liège University, Dr Ernst Fuchs, be appointed Professor and Director of Vienna's 2nd Eye Clinic.

This is not to say that Professor Dr. Mauthner, who was part of the initial shortlist alongside Professor Fuchs, whose style of delivery has been described as especially brilliant and who has an excellent reputation as a surgeon, would not be qualified for the role of professor at [the University of] *Vienna.*

If I nevertheless give preference to Professor Fuchs, I do so in light of the fact that Mauthner has hardly been active at all in the field of [microscopic] *pathological anatomy of the eye, which is so important nowadays.*

In addition to the conviction that Professor Fuchs is fully qualified to acquit himself honourably of his tasks as teacher and director in charge of a major eye clinic, I was also guided by the thought that it is incumbent on the Ministry of Education to make sure, in view of the brilliant tradition of Arlt's school, that the latter continues to be represented in times to come at Vienna's University by one of its most capable representatives.[631]

A brief summary of Ernst Fuchs's CV was followed by a description of his academic merits and his impeccable lifestyle:

Both in respect of his teaching and of his scientific work [Ernst Fuchs's] *record to date is considered to be deserving of the highest praise. He reorganised the Department of Ophthalmology and the Eye Clinic in Liège and his didactic skills, his medical successes and his demeanour, bespeaking humanity, tact and strength of character, soon won him the respect and the hearts both of his colleagues and students and of those who turned to him for help.*

His contributions to specialist literature cover a wide range of topics. He has published 37 minor and major works to date, some in French, others in English, partly pertaining to descriptive anatomy and normal histology, partly

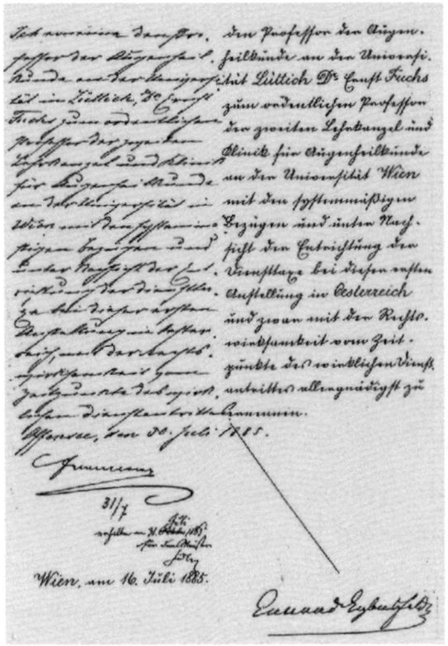

Fig. 37 Certificate of Ernst Fuchs's appointment as Full Professor at the University of Vienna on 30 July 1886

to the physiology of the eye; several of his works deal with purely clinical questions, but the majority are devoted to the pathological anatomy of the eye.

What deserves special mention is his monograph on the Sarcom des Uvealtraktes [The Sarcoma of the Uveal Tract], *generally agreed to be a thoroughly competent work, for which the author has zealously digested the huge relevant literature and has rearranged it to form a new, readily understandable whole. He makes use of his own research on the macro- and microscopic structure of sarcoma and its many different varieties, on its development, growth and spread via the blood vessels, on its clinical significance, the causes of tumour formation and, finally, on its operative treatment, to bridge in the most commendable manner existing gaps as far as possible. The core of this work, which is supplemented by several works of the same category, belongs to pathological anatomy. The many* [additional] *contributions Fuchs has published are partly case studies, partly devoted to the pathogenetic foundations of ametropia. They include papers on the congenital anomalies of the optic nerve and on anomalies of refraction and accommodation, and his clinical miscellanea.*[632]

Enquiries made in Brussels in December 1884 with regard to Fuchs's political record had resulted in a clean sheet:

M. Fuchs, who is married and has a family, is considered to be above reproach in both his lifestyle and his morals. He has the reputation of being a man of science thoroughly proficient in his chosen specialty.

As for his political and social opinions, information from [relevant] *sources leaves no doubt that this scholar is completely indifferent to politics and cannot be classed as belonging to any specific* [political] *party.*[633]

The imperial decree appointing Ernst Fuchs as Professor of Ophthalmology and Director of the Second Eye Clinic of Vienna University was issued on July 30, 1885.[634] (Fig. 37) In keeping with the academic traditions of the time, Fuchs did not himself put forward his name. Political considerations, as one might call them for want of a better term, nearly scuppered Fuchs's appointment:

I had received a telegram from Mracek,[635] *to the effect that I had been nominated for the vacancy in Vienna. I had not heard anything from the people in Prague and then the position in Vienna became vacant. The appointment committee had put forward the proposal Fuchs, Sattler, Mauthner, a ranking the plenum changed to Mauthner, Sattler, Fuchs, mainly due to the philosemitic influence of Stricker,*[636] *with whom Albert and Ludwig*[637] *had always made common cause. I had therefore given up all hope concerning Vienna. In Vienna, the nomination of Mauthner was considered a done deal and the* Neue Freie Presse *released a triumphant editorial about yet another of their coreligionists who had gained entry to the faculty. This editorial was said to have brought about Mauthner's downfall. A member of parliament from the Tyrol, Father Greuter,*[638] *an exceedingly combative gentleman, who for this reason went under the name of the "battle steed of Hippach", delivered a flaming speech in parliament in which he claimed that a disproportionate number of Jews were being appointed to professorial chairs. This is said to have come as a shock to the then Minister of Education,* [...] *so much so that he substituted my name for the one in the nomination decree, which had not yet been signed by the Emperor. I learnt this later from hearsay in Vienna and cannot vouch for its accuracy.*[639]

Fuchs was right in sounding that note of warning. Instead of a *Neue Freie Presse* editorial on that topic in the period in question there is only a brief, neutral note on p. 5 of the edition dated August 2, 1885:

(Filling the Vacancy at the Ophthalmological Clinic in Vienna.)
As the Medicinische Presse *has learnt, the appointment to the Chair of Ophthalmology, which has become vacant due to the death of Professor v. Jaeger, is now imminent. According to the same source, it appears that instead of Professor Dr. Mauthner, who was ranked primo loco by the Professorial College, Professor Dr. Fuchs from Liège (a native of Vienna and one of Arlt's students) will be appointed; he had been ranked secundo loco. Originally, Professor Fuchs had been a candidate for the clinic in Prague, which had fallen vacant through v. Hasner's retirement.*[640]

More to the point is Fuchs's mention of a speech the Conservative Catholic priest Father Joseph Greuter contributed to a debate on university matters on March 10, 1985 in the Reichsrat. Greuter argued as follows:

If things are allowed to go on at Vienna University in the present style, Vienna University will stop being a university, being transformed into a second oriental academy instead […] *Kindly let me finish, gentlemen, I will cite evidence. What I mean is the way professors are being replaced at this university. I am not basing my remarks on my own confessional point of view, I am basing them on the point of view of compensatory justice and of fairness towards men of an occidental ancestry.*

What is the [numerical] *relationship between Semites and Christians? I have to spell this out so that the peoples of Austria know it: according to the statistics, the relationship between Israelites and the rest of the population is four point five* [out of one hundred].

If I base my calculation on this proportion, I find that at the two […] *faculties of medicine and law there are altogether 159 professors and lecturers. 4½ out of 159: what would be a fair quota in the context of overall population figures?* […]

At the University of Vienna, if fairness is used as a guiding principle and if no one insists on being disproportionately represented there could be no more than 7, or at most 8 […] *Semitic professors.*

What we are finding in the catalogue now, gentlemen, is not 7, but 64 teachers of Semitic extraction. […] *In one faculty they account almost for one half, and in another the same situation will prevail soon if things are allowed to run their course unchecked. Then the representatives of the occidental culture – I won't even say, Christians – will be outstripped* [for good], *and therefore I am justified in saying if things go on unchecked, the University of Vienna will stop being a University, it will be transformed into a second oriental academy.* […]

I know what [my opponents] *will say. They will say: it so happens that our constitution does not allow for any difference to be made between denominations, let alone between races. That is correct. But it is not on the basis of our constitution that I am opposed to this way of doing things. Even if the constitution allows this and even if the Ministry does not infringe the constitution by ousting all Christians and employing Semites only, then at least this is not part of the constitution that you have to proceed so exclusively, that these are the choices that have to be made. I won't even mention that the majority of our present universities were founded by the ancestors of our most illustrious Emperor as Catholic institutions, endowed with Catholic funds, I don't want to discuss this today; the foundation deeds have simply been filed away and forgotten and the Catholic deeds have been made over into an entirely "kosher" affair* […], *and in this respect there is no discrimination against any religious or racial group according to our constitution.* […]

What is so striking, however, is the fact that the Ministry has never rejected an application [filed by a Jewish applicant] *in favour of a Christian.* […] *Whenever it rejected an application, this was always done in favour of a Semite.* […]

All I am demanding is that the principle be adhered to which has been upheld over centuries, including by the likes of Goethe and Herder, that the core of the entire occidental civilisation rests on Christianity. *It is deeply painful to us that the Ministry seems to be about to abandon this ancient principle.*[641]

Minister Conrad v. Eybesfeld responded to Greuter's charges the very next day:

If the Honourable Member continues to concern himself with the appointments to the various chairs at Vienna University and to find a special characteristic in the religious affiliation of the appointees, most of us are surely susceptible to the witticism with which the Honourable Member predicts that the University of Vienna will, all things remaining the same, be transformed into an oriental academy. This, according to the Honourable Member, will be effected through the nomination of individual professors of non-Christian religion. It is with great regret that I declare myself unable to make use of the well-intentioned friendly warning, which the Honourable Member has attached to his vignette, for the simple reason that the numerical data the Honourable Member has cited with regard to religious affiliation are beyond my control. I do not keep lists of professors according to the religion they belong to […] *and, what is more, I am not aware today of what religion individual teachers profess allegiance to because the selection of candidates is governed by* [an assessment of] *their didactic skills, scientific talents and merits* […] *and not by their religion.*[642]

As is evident from the sources cited above, this debate, unfolding against the backdrop of the rise of nationalism and of clerical-confessional (as opposed to racially motivated) antisemitism[643] at the time, was primarily concerned with the religious affiliation of candidates for appointments at Vienna University, rather than with the question at hand of who was to succeed v. Jaeger as Director of the Second University Eye Clinic – or to put it more pointedly – the choice between Mauthner (Mosaic) and Fuchs (Catholic). Greuter, a Catholic priest, forcefully demanded that in the appointment of professors the relative percentages of religious affiliation in the overall population be taken into account, charging the competent minister, Conrad v. Eybesfeld, with giving undue preference to candidates of Mosaic affiliation, a charge he backed up with his own statistics. The Minister in turn sought to rebut this by pointing out that the only decisive criterion was a candidate's scientific and didactic qualification.[644] It should also be noted that, as the appointment struggle concerning the vacancy at the Second University Eye Clinic unfolded in Vienna's leading medical print media, Greuter abstained from seeking to exert any sort of verbal pressure on the Minister. That Fuchs himself had remained pointedly reserved in the matter of the call to Vienna and had not lobbied anyone either at the Faculty, at court or in political or clerical circles is also evident from the following remark:

After my appointment had gone through various people came to see me whom I had not met before, who claimed they had contributed in one way or another [to my appointment] *and wanted to be reimbursed. I threw them all out; the only one who may in fact have made a difference was Father Greuter, who never turned up.*[645]

The Ministerium für Cultus und Unterricht informed Fuchs on August 1, 1885 of his appointment as follows:

His Imperial and Royal Apostolic Majesty has, by decree of July 30, 1885, graciously deigned to appoint you Full Professor at the 2nd Chair and Clinic of Ophthalmology of the k.k. University of Vienna. Your salary will correspond to the regular pay scales. As this is your first employment in Austria, no employment tax will be levied. Your appointment enters into force with your actual entry into service.

In light of His Majesty's decree I would ask Your Excellency to take up your position at the beginning of the next academic year and to contact in good time the Deanery of the Medical Faculty of the University of Vienna with regard to the announcement and realisation of lectures at the clinic, which during the last academic year was provisionally headed by private lecturer Dr. von Reuss. As for your teaching obligations, I would like to point out that your full professorship at the said clinic is governed by the applicable laws and regulations.

The Governor of Lower Austria, whom Your Excellency will contact upon your arrival in Vienna to arrange for the taking of the oath, has been requested, on condition you enter into service at the date mentioned above, to make your salary available, two thousand two hundred (2,200) fl, plus the activity allowance of eight hundred (800) fl from October 1, 1885.

I would like to add that appointment to a professorship in Austria is contingent on the acquisition of Austrian citizenship, which means that Your Excellency will kindly take whatever steps are required to renounce your present citizenship.[646]

Vienna, August 1, 1885.
Der Minister für Cultus und Unterricht
Frh Conrad Eybesfeld[647]

On the very next day, Sunday, August 2, 1885, the *Wiener medizinische Presse*, edited by Johann Schnitzler (1835–1893), a Jewish laryngologist at the Allgemeine Poliklinik and father of Arthur Schnitzler (1862–1931), carried the following highly instructive comment:

We have just learned that the vacancy at the Eye Clinic caused by JAEGER's death is about to be filled at last. The decision, as is well known, has been in the balance for about a year between Prof. FUCHS, Liège, who was nominated primo loco by a committee *expressly convened for the purpose, and Prof. MAUTHNER, Vienna, who was in turn nominated primo loco by a* Professorial College. *A decision now appears to have been made but is still being kept under strict wraps for the time being. Anyone familiar with existing conditions and especially with the momentarily prevailing trend must have seen quite clearly from the very first beginnings which way the decision was likely to go.* We *at least felt from the word go that the appointment of Prof. FUCHS was, while not more desirable, more probable. – It was, incidentally, not, as will in all probability be generally claimed now, only Father GREUTER's much discussed speech on the University of Vienna that turned the tables* against *MAUTHNER; rather it was powerful personal interventions that were responsible for the decision* in favour of *Prof. FUCHS. – By appointing Prof. FUCHS from Liège,* Vienna *arguably stands to gain an excellent new ophthalmologist, while our* University *at the same time stands to lose an excellent teacher due to the downgrading of Prof. MAUTHNER; the latter will hardly be inclined to continue to work here as a "private lecturer". – Perhaps a solution can be found to make sure that our faculty may in some way retain Prof. MAUTHNER; it would be a matter of great regret should this prove impossible. – Dr. von REUSS, who deputised at the Chair of Ophthalmology for a year, should be appointed Associate Professor in recognition of his merits, without, incidentally, waiting for a proposal to be submitted by the Professorial College, but simply on the basis of the Ministry of Education's own initiative.*[648]

The "Wochen-Chronik" [Weekly Digest] of the *Allgemeine Wiener medizinische Zeitung* of August 3, 1885, edited by Bernard Kraus (1828–1887), a medical doctor at the Allgemeines Krankenhaus, commented on the appointment as follows:

According to the latest report, Prof. Fuchs *from Liège is due to be appointed to this clinic within the next few days. With regard to the question of a successor to the late* [Professor] Jaeger *and the shortlist submitted in that context by the Professorial College, we have expressed our conviction that all three candidates, Professors* Mauthner, Fuchs, *and Schnabel, are eminently qualified to succeed to the vacant chair at Vienna's University. The Ministry of Education has therefore been able to submit all three to the Crown – without there being any need to impute to Father* Greuter *the influence that would have enabled him [single-handedly] to abort* Mauthner*'s appointment. Austria would be in a sorry state indeed if the government, having gone into shock at an outburst of animosity in Parliament by a run-of-the-mill MP, felt called upon to curtail the rights of dissenters that are guaranteed to them by the constitution. While we are not blind to confessional agitation cropping up everywhere in social life, even in academic circles, we are not prepared to credit Father* Greuter *with omnipotence, even if he has managed to give the Education Minister a hard time, given that the appointment issue has attracted keen attention at the highest level of the state, where no distinction is made between nations and confessions.*[649]

On August 9, 1885, the *Wiener medizinische Presse* continued its coverage of the appointment procedure in its column "Ex urbe et orbe":

With regard first of all to the appointment to the 2nd Chair of Ophthalmology, we will gladly abstain from regarding as factually correct the frequently uttered conjectures concerning the allegedly inevitable link between the choice of the candidate and Father Greuter*'s capital speech. Personnel and appointment decisions are hardly ever made in a way that is satisfactory to all concerned; everyone knows this from experience. One thing, though, can be demanded – and, we hasten to add – can also safely be expected, in light of the well-known and frequently demonstrated love of justice on the part of the decisive factors: that for appointments, all other things being equal, it will only ever be scientific merits* *and didactic skills that tilt the scales and that, whenever the reputation and the fame of our* alma mater *is at stake, those same decisive factors will always have their eyes on the* "mother" [mater] – *and never on the* "father" [pater].[650]

The same issue of the *Wiener medizinische Presse* carried in its "Kleine Chronik" [Diary] this additional report:

Our report last week on the appointment to the Chair of Ophthalmology, which has fallen vacant due to JAEGER's death, has caused quite a stir all round – understandably, since over the last few months the appointment of Prof. MAUTHNER was considered a foregone conclusion. – We have hinted at what caused the turnabout and did not believe it permissible to be more explicit. Today's Wiener Zeitung *will remove all doubts by affirming the news we were the first to break. The* Wiener Zeitung *of August 8 carries the following official announcement: His Majesty the Emperor has appointed the Professor of Ophthalmology in Liège, Dr. ERNST FUCHS, Full Professor at the 2nd Chair and Clinic of Ophthalmology of the k.k. University of Vienna by a decree dated July 30,* [1885].[651]

The last in the chorus of Viennese specialist journals to announce Fuchs's appointment was the *Wiener medicinische Wochenschrift*, founded in 1850 by Leopold Wittelshöfer (1818–1889)[652] and edited by him ever since. In early December 1884, as has already been said, the journal had vehemently taken sides for Mauthner and against Fuchs. The tone in this article, published on August 15, 1885, was much more moderate, as indeed was to be expected in view of the unexpected turn events had taken:

The official Wiener Zeitung *of* [August] *8 has announced the appointment of Dr. Ernst* Fuchs, *Professor in Liège, as Full Professor and Director of the Second Eye Clinic in Vienna. On July 5,* [1884], *Prof. von* Jaeger *died and it took a provisional arrangement lasting all of 13 months until a successor was chosen. Our point of view on this crucial appointment is well known: the candidate whom we have supported all along was Prof. L.* Mauthner, *who was ranked primo loco in the shortlist submitted by the Professorial College, whose didactic, scientific and practical-operative merits have not been called into doubt by anyone, not even by his opponents or at least not publicly. It is deeply to be regretted that in the place where the relevant decisions were made it was considered appropriate to allow such great potential to go unused. This is the case all the more since it need not have meant that Prof.* Fuchs *was not recalled to Austria. Prof.* Fuchs, *who has made a name for himself as an ophthalmologist in Liège and is among the most capable younger exponents of the school of von Arlt, may be thought to be entitled to a chair* [in his native country], *but this need not be a chair at the* [country's] *top university, all the more so as he had already declared himself willing to accept a call to the German university in Prague, whence the road to Vienna would have been open for him in a few years' time. It would therefore have been easily possible to assign an appropriate position to him without slighting a man of* Mauthner*'s merits, talent and scientific prestige. This is to commit a grave injustice against the latter, which makes one suspect that the scales were tipped by personal motives and social prejudice, rather than by purely objective considerations.*[653]

In retrospect across four decades, this is how Fuchs himself describes his appointment:

I was simply appointed [to the chair] *in Vienna, without any prior questions being asked and without even the conditions being granted I had stipulated for Prague, namely that my salary was to be at least the same as in Liège and that my time there must be taken into account as years of actual service; now the years one has spent as an assistant are taken into account, which was not the case at the time. I could have told them that my acceptance was contingent on these conditions and, seeing that the Emperor had already signed the decree and always took it in bad part when he had to retract his signature, they would probably have had to take me on my own terms. However, I did not want to do that. I was so glad to be reunited with my parents (my father having suffered a minor stroke briefly before my departure for Liège) and my practice was so lucrative that the smaller salary was not of particular import.* […] *I went* […] *to Vienna to rent a flat and returned to Liège alone. I gave my colleagues the usual farewell dinner and paid my farewell visits.* […] *It was with a heavy heart that I left Liège, where I had been very happy; what a beautiful city, what beautiful surroundings, what good friends and time galore for scientific work!*[654]

Notes

549 UA Wien, Med. Fak. Med S1 ("Normalien") No. 21 from 1812; (Ed.) "Errichtung einer stehenden Klinik für Augenkranke", in: *Med. Jahrb.* II (1814), pp. 8–11; BOECKER-REINARTZ (as in FN 179); KÜCHLE (as in FN 179), pp. 15–23; A. HADWIGER, *Geschichte der k. k. Wiener Augenklinik*. J. B. Wallishauser, Vienna 1836; Ernst FUCHS, "Memories of Vienna Clinics", in: *American Journal of Ophthalmology* [*Am. J. Ophhalmol.*] 9 (1926), pp. 605–607; Isidor FISCHER, "Zur Vorgeschichte der Wiener Augenkliniken", in: *Zeitschr. Augenheilk.* 85 (1935), pp. 326–336; Erna LESKY, "Die Wiener ophthalmologische Schule", in: *Wien. klin. Wochenschr.* 74 (1962), pp. 529–532; LESKY, *Wien. Med. Schule* (as in FN 12), pp. 81ff; Helmut WYKLICKY, "Die Ophthalmologie vor und nach der Begründung der I. Universitäts-Augenklinik", in: *Spektrum Augenheilk.* 2/2A (1988), pp. 2–8; Gabriela SCHMIDT-WYKLICKY, Helmut GRÖGER, "Die Gründung der weltweit ersten Universitäts-Augenklinik in Wien 1812 und ihre Erhebung zum Ordinariat 1818", in: *Spektrum Augenheilk.* 26 (2012), pp. 273–282.

550 Cf. FN 525.

551 ÖSTA/AVA Wien, Studien-Hofkommission 4 Med Augenheilkunde, Augenoperationslehre, Augenkrankheiten u. Assistent. Karton 241, No. 1988/179 from 1818, Dekret v. 13. August 1818; (Ed.) "Errichtung ordentlicher öffentlicher Lehrkanzeln und Kliniken für die Augenheilkunde an den Universitäten zu Wien und Prag", in: *Med. Jahrb.* V/I (1818), pp. 7–9; (Ed.), "Regulirung des Studiums der Augenheilkunde", in: Eduard Vincenz GULDENER Edl. v. LOBES, *Sammlungen der Sanitäts-Verordnungen für das Erzherzogthum Oesterreich unter der Enns, als Fortsetzung der v. Ferro'schen Sammlung*. Fünfter Theil, enthaltend die Verordnungen vom Jahre 1818 bis Ende des Jahres 1824. Gerold, Wien 1825, pp. 46–47; (Ed.), "Errichtung einer ordentlichen öffentlichen Lehrkanzel und Klinik für die Augenheilkunde", in: Johann Nepomuk Frh. v. HEMPEL-KÜRSINGER, *Handbuch der Gesetzeskunde im Sanitäts- und Medicinal-Gebiethe in alphabetisch-chronologisch und materienweiser Zusammenstellung für Sanitäts- und Polizeybeamte im Allgemeinen und insbesondere für Aerzte, Wundärzte, Geburtshelfer, Hebammen und Apotheker.* First volume A–I, Vienna 1830, pp. 114–117.

552 Ophthalmology had until then been considered to be part and parcel of surgery because of the leading role played by cataract surgery.

553 Friedrich Jaeger von Jaxtthal (1784–1871). Originally from Württemberg. Studied at Würzburg, at the med.-surg. Josephs-Akademie in Vienna and at Vienna Univ.; 1808 Dr. med. et chir. Univ. Landshut. Moved to Vienna. Student of Georg Josef Beer; 1812 ophthalmol. dissertation (MA in Ophthalmol.) at Vienna Univ. and licentia practicandi for foreigners. Beer's private assist. and son-in-law. 1826–1848 Prof. of Ophthalmol. at the Med.-Surg. Josephs-Akademie (Josephinum). Physician and friend of Austria's State Chancellor Metternich. Made a significant contribution to the establishment of a med.-surg. school according to Europ. standards in Istanbul. Cf. GERABEK et al. (as in FN 13); HIRSCHBERG, *Geschichte der Augenheilkunde* (as in FN 18), 2nd ed., W. Engelmann, Leipzig 1911, vol. 14/I (= Reprint, G. Olms, vol. II, Hildesheim/New York 1977), pp. 551–557; IBBO (as in FN 18); Wilhelm SCHLESINGER, "Erinnerung an Friedrich Jaeger", in: *Wien. med. Wochen-*

schr. 22 (1872), cols. 15–17; Wilhelm v. ZEHENDER (ed.), "Friedrich Jäger, Ritter von Jaxtthal", in: *Klin. Monatsbl. f. Augenheilk.* 10 (1872), pp. 177–181; Louis de WECKER, "Notice nécrologique sur Frédéric Jaeger. Chevalier de Jaxtthal", in: *Annales d'oculistique [Ann. oculist.]* 69 (1873), pp. 85–93; Georg PREYSS, *Das Leben und Wirken des k. k. Raths, Stabsfeldarzts und Professors der Augenheilkunde am Josefinum Dr. Friedrich Jaeger Ritter von Jaxtthal.* Gedächtnisrede ..., Gesellschafts-Buchdruckerei, Vienna 1877; Theodor PUSCHMANN, *Die Medicin in Wien während der letzten 100 Jahre* [= PUSCHMANN, *Wien. Med. 100 J.*], Moritz Perles, Vienna 1884, pp. 167–169; KIRCHENBERGER, *Lebensbilder* (as in FN 165), pp. 83ff.; LESKY, *Wien. Med. Schule* (as in FN 12), pp. 87–88; WYKLICKY, *Josephinum* (as in FN 165), pp. 103–105; WYKLICKY, "Ergänzungen zur Kenntnis des Stammvaters der medizinischen Schule von Galatasaray (Über unveröffentlichte Briefe Metternichs an Friedrich Jaeger)" [= "Stammvater"], in: Erwin LUCIUS, Arslan TERZIOGLU (eds.), Österreichisch-Türkische medizinische Beziehungen. Berichte d. Symposions v. 28. u. 29. 4. 1986 in Istanbul. Istanbul 1987, pp. 78–86; Maria SCHNEIDER, *Dr. med. Friedrich Jäger Ritter von Jaxtthal (1784–1871) – Augenarzt zu Wien und Leibarzt des Fürsten Metternich – Autobiographie mit Kommentar.* Diss. Techn. Univ. München 1988. [= *Medizin & Gesellschaft* vol. 4]. Münster 1989.

554 Friedrich Jaeger had fallen foul of Protomedicus Andreas Joseph Freiherrn v. Stifft (1776–1836), because he had rejected a call to the Chair of Ophthalmol. at Pest Univ. in 1812. Cf. WYKLICKY, *Josephinum* (as in FN 165), p. 103.

555 Ibid., p. 104.

556 Arno DUSINI (ed.), *Franz GRILLPARZER, Selbstbiographie.* Residenz Verlag, Salzburg/Wien 1994, pp. 102–103.

557 WYKLICKY, "Stammvater"; SCHNEIDER, *Friedrich Jäger.*

558 ÖSTA/AVA Wien. Box 874 4 G Medizin Augenklinik No. 3189/415 of 21 April 1849.

559 Dieter HALBWIDL, "Life and Times of Count Thun", in: *Mensch–Wissenschaft–Magie.* Mitteilungen der Österreichischen Gesellschaft für Wissenschaftsgeschichte (ÖGW) 30 (2013), pp. 111–131.

560 Cf. FN 558, No. 5492/752 of 27 July 1849.

561 Ibid., reply of 6 August 1849.

562 Carl Graf VASQUEZ, *Grundriss der inneren Haupt- und Residenzstadt Wien, nebst 14 Ansichten der vorzüglichsten Gebäude.* See ÖHLINGER, *Pläne* (as in FN 71), p. 11.

563 LESKY, *Wien. Med. Schule* (as in FN 12), p. 87.

564 Eduard Jaeger von Jaxtthal (1818–1884). Cf. HIRSCHBERG, *Geschichte der Augenheilkunde* (as in FN 18), vol. 15/2, pp. 380–398; Ludwig MAUTHNER, "Gedenkrede auf Prof. Eduard Jaeger", in: *Wien. med. Bl.* 7 (1884), pp. 1407–12; Salomon KLEIN (BÄRINGER), "Gedenkrede zu Ehren Prof. Eduard v. Jaegers anläßlich der Enthüllung seines Denkmals in der Universität am 28. Februar 1910", in: *Wien. klin. Wochenschr.* 23 (1910), pp. 410–413; Gabriela SCHMIDT-WYKLICKY, Helmut GRÖGER, "Die Gründung der II. Universitäts-Augenklinik in Wien 1883 und ihr erster Vorstand Eduard Jaeger von Jaxtthal 1883 bis 1884", in: *Spektrum Augenheilk.* 26 (2012), pp. 296–302.

565 Eduard JAEGER, *Ueber die Behandlung des grauen Staares an der ophthalmologischen Klinik der Josephs-Akademie.* Carl Ueberreuter, Wien 1844.

566 UA Wien, Med. Fak. Sonderreihe Lehrkanzelbesetzungen, Augenklinik (1) (1821–1831), Box 117, pp. 17.12.1 to 17.12.37.

567 Anton von Rosas (1791_1855). Originally from Fünfkirchen (today: Pécs/Hungary). Studied at the Univ. of Pest (1806–1811) and Vienna (Dr. med., Mag. ophthalm. 1814, Dr. chir. 1816). Assist. under Beer at the Vienna University Eye Clinic, 1819–1921 Director of the Eye Clinic in Padua, then part of Austria, where he performed highly appreciated foundational work. 1821–1855 Succeeded Beer as Full Prof. and Dir. of the University Eye Clinic Vienna, where he introduced many improvements. Excellent reputation as clinical teacher and surgeon. His three-volume *Handbuch der theoretischen und praktischen Augenheilkunde* (1830) met with great acclaim as did his *Lehre von den Augenkrankheiten* (1834). He also concerned himself with the history of the University of Vienna and its medical faculty, which resulted in a seminal work (1843–1847). Cf. CZEIKE (as in FN 13); HEID *Personalbibliographien* (as in FN 165); HIRSCHBERG, *Geschichte der Augenheilkunde* (as in FN 18), vol. 14/1, pp. 557–561; IBBO, Part 2; Heid (as in FN 165), pp. 20–25; LESKY, *Wien. Med. Schule* (as in FN 12), pp. 86–87; Karl HOLUBAR, "Anton von Rosas (1791–1855): On the occasion of the bicentennial of his birth. Part 1": *Wien. klin. Wochenschr.* 103 (1991), pp. 470–472; Edoardo MIDENA, "Anton von Rosas (1791–1855): On the occasion of the bicentennial of his birth. Part 2: A survey of his scientific works with special emphasis on specific topics", in: *Wien. klin. Wochenschr.* 103 (1991), pp. 473–476; Gabriela SCHMIDT-WYKLICKY, Helmut GRÖGER, "Anton von Rosas. Vorstand der Universitäts-Augenklinik in Wien 1821 bis 1855", in: *Spektrum Augenheilk.* 26/6 (2012), pp. 283–289.

568 On Arlt as a person, cf. FN 18. On filling the vacancy at the top of the Vienna Univ. Eye Clinic in 1856, cf. AVA Wien. AVA Unterricht Allgemein (1848–1940) Universität Wien, Medizin Lehrkanzeln: in genere u. A–G Anatomie–Gewerbekrankheiten. Box 617: 4 Med Augenheilkunde No. 2869 from 1856 *Wiederbesetzung des Lehramtes der Augenheilkunde an der Universität in Wien*; Heid (as in FN 165); HIRSCHBERG, *Geschichte der Augenheilkunde* (as in FN 18), 15/2, pp. 352–376; IBBO (as in FN 18); LESKY, *Wien. Med. Schule* (as in FN 12), pp. 220–226; Ernst FUCHS, "Ferdinand von Arlt †", in: *Wien. med. Bl.* 10 (1887), pp. 317–321; Hubert SATTLER, "Ferdinand von Arlt", in: *Klin. Monatsbl. Augenheilk.* 25(1887), pp. 133–146; Friedrich DIMMER, "Ferdinand Ritter von Arlt. Zu seinem hundertsten Geburtstag", in: *Wien. klin. Wochenschr.* 25 (1912), pp. 607–608, Gabriela SCHMIDT-WYKLICKY, Helmut GRÖGER, "Ferdinand Ritter von Arlt, Vorstand der Universitäts-Augenklinik in Wien 1856 bis 1883. Eine Würdigung zum 200. Geburtstag", in: *Spektrum Augenheilk.* 26 (2012), pp. 290–295.

569 Cf. ÖSTA/AVA Wien. Karton 874 4 G Medizin Augenklinik No. 7054/313 of 4 May 1856; ARLT, *Meine Erlebnisse*, pp. 64–65.

570 Even influential pathologist Carl v. Rokitansky, who represented the Faculty's interests in the Ministerium f. Cultus u. Unterricht, could do nothing to increase the number of beds at Arlt's disposal. Cf. ÖSTA/AVA Wien, Karton 874, 4 G Medizin Augenklinik No. 12582/432 of 26 July 1857. In 1858, however, the so-called spare room with another thirty beds, which were not considered to be clinical beds, was added to Arlt's clinic. (Cf. LESKY, *Wien. Med. Schule* [as in FN 12], p. 224). Arlt himself wrote in his autobiography: *"I remained frustrated for quite a long time in my efforts to gain*

access to a greater number of beds (it was always the hospital director who got in the way) until in late February 1858 Professor Hebra [cf. FN 163, A/N] *ceded one of his larger hospital rooms, which was adjacent to my clinic, to be used by the clinic as an additional room. It was divided into two by a wooden partition, thus creating space for thirty beds."* Cf. ARLT, *Meine Erlebnisse*, p. 67.

571 ÖSTA/AVA Wien, 4 G Med Augenheilkunde, Karton 874, No. 12582/432 of 26 June 1857.

572 At this stage, Eduard Jaeger v. Jaxtthal had already published his innovat. studies mainly in the following monographs: *Ueber Staar und Staaroperationen nebst anderen Beobachtungen und Erfahrungen aus seines Vaters Dr. Friedrich Jaeger, k. k. Professors etc. etc. und aus der eigenen ophthalmologischen Praxis*. L. W. Seidel, Vienna 1854 (Habilitation thesis); JAEGER v. JAXTTHAL, *Beiträge zur Pathologie des Auges*. Mit Abbildungen im Farbendruck. Kaiserlich-Königliche Hof- und Staatsdruckerei, Vienna 1855; JAEGER v. JAXTTHAL, *Ergebnisse der Untersuchung des menschlichen Auges mit dem Augenspiegel*. Braumüller, Vienna 1855.

573 Cf. ÖSTA/AVA Wien. Unterricht Allgemein (1848–1940) Universität Wien, Medizin Lehrkanzeln: in genere u. A–G Anatomie–Gewerbekrankheiten. Karton 617: 4 Med Augenheilkunde No. 13.316 from 1863.

574 Cf. ibid., 4 Med Augenheilkunde No. 17750 from 1856.

575 Cf. ARLT, *Meine Erlebnisse*, p. 65.

576 Cf. ÖSTA/AVA Wien 4 G Medicin. II. Augenklinik Errichtung, No. 9714 of 21 May 1883.

577 Ibid., 4 G Medicin Eye Clinic, No. 7954 of 11 June 1874 and No. 8972 of 1 July 1874.

578 Reports differ with regard to the number of rooms allotted to Jaeger. The original file mentions *"7 rooms, some larger, some smaller"*. In a list compiled by the then manager of the Allgem. Krankenhaus from 1965 these 81 beds were, during the period in question, dispersed over only five rooms: 1. Men: Room 44a (19 beds), Room 44b (17 beds), Room 45 (9 beds), 2. Women: Room 43 (19 beds) and Room 46 (17 beds). Cf. Bernhard GROIS, *Das Allgemeine Krankenhaus in Wien und seine Geschichte*. Wilhelm Maudrich, Wien 1965, p. 117.

579 Ibid. This proposal involved a reference to its implementation at the Clinic and Department of Syphilis. Furthermore, an additional motif was the possibility of cutting back expenses by making do without a junior doctor, as the new clinic would have an assistant anyway.

580 FUCHS, *Augenarzt* (as in FN 2), p. 80. The institution Fuchs refers to, first, as Skin Clinic and immediately afterwards as Department of Skin Diseases was the II. Abteilung für Syphilis at the Allgem. Krankenhaus, headed by the Hebra disciple Hermann Zeissl (1817–1884). This ward, which was reserved for women, comprised the two hospital rooms 57a and 57b with 24 beds apiece. Cf. GROIS (as in FN 578), *Allgemeines Krankenhaus*, p. 118.

581 ÖSTA/AVA Wien 4 G Medicin II. Eye Clinic Nr. 14953 of 3 August 1883 and No 16930 of 5 September 1883.

582 J. F. WAGNER, *Orientirungs-Plan des Wiener k.k. allgemeinen Krankenhauses nebst Daten über dasselbe, über das Gebärhaus und die pathologisch-anatomische Anstalt in Wien*. Josef Šafář, Vienna 1886, p. 17.

583 ÖSTA/AVA Wien, 4 G Medicin II Eye Clinic u. 4 Medicin Jäger, Z. 18.239 ex 1883. Imperial decree regard. the systemising of a Second Eye Clinic at Vienna Univ. and the appointment of Eduard Jaeger as Full Prof. and Director of this Clinic of 26 September 1883.

584 FUCHS, *Augenarzt* (as in FN 2), pp. 80–81.

585 Eduard von JAEGER, *Ophthalmoskopischer Hand-Atlas.* K. K. Hof- und Staatsdruckerei, Vienna 1869; Louis de WECKER, Eduard de JAEGER, *Traité des maladies du fond de l'œil et atlas d'ophtalmoscopie.* Delahaye, Paris 1870.

586 Eduard von JAEGER, Über die Einstellungen des dioptrischen Apparates im menschlichen Auge. Seidel, Vienna 1871.

587 Eduard JAEGER, *Staar- und Staaroperationen* (1854), cf. FN 572. Appended to the 1st edition was what has become known as the Jaeger chart, text passages from world literature with fonts gradually increasing in size, in German, French and English. Only three years later a second, stand-alone edition of these reading samples was published: (Eduard JAEGER), *Schrift-Scalen des Prof. Jaeger jun.* 2nd aug. ed., K. K. Hof- und Staatsdruckerei. Vienna 1857. How extensively the Jaeger chart was used is apparent from its translation into Spanish, Portuguese, Russian, Polish, Italian, Modern Greek and Hebrew. In 1895 Fuchs published a revised version of the Jaeger chart: Ernst FUCHS, *Leseproben für die Nähe. Jäger's Schriftscalen modifiziert von Professor Dr. E. Fuchs.* Fritsch, Vienna 1895. Cf. HIRSCH, *Geschichte der Augenheilkunde*, p. 528; HIRSCHBERG, *Geschichte der Augenheilkunde* (as in FN 18), vol. 15/2 [= Reprint vol. VI], § 1240, p. 389; Arthur LINKSZ, "The Development of Visual Standards: Snellen, Jaeger, and Giraud-Teulon", in: *Bulletin of the New York Academy of Medicine* [*Bull. N. Y. Acad. Med.*] 51/2 (1975), pp. 277–285; Paul E. RUNGE, "Eduard Jaeger's Test-Types (Schrift-Scalen) and the Historical Development of Vision Tests", in: *Transactions of the American Ophthalmological Society [= Trans. Am. Ophthalmol. Soc.*] 98 (2000), pp. 375–438.

588 Hans ADLER, "Eduard Jaeger, † 5. Juli 1884", in: *Mittheil. Wien. med. Doct. Coll.* 10 (1884), p. 212.

589 August Leopold Ritter v. Reuss (1841–1924). Studied at the Univ. of Prague and Vienna (Dr. med. 1865, Dr. chir. 1867). Ophthalmol. specialist training under Eduard Jaeger v. Jaxtthal and as clin. assist. and private assist. under Arlt. 1870 Habilitation. 1872 Founding member of Vienna's Allgem. Poliklinik. 1872–1922 Head physician of its Eye Dept. 1909 Hospital Director of the Poliklinik. Cf. DEIMER, *Poliklinik* (as in FN 200), pp. 155–157. Obituaries, in: *Die feierl. Inauguration d. Rektors d. Wiener Universität für d. Studienjahr 1924/25.* Eigenverlag Vienna Univ. 1924, pp. 33–34 (Viktor Hanke); *Jahresbericht der Allgem. Poliklinik für 1924.* Eigenverlag Poliklinik 23 (1925), pp. 4–6 (Julius Mannaberg); *Wien. klin. Wochenschr.* 37 (1924), pp. 1171–72 (Julius Mannaberg).

590 August v. REUSS, "Ophthalmologische Mittheilungen. Aus der zweiten Universitäts-Augenklinik in Wien. I. Abtheilung", in: *Wien. med. Presse* 26 (1885), p. 2.

591 Carl (Karl) Koller (1857–1944). Originally from Bohemia. Dr. med. univ. 1882 Vienna Univ.; collaborator of the Viennese experimental pathol. Salomon Stricker (cf. FN 610). Junior doctor at the 1st (Arlt) and at the 2nd Univ. Eye Clinic (Jaeger, Reuss). Having been alerted by his friend Sigmund Freud (1856–1939) to the superficially anaesthetising effect of cocaine on lingual mucosa, Koller applied an aqueous

solution of 2 % cocaine to painful diseases of the eye and to eye operations. In this way he discovered local anaesthesia. As he had not yet completed his training as an ophthalmologist, he asked the Triestine eye specialist Josef Brettauer (cf. FN 303) to announce his epoch-making discovery at the annual conference of the Dt. Ophthalmol. Gesellsch. in Heidelberg on 15. September 1884. Having been insulted because of his Jewish descent, he engaged in a duel. With duels already on the verge of illegality, Koller was forced to leave Austria in September 1885. [Cf. Carl Koller's handwritten letter to the Directorate of the Wiener Allg. Krankenhauses, dated Cologne 28 September 1885, in which K. informed the hospital of his resignation from his position as junior doctor (Private collection). K. also mentions his intention of writing in a private capacity to the hospital director, Obersanitätsrat Dr. Hoffman. It may be presumed that in this letter K. put forward his personal views on why the duel was justified and on his subsequent resignation.] 1885–1887 Assist. under Donders (cf. FN 38 and 291) and Snellen (cf. FN 292) in Utrecht. 1888 Emigration to New York. Highly respected as a doctor at Mount Sinai and Montefiore Hospitals. 1929 Kussmaul Medal (Adolf Kussmaul (1822–1902, German clinician) awarded by Heidelberg Univ. Cf. FISCHER (as in FN 28); NDB (as in FN 15); ÖBL (as in FN 11); Obituaries: *Arch. Ophthalmol.* 31 (1944), pp. 344–345; LESKY, *Wien. Med. Schule* (as in FN 12), pp. 486–490; *Austrian Ophthalmologists*, pp. 12–13; *Jewish Telegraphic Agency* Febr. 25, 1929.

592 Carl KOLLER, "Vorläufige Mittheilung über lokale Anästhesirung am Auge", in: *Klin. Monatsbl. Augenheilk.* 22 (1884), Beilageheft [= Bericht über d. XVI. Versammlg. d. Ophthalmol. Gesellschaft Heidelberg 16 (1884)], pp. 60–63, Sitzung v. 15. Sept. 1884; KOLLER, "Ueber die Verwendung des Cocaïn zur Anästhesirung am Auge", in: *Wien. med. Wochenschr.* 34 (1884), cols. 1275–1278 and cols. 1309–11 (Sitzung d. k. k. Gesellschaft d. Ärzte v. 15. Oktober 1884, see also: *Anzeiger d. k. k. Gesellsch. d. Aerzte in Wien*, No. 2, 23 October 1884; KOLLER, "Historische Notiz über die ersten Anfänge der lokalen Anästhesie", in: *Wien. med. Wochenschr.* 78 (1928), cols. 601–602 [Reprint ibid. 84 (1934), cols. 1179–80]; KOLLER, "Nachträgliche Bemerkungen über die ersten Anfänge der Lokalanästhesie", in: Ibid. 85 (1935), cols. 7–8.; GARRISON/MORTON (as in FN 124), HIRSCHBERG, *Geschichte der Augenheilkunde* (as in FN 18), vol. 14/2 [= Reprint vol. III], § 489, p. 83, 85 and pp. 87–88 (Literature)]; IBBO (as in FN 18); Sigmund FREUD, "Beitrag zur Kenntnis der Cocawirkung", in: *Wien. med. Wochenschr.* 35 (1885), cols. 129–133; Gustav GAERTNER, "Die Entdeckung der Lokalanästhesie", in: *Der neue Tag* Yr 1, No. 137, Vienna, Saturday 9 August 1919, p. 6; Wilhelm COMBERG, "Fünfzig Jahre Lokalanästhesie des Auges", in: *Münchener medicinische Wochenschrift* [= *Münch. med. Wochenschr.*] 81 (1934), p. 1649; Josef MELLER, "Gedenkworte zum 50. Jahrestage des Vortrages von Dr. Karl Koller über das Kokain vor der Gesellschaft der Ärzte in Wien", in: *Wien. klin. Wochenschr.* 47 (1934), pp. 1313–17; Hortense KOLLER BECKER, "Carl Koller and Cocaine", in: *Psychoanalytic Quarterly* 32 (1963), pp. 309–373; James E. LEBENSOHN, "The Application of Cocaine to the Eye as an Anesthetic", in: James E. LEBENSOHN, *An Anthology of Ophthalmic Classics*. Williams & Wilkens Co., Baltimore 1969, pp. 324–32; Heinrich HONEGGER, Herbert HESSLER, "Die Entdeckung der Lokalanästhesie durch Karl Koller (I–III)", in: Klin. *Monatsbl. Augenheilk.* 157 (1970), pp. 428–438, 569–578 and 714–723; Wolfgang MÜN-

CHOW, "Geschichte der Augenheilkunde", in: Karl VELHAGEN, *Der Augenarzt.* vol IX, 2nd ed., Georg Thieme, Leipzig 1983, pp. 618–623; Helmut WYKLICKY, *Zur Geschichte der Augenheilkunde*, p. 22; WYKLICKY, "Hundert Jahre Lokalanästhesie", in: *Wien. klin. Wochenschr.* 97 (1984), pp. 449–450; WYKLICKY – Manfred SKOPEC, "Carl Koller (1857–1944) and his time in Vienna", in: D. B. SCOTT, J. Mc CLURE, J. A. W. WILDSMITH (eds.), *Regional Anesthesia 1884–1984.* Centennial Meeting of Regional Anesthesia. European Society of Regional Anaesthesia in Association with the American Association of Regional Anesthesia. Vienna, September 12–15, 1984, pp. 12–23; Karl HRUBY, "Wurde Dr. Carl Koller 1885 aus Wien vertrieben?", in: *Wien. klin. Wochenschr.* 98 (1985), pp. 155–156; Hubert BODAMMER, *Die Anfänge der Lokalanästhesie in der Augenheilkunde.* Diss. Med. Hochschule Hannover 1988; Helmut GRÖGER, Gabriela SCHMIDT-WYKLICKY, "Carl Koller und die Entdeckung der Lokalanästhesie 1884", in: *Spektrum Augenheilk.* 26 (2012), pp. 309–311; M. GOERIG, "Aus dem Nachlass von Carl Koller. Aufzeichnungen zu seinen Experimenten mit Kokain", in: *Der Anaesthesist* 64/6 (2015), pp. 469–477.

593 Cf. REUSS, *Mittheilungen* (as in FN 590), I. Abth., pp. 3–6.

594 Ernst FUCHS, "Ueber Cocain", in: *Wien. klin. Wochenschr.* 15 (1902), pp. 962–964.

595 Cf. Gabriela SCHMIDT-WYKLICKY, Helmut GRÖGER, "Carl Stellwag von Carion. Vorstand der I. Universitäts-Augenklinik in Wien 1884 bis 1894" (as in FN 165), pp. 303–308.

596 Cf. FN 17.

597 Hans Kundrat (1845–1893). While still a student at Vienna Univ. (Dr. med. 1868), demonstrator under anatomist Joseph Hyrtl (cf. FN 13) and pathologist Carl v. Rokitansky (cf. FN 15). As Rokitansky's assist. 1873 habililitation in Pathol. Anat. at Vienna Univ. (1875 Assoc. Prof.). 1877 Chair of Pathol. Anatomy at Graz Univ., 1882 Assoc Prof. of Pathol. Anatomy at Vienna Univ.; 1887/88 Dean of the Med. Fac.; initial description of lymphosarcoma. Cf. CZEIKE (as in FN 13); EISENBERG 2 (as in FN 13); HIRSCH (as in FN 13); NDB (as in FN 15); ÖBL (as in FN 11); PAGEL (as in FN 13); LESKY, Wien. Med. Schule (as in FN 12), pp. 566ff; Obituaries: *Wien. klin. Wochenschr.* 6 (1893), pp. 323ff.; *Wien. med. Wochenschr.* 43 (1893), cols. 810–811.

598 Hermann Nothnagel (1841–1905). Originally from Alt-Lietzegöricke in what was then Mark Brandenburg (since 1945 Stare Łysogórki, Poland). Stud. at the Med.-Chirurg. Friedrich Wilhelm-Inst. at the Pépinière in Berlin (Dr. med. 1863). Initially military doctor, 1865 Assist. under the internal clinician Ernst v. Leyden (1832–1910) at Königsberg (Habilitation 1866). 1872 Prof. of Pharmacology and Med. Clinic in Freiburg/Breisgau. 1874 Prof. of Special Pathol. and Therapy in Jena. 1882–1905 Full Prof. and Director of the 1st. Med. Univ. Clinic in Vienna. His *Handbuch d. Arzneimittellehre* (1870) remained in use for decades and was translated into several languages. Main area of interest: Neurol. (then still considered to be part of internal medicine). Another widely respected work was *Topische Diagnostik der Gehirnkrankheiten* (1879). In it, he describes the upper syndrome of the nucleus ruber as a complex of neurolog. symptoms typical of tumours of the colliculi. Definition of acroparesthesia, which is associated with his name to this day. Initial description of angina pectoris vasomotorica and identification of the pain as a spasm of the coronary vessels. Explored the causes of arrhythmias. During his time in Vienna focus on gastroenterology. Main

area of interest: description of the bacillus subtilis and bac. butyrcus. Studied the functions of intestinal bacteria in digestion and bowel motility. Described the fatty degeneration of digestive tract muscles and colitis membranacea. One of the most outstanding internists of his time, he was also much appreciated as a teacher. Cf. CZEIKE (as in FN 13), EISENBERG 2 (as in FN 13); FISCHER (as in FN 28); ÖBL (as in FN 11); PAGEL (as in FN 13); "Feierl. Inauguration d. Rektors 1905/06", *Almanach d. Akad. Wiss.*, Vienna 1906; Max NEUBURGER, *Hermann Nothnagel. Leben und Wirken eines deutschen Klinikers*. Rikola, Vienna/Berlin/Leipzig/Munich 1922; LESKY, *Wien. Med. Schule* (as in FN 12), pp. 313 ff.

599 Carl Toldt (1840–1920). Originally from South Tyrol. Studied at the med.-chir. Josephs-Akademie (Josephinum) in Vienna (Dr. med. 1864), Assist. under the physiologist Ewald Hering (cf. FN 296) at the Josephinum, 1869 Habilitation in Microscop. Anat; after the dissolution of the Josephinum (1874) assist. under the anatomist Carl Langer v. Edenberg (cf. FN 616) at the Med. Fac. of Vienna Univ. (1875 Assoc. Prof.). 1876–1884 Full Prof. at Prague Univ., where he rebuilt his Institute and established an anat. museum. 1884–1908 Full Prof. of Descript. and Topograph. Anatomy (2nd Chair of Anat.) at Vienna Univ., where he established a museum and a library. Highly respected also as a histologist and anthropologist. Cf. CZEIKE (as in FN 13); EISENBERG 2 (as in FN 13); HIRSCH (as in FN 13); LESKY, *Wien. Med. Schule* (as in FN 12), pp. 505–507; Obituaries: *Wien. klin. Wochenschr.* 33 (1920), pp. 1041ff.; *Wien. med. Wochenschr.* 70 (1920), col. 2045; *Feierl. Inauguration … Studienjahr 1921/22*, pp. 30ff.; Carl TOLDT, *Autobiografie*. Urban & Schwarzenberg, Berlin/Wien 1922; Helmut GRÖGER, "Carl Toldt. Hervorragender Anatom und Anthropologe der Wiener medizinischen Schule", in: *APIS* [= *Arzt und Patient in Südtirol*] 3 (1990), pp. 44ff.

600 Cf. FN 200.

601 Cf. FN 220.

602 Isidor Schnabel (1842–1908). Alongside Mauthner one of the students closest to Eduard Jaeger v. Jaxtthal. 1871 Habilitation in Vienna. One of his achievements was the introduction of object lessons in the use of the ophthalmoscope at Austria's universities. 1877–1887 Full Prof. at Innsbruck (as Mauthner's successor); 1887–1891 Full Prof. at Graz; 1891–1895 Full Prof. in Prague; 1895–1908 Full Prof. at the 1st Univ. Eye Clinic in Vienna. Cf. CZEIKE (as in FN 13); FISCHER (as in FN 28); KÜCHLE (as in FN 179); ÖBL (as in FN 11); PAGEL (as in FN 13); IBBO, Part 2; LESKY, *Wien. Med. Schule* (as in FN 12), pp. 482–485; Obituaries: *Klin. Monatsbl. Augenheilk.* 47 (1909), pp. 168–171; *Wien. klin. Wochenschr.* 22 (1909), pp. 32–34 (Anton Elschnig); *Wien. klin. Rundschau* 22 (1908), pp. 815–816; *Zeitschr. Augenheilk.* 21 (1909), pp. 90–93 (Hans Lauber); Appreciation: Helmut GRÖGER, Gabriela SCHMIDT-WYKLICKY, "Isidor Schnabel. Vorstand der I. Universitäts-Augenklinik in Wien von 1895 bis 1908", in: *Spektrum Augenheilk.* 26 (2012), pp. 321–324.

603 Cf. ÖSTA/ AVA Wien. Unterricht Allgemein (1848–1940) Universität Wien, Medizin Lehrkanzeln: in genere u. A–G Anatomie–Gewerbekrankheiten. Karton 617: 4 Medicin Augenheilkunde No. 23518 of 2 December 1884, fol. 1–14.

604 August Emil Vogl (1833–1909). Pharmacologist and pharmacognosist. 1860 the first physician to graduate from the med.-chir. Josephs-Akademie during the third study period (relaunch in 1854 after the closure in 1848) as Dr. med. univ. (Vienna

Univ. introduced this degree in 1873 in keeping with the new study regulations.) Prof. of Pharmacognosy at the Josephinum until its final closure in 1874, then Prof. of Pharmcogn. at Vienna Univ. until 1904. Pioneering work in the microscop. and microchem. examination of foodstuffs and luxury food. Dean of the Med. Fac. 1876/77, 1881/82, 1882/83, 1884/85, 1889/90, 1893/94. Rector of Vienna Univ. 1887/88. Cf. CZEIKE (as in FN 13); HIRSCH (as in FN 13); PAGEL (as in FN 13); LESKY, *Wien. Med. Schule* (as in FN 12), pp. 583–588; WYKLICKY, *Josephinum*; p. 121; Johann JURENITSCH, Claudia MÜLLER, Kurt SCHNEIDER, Wolfgang KUBELKA, *200 Jahre Pharmakognosie in Wien. Eine Wissenschaft im Dienst der Arzneimittelsicherheit*. Facultas Universitätsverlag, Wien 1998, pp. 27–41.

605 ÖSTA/AVA Wien. K. K. Ministerium für Cultus u. Unterricht, 4 Medicin Fuchs No. 14313 from 1885, fol. 15.

606 Nothnagel's declaration of support, which is mentioned in the original file, is missing.

607 Hermann NOTHNAGEL, *Topische Diagnostik der Gehirnkrankheiten*. Eine klinische Studie. A. Hirschwald, Berlin 1879; Ludwig MAUTHNER, *Gehirn und Auge*. Bergmann, Wiesbaden 1881(= MAUTHNER, *Vorträge aus dem Gesammtgebiete der Augenheilkunde für Studirende und Aerzte*. Heft IX–XI, 1881–1882). Cf. EISENBERG 2 (as in FN 13) (with bibliography); SEYFARTH/ZOTTOLI (as in FN 200).

608 The Viennese medical historian Max Neuburger (1868–1955) characterised Nothnagel's outlook in his own inimitable way: *Without being a member of any one political party – his mindset made him sympathise by and large with Germany's National Liberals – Nothnagel reacted with unease and sadness to the rise of some of the movements that surfaced soon after the establishment of the German Empire, especially the rise of antisemitism, which of all political and cultural movements was most offensive to his unchanging, rock solid sense of justice. He not only denied the justification of its loudly proclaimed catchphrases, he believed that this, in his eyes, thoroughly ignoble and inhumane movement was based on motifs that differed entirely from the ethnic, religious, ethical and economic concerns it professed. What appalled him most of all was the spectacularly rude aggression of the sort he had had occasion to observe especially in Vienna. Unlike other likeminded people, who were equally pure of heart and mind, he felt he could not pass these things over in silence; wherever humanity was at stake, he considered it to be his duty to express his conviction publicly, loudly and unreservedly. It is owing to his initiative, which soon resonated in noble, educated circles of the imperial capital, that in conjunction with Friedr. Freiherr v. Leitenberger* [1837–1899, Austrian industrialist, A/N] *and Arthur Gundaccar Freiherrn v. Suttner* [1850–1902, Austrian writer, married Bertha, née Gräfin Kinsky v. Wchinitz u. Tettau in 1876, A/N] *the* Verein zur Abwehr des Antisemitismus *was founded in 1891.* Max NEUBURGER, *Hermann Nothnagel. Leben und Wirken eines deutschen Klinikers*. Rikola, Vienna/ Berlin/Leipzig/Munich 1922, pp. 235–236. For political movements in fin-de-siècle Austria, see Albert FUCHS, *Geistige Strömungen in Österreich 1867–1918*. Mit einem Essay von Friedrich Heer. Löcker, Vienna 1996; Kathrin McEWEN, *Antisemitismus in Wien um 1900: Eine Diskursanalyse der christlich-sozialen und deutschnationalen Presse*. VDM Verlag Dr. Müller 2010; Gerhard BOTZ, Ivar Michael POLLAK, Nina SCHOLZ (eds.), *Eine zerstörte Kultur. Jüdisches Leben und Antisemitismus in Wien seit dem 19. Jahrhundert*. Czernin Verlag, Vienna 2002.

609 Eduard Albert (1841–1900). Originally from Senftenberg in Bohemia (today Žamberk, Czech Republic). 1867 Dr. med. Vienna Univ., trainee surgeon (from 1869 assistant) at the 1st Surg. Univ. Clinic of Vienna's Allgem. Krankenhaus under Johann Dumreicher Frh v. Österreicher (1815–1880). 1872 Habilitation in Surgery, 1873 Full Prof. and Director of the Surg. Univ. Clinic Innsbruck, 1881 Full Prof. and Director of 1st Chir. Univ. Klinik in Vienna. 1876 First human nerve graft. Cf. CZEIKE (as in FN 13); EISENBERG 2 (as in FN 13); EULNER (as in FN 13); HIRSCH (as in FN 13); NDB (as in FN 15); ÖBL (as in FN 11); LESKY, *Wien. Med. Schule* (as in FN 12), pp. 449–454; Obituary: *Wien. klin. Wochenschr.* 13 (1900), pp. 995ff. (K. Gussenbauer); Julius v. HOCHENEGG, Dem Andenken Eduard Alberts. Wien 1909; Karl EWALD, "Eduard Albert (20. 1. 1841 bis 25. 9. 1900) und die Chirurgie seiner Zeit", in: *Wien. med. Wochenschr.* 91 (1941), cols. 79ff. and cols. 121ff.; Gabriela SCHMIDT, "Eduard Albert and the Beginning of Human Nerve Grafting", in: *Acta chir. Austriaca* 25 (1993), pp. 287–288.

610 Salomon Stricker (1834–1898). Studied medicine in Vienna (Dr. med. 1858). While still a student, first experimental research in the lab of the Physiolog. Institute under Ernst Wilhelm v. Brücke (cf. FN 14). 1859–1862 Training in Vienna's Allgem. Krankenhaus. 1862 Habilitation in Embryology at Vienna Univ. 1863 Back in Brücke's lab (aspirant, assistant). Discovery of the diapedesis of erythrocytes and first microscopic observation of a complete cycle of cell division. Clin. assistant in experimental research at the 2nd Med. Univ. Clinic under Johann R. v. Oppolzer (1808–1871). 1868 Assoc. Prof. and transformation of this lab into the Institute of Experiment. Pathology of Vienna Univ. At the instigation of his teacher Carl Frh. v. Rokitansky 1873 creation of the Department of Gen. and Experiment. Pathology of Vienna Univ., which was at that stage unique to Austria and served as a hotbed of world class clinical-experiment. research of the Viennese Med. School. Cf. CZEIKE (as in FN 13); EISENBERG 2 (as in FN 13); HIRSCH (as in FN 13); PAGEL (as in FN 13); ÖBL (as in FN 11); WURZBACH (as in FN 15); "Feierl. Inauguration d. Rektors ... 1898/99", pp. 33ff.; LESKY, *Wien. Med. Schule* (as in FN 12); pp. 549–558; Obituaries: *Münch. med. Wochenschr.* 45 (1898), pp. 568–569; *Wien. med. Wochenschr.* 48 (1898), cols. 712–713 and pp. 911ff.; Helmut WYKLICKY, "Zur Geschichte des Instituts für allgemeine und experimentelle Pathologie der Wiener Univ.", in: *Wien. klin. Wochenschr.* 97 (1985), pp. 346ff.; Karl HOLUBAR, "Salomon Stricker (1834–98) pioneer experimental pathologist", in: *American Journal of Dermatopathology* [= *Americ. J. Dermatopathol.*] 9 (1997), pp. 147ff.

611 Theodor Meynert (1833–1892). Originally from Dresden. Studied at Vienna Univ. (Dr. med. 1861); 1865 Habilitation in Neuropathol. at Vienna Univ.; 1866 Creation of the position of prosector for Meynert at the k. k. Niederösterr. Landesirrenanstalt (Inauguration as the K. K. Irren-, Heil- und Pflegeanstalt in 1853) at the Brünnlfeld in the immediate vicinity of the Allgem. Krankenhaus at the instigation of pathologist Rokitansky (cf. FN 15), whose word had great weight both in the Vienna's Med. Fac. and the Ministry of Education. 1868 Extension of Meynert's venia legendi at Vienna Univ. to psychiatry. 1870 Assoc. Prof. 1870–1875 Director (Full Prof. 1873) of the 1st Psychiatr. Univ. Clinic. 1875–1892 Full Prof. and Director of the 2nd Psychiatr. Univ. Clinic. Exponent of clin. psychiatry based on findings in the anatomy of the brain, in sharp opposition to the psycholog. humanit. orientation of asylum

psychiatry. See CZEIKE (as in FN 13); EISENBERG 2 (as in FN 13) (with comprehens. bibliogr.); HIRSCH (as in FN 13); LESKY, *Wien. Med. Schule* (as in FN 12), pp. 373–379; NDB (as in FN 15); ÖBL (as in FN 11); PAGEL (as in FN 13); WURZBACH (as in FN 15); *Feierl. Inauguration d. Rektors … 1892/93*, pp. 13–14; Obituaries: *Wien. klin. Wochenschr.* 5 (1892), pp. 333–334; *Wien. med. Wochenschr.* 42 (1892), cols. 938–939; *Münch. Med. Wochenschr.* 39 (1892); pp. 495–496; Appreciations: Theodor KIRCHHOFF; Gabriel ANTON, "Theodor Meynert, seine Person und sein Werk", in: *Journal für Psychologie und Neurologie* [*J. Psych. Neurol.*] 40 (1930), pp. 256ff.; Dora STOCKERT-MEYNERT, *Theodor Meynert und seine Zeit.* Wien/Leipzig 1930; Max de CRINIS, "Meynert in seinem Einfluß auf die moderne psychiatrische Forschung", in: *Wien. klin. Wochenschr.* 55 (1942), pp. 781ff.; Peter BERNER, Walter SPIEL, Hans STROTZKA, Helmut WYKLICKY, *Zur Geschichte der Psychiatrie in Wien/Psychiatry in Vienna.* Eine Bilddokumentation/An Illustrated Documentation. Brandstätter, Wien 1983, pp. 7ff., pp. 46ff.; Helmut GRÖGER, Eberhard GABRIEL, Siegfried KASPER (eds.), *Zur Geschichte der Psychiatrie in Wien.* Brandstätter, Wien 1997, pp. 38–39.

612 Cf. FN 603, fol. 1v. There this group was referred to as *"Prof. Albert mit 4 Genossen"* [Prof. Albert with 4 colleagues].

613 Ibid., fols. 11 and 12.

614 Ernst FUCHS, *Die Ursachen und die Verhütung der Blindheit* (as in FN 506). – Compare this assessment with the appreciation Ernst Fuchs met with when he was awarded the Leslie Dana Medal for the Prevention of Blindness in the United States (1929). See Ch. 11.

615 (Ed.), "Zur Besetzungsfrage der Augenklinik", in: *Wien. med. Wochenschr.* 34 (1884), col. 1477.

616 Carl (Karl) Langer Ritter v. Edenberg (1819–1887). 1842 Dr. med. Vienna Univ.; as a student of physiologist Joseph Julius Czermak (Čermák) (1799–1851) introduction to microscop. anat.; 1845–1847 prosector, then until 1850 assist. of the internation. renowned anatomist Joseph Hyrtl (1810–1894, Cf. FN 13). Helped to establish Hyrtl's Museum of Comp. Anat., specialising in zoology. 1851 Prof. of Zoology at Pest Univ.; 1856–1870 Prof. of Anat. at the Med.-Chir. Josephs-Akademie (Josephinum). 1870–1874 Full Prof. at the newly founded 2nd Departm. of Anatom. of Vienna Univ.; 1874–1887 Hyrtl's successor at the 1st Department of Anatom. Cf. CZEIKE (as in FN 13); HIRSCH (as in FN 13); ÖBL (as in FN 11); PAGEL (as in FN 13); WURZBACH (as in FN 15); LESKY, *Wien. Med. Schule* (as in FN 12), pp. 246–248 and p. 504; WYKLICKY, *Josephinum*, pp. 118–119; Obituaries: *Wien. med. Wochenschr.* 37 (1887), col. 1657 (Carl Toldt); *Wien. med. Blätter* 10 (1887), p. 1597 (Ferdinand Hochstetter); *Almanach Akad. Wissensch.* 38 (1888), pp. 185ff. (Eduard Sueß).

617 The reference is to Leopold Hasner von Artha (1818–1891). Studied in Prague (Dr. iur. 1842). Habilitation 1849, Assoc. Prof. of Philosophy of Law. 1853–1863 Full Prof. of Economics at Prague Univ., 1865–1867 Full Prof. of Polit. Economy at Vienna Univ.; 1867–1870 Minister f. Cultus u. Unterricht. 1869 Reopening of the Med. Fac. of the Leopold-Franzens Univ. Innsbruck (since 2004 Med. Univ. Innsbruck). Cf. CZEIKE (as in FN 13); ÖBL (as in FN 11), WURZBACH (as in FN 15); Franz HUTER (ed.), *Hundert Jahre Medizinische Fakultät Innsbruck 1869 bis 1969* [= Veröffentlichungen der Universität Innsbruck 17, *Forschungen zur Innsbrucker*

Universitätsgeschichte, vol. 7]. Österr. Kommissionsbuchhandlung, Innsbruck 1969; Heinz HUBER, *Geschichte der Medizinischen Fakultät Innsbruck und der medizinisch-chirurgischen Studienanstalt (1673–1938)*. Böhlau, Wien 2010; Franz DAXECKER, "Geschichte der Innsbrucker Medizinischen Schule. Von Claudia de' Medici bis zur ersten Rektorin 2013", in: *Die Innsbrucker Medizinische Schule*, 2nd ed., Medical University Press, Innsbruck 2013. His brother, Joseph Hasner v. Artha (1819–1892), was Professor of Ophthalmology at the Charles University in Prague between 1856 and 1883 (successor of v. Arlt). Cf. FN 473.

618 Cf. ÖSTA/AVA Wien. K. K. Ministerium f. Cultus u. Unterricht, 4 Medicin Fuchs No. 14313 from 1885 fols. 10 and 13.

619 The reference is to Albrecht von Graefe (1828–1870). Cf. FN 236.

620 In the margin of the last two pages of this memorandum Arlt had noted the names of 68 foreign medical doctors. Their countries of origin, also noted in the margin, were Egypt, Brazil, Chile, Germany, England, Finland, Greece, Ireland, Cuba, Macedonia, North America, Norway, Poland, Russia, Silesia, Sweden and Switzerland.

621 "*Audacter calumniare, semper aliquid haeret*": Slander boldly, something always sticks. Originally conceived by the Greek writer Plutarch (ca. 45–125), this piece of advice from what might be called the devil's toolbox has gained currency in the form Francis Bacon (1561–1626) gave it in *De Augmentis Scientiarum* (1623).

622 Arlt's handwritten memorandum (private collection).

623 Cf. FN 618, fol. 13v. The expert opinion Arlt mentions in the context of Ernst Fuchs's candidacy for the chair at the Eye Clinic in Prague is unaccounted for and must be presumed lost. For more details, see the previous chapter.

624 Ibid.

625 Ibid., fol. 14ff.

626 Cf. FN 352.

627 Frank KROGMANN, "Ferdinand von Arlt (1812–1887) unter dem Aspekt seiner Beziehungen zu deutschen Wissenschaftlern", in: Würzburger medizinhistorische Mitteilungen [Würzb. medizinhist. Mitteil.] 13 (1995), pp. 60–66; KROGMANN, "Streifzug durch die Geschichte der Augenheilkunde in Wien", in: *Mitteilungen der Österreichischen Gesellschaft für Wissenschaftsgeschichte* [*Mitteil. Österr. Gesellsch. Wissenschaftsgesch.*] 16 (1998), pp. 125–152.

628 Cf. Sammlungen d. Med. Univ. Wien, Handschriftenarchiv, No. 2.163.

629 Ibid.

630 In the period in question until Fuchs's call to Vienna by Imperial decree dated 30 July 1885 there is no evidence of Arlt having applied for an audience with Francis Joseph. Cf. ÖSTA/Haus-, Hof- und Staatsarchiv [HHSTA], Obersthofmeisteramt. Neuere Zeremonialakten [Neu. Zerem. A.], Karton Nr. 288 R(ubrik) XIV Audienzen etc. aus 1885.

631 Cf. FN 618, fol. 6v to 7v.

632 Ibid., fols. 8v to 10v.

633 *M. Fuchs, qui est marié et père de famille, est considéré comme étant d'une honorabilité et d'une moralité à l'abri de tout reproche. Il a la réputation d'un homme de science capable dans sa spécialité. Quant à ses opinions politiques et sociales, il resulte de renseignements pris à des sources donnant toute confiance que ce savant est assez indifférent à la politique et qu'il n'est pas possible de le classer dans l'un ou l'autre parti.* Ibid., fol. 19. Confiden-

tial, personal letter from Brussels' Police President, dated 27 December, in reply to an enquiry made by envoy extraordinary and minister plenipotentiary, Graf Chotek, of 3 December 1884. Bohuslav Graf Chotek von Chotkow und Wognin (1829–1896) was Austria-Hungary's ambassador in Brussels between 1872 and 1888. Cf. Erwin MATSCH, *Geschichte des Auswärtigen Dienstes von Österreich (-Ungarn) 1720–1920.* Böhlau, Vienna/Graz/Cologne 1980, p. 110. – On 30 December 1884, this character reference was sent to the Ministry of Foreign Affairs in Vienna and passed on to the Ministerium für Cultus u. Unterricht on 3 January 1885.

634 Cf. FN 618, fol. 11v.

635 Franz Mraček (1848–1908). Studied at Vienna Univ. (Dr. med. univ. 1876). Specialist training under Ferdinand Ritter v. Hebra (dermatol., cf. FN 163) and Carl Ludwig Sigmund Ritter v. Ilanor (1810–1883, syphilidologist) at the relevant University Clinics at Vienna's Allgem. Krankenhaus. Habilitation at Vienna Univ. 1880 (syphilidol.) and 1884 (dermatol.). 1896 Assoc. Prof., 1904 tit. Full Prof.; 1880–1908 Head physician at the Krankenanstalt Rudolfstiftung in Vienna. Cf. CZEIKE (as in FN 13); EISENBERG 2 (as in FN 13); FISCHER (as in FN 28); ÖBL (as in FN 11); PAGEL (as in FN 13); Obituaries: *Feierl. Inaug. … 1908/09*, pp. 29–30; *Wien. klin. Wochenschr.* 21 (1908), p. 633; *Münch. med. Wochenschr.* 55 (1908), p. 832.

636 Cf. FN 610.

637 Ernst Ludwig (1842–1915). Studied chemistry at Vienna Univ. (Dr. phil. 1864). 1865 Habilitation in Analyt. and Organ. Chemistry under his former teacher, Joseph Redtenbacher (1810–1870), at the Phil. Fac. of Vienna Univ. (1872 Assoc. Prof.). 1874–1912 Full Prof. of Med. Chemistry (a newly establ. dept.) at the Med. Fac. of Vienna Univ. (1882 Dr. med. h. c.). 1892/93 Rector of Vienna Univ.; Ludwig thus gained the recognition that had been denied to the chemist at the Allgem. Krankenhaus Johann Florian Heller (1813–1871). It is highly likely that Ernst Ludwig was one of the two professors not mentioned by name in the report on Albert's additional shortlist (*"Prof. Albert mit 4 Genossen"*; cf. FN 612). Cf. CZEIKE (as in FN 13); EISENBERG 2 (as in FN 13); FISCHER (as in FN 28); NDB (as in FN 15); ÖBL (as in FN 11); PAGEL (as in FN 13); LESKY, *Wien. Med. Schule* (as in FN 12), pp. 522–555; Appreciations: *Wien. med. Wochenschr.* 62 (1912), cols. 353ff.; Obituaries: *Wien. med. Wochenschr.* 65 (1915), cols. 1593–94 and 1825ff.; *Almanach Akad. Wissensch.* 66 (1916), pp. 323ff.

638 Joseph Greuter (1817–1888), OFMCap. Tyrolean Conservative MP both in Tyrol's diet and the Reichsrat. A vociferous opponent of the Liberals in Parliament, a significant proportion of whom were Jewish, already in the days of the struggle of Concordat versus Constitution and the conflict focused on the religious laws in 1868. No evidence has yet been found of any personal contacts between Greuter and Ernst Fuchs. Cf. ÖBL (as in FN 11); Gertrud KRETSCHMAR, *Monsignore Joseph Greuter und die Tiroler Konservativen.* Diss. Vienna Univ. 1949; Hugo HANTSCH, *Die Geschichte Österreichs.* Vol. 2. Styria, Graz/Vienna/Cologne. 2nd ed. 1955, pp. 389–390 and p. 408; Karl VOCELKA, *Verfassung oder Konkordat? Der publizistische und politische Kampf der österreichischen Liberalen um die Religionsgesetze des Jahres 1868* [= *Studien zur Geschichte d. österreichisch-ungarischen Monarchie* Vol. XVII]. Verlag d. ÖAW, Wien 1978; Helmut RUMPLER, "Eine Chance für Mitteleuropa. Bürgerliche Emanzipation und Staatsverfall in der Habsburgermonarchie", in: Herwig WOLF-

RAM (ed.), Österreichische Geschichte 1804–1914. Ueberreuter, Wien 1997, pp. 419–422.

639 FUCHS, *Augenarzt* (as in FN 2), pp. 79–80.

640 *Neue Freie Presse* No. 7516, morning edition, Sunday, 2 August 1885, p. 5.

641 *Stenographisches Protokoll.* Haus der Abgeordneten. IX. Session 409. Sitzung, am 10. März 1885, in: *Stenographische Protokolle über die Sitzungen des Hauses der Abgeordneten des österreichischen Reichsrathes.* IX. Session. XIV. vol. 400–430. Sitzung (pp. 13891–15185). K. K. Hof- und Staatsdruckerei, Wien 1885, cols. 14270–14271. Cf. Kamila STAUDIGL-CIECHOWICZ, *Das Dienst-, Habilitations- und Disziplinarrecht der Universität Wien 1848–1918.* Eine rechtshistorische Untersuchung zur Stellung des wissenschaftlichen Universitätspersonals [= *Schriftenreihe d. Archivs d. Wiener Univ.* 22]. Vienna University Press bei V&R unipress, Göttingen 2017, pp. 114–115.

642 Ibid. *Stenograph. Protokoll.* Sitzung der 9. Session am 11. März 1885, pp. 14282–14283.

643 McEWEN, *Antisemitismus* (as in FN 608).

644 For details on this confessional debate, cf. Gustav KOLMER, *Parlament und Verfassung in Österreich.* Vol. 3 1879–1885. Carl Fromme, Vienna/Leipzig 1905, pp. 303–304.

645 FUCHS, *Augenarzt* (as in FN 2), p. 82.

646 The reference is to Fuchs's Belgian citizenship, which he had been forced to adopt for his professorship in Liège.

647 Cf. Family archive.

648 (Ed.), "Zur Besetzung der ophthalmologischen Klinik an der Wiener Universität", in: *Wiener medicinische Presse [= Wien. med. Presse]* 26 (1885), p. 1011.

649 (Ed.), "Zur Besetzung der II. Klinik für Augenheilkunde in Wien", in: *Allgemeine Wiener medicinische Zeitung* [*Allg. Wien. med. Zeitg.*] 30 (1885), p. 367.

650 "Notiz", in: *Wien. med. Presse* 26 (1885), p. 1037.

651 (Ed.), "Zur Besetzung der ophthalmologischen Klinik in Wien", in: ibid., p. 1041.

652 Leopold Wittelshöfer (1818–1889). Originally from Hungary. Studied at Vienna Univ. (Dr. med. 1841). Practised for several years in Hungary. 1850 Moved to Vienna, where he founded the *Wiener medicinische Wochenschrift.* Cf. PAGEL (as in FN 13); WURZBACH (as in FN 15).

653 "Notiz", in: *Wien. med. Wochenschr.* 35 (1885), col. 1025.

654 See FUCHS, *Augenarzt* (as in FN 2), pp. 80–81.

5. Relaunching the Clinic: Teaching and Research Activities as Chair at Vienna's Medical Faculty, 1885–1915

Before Fuchs returned to Vienna for good to take over the chair he had been appointed to on 1 October 1885, he embarked on a tour d'horizon of his new workplace at the Allgemeines Krankenhaus in early September 1885:

The newly appointed Professor of Ophthalmology at the University of Vienna, Dr E. Fuchs, has arrived in Vienna to inspect his clinic and submit several adaptation proposals to the Ministry of Education. Prof. Fuchs will not move to Vienna for good until October 15, as official commitments such as examinations require his presence in Liège until then.[655]

It was during this brief visit that Fuchs took the required oath of office[656] on September 6, 1885.

As the Second University Eye Clinic had only been founded in 1883 and its first director, Eduard Jaeger von Jaxtthal, had died a few months later, Fuchs's takeover at the beginning of the winter semester of 1885/86 required an organisational relaunch. The rooms of the clinic, both the outpatient clinic facilities and those of the clinic itself, and the venues for clinical tuition and scientific research all had to be reorganised from scratch.

On September 7, only one day after he had taken the oath of office, Fuchs submitted a list of the changes that needed to be made. Reprinted here for the first time, it reads as follows:

Löbliche Direction des K. K. allgem. Krankenhauses!
The 2nd Eye Clinic, which has been given into my charge by Imperial Decree, urgently requires several changes in its facilities. These are necessary for three reasons: first, to allow as wide-ranging a scope to clinical tuition as possible; second, to provide the foundations for autonomous clinical research; and, third, to facilitate the treatment of a great number of patients. The required changes concern the refitting of the lecture hall, its side rooms and the hospital rooms, and the creation of a workroom.
1. In the lecture hall: the blackboard must be mounted differently. One of the staircases leading to the upper rows of benches has to be relocated from the side to the centre.

2. In the hall adjacent to the lecture hall, which will serve as the outpatient clinic: the side windows must be enlarged. Stud walls must be put in place to divide the hall into two sections, each with its own entrance and exit.
3. In the ophthalmoscopy room: the door needs to be replaced by a double portière. Three low, wooden partitions are to be installed, the gas outlets changed and the entire ophthalmoscopy room to be redecorated in black.
4. In the foyer (waiting room): this room is to be divided into two sections by a partition made of wood up to the mean height of a man and topped with glass. It should have a door in the centre and on one of its sides a bench attached to the partition. The stove needs to be moved to the other corner of the room, into a recess in the wall. The hose running down one of the windows is to be removed and both windows are to be fitted with mirror panes.
5. In the hospital rooms: The rooms are to be connected to the gas main, with one outlet per room.
6. The staircase that used to exist between Rooms 44a and 43 is to be restored.
7. The antechamber off Staircase III outside Room 43 is to be partitioned off from the staircase by means of a wall made of wood and glass.
8. The apartment of Assistant Dr Bochner,[657] *Room No....*[658]*, is to be transformed into a workroom. To this end it needs to be connected to the gas and the water mains.*

I take the liberty of submitting to the esteemed Directorate my request that these structural changes be approved and duly realised. It is highly desirable for these changes to be initiated and carried out as swiftly as possible so that they may be finished before lectures start. In this way it will be possible not only to prevent a disturbance of activities and teaching but to ensure that the workroom is available for use when clinical tuition starts.

Wien 7. September 1885.
Dr Ernst Fuchs
Vorstand der II. Augenklinik[659]

The Medical Director of the Allgemeines Krankenhaus, Dr Joseph Raimund Hoffmann (1823–1892),[660] in office since 1869, dealt with Fuchs's request on November 29, 1885 with the memo that an identical request had been submitted to the Ministry of Education, that the matter was under ongoing consideration and that some of the proposed changes had already been made.[661]

Inaugural Lecture

On October 19, 1885, four days after Fuchs had officially taken up his position of Professor of Ophthalmology and Director of the Second University Eye Clinic he delivered his inaugural lecture.[662] (Fig. 38) Unlike today, inaugural lectures were delivered at that time to a small audience of students rather than to the entire faculty.[663] Having identified himself as a "new recruit", Fuchs first of all paid homage to his predecessor, Eduard Jaeger von Jaxtthal.[664] His own teaching objectives Fuchs described as follows:

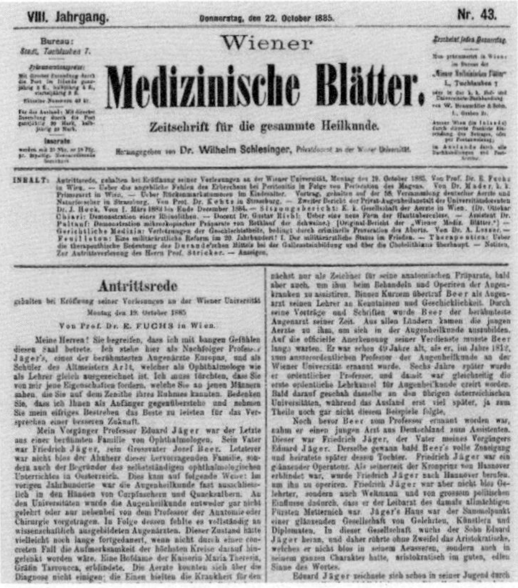

VIII. Jahrgang. Donnerstag, den 22. October 1885. Nr. 43.

Bureau: Stadt, Tuchlauben 7.

Wiener
Medizinische Blätter.
Zeitschrift für die gesammte Heilkunde.
Herausgegeben von Dr. Wilhelm Schlesinger, Privatdocent an der Wiener Universität.

Erscheint jeden Donnerstag.

INHALT: Antrittsrede, gehalten bei Eröffnung seiner Vorlesungen an der Wiener Universität, Montag den 19. October 1885. Von Prof. Dr. E. Fuchs in Wien. — Ueber das angebliche Fehlen des Erbrechens bei Peritonitis in Folge von Perforation des Magens. Von Dr. Mader, k. k. Primararzt in Wien. — Ueber Rückenmarkstumoren im Kindesalter. Vortrag, gehalten auf der 58. Versammlung deutscher Aerzte und Naturforscher in Strassburg. Von Prof. Dr. Kohts in Strassburg. — Zweiter Bericht der Privat-Augenheilanstalt des Universitätsdocenten Dr. J. Hock. Vom 1. März 1884 bis Ende December 1884. — Sitzungsbericht: K. k. Gesellschaft der Aerzte in Wien. (Dr. Ottokar Chiari: Demonstration eines Rhinolithen. — Docent Dr. Gustav Riehl: Ueber eine neue Form der Hauttuberculose. — Assistent Dr. Paltauf: Demonstration mikroskopischer Präparate von Rothlauf der Schweine.) [Original-Bericht der „Wiener Mediz. Blätter."] — Gerichtliche Medizin: Verletzungen der Geschlechtstheile, bedingt durch criminelle Provocation des Aborts. Von Dr. A. Lesser. — Feuilleton: Eine militärärztliche Reform im 20. Jahrhundert! I. Der militärärztliche Status im Frieden. — Therapeutica: Ueber die therapeuthische Bedeutung des Durande'schen Mittels bei der Gallensteinbildung und über die Cholelithiasis überhaupt. — Notizen. Zur Antrittsvorlesung des Herrn Prof. Stricker. — Anzeigen.

Antrittsrede
gehalten bei Eröffnung seiner Vorlesungen an der Wiener Universität
Montag den 19. October 1885
Von Prof. Dr. E. FUCHS in Wien.

Meine Herren! Sie begreifen, dass ich mit bangen Gefühlen diesen Saal betrete. Ich stehe hier als Nachfolger Professor Jäger's, eines der berühmtesten Augenärzte Europas, und als Schüler des Altmeisters Arlt, welcher als Ophthalmologe wie als Lehrer gleich ausgezeichnet ist. Ich muss fürchten, dass Sie von mir jene Eigenschaften fordern, welche Sie an jenen Männern sahen, die Sie auf dem Zenithe ihres Ruhmes kannten. Bedenken Sie, dass ich Ihnen als Anfänger gegenüberstehe und nehmen Sie mein eifriges Bestreben das Beste zu leisten für das Versprechen einer besseren Zukunft.

Mein Vorgänger Professor Eduard Jäger war der Letzte aus einer berühmten Familie von Ophthalmologen. Sein Vater war Friedrich Jäger, sein Grossvater Josef Beer. Letzterer war nicht blos der Ahnherr dieser hervorragenden Familie, sondern auch der Begründer des selbstständigen ophthalmologischen Unterrichtes in Oesterreich. Dies kam auf folgende Weise: Im vorigen Jahrhunderte war die Augenheilkunde fast ausschliesslich in den Händen von Curpfuschern und Quacksalbern. An den Universitäten wurde die Augenheilkunde entweder gar nicht gelehrt oder nur nebenbei von dem Professor der Anatomie oder Chirurgie vorgetragen. In Folge dessen fehlte es vollständig an wissenschaftlich ausgebildeten Augenärzten. Dieser Zustand hätte vielleicht noch lange fortgedauert, wenn nicht durch einen concreten Fall die Aufmerksamkeit der höchsten Kreise darauf hingelenkt worden wäre. Eine Hofdame der Kaiserin Maria Theresia, Gräfin Tarroucca, erblindete. Die Aerzte konnten sich über die Diagnose nicht einigen; die Einen hielten die Krankheit für den

nächst nur als Zeichner für seine anatomischen Präparate, bald aber auch, um ihm beim Behandeln und Operiren der Augenkranken zu assistiren. Binnen Kurzem übertraf Beer als Augenarzt seinen Lehrer an Kenntnissen und Geschicklichkeit. Durch seine Vorträge und Schriften wurde Beer der berühmteste Augenarzt seiner Zeit. Aus allen Ländern kamen die jungen Aerzte zu ihm, um sich in der Augenheilkunde auszubilden. Auf die officielle Anerkennung seiner Verdienste musste Beer lange warten. Er war schon 49 Jahre alt, als er, im Jahre 1812, zum ausserordentlichen Professor der Augenheilkunde an der Wiener Universität ernannt wurde. Sechs Jahre später wurde er ordentlicher Professor, und damit war gleichzeitig die erste ordentliche Lehrkanzel für Augenheilkunde creirt worden. Bald darauf geschah dasselbe an den übrigen österreichischen Universitäten, während das Ausland erst viel später, ja zum Theile noch gar nicht diesem Beispiele folgte.

Noch bevor Beer zum Professor ernannt worden war, nahm er einen jungen Arzt aus Deutschland zum Assistenten. Dieser war Friedrich Jäger, der Vater meines Vorgängers Eduard Jäger. Derselbe gewann bald Beer's volle Zuneigung und heiratete später dessen Tochter. Friedrich Jäger war ein glänzender Operateur. Als seinerzeit der Kronprinz von Hannover erblindet war, wurde Friedrich Jäger nach Hannover berufen, um ihn zu operiren. Friedrich Jäger war aber nicht blos Gelehrter, sondern auch Weltmann und von grossem politischen Einflusse dadurch, dass er der Leibarzt des damals allmächtigen Fürsten Metternich war. Jäger's Haus war der Sammelpunkt einer glänzenden Gesellschaft von Gelehrten, Künstlern und Diplomaten. In dieser Gesellschaft wuchs der Sohn Eduard Jäger heran, und daher rührte ohne Zweifel das Aristokratische, welches er nicht blos in seinem Aeusseren, sondern auch in seinem ganzen Charakter hatte, aristokratisch im guten, edlen Sinne des Wortes.

Eduard Jäger zeichnete sich schon in seiner Jugend durch

Fig. 38
Ernst Fuchs's Inauguration Lecture as Full Professor at the University of Vienna on 19 October 1885

The primary objective of this course is to provide you with a training in ophthalmology that will enable you in your later practice to treat eye patients on your own. Those among you who intend to establish themselves later in a major town may point out that they will be able to refer their eye patients to a specialist. I would reply to this that a knowledge of ophthalmology is necessary for you not only to treat eye patients but almost to the same extent for your internal practice. A great number of diseases of the eye, especially of its deeper parts, are only the result or a collateral consequence of a general illness. You will have to treat the latter in conjunction with the eye disease and, what is more, you will often be led to the correct diagnosis of the general illness by examining the eye.[665]

Having enumerated cases in point, such as retinitis albuminurica, diabetic lens opacification, atrophy of the optic nerve as a complication of tabes, and eye diseases in the context of scrofulosis, tuberculosis and syphilis, Fuchs summed up the topic by asserting that *"ophthalmological expertise is almost as necessary for the internist as is an expertise in internal medicine for the eye specialist."*[666]

Fuchs sought to kindle a similar spirit in his students:

I cannot help expressing the hope that another, even higher motive will fire you up in the study of ophthalmology and that I will succeed in awakening your scientific interest in this specialty. I do not hesitate to claim that, among all the medical specialties, it is ophthalmology that has reached the highest level of refinement and exactitude.[667]

Fuchs argued this point by demonstrating how ophthalmology was firmly grounded in physical and mathematical laws. He paid homage to Helmholtz's invention of the ophthalmoscope, which made the parts of the eye underneath the pupil accessible for direct inspection:

By consequence of this it is possible in the majority of cases to arrive at a reliable diagnosis. Those uncertain cases, which are so common especially in internal medicine where one is more or less reduced to guesswork, have become relatively rare in ophthalmology.[668]

Having outlined his teaching objectives, Fuchs gave a graphic overview of the methods of scientific investigation current at the time to illustrate the scientific challenge he expected his students to meet:

The transparency of the refracting media makes the eye appear especially suited for many physiological and pathological experiments. Injections of fluorescein, which cause the blood plasma secreted into the eye to become strongly fluorescent and thereby visible, allow us to observe the circulation of fluids in the living eye. The doctrine of inflammation was formulated in large part on the basis of experiments that took place on the cornea. The anterior chamber of the eye provides us with an ideal moist chamber for experiments. Fresh tissue samples transplanted into it continue to live and to grow and you can observe the changes as though the whole process was under a bell jar. By the same token, the anterior chamber is ideal for the cultivation of certain microorganisms, among which I would like to single out tuberculosis bacteria. It was experiments involving injections of tubercular matter into the anterior chamber that have cast the most light on the nature of tuberculosis. Owing to the favourable conditions the eye offers for such experiments, ophthalmologists have been able to focus on both the normal and the pathological anatomy of the eye, and science has greatly profited from their efforts. Nothing is more instructive than concentrating on the underlying anatomical changes as any given pathological process unfolds before us.[669]

In the peroration of his inaugural address Fuchs affirmed to his future students his resolve to allow them as much scope as possible for investigating and getting to "see" things on their own. His principal aim would be to teach them to see things from the clinical point of view. In addition to examining patients they would be given ample opportunity to be present during a wide range of operations on the eye. To this end, Fuchs planned to divide the students in his courses into groups of six, who would not only witness operations at close quarters but be involved on the periphery in the operations themselves on a learning-by-doing basis. The instruction and supervision required for this Fuchs planned to delegate to his assistants, who were also to be in charge of the day-clinic patients. Radiating youthful enthusiasm, the last sentence of his programmatic inaugural address encapsulates Fuchs's entire personality as a teacher and researcher:

I hope our relationship will become closer the deeper we advance together into our field of science and that finally we will be friends and colleagues rather than teacher and students.[670]

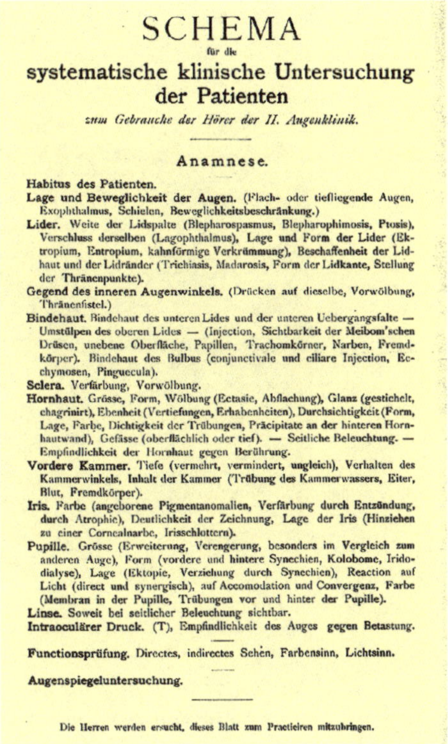

SCHEMA

für die

systematische klinische Untersuchung der Patienten

zum Gebrauche der Hörer der II. Augenklinik.

Anamnese.

Habitus des Patienten.

Lage und Beweglichkeit der Augen. (Flach- oder tiefliegende Augen, Exophthalmus, Schielen, Beweglichkeitsbeschränkung.)

Lider. Weite der Lidspalte (Blepharospasmus, Blepharophimosis, Ptosis), Verschluss derselben (Lagophthalmus), Lage und Form der Lider (Ektropium, Entropium, kahnförmige Verkrümmung), Beschaffenheit der Lidhaut und der Lidränder (Trichiasis, Madarosis, Form der Lidkante, Stellung der Thränenpunkte).

Gegend des inneren Augenwinkels. (Drücken auf dieselbe, Vorwölbung, Thränenfistel.)

Bindehaut. Bindehaut des unteren Lides und der unteren Uebergangsfalte — Umstülpen des oberen Lides — (Injection, Sichtbarkeit der Meibom'schen Drüsen, unebene Oberfläche, Papillen, Trachomkörner, Narben, Fremdkörper). Bindehaut des Bulbus (conjunctivale und ciliare Injection, Ecchymosen, Pinguecula).

Sclera. Verfärbung, Vorwölbung.

Hornhaut. Grösse, Form, Wölbung (Ectasie, Abflachung), Glanz (gestichelt, chagrinirt), Ebenheit (Vertiefungen, Erhabenheiten), Durchsichtigkeit (Form, Lage, Farbe, Dichtigkeit der Trübungen, Präcipitate an der hinteren Hornhautwand), Gefässe (oberflächlich oder tief). — Seitliche Beleuchtung. — Empfindlichkeit der Hornhaut gegen Berührung.

Vordere Kammer. Tiefe (vermehrt, vermindert, ungleich), Verhalten des Kammerwinkels, Inhalt der Kammer (Trübung des Kammerwassers, Eiter, Blut, Fremdkörper).

Iris. Farbe (angeborene Pigmentanomalien, Verfärbung durch Entzündung, durch Atrophie), Deutlichkeit der Zeichnung, Lage der Iris (Hinziehen zu einer Cornealnarbe, Irisschlottern).

Pupille. Grösse (Erweiterung, Verengerung, besonders im Vergleich zum anderen Auge), Form (vordere und hintere Synechien, Kolobome, Iridodialyse), Lage (Ektopie, Verziehung durch Synechien), Reaction auf Licht (direct und synergisch), auf Accomodation und Convergenz, Farbe (Membran in der Pupille, Trübungen vor und hinter der Pupille).

Linse. Soweit bei seitlicher Beleuchtung sichtbar.

Intraoculärer Druck. (T), Empfindlichkeit des Auges gegen Betastung.

Functionsprüfung. Directes, indirectes Sehen, Farbensinn, Lichtsinn.

Augenspiegeluntersuchung.

Die Herren werden ersucht, dieses Blatt zum Practiciren mitzubringen.

Fig. 39
Medical evaluation schema in use at the 2nd University Eye Clinic

To standardise the eye examination procedure at his clinic, a set of schematic instructions prepared by Fuchs was handed to the members of his audience with the request to bring it along to all practice sessions.[671] (Fig. 39)

Positioning the Second Eye Clinic within Vienna's Medical Faculty

As Ernst Fuchs was only 34 when he was given charge of the Second University Eye Clinic in 1885 as Full Professor, which was extremely young by the standard of the time, he was referred to as "the young gentleman from Courtyard 1"[672] both by his former teacher and mentor, Carl Ferdinand von Arlt, and the Director of the First University Eye Clinic, Carl Stellwag von Carion.[673] The sobriquet reflects both the ongoing surprise on the part of these two men and the expectations Vienna's medical faculty had formed of Fuchs. When Fuchs joined it, it still retained several of his own former teachers, such as Brücke[674] and Billroth,[675] who had contributed significantly to the training and the scientific formation of this ambitious "young gentleman".[676]

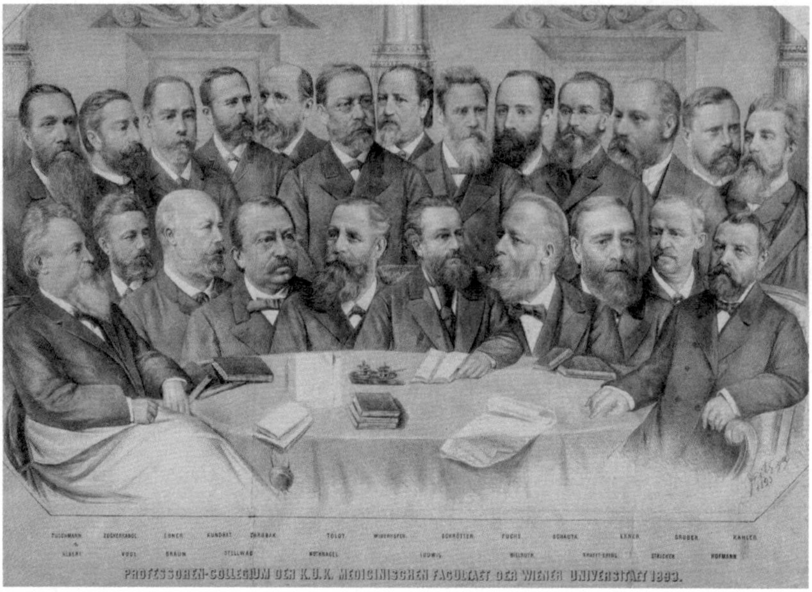

Fig. 40
The Medical Faculty in 1893 (Fuchs: 2nd row, 5th from right)

As a newcomer to the faculty (Fig. 40) Fuchs first had to learn the ropes and familiarise himself with existing factions before he could set about consolidating his own position. The faction that pulled the strings at the medical Professorial College at the time consisted of the surgeon Eduard Albert[677] and forensic pathologist Eduard Ritter von Hofmann (1837–1897),[678] both of whom Fuchs characterised as "scheming Czechs".[679] The two could rely on the support of experimental pathologist Salomon Stricker[680] and medical chemist Ernst Ludwig.[681]

After Fuchs's former teacher and mentor Carl Wedl[682] had retired as Head of the Department of Histology, the Albert-Hofmann faction sought to have this department abolished, because Stricker taught histology in addition to experimental pathology. Convinced that histology was an integral part of the study of medicine, Fuchs, anatomists Carl Toldt (1840–1920)[683] and Emil Zuckerkandl (1849–1910)[684] submitted a minority vote,[685] which provided the basis for the Minister of Education to overturn the negative majority vote passed by the Faculty. Histology remained an autonomous specialty at Vienna University and in 1888 Viktor Ebner Ritter von Rofenstein (1842–1925)[686] was appointed Head of Department.

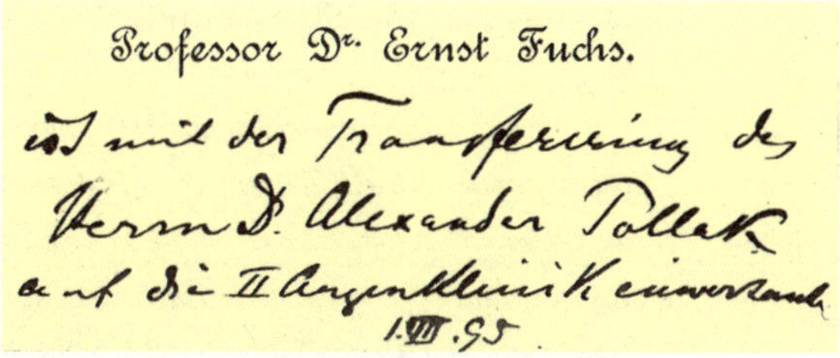
Professor Dr. Ernst Fuchs.
ist mit der Transferierung des
Herrn Dr. Alexander Pollak
auf die II Augenklinik einverstanden
1.VIII.95.

Fig. 41 Ernst Fuchs's card

The group in the faculty that befriended Fuchs comprised Ebner, Toldt, physiologist Sigmund Exner von Ewarten (1846–1926),[687] gynaecologist Rudolf Chrobak (1843–1910),[688] and, later, psychiatrist Julius Wagner Ritter von Jauregg (1857–1940),[689] paediatrician Theodor Escherich (1857–1911)[690] and laryngo-rhinologist Ottokar Freiherr von Chiari (1853–1918).[691] The pathologist Hans Frh. von Chiari (1851–1916),[692] Ottokar's brother, had been Fuchs's close friend ever since their schooldays at the Schottengymnasium.[693]

Reorganising the Second University Eye Clinic

The most urgent task awaiting Fuchs was to bring the Second University Eye Clinic up to speed; even the most basic adaptations had been omitted after its foundation in 1883 owing to the rapidly deteriorating state of health of his predecessor, Eduard Jaeger. Looking back, Fuchs described the situation in 1883 as follows:

Most people believe I had succeeded Arlt as Chair. This was never the case. On the occasion of the abolition of the Josephinum [in 1874], *Stellwag was assigned a couple of rooms above the Dermatological Clinic; Jaeger had at that stage been Director of the Eye Department for quite some time. His department was located in the same place my own clinic occupied later. After Arlt's departure Stellwag took over his clinic, and Stellwag's rooms were returned to the Skin Clinic; Eduard Jaeger, who had only been an Associate Professor up until then, was now appointed the second Full Professor, and Rooms 44 and 46 were designated as clinical rooms. (Room 45 had already been transformed into a lecture hall and an outpatient clinic; Room 46 was transformed at my request into an ophthalmoscopy room, an optotype room and an operation room after I had been assigned Room 47, which used to be part of Pal's*[694] *department.) Jaeger was already seriously ill at the time and died soon thereafter; up until my appointment Reuss had deputised for him. When Koller first experimented with cocaine, he was an aspirant under Reuss.*[695]

Fuchs's clinic therefore comprised the following rooms (see Fig. 36, p. 181):

Courtyard 1, Staircase No. 2, 1st Floor, rooms No. 44 b and 46. Connected to this was the clinical department in Courtyard 1, Staircase No. 3, rooms No. 43 and 44a.
Lecture Hall: Courtyard 1, Staircase No. 2, 1st Floor.
Out-patient Clinic: Courtyard 1, Staircase No. 1 (to the right of the main entrance in Alserstrasse), 1st Floor, room No. 45. [696]

In the presence of Dean Toldt, Reuss handed to Fuchs in his capacity of newly appointed Director (Fig. 41) what little inventory the Clinic had and the sum of 168 gulden and 3 kreuzer as the Clinic's remaining dotation from the period 1 January to 30 September 1885.[697]

Given that the Ministerium für Cultus und Unterricht had failed to respond to the request Fuchs had submitted in September 1885, in which he had outlined the changes that needed to be made to his clinic,[698] Fuchs wrote again in the spring of 1886 to remind them of unfinished business:

Hohes K. K. Ministerium für Cultus und Unterricht!
The undersigned submitted a request to the Ministry at the beginning of this winter semester asking for certain changes to be made to the Second Eye Clinic and to approve the release of the necessary funds. As this request has not yet been dealt with, the undersigned takes the liberty of singling out the most pressing of the proposals outlined in the original request and to resubmit it for consideration. It concerns the establishment of a workroom (laboratory) connected to the Clinic.

It will be seen as superfluous here to elaborate at length on how it behoves the professor of a specialty more than anyone else to keep abreast with progress in his chosen field. He can only do so if he himself is permanently involved in furthering science. It is an equally well-established truth that nowadays even what may look like purely practical aspects of medicine owe as much – or even more – to work in the laboratory as to observations made at the sickbed. In fact, the two preoccupations must always go hand in hand. Nor is it a question of the professor alone being able to carry out such work in the laboratory. Assistants and students need to be offered the opportunity to take part in such work under the guidance of the professor. These reasons seem sufficient in the eyes of the undersigned to mark the establishment of a workroom in the Second Eye Clinic as one of the most pressing desiderata. What makes it especially urgent is the fact that up until now tuition has palpably suffered and has indeed remained deficient because of the lack of a laboratory. In light of the principle generally observed today that teachers must aim above all to provide object lessons, it is absolutely imperative for the teacher not only to describe the pathological changes underlying the different diseases but to make them visible by means of pertinent preparations. This is necessary all the more for diseases of the eye as opposed to other illnesses of the human body since the pathological anatomy of the eye is given no more than cursory treatment either in the textbooks or in lectures on pathological anatomy. Up to this point the undersigned has been unable to show even a single preparation to his students, partly for lack of the required instruments, partly for lack of a workroom. The former grievance is now about to be at least partially remedied, as the Ministry has recently approved the release of 1,000 gulden[699] *for the purchase of instruments. However, a work room where such preparations can be made is still conspicuous by its absence.*

At the beginning of the winter semester, the Director[700] *of the k. k. Allgemeines Krankenhaus allocated*[701] *two – albeit very small – rooms at the Allg. Krankenhaus to the undersigned, to be transformed into a work room, provided the Ministry and the Governor* [Statthalterei] *give their approval. What is still missing is any adaptation of these two rooms as a laboratory. All this requires is the enlargement of the two very small windows, the installation of a door to make the two adjacent rooms accessible from either side and their connection to the gas and water mains. A building committee has inspected the rooms in question, has classified the changes as easy to carry out and has submitted a report on the matter.*

The undersigned therefore submits to the Ministry the request that the two rooms mentioned above be assigned to the undersigned as soon as possible and that the requisite adaptation measures be approved.
Vienna, 23 March 1886

Dr Ernst Fuchs
o. ö. Professor der Augenheilkunde und
Vorstand der II. Augenklinik[702]

Despite its rather stop-go nature, the relaunch of the Second University Eye Clinic under Fuchs was ultimately a success. The Clinic comprised a clinical and a supplementary department with forty beds each and had additional rooms for ophthalmoscopy and for eyesight testing, several small rooms for

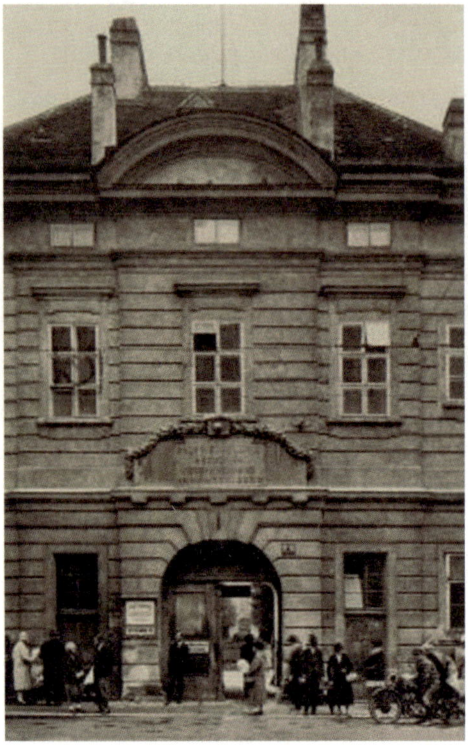

Fig. 42 Main entrance of the Allgemeines Krankenhaus, Alserstrasse 4

histological and bacteriological work and, in the loft above the Clinic, which was located directly above the main entrance of the Allgemeines Krankenhaus, a workroom that had been adapted for Fuchs himself. (Fig. 42) Attendance at the outpatient clinic rose steadily, reaching more than 15,000 patients a year in the latter half of the 1890s – amounting to a daily volume of about forty patients. In addition to this, Fuchs, like all other clinical professors of the Medical Faculty, made himself available for an hour a day to treat indigent patients for free. (Figs. 43, 44) Given that there were only two salaried assistants in addition to several junior doctors, the Second University Eye Clinic outperformed all other clinics both in Austria and abroad,[703] with the exception of the Hôpital des Quinze-Vingts in Paris and London's Moorfields Hospital. Their greater attendance was balanced by a greater number of senior specialists and junior doctors.

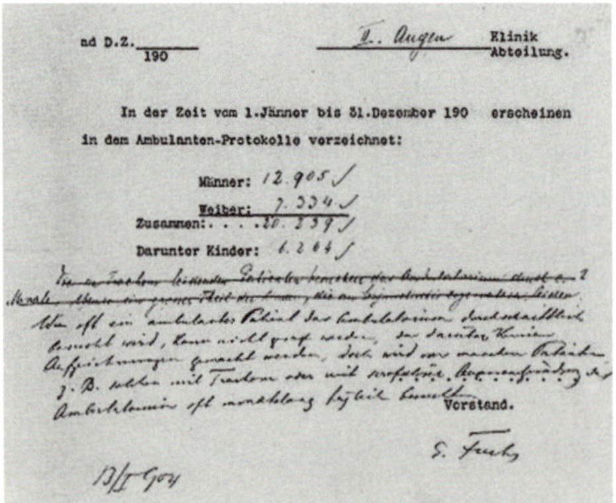

ad D.Z. ______ 190 II. Augen Klinik Abteilung.

In der Zeit vom 1. Jänner bis 31. Dezember 190 erscheinen in dem Ambulanten-Protokolle verzeichnet:

Männer: 12.905

Weiber: 7.334

Zusammen: 20.239

Darunter Kinder: 1.264

[illegible]

Vorstand.

E. Fuchs

13/II 904

Fig. 43 Ambulance statistic of the 2nd University Eye Clinic for 1903

Ludwig Lazarus Zamenhof as a Guest Student in 1886

In his early years as Full Professor in Vienna Fuchs had a student who was to rise to world fame, though admittedly in a field that had nothing to do with medicine: Ludwig Lazarus Zamenhof (1859–1917),[704] who went on to create Esperanto as a language of international communication. Zamenhof had studied medicine first in Moscow and then in Warsaw, where he graduated in 1884 and received his medical licence in 1885. Having briefly practised among the predominantly Lithuanian rural population, he decided to specialise in ophthalmology. Zamenhof began his specialist training at Warsaw's Jewish hospital. Keen on perfecting his expertise and skills, he came to Vienna in May 1886 and took up residence in the hotel "Zum goldenen Schlössel", Florianigasse 8, in Vienna's 8th District, not far from the University Clinics of the Allgemeines Krankenhaus. In the summer of 1886, he attended several courses given by Fuchs at the Second University Eye Clinic. He is said to have translated one of Fuchs's texts into Esperanto and to have published it. According to an unverified report by his brother, Zamenhof attended one more vacation course in Vienna in 1897.

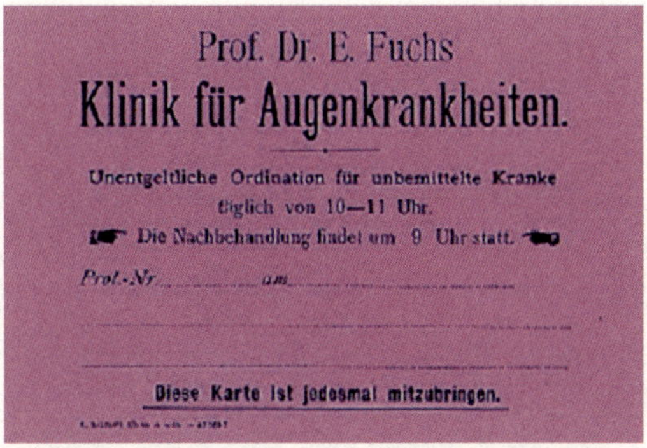
Prof. Dr. E. Fuchs
Klinik für Augenkrankheiten.
Unentgeltliche Ordination für unbemittelte Kranke
täglich von 10—11 Uhr.
Die Nachbehandlung findet um 9 Uhr statt.
Prot.-Nr. .... am ....
Diese Karte ist jedesmal mitzubringen.

Fig. 44 Ambulance card of the 2nd University Eye Clinic under Ernst Fuchs

In the autumn of 1886 Zamenhof returned to Warsaw and opened a private ophthalmological practice in the house of his parents, where he made himself available free of charge to indigent patients. His real passion, however, was the realisation of a dream he had first conceived while still in his teens: the creation of a language that would be easy to acquire and readily understood, facilitating communication among the speakers of a host of different national languages. Having mastered ancient Greek, Latin, German, English, French, Russian, Polish, Yiddish and Hebrew, Zamenhof, the son of a language teacher, had come forward in 1878, when he was barely 18, with his first version of a generally intelligible artificial language, which he called "Lingwe Uniwersala". In around 1885 Zamenhof had completed his linguistic system and published it in 1887 under the pseudonym Doktoro Esperanto – Dr Hopeful – in several languages. The pseudonym was soon adopted as the name of Zamenhof's universal language.[705]

1888: Fuchs as the Co-Founder of the Wiener Klinische Wochenschrift

Fuchs felt that the coverage of the appointment procedure[706] to fill the vacancy at the Second University Eye Clinic by Vienna's two leading medical journals, the *Wiener medicinische Wochenschrift* and the *Wiener medicinische Presse*, had been distinctly biased against him. This feeling was exacerbated by several appointments at the Medical Faculty, which were in his view unjustified. Consequently, a high priority item on his agenda as newly appointed Full Professor and Director of the Clinic was to put medical publishing on a new, objective basis:

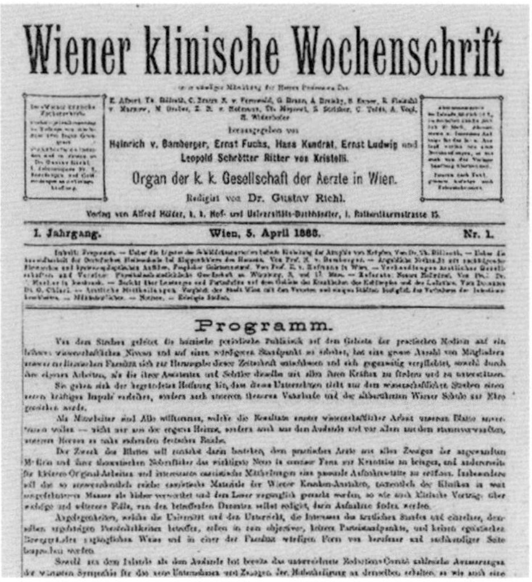
Wiener klinische Wochenschrift

herausgegeben von

Heinrich v. Bamberger, Ernst Fuchs, Hans Kundrat, Ernst Ludwig und Leopold Schrötter Ritter von Kristelli.

Organ der k. k. Gesellschaft der Aerzte in Wien.

Redigirt von Dr. Gustav Riehl.

I. Jahrgang.	Wien, 5. April 1888.	Nr. 1.

Programm.

Fig. 45 Title page of the first issue of the *Wiener klinische Wochenschrift*, 1888 (detail)

I believe it was in the second year after my appointment that indignation at the attitude of the two chief medical journals, the Wiener med. Wochenschrift *and the* Wiener med. Presse, *got the better of me. Whenever there was a vacancy or a lectureship to be filled, these journals carried all sorts of personal stories for and against* [various candidates] *from a strictly Jewish point of view, since both journals were in Jewish hands. I wrote first to Bamberger,*[707] *one of the most highly respected men in the* [Professorial] *College, outlining these facts and a proposal that the Faculty as such publish a respectable medical journal. This proposal was accepted by the Faculty, with only Stellwag voting against it. All Faculty members listed as editors on the title page committed not to pass on any of their own papers or the papers written by their students that were suitable for the new weekly to any of the other Viennese periodicals, a commitment that ceased to be honoured later by quite a few. Riehl*[708] *was the first editor. The journal was the official organ of the Gesellschaft der Ärzte, whose members were each entitled to a free subscription.*[709]

Heinrich von Bamberger,[710] Hans Kundrat (1845–1893),[711] Ernst Ludwig,[712] Leopold Schrötter Ritter von Kristelli (1837–1908),[713] and Fuchs together formed the editorial committee that oversaw the launch of the *Wiener klinische Wochenschrift*; Fuchs was its editor-in-chief for many decades.[714] (Fig. 45) As the official organ of the K. K. Gesellschaft der Ärzte, then the most prestigious medical association in Austria, the *Wiener klinische Wochenschrift* immediately established itself as a highly respected scientific journal. Fuchs regularly contributed original research to it, such as a paper on traumatic lens opacification[715] and on inflammations of the edge of the eyelid[716] in the first year of the journal. Ernst Fuchs's merits as initiator and co-founder of the *Wiener klinische Wochenschrift* were the subject of special appreciation even twenty-five years later.[717]

Ernst Fuchs as a Teacher

As he had announced in his inaugural address, Fuchs set great store by setting up object lessons for his students. He taught his course five times a week from 10 to 12 noon in the clinic, the lecture hall and the outpatient clinic. During the winter term of 1885/86, his first semester as a newly appointed professor, the printed course directory still listed the name of Jaeger's former deputy Reuss[718] instead of Fuchs, presumably for organisational-technical reasons. This was corrected for the summer semester 1886. The number of hours and the times coincided with those of Stellwag, the Head of the First University Eye Clinic,[719] just as had been the case under Reuss.

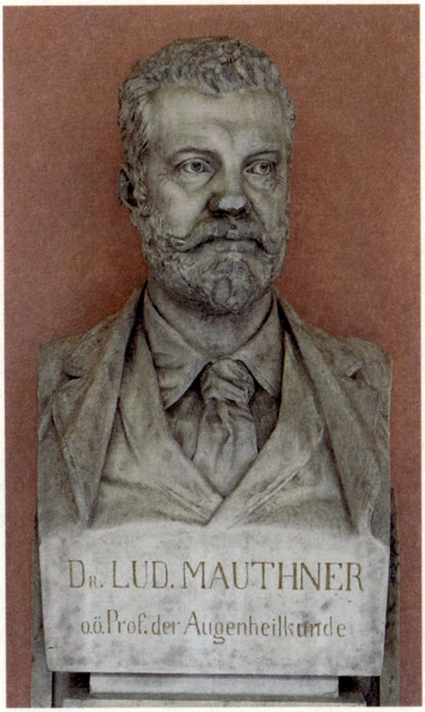

Fig. 46 Monument bust of Ludwig Mauthner by Rudolf Weyr 1898. Arkadenhof of the University of Vienna

It was a high-priority concern for Fuchs to produce a comprehensive textbook[720] of his specialty as early in his tenure as possible. First published in 1889, it was to see eighteen editions in German until 1945 and translations into Chinese, English, French, Italian, Japanese, Russian and Spanish.[721] It retained its global significance for more than half a century, thus making a crucial contribution to popularising the principles of the Vienna Ophthalmological School[722] worldwide.

The Academic Relationship between Fuchs and Mauthner after Fuchs's Appointment

Ludwig Mauthner[723] (Fig. 46), as has already been said, was noted for his eminent didactic skills. Having been disappointed in the succession of Jaeger as Director of the Second University Eye Clinic, he was forced to cast about for a suitably independent context within the Medical Faculty where he could exercise this talent. As he belonged to neither of the two Eye Clinics, his chief aim was to be assigned a lecture hall and a time slot for his lectures. It was Fuchs who granted his former co-competitor and main rival for the chair of ophthalmology the continued use of the Second University Eye Clinic's lecture hall for his one-hour lectures immediately after Fuchs's own course.[724] Had Fuchs nurtured professional or antisemitically motivated animosities against Mauthner, whom he had first met as an assistant at Innsbruck University,[725] this gesture of goodwill would in all likelihood not have been forthcoming.

Mauthner, however, sought to broaden his field of activity by making his course part of the obligatory curriculum of the study of ophthalmology. As he wanted to combine his lectures with practical demonstrations involving patients, the logical next step, as he conceived it, was the establishment of an ophthalmological outpatient clinic. In January 1887 the Professorial College began its deliberations on this matter.[726] As a unanimous consensus was not in sight, a committee comprising Professors Albert, Bamberger, Billroth, Fuchs, Stellwag and Toldt was formed and tasked with presenting and arguing the reasons that spoke against Mauthner's proposal. As the committee's secretary, Fuchs delivered a summary of those reasons on February 26, 1887. While taking its cue from Mauthner's proposal, his argument went much further than was required by the occasion in that it provided an objective, principled analysis of what constituted responsible and comprehensive teaching in ophthalmology. Teaching of this kind, Fuchs declared as the spokesman of a committee embodying the Faculty's commitment to the highest standards, required a clinic with in-patients and could not possibly be delivered by an isolated outpatient establishment.

Expert Opinion concerning the ministerial decree of January 7, 1887, No. 403 relating to the establishment of an oculist outpatient clinic and its use for teaching obligatory courses in ophthalmology by Professor Dr L. Mauthner.

There can be no question that in his capacity of lecturer Herr Professor Mauthner is entitled to deliver lectures of whatever length on ophthalmology, with or without the additional use of an outpatient clinic; he is equally entitled to deliver theoretical or practical lectures on eye operations. What the Professorial College would like to see is for Professor Mauthner to become more intensely involved in teaching in this way. It needs to be pointed out, though, that an ophthalmological outpatient clinic, which is non-existent at present, cannot be created for him by fiat. Such an outpatient clinic can only be established by the person in question himself, on the strength of his reputation and with the input of a great deal of time and energy; this can only be done step by step and will require years of effort.

What does need to be addressed about the request put forward by the Ministry is the question whether such lectures can be seen as equivalent to regular clinical tuition of the kind that is offered at both University Eye Clinics as required by law. The question, which is to be answered regardless of the person concerned, must be phrased like this: Is it possible to provide complete clinical tuition in ophthalmology based on an outpatient clinic rather than a clinic?

Those sections of ophthalmology that students can only acquire by personal experience and never from a textbook or a theoretical lecture concern diagnostics and therapy. Let us consider therapy first.

Therapy comprises the entire field of ophthalmic operations. Those diseases of the eye that threaten people with blindness most often and most seriously, such as cataract, glaucoma or the closure of the papilla, are only curable by surgery. Surgery is the most promising aspect in the activity of both eye clinics and the eye specialist. – All major eye operations can only be performed on in-patients, often on the hospital bed itself. No self-respecting ophthalmologist would even think of performing such an operation on an outpatient. Students who receive their clinical training at an outpatient clinic would never be given the opportunity of seeing such an operation performed on a living human being nor would they be able to see with their own eyes the healing process, the postoperative treatment and the final result. The most significant and the most successful part of ophthalmologic therapy would in this type of training be reduced to theoretical lectures. The diploma entitles the young physician to perform all types of operations. What can be expected from a physician who has derived the sum total of his knowledge of the surgical aspect of ophthalmology from lectures and perhaps from the dissection of cadavers. Should he dare to perform such surgery, as someone who has never seen surgery performed on a living human being? Only those who have surgical experience know that there is a multitude of things the surgeon needs to be aware of, things that relate not only to the positioning of the patient, to anaesthesia, assistance, antisepsis, bandaging, etc. All of this is not even mentioned in practical surgical courses; this can only be learnt from fastidious observation at the operating table and the hospital bed. Should anyone be given the legal entitlement to perform such operations who has himself never seen them performed on a living human being?

In addition to surgical cases there are other cases of serious illnesses of the eye (such a purulent inflammations of the retina and the cornea, practically all serious injuries and acute inflammations of the interior part of the eye) that cannot be treated in outpatients. All this would be missing from this type of training. It would have to confine itself mainly to less serious cases.

As far as the second part of ophthalmology is concerned, the diagnostics of diseases of the eye, it might appear at first sight that an outpatient clinic is not significantly inferior to a clinic proper. At both Eye Clinics the outpatient clinics that are attached to them are extensively used for teaching purposes. It would, however, be a grave error to consider an outpatient clinic that is not attached to a clinic as equivalent to one that is. The patient material the two types of outpa-

tient clinics deal with is radically different. The serious cases in need of hospital treatment gravitate towards the clinics, the only places where they are likely to find help; the same is true of the majority of surgical cases. An outpatient clinic without beds for in-patients will invariably attract almost exclusively the less serious cases. This means that students are likely to get to see only very few of the most important cases; they would be afflicted with a major deficit in their diagnostic expertise that cannot be filled by lectures or by the study of a textbook. – A second drawback of an outpatient clinic that weighs at least as heavily is that the teacher can never be sure of his material. He may have a surfeit of patients one day and the next day not a single case may present at the outpatient clinic that is suitable for demonstration. A teacher who does not want to be completely at the mercy of chance must be able to rely on an in-patient clinic whose patients are always at his disposal.

It has arguably been established beyond doubt that clinical training can only take place at a full clinic and never at an outpatient clinic.

The question that has been raised is of far-reaching significance, as it is a question of principle. As far as training is concerned, there is no substantial difference between ophthalmology and other clinical disciplines. If an ophthalmologist believes he can offer comprehensive clinical training in ophthalmology at an outpatient clinic, the same claim may be made by a surgeon, an internist, an obstetrician or a gynaecologist. Perhaps one day someone will come along and offer to demonstrate to his students on an outpatient the course taken by pneumonia or typhus.

The clinic plays the same role for clinical training [in ophthalmology] *as the dissecting room for the anatomist and the laboratory for the chemist.*
Vienna, February 26, 1887.

Professors Bamberger, Stellwag, Albert,
Dr Th. Billroth, Professors C. Toldt and
E. Fuchs[727]

From the winter semester 1887/88 Mauthner made the Academic Hall in the building of the Directorate of the Allgemeines Krankenhaus the venue for his teaching activities, which he took the opportunity of broadening at the same time.[728] The negative expert opinion of the committee notwithstanding, he succeeded in establishing an outpatient clinic in the same locale. It is also noteworthy that Mauthner chose a time for his course, scheduled on five days a week as previously, that coincided at least in part with the main series of lectures given by the Directors of the two University Eye Clinics at the Allgemeines Krankenhaus, Stellwag v. Carion and Fuchs. Arguably the result of a deliberate choice, this seems to point to a situation fraught with competition. In 1890, Mauthner was appointed Head of Department at the Allgemeine Poliklinik round the corner from the Allgemeines Krankenhaus, where he taught from the summer semester of 1891.[729]

In the thirty years Fuchs taught at the clinic of the University of Vienna he regularly lectured, over and above his main courses, on specialist topics such as "Refraction and Accommodation of the Eye,"[730] "Functional Vision Assessment"[731] and "Pathological-Anatomical Demonstrations in Ophthalmology",[732] his main area of research.

1894: Creation of a Surgical Institute

The Minister für Cultus und Unterricht had asked Ernst Fuchs for an expert opinion on the proposed creation of a training facility for surgeons at the Eye Clinic of Graz University. In the summer of 1893 Fuchs submitted a similar proposal to the Ministry, suggesting the creation of a training facility for ophthalmic surgeons, an *oculistisches Operations-Institut*, with three places for his own Eye Clinic. In a ministerial decree of June 9, 1893, the Minister instructed the Dean of the Medical Faculty, Eduard Hofmann, to put this proposal to the vote at the Professorial College. In the meeting convened by Hofmann on July 8, 1893 Fuchs's proposal was unanimously accepted and subsequently implemented at the two University Eye Clinics.[733]

Fuchs's initiative brought about a significant improvement in the clinical-surgical training of future ophthalmologists, modelled not least on the surgical training institutions that had existed in Vienna since 1804 at the Medical-Surgical Military Academy (Josephinum) and, since 1807, at the two Surgical University Clinics of Vienna's Medical Faculty.[734]

Applications for a spell as trainee surgeon at the Surgical Institute of the Second Eye Clinic could be submitted from anywhere within the Austro-Hungarian Monarchy until the end of the summer semester. The only requirement was a general practitioner's diploma. Applicants had to prove their manual skill in an entrance exam, which consisted in operating on the eye of a cadaver. The final selection of applicants was left to the Professorial College of the Medical Faculty acting on recommendations given by the Head of the Clinic. All other things being equal, hospital doctors already active at the Allgemeines Krankenhaus were given precedence over applicants from outside. The candidates' final acceptance lay with the Ministerium für Cultus und Unterricht. In general, the course lasted one year, starting on October 1, but it was up to the Director of the Clinic to recommend an extension of the course to two or even three years.[735] (Fig. 47)

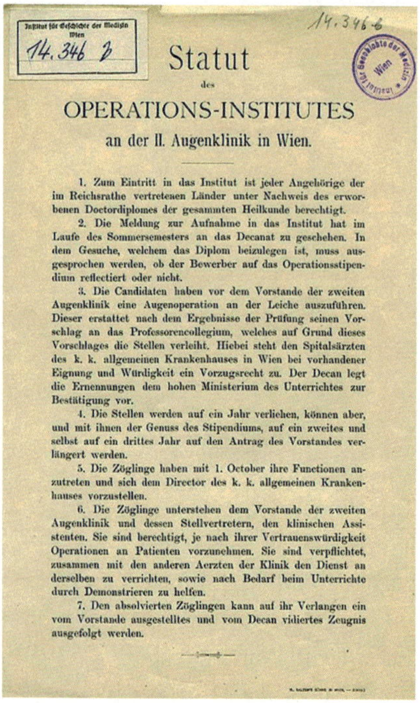

Statut
des
OPERATIONS-INSTITUTES
an der II. Augenklinik in Wien.

1. Zum Eintritt in das Institut ist jeder Angehörige der im Reichsrathe vertretenen Länder unter Nachweis des erworbenen Doctordiplomes der gesammten Heilkunde berechtigt.

2. Die Meldung zur Aufnahme in das Institut hat im Laufe des Sommersemesters an das Decanat zu geschehen. In dem Gesuche, welchem das Diplom beizulegen ist, muss ausgesprochen werden, ob der Bewerber auf das Operationsstipendium reflectiert oder nicht.

3. Die Candidaten haben vor dem Vorstande der zweiten Augenklinik eine Augenoperation an der Leiche auszuführen. Dieser erstattet nach dem Ergebnisse der Prüfung seinen Vorschlag an das Professorencollegium, welches auf Grund dieses Vorschlages die Stellen verleiht. Hiebei steht den Spitalsärzten des k. k. allgemeinen Krankenhauses in Wien bei vorhandener Eignung und Würdigkeit ein Vorzugsrecht zu. Der Decan legt die Ernennungen dem hohen Ministerium des Unterrichtes zur Bestätigung vor.

4. Die Stellen werden auf ein Jahr verliehen, können aber, und mit ihnen der Genuss des Stipendiums, auf ein zweites und selbst auf ein drittes Jahr auf den Antrag des Vorstandes verlängert werden.

5. Die Zöglinge haben mit 1. October ihre Functionen anzutreten und sich dem Director des k. k. allgemeinen Krankenhauses vorzustellen.

6. Die Zöglinge unterstehen dem Vorstande der zweiten Augenklinik und dessen Stellvertretern, den klinischen Assistenten. Sie sind berechtigt, je nach ihrer Vertrauenswürdigkeit Operationen an Patienten vorzunehmen. Sie sind verpflichtet, zusammen mit den anderen Aerzten der Klinik den Dienst an derselben zu verrichten, sowie nach Bedarf beim Unterrichte durch Demonstrieren zu helfen.

7. Den absolvierten Zöglingen kann auf ihr Verlangen ein vom Vorstande ausgestelltes und vom Decan vidiertes Zeugnis ausgefolgt werden.

Fig. 47 Ernst Fuchs's Statutes for the Surgical Institute at his Clinic

1896: Plaque in Commemoration of Ferdinand von Arlt

Given his wish to honour the memory of his revered teacher Ferdinand von Arlt,[736] Ernst Fuchs informed the then Rector of Vienna University, Adolf Exner (1841–1894),[737] in March 1892 of his intention to present the University with the gift of a bronze medallion featuring Arlt's portrait. This was to serve as a model for a marble plaque with Arlt's bronze relief to be installed in the University's Arcade Court. The university was to defray the cost of the execution of the plaque by the sculptor Hans Bitterlich (1860–1940)[738] and its installation in the Arcade Court. Having overcome several hurdles,[739] Bitterlich finally realised the project.[740] The plaque was solemnly unveiled on July 9, 1896,[741] with Fuchs delivering a speech focussed on Arlt's merits.[742] The lower edge of the marble plaque bears a Latin inscription outlining Arlt's significance for Vienna's School of Ophthalmology: FERDINANDO EQUITI DE ARLT – OPHTHALMOLOGIAE PROFESSORI – SUAE ARTIS PRINCIPI – FLORENTIS SCHOLAE CONDITORI [In honour of Ferdinand Ritter von Arlt, professor of ophthalmology, master practitioner of his specialty, and founder of a flourishing school].

1909: Inauguration of the First Trachoma Ward at a University Eye Clinic

In the wake of the resignation of Albert Mosetig Ritter von Moorhof (1838–1907),[743] Director of the 2nd Surgical Department of the Allgemeines Krankenhaus in 1906, the Directors of the two Surgical University Clinics, Julius Hochenegg (1859–1940)[744] and Anton Freiherr von Eiselsberg (1860–1939),[745] proposed to the Ministerium für Cultus und Unterricht in 1907 that this ward with its 80 beds that had now fallen vacant be abolished and that a casualty ward be created instead, attached to the two Surgical University Clinics. Ernst Fuchs supported this initiative, adding the urgent request that as part of the restructuring of "his" Second University Eye Clinic a new department be created for the isolated in-patient treatment of trachoma patients. As this well-argued proposal, although flagged as urgent, elicited no response for more than a year, Eiselsberg, Fuchs and Hochenegg brought the matter to the attention of the public by making their case in the *Neue Freie Presse* on August 30, 1908. The part relating to the creation of the trachoma ward reads as follows:

The intransigence of the competent authorities is all the more contrary to all reason since the abolition of the old ward and the creation of a casualty ward creates an opportunity to meet another urgent need. The beds that will no longer be needed after the transformation of the large surgical ward into a casualty ward should be pooled to create a small trachoma ward. While trachoma (Egyptian ophthalmia) was initially not endemic in Vienna and Lower Austria, a great number of people afflicted with the disease come to Vienna every year from the north and the east, mostly from Galicia, Hungary, and Russia, partly as workers, partly in search of material assistance. Once here, they pass on the disease to the indigenous population, as they subsist in conditions marked by poverty, mostly in mass accommodation. This is why trachoma has gained such a foothold among the indigenous population; even in the countryside, which used to be absolutely trachoma free, many isolated trachoma cases can be found alongside a number of larger concentrations. The only step taken so far by the public health authorities is to make it mandatory to report cases of trachoma. Apart from the generation of a great deal of red tape, this makes absolutely no sense. On the contrary. When a case has been reported and a public health officer turns up at the abode of the trachoma patient, who is usually a lodger, his fellow lodgers learn about the infectiousness of the disease and kick him out. He will then look for new accommodation, where he will proceed to infect a new set of fellow lodgers.

The spread of trachoma is effected by the transfer of secretions, most commonly by jointly used washing utensils. The only measure to stop the disease from spreading would be the hospitalisation of all patients or the provision of one room per person. Both measures are impracticable not only because of the absence of the appropriate legal means but also because of the large number of patients. In the Second Eye Clinic (Hofrat Fuchs), at times between 60 and 80 trachoma patients a day are receiving outpatient treatment. If such patients, as happens only in the most desperate cases, are transferred to the clinic, they constitute a danger for other patients who share the room with them. Regardless of the strictest precautions enforced by the medical and the nursing staff, it is impossible to ensure against all transmission, and it is a fact that cases of infection occur from time to time in the clinic itself. Petitions submitted to the Governor in the course of almost twenty years have pointed out this unsatisfactory state of affairs and have called for the creation of a dedicated trachoma ward at a hospital of the government's choice. It is a matter of the gravest reproach for the authorities that at first they failed to respond at all to these submissions and that more recently they have kept asking for proposals to improve the existing situation, while at the same time consistently rejecting the detailed proposals submitted to them. In view of the great number of patients, the creation of a small trachoma ward would admittedly not make a great difference, but it would at least be a start. The Eye Clinic would at least be in a position to isolate the trachoma patients in its ward, as opposed to the present situation where they are placed among all the other eye patients. The Director [of the 2nd Eye Clinic], *Hofrat Fuchs, has pointed out repeatedly that any patient infected with trachoma* [at the Clinic] *would be entitled to file a claim for significant damages, which may involve at one blow a much greater financial expense than would be needed at present for the transformation of the room in question.*[746]

Involving the public in this way increased the pressure on the education authorities, who in June 1909 finally authorised the establishment of the globally first trauma ward and the first ward for trachoma patients at a university.[747]

The trachoma ward newly established at the Second University Eye Clinic was assigned hospital rooms 8 (19 beds) and 9 (10 beds) and the two Surgical University Clinics were assigned rooms with 30 beds each. The trachoma ward made it possible for outpatients suffering from the disease to be treated separately from the general body of outpatients. The joint inauguration of the two trauma wards and the trachoma ward took place on November 3, 1909.[748]

In addition, an antiseptic operating room and a customised washing facility were installed. The washing facility enabled trachoma patients to rinse their eyes. For reasons of prophylactic hygiene, it was equipped with an upward water jet, which rendered the use of gauze pads unnecessary. An isolation room was attached to room 8, which was predominantly used for children suffering from highly infectious blennorrhoea.[749]

At Fuchs's explicit wish it was made quite clear that *"the Director of the Second Eye Clinic is at the same time in full charge of the ward for eye patients which is linked to a trachoma ward".*[750]

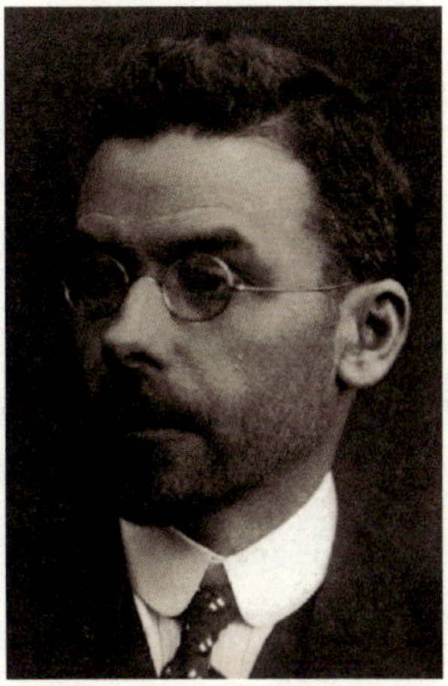

Fig. 48.
Karl David Lindner (1883–1961)

Fuchs put Karl David Lindner (1883–1961),[751] (Fig. 48) in charge of the trachoma ward. Having been instructed by Fuchs to concentrate on trachoma research when he joined the Second University Eye Clinic immediately after his graduation in 1907 as a trainee surgeon, Lindner was ideally qualified for the task. When he stepped up to it, he was still a junior doctor at Fuchs's Clinic. The eye diagnosis of a female trachoma patient which Lindner made and documented in 1909, the foundation year of the trachoma ward, has come down to us in his private clinical log. (Fig. 49)

Even four and a half decades after Fuchs's creation of the trachoma ward Lindner still vividly remembered those pioneering days:

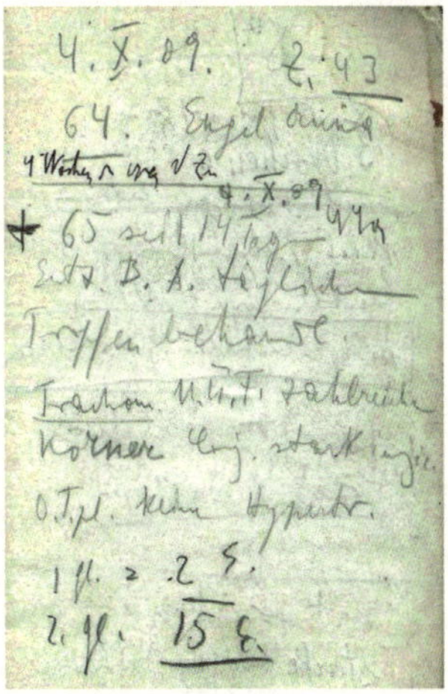

Fig. 49
Lindner's handwritten entry concerning a female trachoma patient, 4 Oct. 1909

In 1908, when I began doing bacteriological work at the Institute of Prof. Paltauf [cf. FN 1228] *in addition to my work at E[rnst] Fuchs's Clinic, we had a plethora of cases of infectious conjunctivitis. There were many cases of trachoma and the same was true of the many types of bacterial conjunctivitis, caused by gonococci, Koch-Weeks bacilli, influenza bacteria, pneumococci und diplo bacteria. Cases of diphtheria of the conjunctiva were already very rare at that time nor were there many cases of gonoblennorrhoea among adults. But it was possible each term to present isolated cases.*

There was not yet a ward exclusively dedicated to trachoma. Serious cases of corneal abscesses had to be put up in the same room as other patients but to my knowledge no infection ever occurred. Less serious cases of trachoma were treated in the outpatient clinic. Every morning at 8, before the general outpatient clinic for external eye diseases came to life, a trachoma surgery was held in the same outpatient room and in order to prevent infection via medicines, the dropper bottles for the use of trachoma patients were painted red.

It took E[rnst] Fuchs until 1909 to succeed in establishing a ward dedicated to trachoma, complete with its own outpatient clinic. With its small isolation ward it had thirty beds. It needs to be said that at that time Vienna was the capital of the far-flung Austro-Hungarian Monarchy and that trachoma was especially common in the east. Special trachoma courses were put on for some time for public health officers.

After the disintegration of the Monarchy the numbers of trachoma patients at the Clinic declined rapidly, but we had no problem with the teaching of trachoma up until the beginning of World War II. Both isolated cases and clusters of trachoma were still to be found everywhere. Improvements in general hygiene and continuous information campaigns resulted in a reduction of the incidence of trachoma and in 1934 the trachoma ward had to be reduced to ten beds.752

In 1909, Lindner had succeeded in clarifying the morphology of the inclusions in the conjunctiva of trachoma patients that had been discovered in 1906 by the Austrian-Bohemian zoologist and biologist Stanislaus Prowazek Edler von Lanow (1875–1915)[753] together with the German dermatologist and radio therapist Ludwig von Halberstätter (1876–1949)[754] during a research trip to Java.[755] Lindner called the free form of the suspected trachoma pathogen "initial bodies" and developed a special technique for dyeing them.[756] In addition, Lindner compiled a detailed report in 1909 on the current state of trachoma research.[757] In 1911 he provided an exact description of the clinical pictures presented by gonoblennorrhea, inclusion blennorrhea and trachoma,[758] with inclusion blennorrhea being a term he had coined himself. A decade and a half later Lindner focused on existing problems of trachoma research,[759] which he did by paying special attention to the difference between trachoma and folliculosis of the conjunctiva. A globally recognised expert on trachoma, he received an invitation to the United States in 1928, one year after being appointed Director of the Second University Eye Clinic. The purpose of the invitation was an assessment of the research results of the microbiologist Hideyo Noguchi (1876–1928), who on the basis of work he had been carrying out at the Rockefeller Institute in New York since 1904 claimed to have identified the pathogen that caused trachoma. Lindner showed that Noguchi's candidate, bacterium granulosis, was not the causative agent. Rather than classic trachoma it only caused folliculosis of the conjunctiva. He first presented his findings on February 18, 1929 at a meeting of the Vienna Ophthalmologische Gesellschaft.[760]

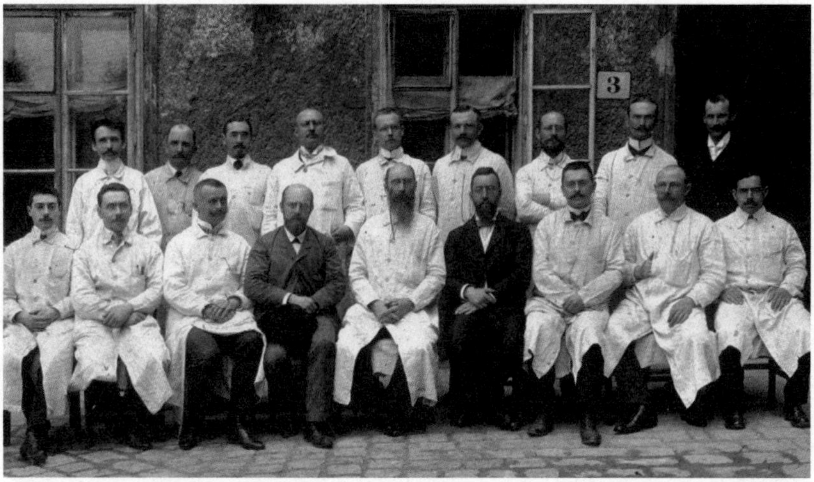

Fig. 50
Ernst Fuchs with assistants and visiting doctors at the 2nd University Eye Clinic, in the courtyard of the Allgemeines Krankenhaus

In 1935 Lindner coined the term "paratrachoma" for the less infectious variant of the disease.[761] In recognition of his many achievements in trachoma research he was honoured in the following year with the commission of contributing the chapter on trachoma to a renowned ophthalmological American textbook.[762]

Ernst Fuchs in turn concerned himself with trachoma in at least four publications[763] between 1894 and 1927 and contributed several presentations and interventions to various conferences on the topic.

Modernisation of the Second University Eye Clinic

Putting "his" Clinic on a proper footing was paramount to Fuchs once he had been appointed. One of Europe's leading ophthalmologists and about to give the reputation of the Vienna School of Ophthalmology a boost worldwide, he set the bar as high as possible for himself and his collaborators (Fig. 50) in quest of the very best care for his patients and the advancement of science at his Clinic.

In addition to the Trachoma Ward (Room 8), the Fuchs Clinic had at its disposal, after a series of conversions and adaptations, two clinical rooms (44a & b), two department rooms (43, 47), a lecture hall, outpatient clinic rooms, a room for vision tests and ophthalmoscopy, a room for the Director of the Clinic and an operating room for patients with non-infectious eye diseases.

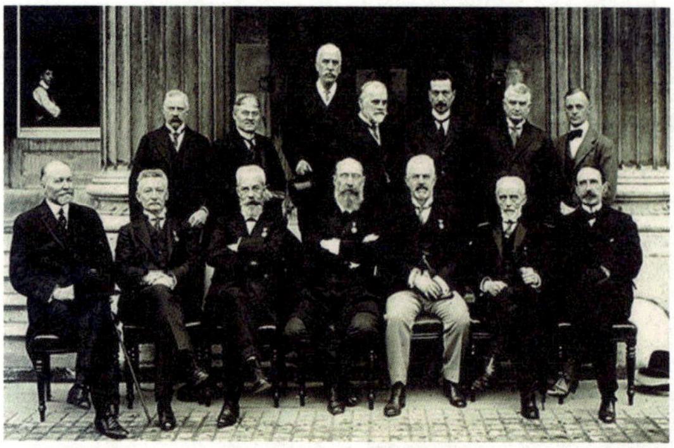

Fig. 51
Award of an honorary membership by the Royal Coll. of Phys. and Surgeons to Ernst Fuchs (1st row, centre) and Anton von Eiselsberg (next to Fuchs on the right)

1913: Award of an Honorary Membership of the Royal College of Surgeons of England, and the Seventeenth International Congress of Medicine in London

The Royal Society of Surgeons of England is an independent professional body and a registered charity, with its beginnings in the fourteenth century. Honorary memberships awarded to outstanding non-British surgeons are much coveted marks of distinction. In 1913, Ernst Fuchs and the surgeon Anton Freiherr von Eiselsberg[764] were the only Austrians to be honoured in that way. The award ceremony took place on August 6, 1913. (Fig. 51)

Immediately after this ceremony Ernst Fuchs took part in the 17th International Congress of Medicine in London. In the Ophthalmological Section (Fig. 52), which was convened from 7 to 12 August 1913, Fuchs and the renowned American ophthalmologist George Edmund de Schweinitz (1858–1938)[765] were in charge of the opening session on August 7, 1913, where the topic of chronic uveitis was discussed.[766] Fuchs presented his point of view, which was at that stage considered state of the art in the world of ophthalmology, in a lengthy paper published in the same year.[767]

Retirement

In early November 1912 Ernst Fuchs applied to the Ministerium für Cultus und Unterricht for early retirement for health reasons. When his teaching load was reduced to nil for the ensuing summer semester, he withdrew the application.[768] Two years later, however, when he was about to turn 63 and had therefore not yet completed the 30 years' period of service required for a full pension, he again submitted an application for early retirement to the

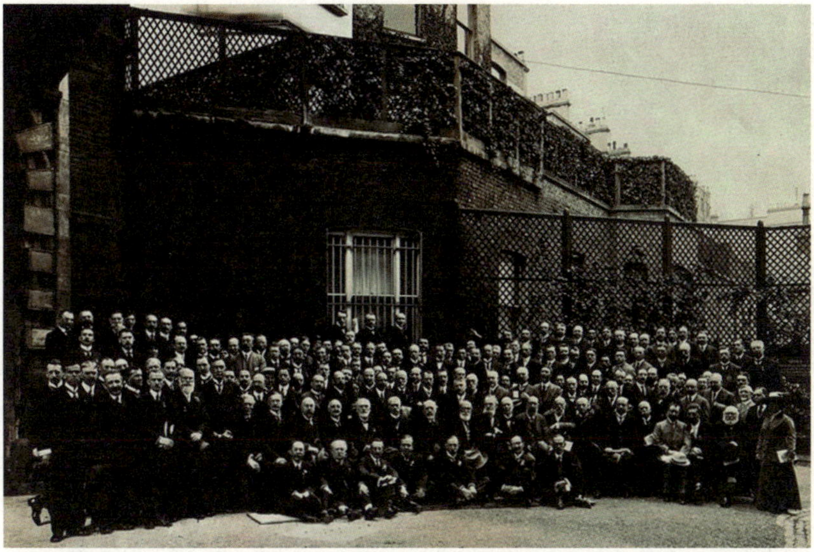

Fig. 52
Ernst Fuchs (2nd row, 9th from right) at the Section of Ophthalmology

Dean of the Medical Faculty, Julius Tandler (1869–1936).[769] The account he gives of this decision in his autobiography reads as follows:

I had at one stage resolved to retire at 60. When the time came, I still felt fit and energetic so I postponed retirement until 63. What had first pushed me in the direction of retirement were excruciating attacks of tachycardia, which I was experiencing with increased frequency at that time. However, if you want to retire before your 30 years' period of service has been completed, you must present a medical certificate. I requested such a certificate from Chvostek,770 who obliged with a certificate according to which my retirement was justified because of my heart and my increasing imbecility. I thanked him for the diagnosis and procured a second certificate, which did not mention imbecility. I submitted it to the Dean, who did not, as normal procedure would have required, pass it on to the Ministry of Education. Instead, he informed the Faculty first, which sent a deputation to ask me to postpone my retirement.[771] *I did so, but only for one year. In 1915,*[772] *when I had completed my 30 years' period of service and was entitled to my full salary as pension, I applied once more for retirement, this time for good and all.*[773]

I retired early even though I was still perfectly fit – I was 65 – because I wanted some time for myself to work through the masses of material that had accumulated – which I did.[774]

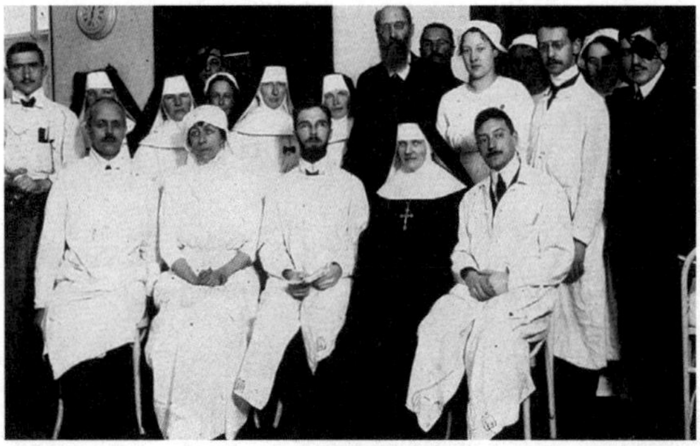

Fig. 53 The last photograph of Ernst Fuchs (2nd row) with the doctors and nurses of his Clinic

There was an additional dimension to Fuchs's decision not to continue in his job for the five years he would have been entitled to. This dimension has to do with his repeatedly mentioned understanding of his professional duties and his sense of responsibility: when World War I broke out in late July 1914, the assistants at his clinic were called up for service one by one. Given the standards Fuchs had set himself in dealing with his organisational, medical and scientific tasks, it now seemed impossible to maintain the commitment to excellence that was associated with his name. Retirement was the only way out. (Fig. 53)

Fuchs's youngest disciple, Karl David Lindner,[775] has left a detailed description of the circumstances that led Fuchs to this decision:

> *Fuchs mentioned in passing once that he had no intention of holding on to his chair until he was 70. However, the cause of his unusually early retirement is little known. Nor does Fuchs mention it in his memoirs. We believe we know it. When the First World War broke out, many foreigners working at the clinic left and the clinic's own medical doctors were called up one after another. This meant that normal clinical work threatened to come to a standstill. Fuchs contacted the Army High Command and declared himself unable to run such a large clinic with so few doctors. The officiating Surgeon General* [Generalstabsarzt], *whose name we will deny a Herostratic mention here, replied that Fuchs was free to close down his clinic. In reaction to this Fuchs submitted his application for retirement five years before the legal age limit, and all interventions by his colleagues and remonstrations citing wartime exigencies were of no avail. However, he continued his research and his teaching. Even during the war he accepted an invitation to lecture in Spain. After the end of the war he went to the United States repeatedly to lecture there and made other such visits to Latin American countries and to Japan and China. In this way Fuchs renewed the* [war-damaged] *links between Vienna and the world and rendered his country arguably a much greater service than he would have done, had he clung to his chair to the end.*[776]

Emperor Francis Joseph accepted Ernst Fuchs's application for retirement on August 16, 1915 with the words:

I approve of the retirement of the Full Professor of Ophthalmology and Director of the Second Eye Clinic of Vienna University, Dr Ernst Fuchs, who has been awarded the title and character of Hofrat, on the basis of his application at the end of September and award him on this occasion the Commander's Cross with Star of my Franz-Joseph Order.[777]

The Ministerium für Kultus und Unterricht made use of the occasion of Fuchs's retirement to express its "*gratitude for and its appreciation of* [his] *dedicated, excellent and successful academic activities over many years*".[778]

His pension – or to give it its Austrian name, his *Ruhegenuss* – amounted to an annual 11,840 crowns,[779] the equivalent roughly of € 40,300 or $ 47,800 in today's (2022) money.

Ernst Fuchs mastered the complex, often heterogeneous tasks that confront the director of a university clinic with outstanding personal commitment, expertise and competence. In the three decades he headed the Second University Eye Clinic he made Vienna the undisputed nerve centre of ophthalmology worldwide.

Notes

655 "Notiz", in: *Wiener medicinische Blätter* [*Wien. med. Bl.*] 8 (1885), col. 1140 of 9 September 1885.

656 Fuchs took his oath in the Presidential Office of the Governor of Lower Austria, Ludwig Freiherr Possinger von Choborski (1823–1905). Cf. Attachment to Ernst Fuchs's certificate of appointment, archive no. Z. 14313 (UA!) in the Family archive.

657 Edmund Bochner. Clin. assist. under the first Director of the 2nd Univ. Eye Clinic, Eduard Jaeger v. Jaxtthal. Continued as assistant under Fuchs for one more year before being appointed Municipal Physician in Brno. Cf. WYKLICKY, *Augenheilkunde*, p. 26, and FUCHS, *Augenarzt* (as in FN 2), p. 96.

658 A blank space in the original.

659 Handwritten letter from Fuchs to the Directorate of the Allgem. Krankenhaus, DZ: 1266–praes 11/9 1885. Original in a private collection.

660 Joseph Raimund Hoffmann (1823–1892). Studied at the Univ. of Prague and Vienna (Dr med., Dr chir. 1847, Mag. obstetr. 1849), junior doctor at the Allgem. Krankenhaus. After several spells as medical officer (e.g. district physician in Korneuburg and

Neunkirchen) 1858 Head physician at the Inquisitenspital of Vienna's Landesgericht [Regional Court]. 1869–1887 Director of the Allgem. Krankenhaus. Cf. EISENBERG 2 (as in FN 13); PAGEL (as in FN 13); GROIS (as in FN 578), *Allgem. Krankenhaus*, pp. 110ff.

661 Cf. FN 659.

662 Ernst FUCHS, "Antrittsrede gehalten bei Eröffnung seiner Vorlesungen an der Wiener Universität Montag den 19. October 1885", in: *Wien. med. Bl.* 8 (1885), cols. 1301–04. When more than forty years later he wrote his autobiography, which was not published until 1946, the topic of his inaugural lecture had obviously slipped his memory: *"I took office with an inaugural lecture about medical doctors in antiquity, especially about ophthalmologists."* (See FUCHS, *Augenarzt* (as in FN 2), p. 85). Nor was he entirely up to speed as regards the organ of publication: *"As far as I remember, the lecture was published in a medical journal."* (Ibid.). That Fuchs was either unable or unwilling to recall the publication details may have had to do with the unpleasant experiences he had been exposed to by the coverage of the appointment procedure by the most widely read Viennese medical journal at the time, the *Wien. med. Wochenschrift*. For the publication of his inaugural lecture Fuchs therefore chose a far less prestigious journal, the *Wien. med. Blätter*.

663 Fuchs therefore says in his autobiography: *"None of my colleagues were present as it was not customary at the time to invite them."* See FUCHS, *Augenarzt* (as in FN 2), p. 85.

664 See also the homage Ernst Fuchs paid to the personalities and the scientific merits of Eduard Jaeger v. Jaxtthal, of his father Friedrich Jaeger v. Jaxtthal and of Eduard Jaeger's grandfather, Georg Joseph Beer, on the occasion of the inauguration of the monument erected in Vienna University's Arkadenhof [Arcade Court] in honour of Eduard Jaeger on 28 February 1910. (Unpublished typescript in private collection).

665 FUCHS, *Inaugural Lecture*, col. 1303.

666 Ibid.

667 Ibid.

668 Ibid.

669 Ibid., cols. 1303–1304.

670 Ibid., col. 1304.

671 Cf. "Schema für die systematische klinische Untersuchung der Patienten zum Gebrauche der Hörer der Zweiten Augenklinik." See Ch. 8.

672 Erna LESKY, *Meilensteine der Wiener Medizin. Große Ärzte Österreichs in drei Jahrhunderten*. Wilhelm Maudrich, Vienna/Munich/Bern 1981, p. 180.

673 FUCHS, *Augenarzt* (as in FN 2), p. 94.

674 Cf. FN 14.

675 Cf. FN 17.

676 See Ch 2.

677 Cf. FN 609.

678 Cf. FN 364.

679 FUCHS, *Augenarzt* (as in FN 2), p. 93.

680 Cf. FN 610.

681 Cf. FN 637.

682 Cf. FN 146.

683 Cf. FN 599.

684 Emil Zuckerkandl (1849–1910). Originally from Hungary. 1874 Dr med. univ. (Vienna Univ.). Demonstrator while still a student under the anatomist Hyrtl (cf. FN 13). 1873/74 Assist. under the pathol. Rokitansky (cf. FN 15). 1874 Assist. under the anatomist Langer. 1880 Assoc. Prof. on the basis of his outstanding scientific achievements without prior habilitation. 1888–1910 Full Prof. of Anatomy at Vienna Univ. as successor of Langer (1st Anat. Department). Z. made anatomy totally subservient to clin. medicine and created seminal topograph. atlases for several specialties, e.g. laryngology, rhinology, and urology. Epochal significance attaches to his four-volume *Atlas d. topograph. Anatomie d. Menschen* (1890–1904), which established itself as a sort of indispensable ordnance survey map for surgeons. Cf. CZEIKE (as in FN 13); FISCHER (as in FN 28); PAGEL (as in FN 13); LESKY, *Wien. Med. Schule* (as in FN 12); pp. 509–512; Obituaries: *Wien. med. Wochenschr.* 60 (1910), cols. 1323–24; *Feierl. Inaug. ... Studienjahr 1910/11*, pp. 39ff. (with bibliography); *Anat. Anzeiger* 37 (1910), pp. 86ff. (J. Tandler); *Wien. klin. Wochenschr.* 23 (1910), pp. 789ff.; *Almanach Akad. Wiss.* 61 (1911), pp. 364ff.; *Archiv f. Ohrenheilk.* 84 (1911), pp. 7–8 (A. Politzer).

685 See FUCHS, *Augenarzt* (as in FN 2), p. 93, and LESKY, *Wien. Med. Schule* (as in FN 12), p. 514.

686 Viktor Ebner Ritter von Rofenstein (1842–1925). Originally from Bregenz. Studied at the Univ. of Innsbruck, Göttingen and Vienna (Dr med. 1866). 1868 Assist. under the physiol. Alexander Rollett (1834–1903) at Graz Univ.; 1870 Habilitation in Histology at Innsbruck. 1873 Assoc. Prof. of Histol. and Embryol. in Graz (Full Prof. 1885). 1888–1922 Full Prof. of Histol. and successor of Wedl at Vienna Univ. It was thanks to his achievements that histol. was established as a specialty in its own right, distinct from anatomy and physiology. 1903 Succeeded in establishing histology as an autonomous examination subject in the new study regulations. Rector of Vienna Univ. 1907/08. Cf. CZEIKE (as in FN 13); EISENBERG 2 (as in FN 13); HIRSCH (as in FN 13); NDB (as in FN 15); ÖBL (as in FN 11); PAGEL (as in FN 13); LESKY, *Wien. med. Schule* (as in FN 12), pp. 513–520; Obituaries: *Wien. med. Wochenschr.* 75 (1925), col. 89; *Wien. klin. Wochenschr.* 38 (1925), pp. 441ff.; *Feierl. Inauguration ... Studienjahr 1925/26*, pp. 28ff; *Anat. Anzeiger 64* (1927), pp. 1ff.

687 Cf. FN 137.

688 Rudolf Chrobak (1843–1910). Originally from Troppau/Austrian Silesia (today Opava/Czech Republic). Studied at Vienna Univ. (Dr med. 1866). Supported by the intern. clinician and Dir. of the 2nd Med. Univ. Clinic Johann Ritter v. Oppolzer (1808–1871), he became a self-taught gynaecologist. 1871 Habilitation in Gynaecology and Obstetrics at Vienna Univ. (1880 Assoc. Prof.). 1889–1908 Full Prof. and Dir. of the 2nd Univ. Women's Clinic. Together with the Dir. of the parallel clinic, Friedrich Schauta (1849–1919, cf. FN 102) significant input in the planning and construction of the new Univ. Women's Clinics. Cf. CZEIKE (as in FN 13); EISENBERG 2 (as in FN 13); NDB (as in FN 15); ÖBL (as in FN 11); PAGEL (as in FN 13); Isidor FISCHER; *Geschichte der Geburtshilfe in Wien.* Franz Deuticke, Leipzig/Vienna 1909; LESKY, *Wien. Med. Schule* (as in FN 12), pp. 471–475; Anton SCHALLER, *Die Wertheim-Klinik. Eine Geschichte der II. Universitäts-Frauenklinik in Wien.* Maudrich, Vienna/Munich/Bern 1992, pp. 53–65.

689 Julius Wagner Ritter von Jauregg (1857–1940). Originally from Wels/Upper Austria. Studied at Vienna Univ. (Dr med. 1880). While still a student, he was introduced (1876) to scientific methodolog. by the experim. pathol. Salomon Stricker. 1880–1882 Assist. under Stricker. 1883 Assistant at the Niederösterr. Landesirrenanstalt under Max Leidesdorf (1816–1889). Specialis. in psychiatry. 1885 Habilitation in Neuropathology and (1887) Psychiatry at Vienna Univ.; 1889–1893 Assoc. Prof. in Graz. 1893–1902 Full Prof. and Dir. of the 1st Psychiatr. Univ. Clinic in Vienna, 1902–1928 Full Prof. and Dir. at the 2nd Psychiatr. Univ. Clinic (1911 Fusion of the two Univ. Clinics). Two pioneering achievements are indelibly associated with his name: 1. The discovery of iodine deficiency as the cause of congenital cretinism and the resulting mental retardation (establishment of a self-funded Institute of Goitre Research in Zeltweg/Styria; 1898 Proposal of the iodination of table salt in rural regions with endemic goitre). 2. The observation that febrile illnesses led to the temporary relief of psychotic symptoms. This inspired the idea of using regular fever bouts to bring about a lasting improvement of psychoses. After initial experiments with tuberculin and other vaccines he achieved the breakthrough with a serum obtained from malaria patients. 1927 Nobel Prize for the malaria therapy of progressive paralysis. Cf. CZEIKE (as in FN 13); EULNER (as in FN 13); FISCHER (as in FN 28); ÖBL (as in FN 11); PAGEL (as in FN 13); LESKY, *Wien. Med. Schule* (as in FN 12), pp. 401–405 (with extensive bibliogr.); Obituary: *Monatsschr. f. Pschiatr. u. Neurol.* 103 (1940), pp. 186ff.; Appreciation: *Wien. med. Wochenschr.* 78 (1928), p. 892; Hans HOFF, "Gedächtnisvortrag zum 100. Geburtstag Wagner-Jaureggs", in: *Wien. med. Wochenschr.* 107 (1957), cols. 168ff.; Helmut WYKLICKY, "Zur Geschichte der Psychiatrie in Österreich", in: Peter BERNER, Walter SPIEL, Hans STROTZKA, Helmut WYKLICKY, *Zur Geschichte der Psychiatrie in Wien. Eine Bilddokumentation / Psychiatry in Vienna. An Illustrated Documentation.* Christian Brandstätter, Vienna 1983; Helmut GRÖGER, Eberhard GABRIEL, Siegfried KASPER (eds.), *Zur Geschichte der Psychiatrie in Wien.* Christian Brandstätter, Vienna 1997.

690 Theodor Escherich (1857–1911). Originally from Franconia. Studied at the Univ. of Würzburg, Strasbourg, Kiel and Berlin (Dr med. Würzburg 1881). 1885 Assist. at the Univ. Children's Clinic in Munich (1886 Habilitation). 1889 Assoc. Prof. (1894 Full Prof.) and Dir. of the Univ. Children's Clinic in Graz, 1902–1911 Full Prof. and Dir. of the Univ. Children's Clinic in Vienna. Main areas of work: infant. metabolism and nutrition. Expanded his clinic by adding wards for new-born babies and infants. Intense lobbying for the protection of infants. Especially noteworthy are his studies on normal intestinal flora. 1886 Recognition of the significance of physiolog. intestinal bacteria for digestion (Escherichia coli). Cf. CZEIKE (as in FN 13); NDB (as in FN 15); ÖBL (as in FN 11); PAGEL (as in FN 13); Obituaries: *Zeitschr. Kinderheilk.* 1 (1911), pp. 423ff.; *Feierl. Inaug. ... Studienjahr 1911/12*; pp. 39ff. (with bibliography. 1882–1909). Appreciation: Franz HAMBURGER, "Theodor Escherich", in: *Wien. med. Wochenschr.* 82 (1932), cols. 1216ff.; LESKY, *Wien. Med. Schule* (as in FN 12), pp. 362–363; Helmut WYKLICKY, "Der Anteil der Wiener medizinischen Schule an der Erforschung und Behandlung von Infektionskrankheiten", in: *Recipe* 4 (1979), pp. 7ff.

691 Ottokar Freiherr von Chiari (1853–1918). Originally from Prague. Studied in Vienna (Dr med. 1877; aspirant at the 2nd Med. Univ. Clinic under Heinrich v. Bamberger

(1822–1888) and at the Univ. Clinic for Dermatol. under Ferdinand R. v. Hebra (cf. FN 163). 1877–1879 Trainee surgeon at the 1st Surg. Univ. Clinic under Johann Dumreicher Frh. von Österreicher (1815–1880) and 1879–1881 at the Laryngolog. Univ. Clinic under Leopold Schrötter von Kristelli (1837–1908). 1882 Habilitation in Rhino-Laryngology. Director of a Day Clinic for Throat and Nose Diseases, initially at the 1st Med. Univ. Clinic under Hermann Nothnagel (cf. FN 598), later in the building of the directorate of the Allgem. Krankenhaus. 1891 Assoc. Prof.; 1893 Head physician of the Department of Oto-Rhinolaryngology at Vienna's Allgem. Poliklinik. 1900 Head of the Laryngol. Univ. Clinic (1907 tit. Assoc. Prof., 1912 Full Prof.). 1911 Inauguration of his newly built clinic. In 1908 he presided over the Internat. Rhino-Laryngol. Congress in Vienna. Cf. CZEIKE (as in FN 13); EISENBERG 2 (as in FN 13); EULNER (as in FN 13); FISCHER (as in FN 28); NDB (as in FN 15); LESKY, *Wien. Med. Schule* (as in FN 12), pp. 419–421; Obituaries: *Internat. Zentralbl. Laryngol. Rhinol.* 34 (1918), pp. 151–152; *Wien. med. Wochenschr.* 68 (1918), pp. 917–918; *Monatsschr. Ohrenheilk. u. Laryngo-Rhinol.* 53 (1919), pp. 81ff.

692 Hans Frh. von Chiari (1851–1916). Studied in Vienna (Dr med. 1875). 1874 Assist. under the patholog. Carl Freiherr v. Rokitansky, 1878 Habilitation in Pathol. Anat. under the latter's successor, Richard Heschl. 1882–1906 Full Prof. at the German Univ. of Prague, which had been hived off from Prague Univ. in 1882. 1900/01 Rector. 1906 Call to Strasbourg Univ. (Rector 1914/15). He has given his name to the Budd-Chiari syndrome and the Chiari malformation. Cf. GERABEK et al. (as in FN 13); HIRSCH (as in FN 13); PAGEL (as in FN 13); ÖBL (as in FN 11).

693 See Ch. 2.

694 Jakob Pál (1863–1936). Originally from Budapest. Studied in Vienna (Dr med. 1886), then active at the Institute of General and Experim. Pathology. 1891 Joined the 1st Med. Department of the Allgem. Krankenhaus. 1888 Habilitation in Internal Medicine, Head physician from 1893 (tit. Assoc. Prof. 1900, Assoc. Prof. 1908, tit. Full Prof. 1922). We owe him a method of dying the myelin sheath fibres of the central nervous system (1886), the discovery of the cancellation of the effect of curare by physostigmine (1900) and the discovery of the spasmolyt. effect of papaverine (1913). Cf. NDB (as in FN 15); Appreciation: Ludwig POPPER, "Jakob Pal 1863–1936. Zur hundertsten Wiederkehr seines Geburtstages", in: *Wien. klin. Wochenschr.* 75 (1963), pp. 606–608.

695 FUCHS, *Augenarzt* (as in FN 2), p. 81.

696 J. F. WAGNER, *Orientirungs-Plan des Wiener k. k. allgemeinen Krankenhauses*, pp. 17–18. Cf. the attached Situationsplan des k. k. allgemeinen Krankenhauses in Wien. See also: HERZIG; Joseph HOFFMANN, *Das Wiener k. k. allgemeine Krankenhaus.* K. K. Hof- und Staatsdruckerei, Vienna 1873; Eugen HOFMOKL, *Wiener Heilanstalten.* [= Supplement of the weekly *Das Österreichische Sanitätswesen*]. Vienna 1910; Adolf KRONFELD (ed.), *Führer durch das Medizinische Wien.* Geschichte und Organisation. Moritz Perles, Vienna 1911, p. 44; and Dieter JETTER, *Wien von den Anfängen bis um 1900* [= *Geschichte des Hospitals*, vol. 5]. Franz Steiner, Wiesbaden 1982.

697 UA Vienna, Z. 183 ex 1885/86. Protocol concerning the takeover of the Second Eye Clinic by Dr Ernst Fuchs.

698 Cf. FN 659.

699 A note has been added here in the left margin by another hand: *Z. Sttth.* [Statthalterei] *Z. 430 ex 1886 bereits flüssig gemacht,* which indicates that the release of funds had been approved by the Governor.

700 Joseph Raimund Hoffmann. Cf. FN 660.

701 In the right-hand margin next to this passage, the same hand that commented on the amount of 1,000 gulden [cf. FN 699] added "blohs versprochen", i. e., a mere promise.

702 Handwritten letter from Ernst Fuchs to the Directorate of the Allgem. Krankenhaus. (Private collection)

703 Cf. Akademischer Senat der Wiener Universität (ed.), *Geschichte der Wiener Universität von 1848 bis 1898. Als Huldigungsfestschrift zum fünfzigjährigen Regierungsjubiläum Seiner k. und k. apostolischen Majestät, des Kaisers Franz Josef I.*, Alfred Hölder, Vienna 1898, p. 236.

704 Ludwig Lazarus Zamenhof (1859–1917), born Eliezer Levi Samenhof, a.k.a. Ludwik Lejzer Zamenhof, Lazar Ludvik Zamenhof; Polish Ludwik Łazarz Zamenhof. Originally from the Polish town Białystok, then part of Tsarist Russia.

705 Cf. Dietmar GRIESER, *Weltreise durch Wien. Lebensstationen berühmter Persönlichkeiten*. Deutscher Taschenbuch Verlag, Munich 2006, pp. 131–136; Reinhard HAUPENTHAL, *Die Wien-Aufenthalte von Lazar Markovic Zamenhof (1859–1917) und seine ophthalmologischen Studien bei Ernst Fuchs (1851–1930): ein Beitrag zum 150. Geburtstag Zamenhofs*. Ed. Iltis, Saarbrücken 2009; Andreas KÜNZLI, *L. L. Zamenhof (1859–1917). Esperanto, Hillelismus (Homaranismus) und die jüdische Frage in Ost und West*. Otto Harrassowitz Verlag, Wiesbaden 2010, pp. 92–94.

706 See the previous chapter.

707 Heinrich von Bamberger (1822–1888). Originally from Zwornarka nr. Prague. Studied at the Univ. of Prague and Vienna (Dr med. 1847). 1851–1854 Assist. of the med. clinician Johann R. v. Oppolzer. 1854 Full Prof. and Dir. of the Med. Clinic in Würzburg, 1872 after the death of his teacher Oppolzer Full Prof. and Dir. of the Med. Clinic in Vienna. Main area of work: cardiac pathologgy. 1886–1888 Pres. of the Gesellsch. d. Ärzte, a capacity that formed the basis for his collaboration with Fuchs. Cf. CZEIKE (as in FN 13); EISENBERG 2 (as in FN 13); EULNER (as in FN 13); HIRSCH, NDB (as in FN 15); ÖBL (as in FN 11*)*; PAGEL (as in FN 13); WURZBACH (as in FN 15); LESKY, *Wien. Med.* Schule (as in FN 12), Reg.

708 Gustav Riehl (1855–1943). Studied in Vienna (Dr med. 1879). 1881–1884 Specialisation in dermatology under Ferdinand R. v. Hebra (cf. FN 163) and assist. under Moriz Kaposi (1837–1902) at the Allgem. Krankenhaus. 1885 Habilitation in Dermatol. and Syphilidol. at Vienna Univ.; 1888–1896 Head physician at the Wiedener Krankenhaus. 1898 Full Prof. at Leipzig Univ.; 1902–1926 Full Prof. and successor of his teacher Kaposi as Head of Clinic at Vienna Univ.; 1921/22 Rector of Vienna Univ.; research on skin tuberculosis, leucaemia and diseases of the skin in close collab. with pathol. Richard Paltauf (1858–1924). One of the pioneers of radiotherapy for skin diseases and of the salvarsan therapy for syphilis. Cf. CZEIKE (as in FN 13), ÖBL (as in FN 11); Appreciations: Leopold ARZT, "Hofrat Professor Dr Gustav Riehl, geb. 10. Februar 1855. Direktor der Klinik für Haut- und Geschlechtskrankheiten, erster Herausgeber der *Wiener Klinischen Wochenschrift*, 1888–1896", in:

Wien. klin. Wochenschr. 67 (1955), pp. 101–103; ARZT, "Hofrat Professor Gustav Riehl zum 100. Geburtstag", in: *Der Hautarzt* 6 (1955), pp. 239–240.

709 FUCHS, *Augenarzt* (as in FN 2), pp. 93–94. See also: Fuchs's handwritten letter to Wagner-Jauregg, dated 4 June 1921. Sammlungen d. Wien. Med. Univ. No. 2855/2 and Helmut WYKLICKY, "Die 'Wiener klinische Wochenschrift' von 1888–1970", in: *Wien. klin. Wochenschr.* 100 (1988), pp. 228–244.

710 Cf. FN 707.

711 Cf. FN 597.

712 Cf. FN 637.

713 Leopold Schrötter Ritter von Kristelli (1837–1908). Originally from Graz. Studied in Vienna (Dr med. et chir. 1861), 1861–1863 Trainee surgeon at the 2nd Chir. Univ. Clinic under Franz Schuh. Until 1869 Assist. at the 1st Med. Univ. Clinic under Joseph Škoda (cf. FN 16). Special. in laryngoscopy (1867 Habilitation in Diseases of the Chest and the Larynx at Vienna Univ.). At his instigation and under his leadership foundation in 1870 of the Laryngolog. Univ. Clinic at the Allgemein. Krankenhaus, a worldwide premiere. 1875 Assoc. Prof. for Diseases of the Chest and the Larynx. 1877/78–1881 Head physician of the 1st Med. Department of the Krankenanstalt Rudolfstiftung, then head physician at the Allgemein. Krankenhaus. 1885 Habilitation in Internal Medicine. 1890 Full Prof. and Dir. of the 3rd Med. Univ. Clinic at the Allgemein. Krankenhaus, which had been created especially for him. Greatly improved the care of tuberculosis patients, for whom he created a first sanatorium in Austria in Alland nr. Vienna (1898 Inauguration). Propagated especially the climatic spas of the Austrian Adriatic. Cf. CZEIKE (as in FN 13); EISENBERG 2 (as in FN 13); HIRSCH (as in FN 13); PAGEL (as in FN 13); NDB (as in FN 15); ÖBL (as in FN 11). Obituaries: *Feierl. Inaug. … Studienjahr 1908/09*, pp. 33 ff.; *Wien. med. Wochenschr.* 58 (1908), cols. 961–962; *Wien. klin. Wochenschr.* 21 (1908), 641–642; *Med. Klinik* 4 (1908), pp. 715–17; *Internat. Centralbl. f. Laryngol., Rhinol, u. verwandte Wiss.* 24 (1908), pp. 281–87 (with bibliography). Appreciations: "Festschr. f. Leopold v. Schrötter", in: *Wien. med. Wochenschr.* 87 (1937), cols. 141–52, 157–60 and 163–164; *Mschr. f. Ohrenheilk. u. Laryngo-Rhinol.* 71 (1937), pp. 1131–1140; LESKY, *Wien. Med. Schule* (as in FN 12), pp. 330–333; E. H. MAJER and Manfred SKOPEC, *Zur Geschichte der Oto-Rhino-Laryngologie in Österreich.* Brandstätter, Vienna^2 1998, pp. 59–64 and 105.

714 "Programm", in: *Wien. klin. Wochenschr.* Yr. 1, No. 1, 5 April 1888, first page without pagination.

715 Ernst FUCHS, "*Über traumatische Linsentrübung*", in: *Wien. klin. Wochenschr.* 1 (1888), pp. 53–57 and 86–88.

716 Ernst FUCHS, "Die Entzündungen des Lidrandes", in: Ibid., pp. 773–776 and 807–810.

717 (Ed.), "Zum fünfundzwanzigsten Jahrestag", in: *Wien. klin. Wochenschr.* 25 (1912), pp. 3–4.

718 "Theoretisch-praktischer Unterricht in der Augenheilkunde," in: *Öffentliche Vorlesungen an der k. k. Universität zu Wien im Wintersemester 1885/86.* Kaiserlich-Königliche Hof- und Staatsdruckerei, Vienna 1885, p. 26. A postscript for the winter semester 1885/86 added by the Deanery of the Med. Faculty correctly identifies Fuchs as the

lecturer of the Main Course in Ophthalmology. Cf. UA Wien, Med. Dekanat 57 aus 1885/86.

719 *Öffentliche Vorlesungen an der K. K. Universität zu Wien im Sommersemester 1886.* Kaiserlich-Königliche Hof- und Staatsdruckerei, Vienna 1886, p. 25.

720 Ernst FUCHS, *Lehrbuch der Augenheilkunde.* Franz Deuticke. Leipzig/Vienna 1889.

721 See the next chapter.

722 Gabriela SCHMIDT-WYKLICKY, Helmut GRÖGER, "Die Wiener Ophthalmologische Schule. Geist und Leistung der ersten 150 Jahre", in: *Spektrum Augenheilk.* 26 (2012), pp. 345–356.

723 Cf. FN 200.

724 *"Über ausgewählte Capitel der Augenheilkunde mit Demonstrationen einschlägiger Fälle"*, in: *Öffentliche Vorlesungen an der k. k. Universität zu Wien im Wintersemester 1886/87.* Kaiserlich-Königliche Hof- und Staatsdruckerei, Vienna 1886, p. 29.

725 See FUCHS, *Augenarzt* (as in FN 2), p. 42.

726 ÖSTA/AVA Wien. Unterricht Allgemein (1848–1940). Universität Wien, Medizin. Lehrkanzeln: in genere u. A–G Anatomie – Gewerbekrankheiten. Box 617 Sign. 4. K. K. Ministerium für Cultus und Unterricht. 4 Medic. Augenheilkunde No. 4822 of 10 March 1887 and Z. 267.

727 Ibid., fols. 3–4.

728 *Öffentliche Vorlesungen an der K. K. Universität zu Wien im Winter-Semester 1887/78.* Kaiserlich-Königliche Hof- und Staatsdruckerei, Vienna 1887, p. 29.

729 *Öffentliche Vorlesungen an der K. K. Universität zu Wien im Sommer-Semester 1891.* Kaiserlich-Königliche Hof- und Staatsdruckerei, Vienna 1891, p. 30; DEIMER, *Poliklinik* (as in FN 200), pp. 158–160.

730 In the summer semesters of 1887, 1889 and 1892.

731 In the summer semester of 1895.

732 In the winter semester (WS) of 1898/99, in the summer semester (SS) of 1899, WS 1899/1900, SS 1900, WS 1900/01, SS 1901, WS 1901/02, SS 1902, WS 1902/03, SS 1903, from the WS of 1903/04 with projection, SS 1904, WS 1904/05, SS 1905, WS 1905/06, WS 1906/07, WS 1907/08, WS 1908/09, WS 1909/10, WS 1909/10, WS 1911/12, WS 1912/13, WS 1913/14, WS 1914/15.

733 UA Wien. Med. Dekanat, Z. 1109 v. 18. 6. 1893, comprising the minist. decree of 9 June 1893, Z. 10.620 and Dean Hofmann's memo regarding the positive settlement. Cf. Adolf KRONFELD (ed.), *Führer durch das Medizinische Wien*, p. 44.

734 Carl Ludwig SIGMUND, *Das k. k. chirurgische Operations-Institut in Wien. Darstellung der Geschichte so wie der innern Einrichtung des Institutes, und Übersicht aller darin bisher gebildeten Operateurs, der hinsichtlich derselben erflossenen Verordnungen und der Vorfälle in der chirurgischen Klinik der Wiener Hochschule während des Operations-Lehrcurses 1839–1841.* Braumüller und Seidel, Vienna 1841, pp. 7ff. Cf. WYKLICKY, *Josephinum*, p. 94, and LESKY, *Wien. Med. Schule* (as in FN 12), pp. 62–63. In general usage and in med. publications the term *Operateur-Institut* was current for this institution. In the course of the 19th cent. the *Operateur-Institut* was repeatedly subjected to reform and used as a model for the new surg. specialties that were hived off from the mother speciality. In 1882, for instance, an obstetrical *Operations-Institut* was established.

Cf. "Erlass des Ministers für Cultus und Unterricht vom 16. Juli 1882, Z. 9642, betreffend die Errichtung eines geburtshilflichen Operations-Institutes an der medizinischen Fakultät der Wiener Universität", in: *Provisorisches Statut für das geburtshilfliche Operations-Institut an der medizinischen Fakultät der Universität Wien*, in: Verordnungsbl. für d. Dienstbereich d. Ministeriums für Cultus u. Unterricht. Redigiert im k. k. Ministerium für Cultus u. Unterricht. Ausgegeben am 15. August 1882, No. 31, Verlag d. k. k. Ministeriums für Cultus u. Unterricht, Vienna 1882, pp. 157–158.

735 *Statut des Operations-Institutes an der II. Augenklinik in Wien*, n. d. – Taking his cue from the seminal initiative of his revered teacher Ernst Fuchs, Wilhelm Czermak (cf. FN 43), active since 1895 as Full Professor of Ophthalmology at the German Karl-Ferdinands Univ. in Prague, established in 1898 an ophthalmic surgical institute at his clinic on the occasion of its reorganisation. The trainee surgeons served as junior doctors at Prague's Univ. Eye Clinic. Cf. *Die Deutsche Karl-Ferdinands-Universität in Prag unter der Regierung Seiner Majestät des Kaisers Franz Josef I.*, Verlag d. J. G. Calve'schen k. u. k. Hof- u. Universitätsbuchhandlung (Josef Koch), Prague 1899, p. 354.

736 Cf. FN 18.

737 Adolf Exner (1841–1894). Originally from Prague. Studied law in Vienna (Dr iur. 1863). 1866 Habilitation at Vienna Univ.; 1868–1872 Full Prof. of Roman Law at Zurich Univ., then return to Vienna as Chair. 1883/84 Dean of the Law Faculty of Vienna Univ., 1891/92 Rector. Cf. ÖBL (as in FN 11).

738 Hans Bitterlich (1860–1949). Son of the painter Eduard Bitterlich (1833–1872). From 1877 training at the Academy of Fine Arts in Vienna. Attended the course given by Caspar v. Zumbusch (1830–1915). 1902–1910 Dir. of the School of Sculptors (1904 Assoc. Prof., 1907 Full Prof.) in Vienna's Academy 1910–1931 Director of an autonomous School of Sculpture. 1930/1931 Rector of the Acad.; created several outstanding monuments for the Arcade Court of Vienna University and a great number of portrait busts. Cf. ÖBL (as in FN 11).

739 Cf. UA Wien, *Akten d. akad. Senats* 92.2 (1892–1896).

740 Thomas MAISEL, *Gelehrte in Stein und Bronze. Die Denkmäler im Arkadenhof der Universität Wien*. Böhlau, Vienna/Köln/Weimar 2007, p. 71.

741 Cf. *Neue Freie Presse*, 23 June 1896, morning edition, No. 11434, p. 5; *Neue Freie Presse*, 9 July 1896, evening edition, No. 11449, pp. 1–2; *Wiener Abendpost*, 9 July 1896, No. 156, p. 2.

742 Ernst FUCHS, *Denkrede auf Arlt*. Gehalten am 9. Juli 1896 bei der Enthüllung seines Denkmals im Arkadenhof der Universität Vienna, in: Anton BETTELHEIM (ed.), *Biographische Blätter*. Jahrbuch für lebensgeschichtliche Kunst und Forschung. Vol. 2. Ernst Hofmann & Co. Berlin 1896, pp. 384–388.

743 Albert Mosetig Ritter von Moorhof (1838–1907). Originally from Trieste. Studied in Vienna (Dr med. et chir. 1861). Trainee surgeon, then assist. at the 1st Surgical Univ. Clinic of the Allgem. Krankenhaus under Johann Dumreicher Freiherr. von Österreicher (1815–1880). 1866 Habilitation in Surg. at Vienna Univ., 1875 Assoc. Prof., 1898 tit. Full Prof. First Head physician at the Krankenanstalt Rudolfstiftung, then at the Krankenhaus Wieden, 1891–1906 Dir. of the 2nd Department of Surgery at the Allgem. Krankenhaus. Cf. EISENBERG 2 (as in FN 13); HIRSCH (as in FN 13); NDB (as in FN 15); PAGEL (as in FN 13); LESKY, *Wien. Med. Schule* (as in FN 12), pp. 456–457; Obituaries, in: *Die feierliche Inauguration des Rektors der Wiener Uni-*

versität für das Studienjahr 1907/1908. Selbstverlag der Universität, Vienna 1908, pp. 45ff.; *Wien. klin. Wochenschr.* 20 (1907), pp. 545–546; *Wien. med. Wochenschr.* 57 (1907), cols. 251–252.

744 Julius Hochenegg (1859–1940). Studied in Vienna (Dr med. 1884). Trainee surgeon at the Allgem. Krankenhaus under Theodor Billroth (2nd Surg. Univ. Clinic, cf. FN 17), Carl Braun R. v. Fernwald (1st Gynaecol. Univ. Clinic, see. FN 702) and Eduard Albert (1st Surg. Univ. Clinic, cf. FN 609). 1886–1890 Assist. under Albert. 1889 Habilitation in Surgery at Vienna Univ.; 1891 Dir. of the Dept. of Surgery at the Allgem. Poliklinik. 1894 Assoc. Prof. 1904–1930 Full Prof. and Dir. of the 2nd Surg. Univ. Clinic at the Allgem. Krankenhaus. Credited with significant progress in carcinoma surgery and the provision of social care to cancer patients. 1910 Initiator and cofounder of the K. & K. Österreichische Gesellschaft für Erforschung und Bekämpfung der Krebskrankheit (later Österr. Krebshilfe). 1914 Knighted. Cf. CZEIKE (as in FN 13); EISENBERG 2 (as in FN 13); NDB (as in FN 15); ÖBL (as in FN 11); PAGEL (as in FN 13); Österr. Krebshilfe (ed.), *100 Jahre Österreichische Krebshilfe 1910–2010*. Verlagshaus d. Ärzte, Vienna 2010.

745 Anton Frh. von Eiselsberg (1860–1939). Studied at the Universities of Vienna, Würzburg, Zurich and Paris (Dr med. Vienna 1884). Surg. specialisation under Theodor Billroth (2nd Surg. Univ. Clinic). 1890 Habilitation in Surg. at Vienna Univ.; 1893 Dir. of the Surg. Univ. Clinic Utrecht, 1896 Full Prof. in Königsberg, 1901–1931 Full Prof. and Dir. of the 1st Surg. Univ. Clinic at the Allgem. Krankenhaus. Pioneer of thyroid surgery and neurosurgery. His exemplary professional ethos shaped the Viennese School of Surgery. Cf. CZEIKE (as in FN 13), NDB (as in FN 15); ÖBL (as in FN 11); Anton EISELSBERG, *Lebensweg eines Chirurgen*. Tyrolia, Innsbruck 1937. Revised edition: *Lebensweg eines Chirurgen. Eine Autobiographie aus der großen Zeit der Wiener Medizin 1860–1937*. Brandstätter, Vienna 1991, Reprint of the first ed.: Severus, Hamburg 2010; Johannes Wolfgang Cornelius WICHT, *Prof. Dr Anton Freiherr von Eiselsberg. Leben und Wirken*. Diplomarbeit. Med. Univ. Innsbruck 2011.

746 Anton Frh. v. EISELSBERG, Ernst FUCHS, Julius HOCHENEGG, "Zur Frage der Unfallstation für die Wiener chirurgischen Kliniken und der Trachomstation für die Augenklinik", in: *Neue Freie Presse* No. 15813 of 30 August 1908, p. 3. Cf. "Wochenschau – Unfall- und Trachomstation", in: *Medicinische Blätter [= Med. Bl.]* 31 (1908), p. 577 of 5 Dec. 1908, Report, in: *Münch. med. Wochenschr.* 55 (1908), p. 1948, and Erna LESKY, "Die Errichtung der beiden Wiener Unfallstationen im Jahre 1909", in: *Acta Chir. Austriaca* 2 (1970), pp. 3–6; Louis OBROWSKY, *Historische Betrachtung der sozialmedizinischen Einrichtungen in Wien vom Beginn des 20. Jahrhunderts bis zum Ende der Ersten Republik*. [= Beiträge zur neueren Geschichte Österreichs, vol. 21]. Peter Lang, Frankfurt am Main/Vienna et al. 2005, p. 209.

747 For more details, see: GROIS, *Allgem. Krankenhaus* (as in FN 578), p. 155; *Brit. Med. J.*, Vol. 2, No. 2544 (Oct. 2, 1909), pp. 978–980.

748 ÖSTA /AVA Wien. K. K. Ministerium für Kultus und Unterricht. 4 G Medizin Chirurgische Kliniken "Unfallstationen" No. 51294 of 16 December 1909.

749 As in FN 747 (GROIS), p. 155.

750 Ministerium für Cultus und Unterricht (ed.), *Unterrichtsanstalten, Wissenschaftliche und Kunst-Institute in Wien und Niederösterreich*. K. K. Schulbücherverlag, 1917, pp. 63 and 65.

751 Karl David Lindner (1883–1961). Studied at the Univ. of Paris and Vienna (Dr med. 1907). Trainee surgeon and junior doctor at the 2nd Univ. Eye Clinic under Ernst Fuchs. 1909 Head of the trachoma ward Fuchs had established at this clinic. Winter semester 1911/12 leave of absence from the clinic to study serology at the Institut Pasteur in Paris. After his return Fuchs's youngest assistant. 1916 Habilitation in Ophthalmology on the basis of his research on trachoma under Fuchs's successor Friedrich Dimmer (cf. FN 44). From 1920 repeatedly in the USA, where he held courses at various universities, such as Chicago, St. Louis, and San Francisco. 1924–1927 Directoir of the Eye Department of the Allg. Poliklinik. 1927–1953 Full Prof. and Dir. of the 2nd Univ. Eye Clinic in Vienna as the successor of Dimmer. 1928 Invitation to the USA as trachoma expert to assess the research results the parasitologist Hideyo Noguchi (1876–1928) had achieved at the Rockefeller Institute for Medical Research (identification of the pathogen causing trachoma). 1935 Invited to the USA to hold one-week courses in Boston, Chicago, Denver, Philadelphia, San Francisco, St. Louis, and Washington. Guest lectures in Budapest, Zagreb, Athens and Paris. 1939 First foreigner to deliver the Montgomery Lecture in Dublin. Main area of work: trachoma research. Contributed major new insights, such as the description of what he termed inclusion blennorrhea; concerned himself with bacteriological problems; developed the shadow test (skiascopy) with cylinder lenses to determine astigmatism (1927); research on retinal detachment (introduction, among other things, of the pinhole glasses named after him). After the publication in 1945 of the 18th and last edition of Fuchs's classic textbook, L. pulled together the teachings of the Vienna Ophthalmological School in a textbook in 1952. After his retirement honorary professor at the Univ. of Cairo and Tabriz and at the Ghandi Eye Hospital in Alligar. Cf. CZEIKE (as in FN 13); FISCHER (as in FN 28); Obituaries: *Wien. klin. Wochenschr.* 73 (1961), pp. *Wien. med. Wochenschr.* 111 (1961), pp. 473–474 (H. Fanta); *Graefes Archiv* 163 (1961), pp. 489–492 (K. Hruby); *Klin. Monatsbl. Augenheilk.* 139 (1961), pp. 383–384 (A. Pillat); Appreciations: DEIMER, *Poliklinik* (as in FN 200), pp. 162ff.; Helmut GRÖGER, Gabriela SCHMIDT-WYKLICKY, "Karl David Lindner. Vorstand der II. Universitäts-Augenklinik in Wien 1927 bis 1953", in: *Spektrum Augenheilk.* 26 (2012), pp. 336–340.429–430. (J. Böck),

752 Karl LINDNER, "Ueber das Verschwinden des Trachoms und die Abnahme der infektiösen Bindehautentzündungen in Oesterreich", in: *Wien. klin. Wochenschr.* 65 (1953), pp. 759–760.

753 Stanislaus Prowazek Edl. von Lanow (1875–1915). Originally from Bohemia. Studied zoology and botany at the Univ. of Prague and Vienna (Dr phil. 1899). 1901/02 Studied one year under the pioneer of the research on infectious diseases, Paul Ehrlich (1854–1915), at Ehrlich's Institut f. Experim. Therapie in Frankfurt/ Main; introduction to modern laboratory methodology. Assist. at the Zoolog. Institut in Munich. Collaborator at the zoolog. station in Rovigno (Istria) and at the Inst. f. Protozoenforschung in Berlin under the man who identified the pathogen causing syphilis, Fritz Schaudinn (1871–1906). 1907 Appointed Schaudinn's successor as Director of Protozoa Research at the Hamburg Tropeninstitut. Research on blennorrhea, trachoma, pocks and rabies. 1913 Discovery of the pathogen causing epidemic typhus (rickettsia prowazekii). Many research trips. 1914 Infection with epidemic typhus, to which he

succumbed in 1915. Cf. GERABEK et al. (as in FN 13); Obituaries, in: *Verhandl. Zoolog.-Botan. Gesellsch. Wien* 65 (1915), pp. 65ff.; *J. Parasitol.* 2 (1915), pp. 51–53.

754 Ludwig von Halberstätter (1876–1949). Studied at the Univ. of Heidelberg and Breslau/Wrocław (Dr med. 1901). Assist. under the dermatol. Albert Neisser (cf. FN 244) at Breslau Univ.; 1905–1907 Research trip to Java with Neisser, where he collaborated with Stanislaus v. Prowazek (cf. FN 753) in research on trachoma. Discovery of the inclusions named after them. 1909 Relocation to Berlin's Charité, where he concerned himself with the radiotherapy of skin diseases. 1922 Habilitation in Dermatol. and Radiotherapy. 1926 Assoc. Prof. 1930 Appointed Dir. of the Dept. of Radiotherapy at the Inst. f. Krebsforschung in Berlin-Dahlem. After the Nazis' accession to power in 1933 dismissed from his academic post. Emigration to Palestine, where he was put in charge of the radiotherapy department of the Hadassah Hospital in Jerusalem. 1935 Prof. of Radiol. at the Hebr. Univ. Jerusalem. Cf. NDB (as in FN 15); Obituaries, in: *Brit. J. Radiol.* 22 (1949), p. 347; *Brit. Med. J.* I (1949), p. 871; *Lancet* I (1949), p. 845; *Zeitschr. Haut- u. Geschlechtskrankh.* 7 (1949), p. 39.

755 Karl LINDNER, "Die freie Initialform der Prowazek'schen Einschlüsse", in: *Wien. klin. Wochenschr.* 22 (1909), pp. 1697–1698, and *Graefes Archiv* 6 (1910), pp. 559–567.

756 Karl LINDNER, "Zur Färbung der Prowazekschen Einschlüsse", in: *Centralbl. Bakt. Parasitenk. Infektionskrankh.* 55 (1910), pp. 429–432.

757 Karl LINDNER, "*Über den derzeitigen Stand der Trachomforschung*", in: *Wien. klin. Wochenschr.* 22 (1909), pp. 1742–46.

758 Karl LINDNER, "Gonoblenorrhoe, Einschlussblenorrhoe, Trachom", in: *Graefes Archiv* 78 (1911), pp. 345–380.

759 Karl LINDNER, "*Über die Schwierigkeiten der Trachomforschung*", in: *Zeitschr. Augenheilk.* 57 (1925), pp. 508–556.

760 Karl LINDNER, "Ist das Bacterium granulosis Noguchi der Erreger des Trachoms?", in: *Graefes Archiv* 122 (1929), pp. 391–414.

761 Karl LINDNER, "Infektionsversuche von Trachom mit Paratrachom des Neugeborenen", in: *Graefes Archiv* 133 (1935), pp. 479–504.

762 Karl LINDNER, "Trachoma", in: Conrad BERENS (ed.), *The Eye and Its Diseases by 82 Authorities*. Saunders, Philadelphia/London 1936, pp. 399–417.

763 Ernst FUCHS, "Die ägyptische Augenentzündung", in: *Wien. klin. Wochenschr.* 7 (1894), pp. 211–214; "Egyptian Ophthalmia", in: *The Medical Age*. A Semi-Monthly Review of Medicine 12 (1894), pp. 262–267; "Die ägyptische Augenkrankheit", in: 1615 *Wien. klin. Wochenschr.* 37 (1924), pp. 564–566; "Die Therapie des Trachoms", in: *Wien. med. Wochenschr.* 177 (1927), cols. –1618.

764 Cf. FN 745.

765 George Edmund de Schweinitz (1858–1938). Originally from Philadelphia. Studied at the Univ. of Pennsylvania (M. D. 1881). Ophthalmol. specialis. under William Fisher Norris (1838–1901), the first Dir. of the Eye Dept. of that Univ. (from 1874). Norris was a disciple of the Viennese ophthalmol. Ferdinand R. v. Arlt, Eduard Jaeger v. Jaxtthal and Ludwig Mauthner and of the exper. pathol. Salomon Stricker. 1892 Clin. Prof. of Ophthalmol. at Jefferson Med. College. 1902–1929 Successor of Norris as Prof. of Ophthalm. at the Univ. of Pennsylvania Med. College, where he established a bacteriol. lab, among other things. Special areas of work: lesions of the pineal gland;

uveitis. Author of a highly respected textbook on diseases of the eye. One of the leading ophthalmologists in the United States alongside Edward Jackson and others. International recognition. Renowned surgeon and charismatic teacher. Pres. of the College of Physicians of Philadelphia (1910), of the Am. Ophthalmol. Soc. 1916, the Am. Med. Assoc. 1922 and the Internat. Congress of Ophthalmol. in Washington 1922. 1945 Establishment of the William F. Norris and George E. de Schweinitz Professorship of Ophthalm. at the Perelman School of Medicine of the Univ. of Pennsylvania, which de Schweinitz endowed in honour of his teacher William Fisher Norris. Cf. IBBO (as in FN 18); ALBERT/SCHEIE (as in FN 334); GORIN (as in FN 38), p. 237; Obituary: *Transact. Am. Ophthalmol. Soc.* 37 (1939), pp. 14.2-21 (John D. Carpenter).

766 Cf. (Ed.), Section of Ophthalmology: "The pathogenesis of chronic uveitis, excluding the syphilitic, tuberculous, and sympathetic varieties", in: *Brit. Med. J.*, June 28, 1913, p. 1375 (announcement); detailed report in: *The Lancet*, Vol. 1882, Issue 4694. pp. 483–484. For more details, see: *Seventh International Congress of Medicine (London 1913)*. Section IX. Ophthalmology. Frowde, London 1914.

767 Ernst FUCHS, "*Über chronische endogene Uveitis*", in: *Graefes Archiv* 84 (1913), pp. 201–292. See Ch. 7.

768 AVA Wien. No. 25.196/15. Beilagen zu dem allerunterthänigsten Vortrage des treugehorsamsten Ministers für Kultus und Unterricht Dr Max Ritter Hussarek von Heinlein. 4 August 1915, Z. 24048, 6v.

769 Julius Tandler (1869–1936). Originally from Iglau/Austrian Crownland Moravia (today Jihlava/Czech Republic). Studied in Vienna (Dr med. univ. 1895). 1895 Assist. under the anatomist Emil Zuckerkandl (cf. FN 684) at the 1st Anatom. Dept. of Vienna Univ. (Habilitation 1909). 1910–1934 Full Prof. and successor of Zuckerkandl as Dir. of Dept. One of Vienna Univ.'s leading anatomists. (Main areas of work: muscle tone, anatomy of the heart, prostate and urethra, topograph. anatomy of vital operations, scientific examination of the skull of Joseph Haydn). 1914–1917 Dean of the Med. Fac. of Vienna Univ.; May 1919–Oct. 1920 Undersecretary of State and Dir. of Public Health. From Nov. 1920 City Councillor for Welfare Affairs. Driving force behind the expansion of Social Democratic health care and youth policy, setting up an example to the world (focus on such areas as youth welfare; combatting infant mortality; tuberculosis pavilion at the municipal hosp. Lainz; pulm. centre Baumgartner Höhe; introduction of radiotherapy with radium to combat carcinoma; prophylact. health care; preschools; crèches; foster care service (inauguration 1925); school doctor system; and free baby care products). Collaborated in the Hygiene Section of the League of Nations. Visited China and the Soviet Union as med. advisor in 1933. In the wake of the 1934 civil war temporary imprisonment and dismissal from his chair. Emigration to the Soviet Union via China. Died in Moscow in 1936. Cf. CZEIKE (as in FN 13); EULNER (as in FN 13); FISCHER (as in FN 28); GERABEK et al. (as in FN 13); NDB (as in FN 15); LESKY, *Wien. Med. Schule* (as in FN 12), see Ind.; Karl SABLIK, *Julius Tandler. Mediziner und Sozialreformer*. 2nd ed., Peter Lang, Frankfurt/Main et al. 2010; Peter SCHWARZ, *Julius Tandler. Zwischen Humanismus und Eugenik*. Edition Steinbauer, Vienna 2017.

770 Franz Chvostek jun. (1864–1944), then Dir. of the 3rd Med. Univ. Clinic.

[771] As was to be expected in light of Fuchs's merits in making the Vienna Ophthalmol. School a brand with worldwide reach, the Professorial College was loth to accede to his wish for early retirement.

[772] Cf. UA Wien, Med. Dekanat Z. 959 of 13 April 1915, *"Betreff: Uebernahme des Hofrates Prof. Dr Fuchs in den dauernden Ruhestand und A[ller]h[öchste] Auszeichnung des Genannten."*

[773] FUCHS, *Augenarzt* (as in FN 2), p. 102.

[774] Ibid.

[775] Cf. FN 751.

[776] Karl LINDNER, "Zum 100. Geburtstage von Ernst Fuchs", in: *Wien. klin. Wochenschr.* 63 (1951), pp. 449–450 (here: p. 450).

[777] ÖSTA/AVA Wien, 4 Medizin Fuchs. K. K. Ministerium für Kultus und Unterricht, No. 25992 of 25 August 1915 and attachment: Sr. K. und K. Apostolischen Majestät Obersthofmeisteramt. Franz-Joseph-Orden. Schreiben a. d. k. k. Ministerium für Kultus u. Unterricht. Wien, am 31. August 1915.

[778] Ibid.

[779] Ibid.

6. The 1889 Textbook:
Eighteen Editions in German up until 1945.
Translations and Worldwide Resonance

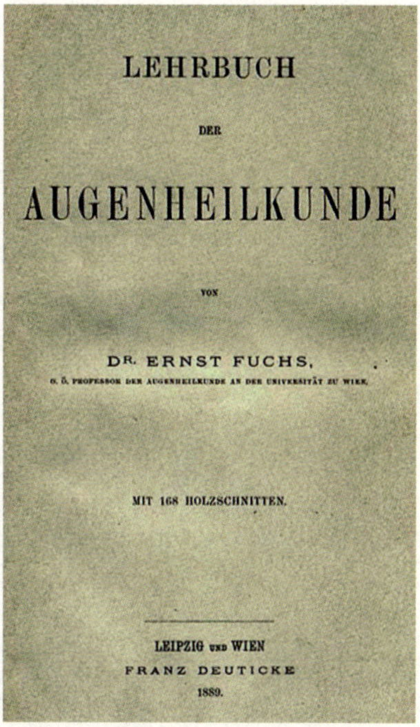

Fig. 54
Ernst Fuchs's *Lehrbuch der Augenheilkunde*, 1889

In nationally and internationally leading places of academic tuition and scientific research it was traditionally incumbent on those in charge of the various departments to sum up the specific doctrines of their respective schools in textbooks that covered their entire specialty. This was especially true of those specialties that owed their emergence and their continued evolution to a particular school of thought. Steadily gaining in acceptance worldwide since the late eighteenth century, the Vienna Medical School provides a wealth of examples for this tradition in several specialties. If one focuses, for example, on the historic leading role of the Vienna School of Ophthalmology[780] since its foundation in the early nineteenth century, it will be seen that there is a remarkable continuity of this particular characteristic, which is of great significance for the identification of graduates from the specific school to which they owe their formation. Since the pioneering establishment of ophthalmology as a specialty in its own right and the resulting foundation of the world's first University Eye Clinic at the Wiener Allgemeines Krankenhaus in 1812,[781] its successive directors, Beer,[782] Rosas[783] (previously University of Padua), Arlt[784] (previously University of Prague) and Stellwag[785] (previously Josephinum, Vienna), had summed up and codified in textbooks whatever had been the Vienna School of Ophthalmology's doctrines at the time. Updated in translations and revised editions, these textbooks remained in circulation for years or even decades and met with international recognition and worldwide resonance.

The Lehrbuch der Augenheilkunde *(1889)*

Four years after Ernst Fuchs had been appointed Director of Vienna's Second University Eye Clinic in the autumn of 1885,[786] he published his textbook,[787] designed in equal measure for students and for practising general physicians (Fig. 54); he was 38 at the time. One of the leading exponents of pathology based ophthalmology, Fuchs described the basis of his teaching as set out in the textbook in all clarity:

The influence of Arlt's school, of which I myself am a product, can clearly be seen in this book. Arlt's particular genius lay in his clinical perspective, which allowed him to see each pathology in the round with all its specific peculiarities and enabled him to describe each one with inimitable accuracy. The textbook he published in 1881 – Klinische Darstellung der Krankheiten der Binde-, Horn- und Lederhaut *– bears brilliant witness to this. If this textbook had been completed, I would have had no cause to write this present book. I have tried to follow Arlt's example by doing my utmost to present the clinical pictures of specific diseases of the eye. I am far from underestimating the significance pathological anatomy and experimental research have for any clinic of eye diseases. Bacteriology in particular can be counted upon to deliver many important insights, which may well bring about revolutions in our way of seeing things. However, what will always remain decisive for the clinician is the insight to be drawn from clinical symptoms.*

I have remained faithful in one more respect to the principles repeatedly enunciated by Arlt. Like him, I put the focus of clinical teaching on the diseases of the anterior section of the eye. These are the most common and they may be diagnosed without instruments – these being both expensive to buy and difficult to use. Likewise, they provide the widest field for therapy and hold out the most promise for success. This is why they must be imprinted above all on students, for whom they will be especially important later on in their practice. Given sufficient application on the students' part, this can be done to an adequate degree within the time allotted to ophthalmology. With the ocular fundus things are different. Acquiring the necessary expertise requires a great deal of practice, and therapy very often lags behind diagnostics. These diseases will remain the domain of specialists for a long time to come. The same applies to anomalies of refraction and to operations.[788]

With his textbook Fuchs sought to shift the focus of his students' attention away from purely mechanical note-taking during his lectures to concentrated clinical observation and the examination of the patient, away from what they heard to what they could see with their own eyes.[789] Fuchs's key objective was a logical consequence of the principles that underpinned his teaching: instructing his students in how to arrive at a correct diagnosis:

Deviations from the usual clinical picture, rare complications, aetiological factors that occur only exceptionally – everything that might occur – had to be mentioned in order to guide non-ophthalmologists along the right path in difficult cases.[790]

Since Fuchs was pursuing two objectives in his textbook at one and the same time – to meet the requirements both of students and of general practitioners – he used two different font sizes:

The basics of ophthalmology, the most important facts whose knowledge is indispensable to every student, are rendered in large print. The small print covers detailed explanations of the various chapters, theoretical disquisitions of general interest and hints for the general practitioner. What has been included on top of all this is the pathological anatomy of eye diseases since textbooks of pathological anatomy pay only scant attention to this as a rule.[791]

The textbook was divided into four sections: Examining the Eye; Diseases of the Eye; Anomalies of Refraction and Accommodation; and a brief Outline of the Basics of Eye Operations. Even in its first edition it ran to 789 pages. Fuchs commissioned a copy of his textbook from his publisher with lots of blank pages for him to jot down mostly stenographic notes to be incorporated in a forthcoming edition.[792] A remarkable feature of this innovative textbook was the number of its illustrations: it contained 168 woodcuts, based on original drawings by his assistant Maximilian Salzmann,[793] which are as accurate as they are aesthetically convincing.

In his review, August von Reuss[794] characterised Fuchs's achievement as follows:

The entire ophthalmological world is deeply indebted to Fuchs for the trouble he has taken, all the more so since he is the most faithful custodian of Arlt's convictions. This is not to say that Fuchs is only the interpreter of these convictions. He has used them as a basis in his book and has continued to build on these foundations by adding a great deal and by seeking to tone down as far as possible the differences that set other schools apart. In his description of pathologies he follows his teacher but he has in no way neglected the anatomical and physiological aspects.[795]

Eighteen German Editions by 1945

No textbook of ophthalmology has ever achieved the same worldwide resonance or a comparable lifespan. In an obituary for his teacher, Josef Meller[796] gave this instructive account for the phenomenal success of the *Lehrbuch*:

What catapulted the name Ernst Fuchs to fame all over the world when he was still young was a masterpiece that made him the most celebrated teacher of his specialty: his Lehrbuch der Augenheilkunde. *It became the Bible of ophthalmology. It may be said quite rightly that decades went by without there being a single eye specialist who had not acquired his knowledge from Fuchs's textbook. It went through twelve editions under his own supervision, was translated into all major languages and reached the most distant lands. The Japanese edition became* the *textbook of ophthalmology in the Far East. If a host of other ophthalmological textbooks has hit the market since then, none has been able to rival its fame, none its reach, none the influence that Fuchs's book has exerted on succeeding generations of medical doctors. It was this textbook that brought Fuchs, who had been appointed to the chair of Vienna's Second University Eye Clinic at the age of only 34, to the attention of the world and that became the reason why doctors eager to learn flocked to his clinic from every country on earth. The clinic soon became a meeting point for eye specialists from all over the world.*[797]

In the German-speaking world, Fuchs's *Lehrbuch* soon received the highest accolade a textbook can hope to be given:

Fuchs's greatest contribution […] *was his textbook, which has been called the Bible of Ophthalmology.*[798]

It was accorded the same accolade in the Anglo-Saxon world:

For half a century it was the Bible of the ophthalmologists throughout the world and Fuchs's department became their Mecca. If ever a book merited the title 'medical classic' it was this work of Fuchs. It is the collection of the scientific life's work of a great physician and it masterfully summarizes in its various editions the ophthalmology of an era.[799]

Only a year and a half after the publication of the first edition strong demand made a second edition imperative,[800] a fact that in the eyes of Reuss, who wrote another short review, constituted *"arguably the best proof of its out-*

standing usefulness".[801] This marked the beginning of what can only be called the textbook's triumphal march, which was to span eighteen editions and more than 50 years. Even by the turn of the century eight editions had been published, following one another at short intervals. The first ten years of the new century saw another four editions.

Julius Hirschberg,[802] unrivalled even today as a historian of ophthalmology in the German-speaking world, linked his homage to Ernst Fuchs's scientific achievements in his monumental *Geschichte der Augenheilkunde* to a detailed assessment of his textbook:

A few words are called for about this textbook, which brilliantly highlights the merits we admire in the author himself, his extensive knowledge, his thoroughness combined with great versatility, his extraordinary talent for providing succinct summaries. Never has a textbook of ophthalmology met with a degree of success that can be compared to Fuchs's and he has every reason to be proud that the resonance his name evokes not only among ophthalmologists but throughout the medical world is owed not least to this work, which means much more to us than a mere textbook in the ordinary sense of the word. What a wealth of facts and original observations is assembled here! How skilfully has the right balance been struck between austere brevity and cumbersome wordiness! Never condescending, it instructs by being entertaining. A judicious selection from the vast material on offer presents what is most pertinent and most significant – and therefore most interesting – to the medical practitioner. Everywhere the unbiased description of facts takes centre stage. Restraint worthy of emulation has led to any insistence on personal convictions in controversial questions being avoided. Each chapter has been dealt with as if it was the author's favourite, and yet the book gives the impression of being a harmonious whole cut from a single cloth. And if the recent twelfth edition appears as modern as the first from 21 years ago, this is due in part to the diligence with which FUCHS takes note of all innovations in our speciality and incorporates them [in his book], *and in part to the above-mentioned strengths evident in the design of the entire work.*[803]

The First World War, the disintegration of the Austro-Hungarian Empire and the drastic economic cutbacks of the postwar years meant that there were no more new editions for the next eleven years. In 1921, however, the 13th edition of the *Lehrbuch* was published in time to coincide with Fuchs's 70th birthday. At the academic ceremony, Friedrich Dimmer[804] assessed Fuchs's achievements as follows:

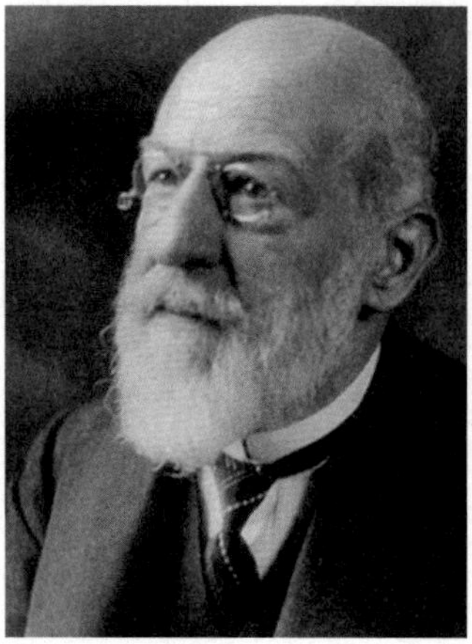

Fig. 55 Maximilian Salzmann (1862–1954)

Fuchs is not only a great augmenter of scientific knowledge, he has also codified the accumulated knowledge in his specialty in an unrivalled way in a textbook that can only be called exemplary in its presentation of the different pathologies. It is a book that both serves as an introduction to the doctrines of ophthalmology and lends a helping hand to already proficient practitioners as a faithful and reliable guide. Here, too, every page resonates with the personality of its author. It is plain to see how everything is anchored in his own experience, in his own observation, in his own critical detachment. The work met with an unparalleled recognition that expressed itself first of all in the number of editions it has gone through. Twelve editions were overseen by Fuchs himself, Number 13, edited by one of his most outstanding disciples, has recently been published. The fact that Fuchs's Lehrbuch *has been translated into the languages of all cultured nations has given it international significance.*

Two qualities of the author's personality are in plain view in the Lehrbuch*: his unfailing attention to scientific progress and his unique didactic gifts.*

A detailed comparison of individual editions will reveal that each chapter takes into consideration what is truly valuable, what represents genuine, lasting progress, having been examined with consummate discernment. Similarly, Fuchs has of course kept abreast of progress in science as a doctor and clinician. He has always shown himself ready to give innovation a try. Some innovations, however, especially operative and therapeutic proposals, Fuchs rejected out of hand or eyed them with great scepticism, and subsequent developments and the clarification of views have proved him right. It will suffice to mention operations to cure shortsightedness and subconjunctival cataract operation methods.

The second quality that is clearly in evidence in Fuchs's Lehrbuch *is his brilliant talent as a teacher. If we survey his activities as a professor – it lies before us in its complete form, being the only type of activity Fuchs no longer pursues –, we will come to the conclusion that hardly ever has there been a better and more successful teacher.*[805]

Following Fuchs's retirement in 1915, his one-time student Maximilian Salzmann[806] (Fig. 55) had taken over the prestigious task of serving as editor. He had been involved in the *Lehrbuch* from its first beginnings by providing the aesthetically satisfying and didactically highly instructive drawings, which served as the basis for the hundreds of woodcuts. In 1911, Salzmann had been

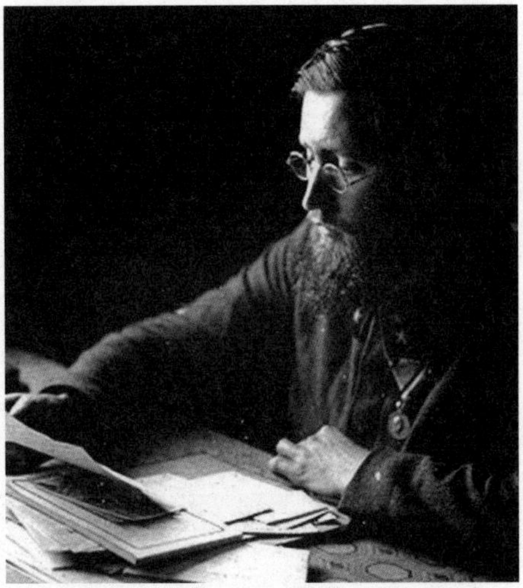
Fig. 56 Adalbert Fuchs (1887–1973)

appointed to the Chair of Ophthalmology at Graz University. All in all, Salzmann was in charge of the revision of editions 13 (1921), 14 (1922) and 15 (1926). After an interval of 13 years, the 16th edition was published in 1939, followed by editions number 17 (1944) and 18 (1945), both braving the turmoil of the Second World War. These three editions were edited by Ernst Fuchs's son Adalbert (1887–1973),[807] (Fig. 56), a clinician sharing his father's focus on ophthalmic pathology.

The Director of the First University Eye Clinic between 1944 and 1963, Arnold Pillat (1891–1975),[808] summed up the historic significance of Ernst Fuchs's *Lehrbuch* on the occasion of the centenary of Fuchs's birthday in 1951 – six years after the publication of its 18th – and last – edition in 1945:

Fuchs's Lehrbuch *has been a model for over fifty years of clear, comprehensive presentation of scientific knowledge. Eye specialists have regarded this classic as the Bible of their specialty for half a century and have drawn instruction, profit and inspiration from it. It stands out in the history of medical textbooks as entirely unique and it is almost up to date in content and presentation even today. It may safely be said that Ernst Fuchs's personality and his* Lehrbuch *have made a decisive contribution to the fame and the worldwide reputation of Vienna's School of Ophthalmology.*

The entire life's work of this great teacher, researcher and medical practitioner is woven into this textbook in such a simple and matter-of-fact way that succeeding generations are hardly aware of the seminal contributions to our speciality Ernst Fuchs made in his other scientific work.[809]

1st edition	1889
2nd edition	1891
3rd edition	1893
4th edition	1894
5th edition	1895
6th edition	1897

7th edition	1898
8th edition	1900
9th edition	1903
10th edition	1905
11th edition	1907
12th edition	1910
13th edition	1921 (Salzmann)
14th edition	1922 (Salzmann)
15th edition	1926 (Salzmann)
16th edition	1939 (A. Fuchs)
17th edition	1944 (A. Fuchs)
18th edition	1945 (A. Fuchs)

Table 1: Ernst Fuchs, *Lehrbuch der Augenheilkunde*, all German editions 1889–1945

International Resonance Fostered by Translations, Revised Editions and Reprints

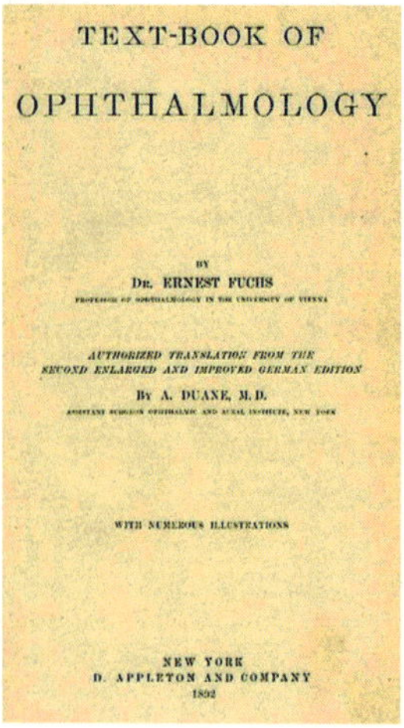
TEXT-BOOK OF
OPHTHALMOLOGY

BY
DR. ERNEST FUCHS
PROFESSOR OF OPHTHALMOLOGY IN THE UNIVERSITY OF VIENNA

AUTHORIZED TRANSLATION FROM THE SECOND ENLARGED AND IMPROVED GERMAN EDITION
BY A. DUANE, M.D.
ASSISTANT SURGEON OPHTHALMIC AND AURAL INSTITUTE, NEW YORK

WITH NUMEROUS ILLUSTRATIONS

NEW YORK
D. APPLETON AND COMPANY
1892

Fig. 57 Ernst Fuchs, *Text-Book of Ophthalmology*, 1892

English

Three years after the publication of the first edition of Ernst Fuchs's *Lehrbuch* in 1889 the first English translation was published in New York in 1892,[810] based on the second German edition of 1891. (Fig. 57) From the third English edition onward a new publishing house was in charge and the *Lehrbuch* was now published both in Philadelphia and in London. This was the start of the unstoppable triumphal march of the *Lehrbuch* across the entire Anglo-American world and beyond. Between 1892 and 1924, New York ophthalmologist Alexander Duane (1858–1926)[811] (Fig. 58), one of Fuchs's friends of many years' standing, was responsible for altogether nine editions, an achievement as tremendous as it was highly acclaimed.[812] Several unrevised editions were published in between newly revised ones. In the introduction to his first translation (1892), Duane, then assistant surgeon at the Ophthalmic and Aural Institute in New York, sums up the impact the very first German edition of the *Lehrbuch* had left in the United States:

No apology seems needed for presenting to American readers the translation of a book so favourably known as Prof. Fuchs's Lehrbuch der Augenheilkunde. *The care and judicious spirit governing the selection and presentation of facts, the thoroughness and freshness of the information, and the scientific accuracy which characterize the original, have won for it the first place among ophthalmological text-books. To these essential properties there is superadded one scarcely less important in a book of this character, namely a clear, concise and pleasing style.*[813]

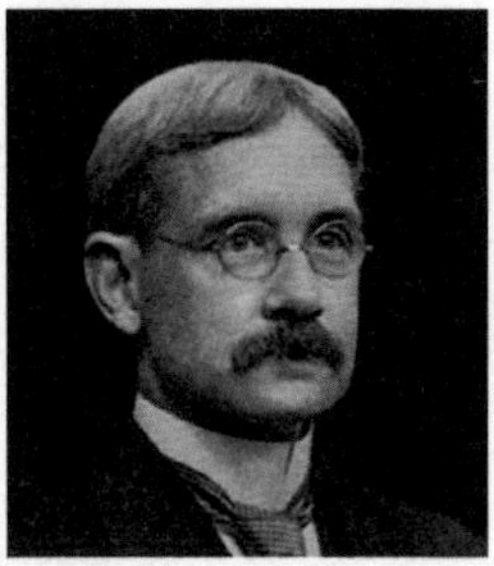

Fig. 58
Alexander Duane
(1858–1926)

Fuchs had given his explicit consent to Duane adding an appendix of eleven instructive woodcuts depicting the instruments most commonly used by American ophthalmologists.[814] For all editions that Duane was in charge of Fuchs gave him practically a free hand in editorial decisions so that Duane was able to add a great number of observations and notes reflecting his own views.

Duane's death in 1926 and Ernst Fuchs's own death in 1930 led to a temporary pause in translation activities so that the 10th revised English edition, based on the 15th German edition overseen by Maximilian Salzmann did not appear until 1933. Its translator, E. V. L. Brown,[815] (Fig. 59), had worked from 1907 at both University Eye Clinics in Vienna. His collaboration and friendship with the ophthalmologic clinicians of the Fuchs school had already borne fruit in 1912 in the English translation of Salzmann's 1912 standard work on the anatomy and histology of the human eye,[816] which the author had dedicated to Ernst Fuchs. In the ensuing decades, when Brown held leading positions at the University of Illinois Medical College and at the University Eye Clinic Chicago, his collaboration with Meller led to a lively academic exchange between Vienna and Chicago to the benefit of budding ophthalmologists on both sides. A prominent example is Peter C. Kronfeld (1900–1980),[817] the son of one of Fuchs's former students, the editor of the *Wiener Medizinische Wochenschrift*, Adolf Kronfeld (1861–1938).[818]

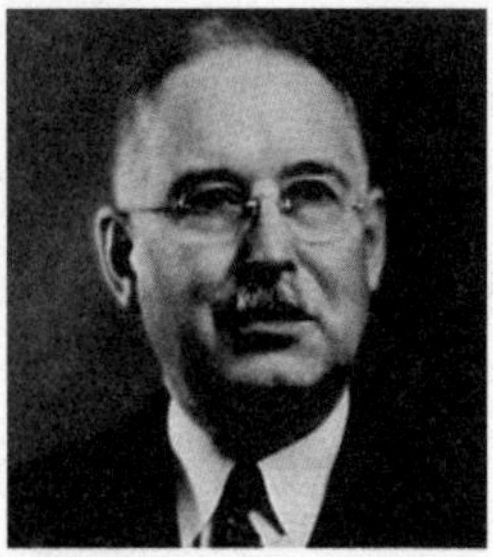

Fig. 59
Edward Vail
Lapham Brown
(1876–1953)

Brown set great store by the fact that he had obtained Fuchs's written consent for the revisions he planned to introduce and reprinted it after his own foreword:

Authorization
It gives me great pleasure to endorse to my English speaking colleagues the tenth edition of my textbook as revised by Prof. Salzmann and translated by Dr. E. V. L. Brown. I do this with special pleasure in view of the fact that the chapters on Refraction and Muscle anomalies, written by our late lamented colleague Dr. Alexander Duane, are to be retained. This will render the book, written as it was primarily for German undergraduate students, more valuable to English-speaking postgraduate students.

Ernst Fuchs[819]

This last, posthumous translation came about by reason of the strong demand for Fuchs's *Lehrbuch* from teachers of ophthalmology in the United States and was conceived primarily with the needs of students in mind. Like Duane before him, Brown had considerable leeway in the design of his translation. For him, great importance attached to usability in combination with an easily accessible and easy-to-memorise style. To reduce the number of pages and therefore the price of the volume, Brown eliminated the introduction and the chapters on the examination of the eye and operation methods plus Duane's chapter on refraction, which Brown felt was too demanding. These eliminations made Brown's translation a textbook on eye diseases and necessitated a change of title. Rather than *Text-Book of Ophthalmology*, he simply called it *Diseases of the Eye*.[820] (Fig. 60)

Number	Year of publication	Publisher	Place of publication
1	1892	D. Appelton & Co.	New York
2 Second Am. edition	1899	D. Appelton & Co.	New York
3	1908	J. B. Lippincott	Philadelphia/London
4	1911		
5	1917		
6	1919		
7	1923		
8	1924		
10 *Diseases of the Eye*	1933	J. B. Lippincott	Philadelphia/ Montreal/London

Table 2: *Lehrbuch der Augenheilkunde* by Ernst Fuchs, all English editions 1892–1933. That there is no ninth edition is due to the different numbering of English and American editions.

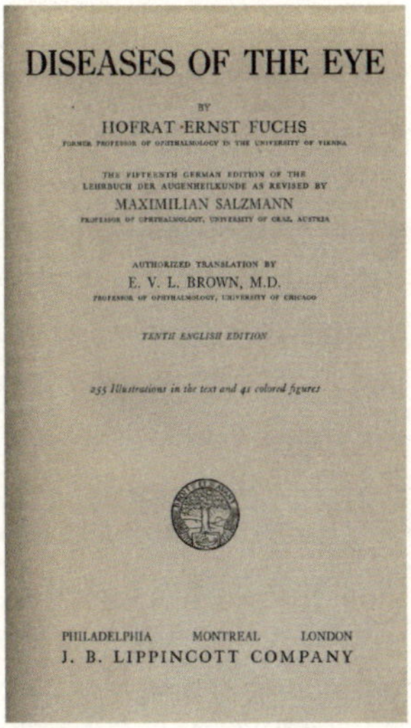
DISEASES OF THE EYE
BY
HOFRAT ERNST FUCHS
THE FIFTEENTH GERMAN EDITION OF THE
LEHRBUCH DER AUGENHEILKUNDE AS REVISED BY
MAXIMILIAN SALZMANN
AUTHORIZED TRANSLATION BY
E. V. L. BROWN, M.D.
TENTH ENGLISH EDITION
PHILADELPHIA MONTREAL LONDON
J. B. LIPPINCOTT COMPANY

Fig. 60
10th English edition of Ernst Fuchs's textbook, 1933

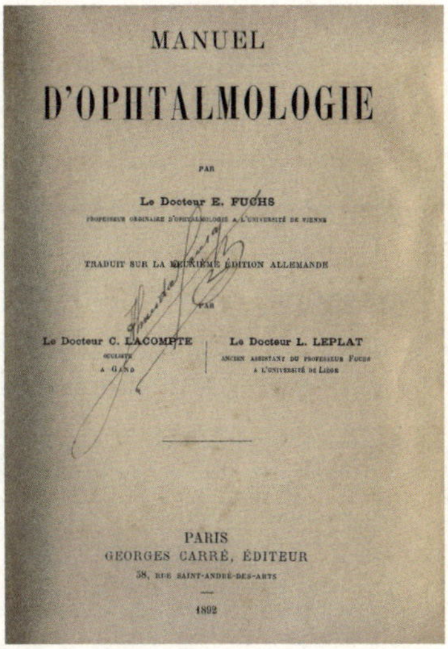
MANUEL
D'OPHTALMOLOGIE
PAR
Le Docteur E. FUCHS
TRADUIT SUR LA DEUXIÈME ÉDITION ALLEMANDE
PAR
Le Docteur C. LACOMPTE
Le Docteur L. LEPLAT
PARIS
GEORGES CARRÉ, ÉDITEUR
1892

Fig. 61
Ernst Fuchs, *Manuel d'ophtalmologie*, 1892

French

The joint translation activities of two Belgian eye specialists, Ghent/Gand ophthalmologist Camille Lacompte[821] and Lucien Leplat,[822] Fuchs's assistant during his spell as professor in Liège, resulted in three French editions (1892, 1897, 1906).[823] (Fig. 61)

Spanish

Ernst Fuchs had many friendly and/or professional contacts with Spanish and Latin-American ophthalmologists. He took part repeatedly in their conferences and gave specialist courses in Spain and in Latin America after his retirement. At the invitation of his former student Manuel Márquez Rodríguez (1872–1962)[824] he spent the winter months of 1919/1920 in Madrid.[825] Regardless of his advanced age and availing himself of his linguistic talent, his undiminished zest for expanding his horizon and his diligence, Fuchs had no problem becoming fluent in spoken and written Spanish, adding yet another language to his English, French and Italian.[826] Fuchs's and Márquez's friendship was in evidence in 1921, when the Spaniard took part in the extraordinary meeting of the Wiener Ophthalmologische Gesellschaft on 4–6 August 1921 to celebrate Fuchs's 70th birthday.[827] Fuchs's extensive travels helped him to cultivate contacts with colleagues in Central and Latin America so that his research – and especially his *Lehrbuch* – were almost as well known in the Hispano-American sphere as in the Anglo-Saxon world.

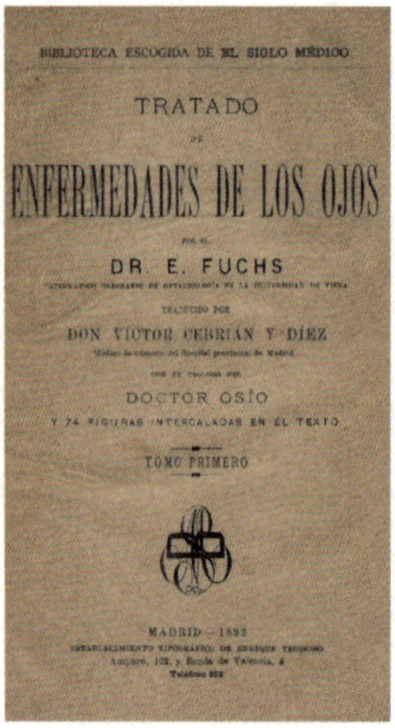

Fig. 62 Ernst Fuchs, *Tratado de enfermidades de los ojos*, 1893

The *Lehrbuch* was translated into Spanish three times. The first translation, a work in two volumes, appeared in 1893, four years after the publication of the first German edition.[828] (Fig. 62) The translator, Víctor Cebrián y Díez (d. 1902) of the University Hospital Madrid, was the author of a monograph on glucosuria[829] and had translated a great number of medical works by German-speaking professors, each of them leading exponents in their respective specialties. The second translation into Spanish[830] was not published until all of 42 years later, in 1935, five years after Ernst Fuchs's death; it was the work of Julián Martín Renedo, who had completed his specialisation in 1922–1924 at the 1st Univ. Eye Clinic in Vienna under Fuchs disciple Josef Meller.[831] During the time he spent working on the translation of the *Lehrbuch*, Renedo was Director of the Eye Department of the Military Hospital Madrid-Carabanchel. His translation was based on the 15th German edition from 1926 – the last one overseen by Salzmann.[832] The appendix dealing with eye operations was contributed by Salvador Viusá of Barcelona University. Great demand made an unrevised reprint necessary in 1936.

It is especially noteworthy that, after an interval of no less than 23 years, a third Spanish translation in two volumes was published in 1958.[833] Based on the revised 18th German edition overseen and published in 1945 by Fuchs's son Adalbert, it was simply entitled *Oftalmología.* It was the work of the Director of the Eye Clinic of the Real Academia de Medicina in Madrid, Santiago Vilahur Pedrals, who, like Víctor Cebrián y Díez six decades earlier, had already translated several German medical monographs.

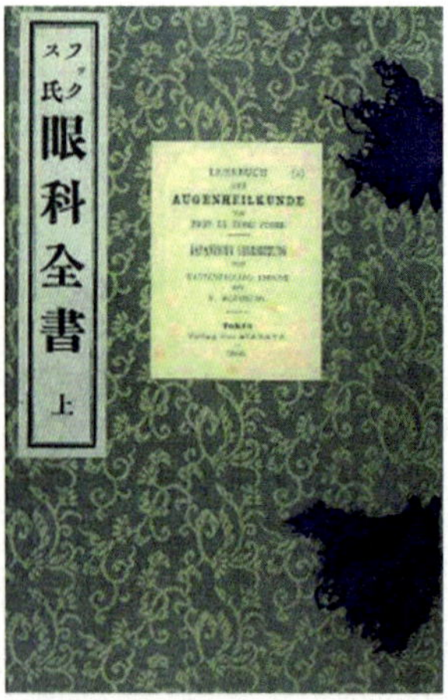

Fig. 63 Japanese translation of Ernst Fuchs's textbook, 1895

Japanese

In 1895, six years after the publication of the first German edition, the *Lehrbuch* was translated into Japanese.[834] (Fig. 63) Historically speaking, this was not the first translation of an ophthalmological work coming out of Austria to be translated into Japanese. Back in 1777 Joseph Jacob Plenck (1738–1807)[835] had published his *Doctrina de morbis oculorum.*[836] A Dutch translation of this work was published in 1787[837] and in 1794 it reached Japan, bringing about a turning point in the development of Japanese medicine. Plenck's work was the very first medical textbook to be transported from Europe to Japan via the country's already existing commercial and scientific relations with the Netherlands.

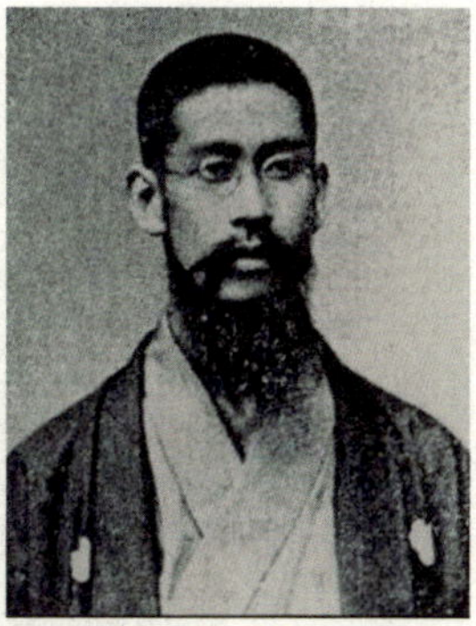
Fig. 64
Tatsushichiro Inouye (1869–1902)

In 1799, the first version of a Japanese translation of Plenck's *Doctrina* was completed by Genshin Udagawa (1769–1834) in the form of a handwritten manuscript.[838] Revised and enlarged by Ruykei Sugita (1786–1845), it was published in 1815.[839] It was the first Western textbook on ophthalmology in Japanese and opened up an entirely new horizon for the development of an independent Japanese school of ophthalmology.

In 1895, 80 years later, a two-volume Japanese translation of the *Lehrbuch* was published,[840] the work of Tatsushichiro Inouye (1869–1902)[841] (Fig. 64) and Y. Morosumi. Inouye's adoptive father Tatsuya Inouye (1848–1895)[842] had established important contacts with the European centres of ophthalmology in 1885/86, when he visited ophthalmic clinician and ophthalmo-historian Julius Hirschberg,[843] who in his turn had stayed in Japan on his world trip,[844] Arlt's former student Hubert Sattler[845] in Leipzig, Herman Snellen[846] in Utrecht and Edmont Landolt[847] in Paris. What has been overlooked in the ophthalmo-historical specialist literature until now is the fact that Tatsuya Inouye had attended the University Eye Clinic under Ferdinand von Arlt. The correspondence between the two men did not end with Arlt's retirement and was continued well into the period when Fuchs was director of the Second University Eye Clinic.[848] The elder Inouye had even planned to translate Arlt's *Operationslehre,*[849] published in 1874.[850]

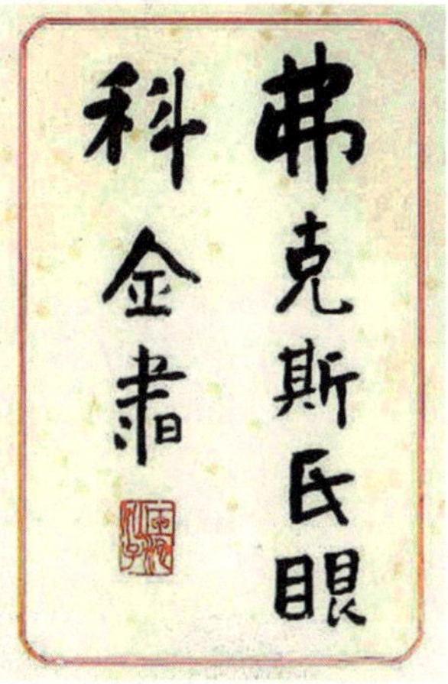

Fig. 65
Japanese title page of the translation of Ernst Fuchs's textbook, 1895

It is highly probable that Ernst Fuchs met Tatsushichiro Inouye in person. When Inouye visited the Eye Clinics in 1895–1897, he had already completed the translation of the *Lehrbuch*. As it was published in early 1895, it must have been completed at some stage in 1894. This is borne out by Fuchs's thank-you letter to the two translators, dated January 9, 1895, which was included, presumably as a mark of respect, in the translation alongside his portrait photograph, his name and the title page in Japanese script (Fig. 65):

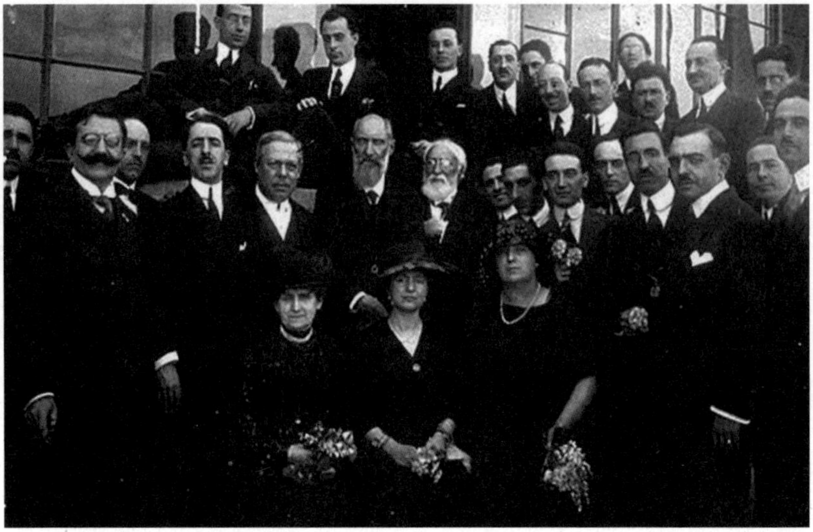

Fig. 66
Ernst Fuchs (2nd row, centre) with Giuseppe Cirincione (5th from left) 1921

Sehr geehrte Herrn Collegen!
Yesterday I received the Japanese translation of my textbook by post. I would like to thank you most cordially for the honour you have shown me by translating my work and for the labour and diligence you have expended on it. The woodcuts that have been made from my figures are excellent, and I hope that your Japanese edition may win ophthalmology many new friends.
Mit dem Ausdruck meiner ausgezeichneten Hochachtung
Ihr ergebenster
E. Fuchs[851]

Four decades after its publication, Meller underscored the influence the *Lehrbuch* was exerting on the development of Japanese ophthalmology along European lines by calling it "*the* textbook in the Far East".[852]

Italian

Ernst Fuchs maintained similarly close ties with leading ophthalmologists in Italy. Pride of place here belongs to Giuseppe Cirincione (1863–1929)[853] (Fig. 66), whose role in the development of modern ophthalmology in Italy is comparable to Fuchs's own significance for the German-speaking world. It was all the more welcome that Cirincione, who was highly regarded by Fuchs, undertook the translation of the *Lehrbuch*,[854] with Cirincione's former teacher Carlo de Vincentiis (1849–1904)[855] supplying the introduction.

The second Italian translation[856] (Fig. 67) appeared after an interval of 35 years. It was based on the 15th edition overseen by Salzmann, published in 1926. Given its date of publication in 1932, a year and a half after Fuchs's death, it was, according to the translator Mario Pagani (1898–1972),[857] designed to show the special esteem in which Fuchs was held by his Italian colleagues:

Soleva dire il Fuchs, con giusto orgoglio, che nulla più aveva contribuito alla sua fama che questo Trattato: ne è testimone la viva attesa fra gli oftalmologi d'Italia.[858]

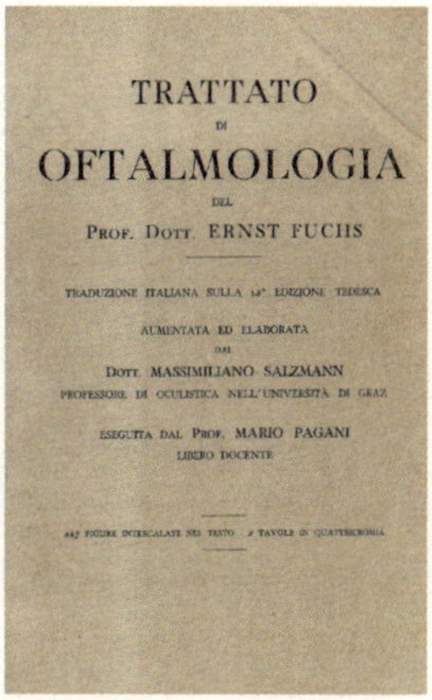

Fig. 67
Second Italian translation of Ernst Fuchs's textbook, 1932

Russian

The *Lehrbuch* was translated into Russian twice.[859] The first translation (1897), the work of Alexander Natanson (1862–1909),[860] was based on the *Lehrbuch*'s fifth edition.[861] It is highly probable that Fuchs and Natanson met in that year in the Ophthalmological Section of the 12th International Medical Conference in Moscow; both men were taking part in an official capacity.[862] The conference took place on 19–26 August 1897 (according to the Gregorian Calendar; 7–14 August according to the Julian Calendar).[863] In the conference's first session on the morning of August 20 (8), the three representatives of the Austro-Hungarian Empire, Fuchs, Hugo Brettauer/Trieste[864] and Jan (Johann) Deyl (Prague),[865] were awarded the title of Honorary Presidents.[866] In the third session of Section XI (Ophthalmology), which was devoted to trachoma, Fuchs was in the chair on the morning of August 21 (9).[867] Natanson was "aide-secrétaire".[868] In the 8th Session of the Section of Ophthalmology Natanson gave a lecture entitled "Zur Wirkung und Anwendung des Holocains".[869] It is noteworthy that, even though he was Russian, he preferred to give his lecture in German. Russian, French and German were the three languages of the Conference.

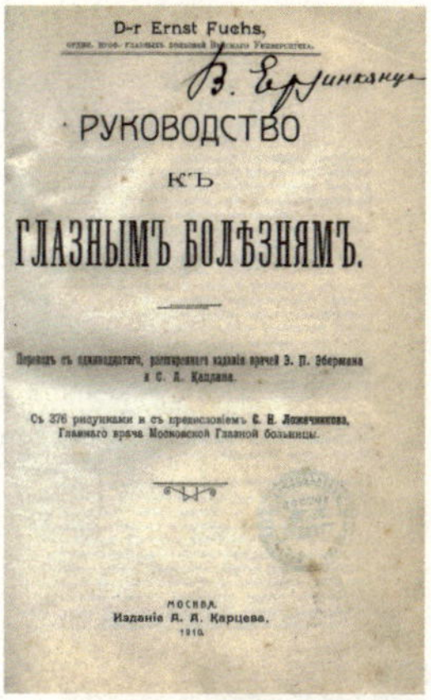

Fig. 68
2nd Russian translation of Ernst Fuchs's textbook, 1910

Thirteen years elapsed after the publication of this first Russian translation before it was followed by the second translation in 1910,[870] based on the 11th edition[871] of the *Lehrbuch*. (Fig. 68) It has proved impossible with regard to the translators, P. Eberman and S. A. Kaplan, to establish any facts other than the participation of Samuel (French: Samouil) Kaplan in the 1897 Inter-

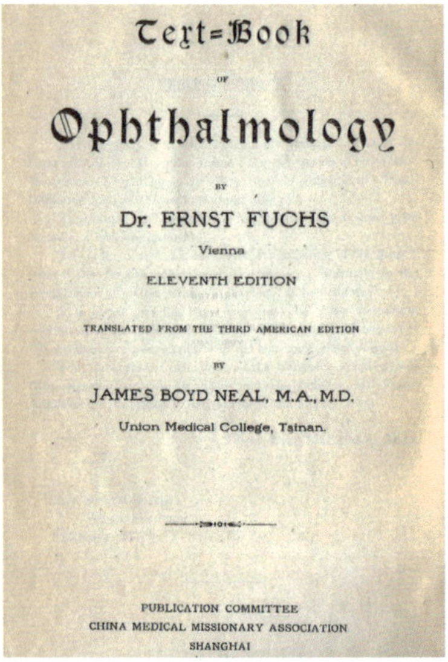

Text-Book
of
Ophthalmology
by
Dr. ERNST FUCHS
Vienna
ELEVENTH EDITION
TRANSLATED FROM THE THIRD AMERICAN EDITION
BY
JAMES BOYD NEAL, M.A., M.D.
Union Medical College, Tsinan.

PUBLICATION COMMITTEE
CHINA MEDICAL MISSIONARY ASSOCIATION
SHANGHAI

Fig. 69 English title page of the Chinese translation of Ernst Fuchs's textbook, 1911

national Medical Conference in Moscow and that he practised in Ufa (French: Oufa), the capital of today's Russian Republic of Bashkortostan.[872]

Chinese

The global dimension of Ernst Fuchs's reputation was again brought to the fore when in 1911[873] his *Lehrbuch* was translated into Chinese,[874] (Fig. 69) with the 11th German edition of 1907 serving, as one might say, as its ultimate source, because this translation was made not directly from any German original but from the third American edition of 1908, as published by the China Medical Missionary Association[875] in Shanghai. The translator, James Boyd Neal (1855–1925),[876] (Fig. 70) focused on the most important parts of the main text of Duane's English original. Only in a few exceptional instances were passages in small print preserved. The order in which Duane had arranged the chapters and their numbering remained unchanged. It is especially noteworthy that Neal added seven coloured illustrations of the normal and the pathological ocular fundus,[877] (Fig. 71) which was a first for Fuchs's *Lehrbuch*. In addition, Neal included a great number of his own drawings and several highly instructive photographs showing Chinese patients having their eyes examined.[878] (Fig. 72) The work was published by the Japanese Fukuin Printing Co. in Yokohama.

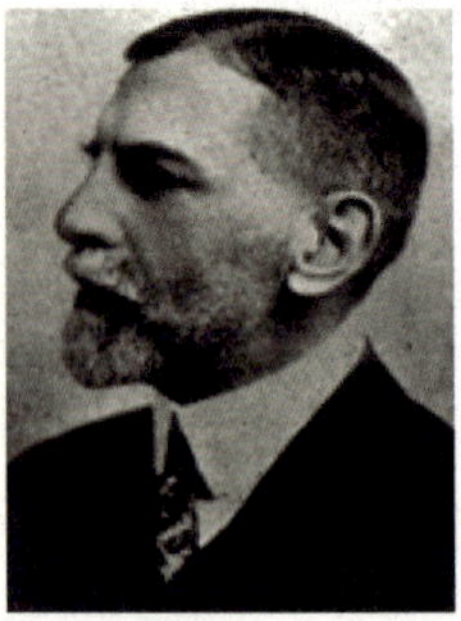

Fig. 70 James Boyd Neal (1855–1925)

In 1922 Fuchs spent several months in China at the initiative of the Rockefeller Foundation.[879] After his death in 1930, Fuchs's academic grandson Arnold Pillat,[880] then Director of the Eye Department of the Peking (today: Peiping) Union Medical College, proposed to have Maximilian Salzmann's 15th edition of the *Lehrbuch* of 1926 translated directly from German into Mandarin by his Chinese collaborators. The project ran into difficulties, as Pillat reported in 1932:

It is regretted that very little progress in the translation of the fifteenth edition of Ernst Fuchs's Lehrbuch der Augenheilkunde *into Chinese by Drs. Pi,*[881] Ling[882] *and Chang*[883] *has been made due to the unusually heavy pressure of work and research activities. It is hoped, however, that this may be completed at an early date.*[884]

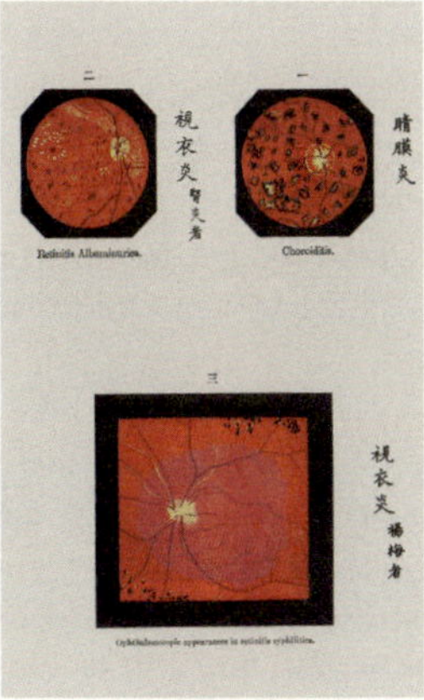

Fig. 71
Colour chart from the Chinese translation of Ernst Fuchs's textbook

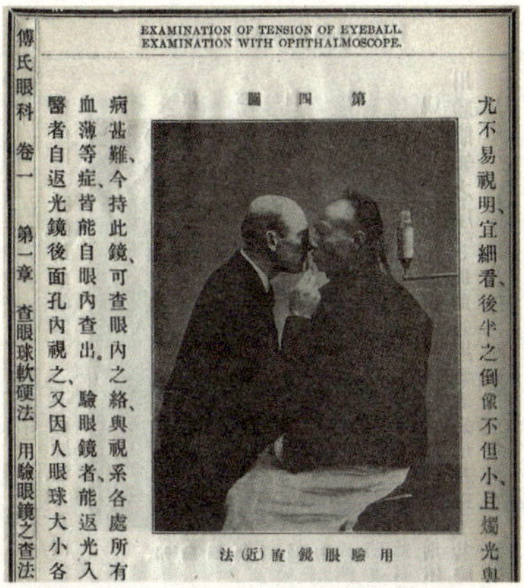

Fig. 72
Examination of an eye patient according to Fuchs's textbook, 1911

Regrettably, it has not yet been possible to ascertain whether the project of a second translation of the *Lehrbuch* was ever brought to fruition.

English	9 editions: 1892, 1899, 1908, 1911, 1917, 1919, 1923, 1924, 1933
French	3 editions: 1892, 1897, 1906
Spanish	3 editions: 1893, 1935, 1958
Japanese	1 edition: 1895
Italian	2 editions: 1897, 1932
Russian	2 editions: 1897, 1910
Chinese	1 edition: 1911

Table 3: Synopsis of all translations of Ernst Fuchs's *Lehrbuch der Augenheilkunde*

Notes

780 Gabriela SCHMIDT-WYKLICKY, Helmut GRÖGER, "Die Wiener Ophthalmologische Schule. Geist und Leistung der ersten 150 Jahre", in: *Spektrum Augenheilk.* 26 (2012), pp. 345–356.

781 Gabriela SCHMIDT-WYKLICKY, Helmut GRÖGER, "Die Gründung der weltweit ersten Universitäts-Augenklinik in Wien 1812 und ihre Erhebung zum Ordinariat 1818", in: *Spektrum Augenheilk.* 26 (2012), pp. 273–282.

782 Georg Joseph BEER, *Lehre von den Augenkrankheiten, als Leitfaden zu seinen öffentlichen Vorlesungen entworfen. Erster Band, welcher die Lehre von der Augen-Entzündung enthält.* Camesina, Vienna 1813; *Zweyter Band, welcher die Lehre von den Nachkrankheiten der Augenentzündung; von dem grauen und schwarzen Staare; und den übrigen in diese Kategorien nicht aufnehmbaren Augenkrankheiten enthält.* Heubner u. Volke, Vienna 1817. Cf. George FRICK, *A Treatise on the Diseases of the Eye; Including the Doctrines and Practise of the Most Eminent Modern Surgeons and particularly those of Professor Beer.* Fielding Lucas Jr., Baltimore 1823.

783 Anton ROSAS, *Lehre von den Augenkrankheiten. Zum Gebrauche für practische Aerzte und Wundärzte, wie auch zur Benutzung als Leitfaden beim klinischen Unterrichte abgefasst.* J. B. Wallishausser, Vienna 1834.

784 Ferdinand ARLT, *Die Krankheiten des Auges, für praktische Ärzte geschildert.* I. Band. Die Krankheiten der Binde- und Hornhaut. F. A. Credner & Kleinbub, Prague 1851; II. Band. Die Krankheiten der Sclera, Iris, Chorioidea und Linse. F. A. Credner & Kleinbub, Prague 1853; III. Band. Die Krankheiten des Glaskörpers, der Netzhaut, der Augenmuskeln, der Augenlider, der Thränenorgane und der Orbita. F. A. Credner & Kleinbub, Prague 1856; ARLT, *Klinische Darstellung der Krankheiten des Auges zunächst der Binde-, Horn- und Lederhaut, dann der Iris und des Ciliarkörpers.* Braumüller, Vienna 1881; ARLT, *Clinical Studies on Diseases of the Eye: Including Those of the Conjunctiva, Cornea, Sclerotic, Iris and Ciliary Body.* Translated by Lyman Ware, Blakiston, Philadelphia 1885.

785 Carl STELLWAG von CARION, *Lehrbuch der praktischen Augenheilkunde.* Wilhelm Braumüller, Vienna 1861; STELLWAG, *Manuale di oculistica pratica. Prima versione italiana sulla seconda edizione tedesca per cura del dott. Antonio Quaglino.* Vallardi, Milano 1865; STELLWAG, *Treatise on the Diseases of the Eye, Including the Anatomy of The Organ. Translated from the third German edition by Charles E. Hackley and D. B. St. John Roosa with an appendix by the editors.* Hadwicke, London/Wood, New York 1868, 2nd ed. 1869/70, 4th ed. 1873; STELLWAG, *A gyakorlati szemészet tankönyve. Írta Carioni Stellwag Károly.* Ford, Pest, 1868.

786 See the previous chapter.

787 Ernst FUCHS, *Lehrbuch der Augenheilkunde*, Franz Deuticke, Vienna 1889.

788 Ibid., Introduction, pp. IV–V.

789 Ibid., p. III.

790 Ibid., p. IV.

791 Ibid.

792 This book had originally ended up in the library of the First University Eye Clinic at an unknown date and was transferred, together with other historically significant items, in 1976 to the library of what was then the Institut für Geschichte der

Medizin der Universität Wien, which then became part of the Central Library of the Medizinische Universität Wien, the entity that replaced the Medizinische Fakultät der Universität Wien in 2004.

793 Cf. FN 45.

794 Cf. FN 589.

795 August REUSS (Rev.), "Lehrbuch der Augenheilkunde. Von Dr. Ernst Fuchs, o. ö. Professor der Augenheilkunde an der Universität Wien." [...] Leipzig and Vienna, Franz Deuticke, 1889, in: *Wien. klin. Wochenschr.* 3 (1890), pp. 256–257.

796 Cf. FN 46.

797 Josef MELLER, "Ernst Fuchs †", in: *Wien. klin. Wochenschr.* 43 (1930), pp. 1493–95 (here: p. 1494).

798 Cited in: Alexander JOKL, "Ernst Fuchs (1851–1930)", in: *Neue Österreichische Biografie (*= NÖB*) ab 1815*. Große Österreicher. Vol. XV. Amalthea, Vienna/Munich/ Zurich 1963, pp. 142–150 (here: p. 148).

799 Erna LESKY, *The Vienna Medical School of the 19th Century*. Translated from the German *Die Wiener Medizinische Schule im 19. Jahrhundert* by L. Williams and I. S. Levij. The William Henry Welch Press, Baltimore/London 1976, p. 447.

800 Ernst FUCHS, *Lehrbuch der Augenheilkunde. 2nd augm. edition*. Franz Deuticke, Leipzig/Vienna 1891.

801 August REUSS (Rev.), "Lehrbuch der Augenheilkunde. Von Dr. Ernst Fuchs, [...]. 2nd augm. edition. Leipzig/Vienna, Franz Deuticke, 1891", in: *Wien. klin. Wochenschr.* 4 (1891), p. 425.

802 Cf. FN 304.

803 Cf. HIRSCHBERG, *Geschichte der Augenheilkunde* (as in FN 18), vol. 15/II (= Reprint vol. VI), pp. 431–432.

804 Cf. FN 44.

805 "Feier des 70. Geburtstages von Ernst Fuchs am 14. Juni 1921 in Wien", in: *Zeitschr. Augenheilk.* 47 (1922), pp. 47–63 (here pp. 50f.). For more details, see the next chapter.

806 Cf. FN 45.

807 Adalbert Fuchs (1887–1973). Studied at the Univ. of Vienna and Innsbruck (Dr. med. univ. 1911 Vienna). Acquired bacteriolog. research methodology under the pathol. anatomist and serologist Richard Paltauf (1858–1924); trainee surgeon at the 1st Chir. Univ. Clinic under Anton Frh. von Eiselsberg (1860–1937) and assist. at the Univ. Eye Clinic Munich under Carl v. Hess (1863–1923). From 1919 Assist. at the 1st Univ. Eye Clinic of the Wr. Allgem. Krankenhaus under Josef Meller. 1922 Habilitation, 1923/24 Visiting Prof. of the Rockefeller Foundation at the Peking Union Medical College. 1924–1927 Return to the 1st Univ. Eye Clinic as Meller's 1st assist.; 1927 (tit. Assoc. Prof.) 1938 Dir. of the Eye Department of the Allgem. Poliklinik. Until 1946 Prof. at Vienna Univ., then at Istanbul. US-funded deployment in China for UNRRA. Call to New York Univ. to give postgraduate courses. Clinician and pathologist at the New York Eye and Ear Infirmary and Morrisania City Hospital. Moved to Merano for the last years of his life. Main works: *Atlas der Histopathologie d. Auges* (German 1923, Engl. 1927), *Die Erkrankungen des Augenhintergrundes* (German 1933, Engl. 1943); in charge of the 16th, 17th and 18th editions (1939, 1944, 1945) of Ernst Fuchs's *Lehrbuch der Augenheilkunde* and of the publication of his

father's autobiography and diary pages (*Wie ein Augenarzt die Welt sah*, 1946), *Clinical Pathology of the Eye* (1952, lead author: Bernard Samuels 1879–1959); *Geography of Eye Diseases* (1962). Cf. UA Vienna (Personalakt); CZEIKE (as in FN 13); IBBO (as in FN 18); DEIMER, *Poliklinik* (as in FN 200), pp. 164f.

808 Arnold Pillat (1891–1975). Originally from Bohemia. Studied at the German Univ. Prague (Dr. med. 1918). Ophthalmol. specialis. at Vienna's 2nd Univ. Eye Clinic Vienna (1927 Habilitation). 1928–1932 Prof. of the Rockefeller Foundation at the Peking Union Med. College. 1933–1936 Head physician of the Eye Department of Krankenhaus Lainz. 1936 Assoc. Prof.; 1936–1944 Dir. of the Univ. Eye Clinic Graz (1940 Full Prof.). 1944–1946 and 1947–1963 Full Prof. and Dir. of the 1st Univ. Eye Clinic. Dean of the Med. Fac. 1957/58. Seminal research on vitamin related diseases of the eye, on iridencleisis antiglaucomatosa Holth (Pillat's modification resulted in the standard procedure applied in cases of chron. glaucoma), on posterior vitreous detachment and on the local application of zytostatic drugs in cases of malignant eye diseases. Cf. Arnold PILLAT, *Lebenslauf von Professor für Augenheilkunde Dr. Arnold Pillat. Meinen Freunden und Schülern gewidmet.* Eigenverlag, Vienna 1971; Obituaries: *Wien. med. Wochenschr.* 126 (1976), pp. 26–27; *Klin. Monatsbl. f. Augenheilk.* 168 (1976), pp. 152–153 (F. C. Blodi); Appreciation: Helmut GRÖGER, Gabriela SCHMIDT-WYKLICKY, "Arnold Pillat. Vorstand der I. Universitäts-Augenklinik in Wien 1944 bis 1963", in: *Spektrum Augenheilk.* 26 (2012), pp. 341–344.

809 Arnold PILLAT, "Der Beitrag der Wiener Schule zur Augenheilkunde", in: *Wien. klin. Wochenschr.* 63 (1951), pp. 614–617 and PILLAT, "The Contribution of the Vienna School to Ophthalmology", in: *Am. J. Ophthalmol.* 36 (1953), pp. 15–25.

810 Ernst FUCHS, *Text-Book of Ophthalmology by Dr. Ernest Fuchs.* Authorized Translation from the Second Enlarged and Improved German Edition by A. Duane, M.D., D. Appleton and Company, New York 1892.

811 Alexander Duane (1858–1926). Originally from New York. Studied at the College of Physicians and Surgeons/New York (today: Columbia Univ. Med. School), M. D. 1881. Ophthalmolog. specialis. under the German émigré Herman(n) Jakob Knapp (1832–1911, cf. FN 1352) at the New York Hospital. 1884 Establishm. of an ophthalmol. practice in New York. Main areas of interest: physiol. optics, movement disorders of the exterior eye muscles, accommodation and refraction. Cf. IBBO (as in FN 18); Obituaries: *Am. J. Ophthalmol.* 9/12 (1926), pp. 917–922 (Conrad Berens); *Arch. Ophthalmol.* 56 (1927), p. 66; *Brit. J. Ophthalmol.* 11/5 (1927), pp. 255–256; *Transact. Am. Ophthalmol. Soc.* 24 (1926), pp. 18–20 (John E. Weeks).

812 The editions were published in 1892, 1899, 1908, 1911, 1913, 1917, 1919, 1923, 1924 and 1933. See the reverse of the title page of FUCHS, *Diseases of the Eye by Hofrat Ernst Fuchs, Former Professor of Ophthalmology in the University of Vienna.* The Fifteenth German Edition of the Lehrbuch der Augenheilkunde as Revised by Maximilian Salzmann, Professor of Ophthalmology, University of Graz, Austria. Authorized Translation by E.V.L. Brown, M.D., Professor Ophthalmology, University of Chicago. Tenth English Edition, Philadelphia/Montreal/London, J. B. Lippincott Company 1933. A review of the 10th edition, published in the translation of E. V. L. Brown (cf. FN 816) in 1933 commented on Duane's merits as follows: *"The original translation of Fuchs by Duane became so much a part of the armamentarium of the ophthalmologist that one could speak of the 'Bible of Ophthalmology' with the knowledge*

that everyone would understand the reference." See also the review by John N. Evans, in: *The Sight-Saving Review* III/4, Dec. 1933, pp. 307–308.

813 FUCHS, *Text-Book*. 1st edition 1892, as in FN 810, Preface, p. III.

814 Ibid., pp. 737–749.

815 Edward Vail Lapham Brown (1876–1953). Studied at Chicago Univ. (M. D. 1902). Ophthalmol. specialis. at Illinois Charitable Eye and Ear Infirmary, Univ. Eye Clinic Berlin and, from 1907 at the 2nd Univ. Eye Clinic in Vienna (Fuchs, Meller). As Meller's collaborator, Brown met Frieda Kirchoff in Vienna in 1911, who copy-edited and redacted the lectures Meller had written in English. In 1912 the two got married. Brown returned to Vienna in 1925, 1926 and 1929. The Vienna Ophthalmolog. School exerted a powerful formative influence on B. both as a doctor and a teacher; he in turn contributed a great deal to the popularisation of the School's teachings. 1917–1926 Prof. and Dir. of the Eye Clinic at the Univ. of Illinois Med. College, and at the Univ. Eye Clinic Chicago. Cf. IBBO (as in FN 18); Obituaries: *Arch. Ophthalmol.* 50/2 (1953), pp. 270–271 (F. Brawley); *Proc. Inst. Med. Chic.* 19/13 (1953), pp. 291–293 (E. B. Fowler); *Trans. Am. Ophthalmol. Soc.* 51 (1953), pp. 3–5 (P. C. Kronfeld); *Am. J. Ophthalmol.* 36 (1953), pp. 865–867 (P. C. Kronfeld); Appreciations: B. MILDER, "As I remember: Edward Vail Lapham Brown", in: *Eye Ear Nose Throat Monthly* 54/12 (1975), pp. 465–467; B. MILDER, "A remembrance of Edward Vail Lapham Brown", in: *Surv. Ophthalmol.* 43/2 (1998), pp. 188–191.

816 Maximilian SALZMANN, *Anatomie und Histologie des menschlichen Augapfels im Normalzustande. Seine Entwicklung und sein Altern.* Franz Deuticke, Leipzig/Vienna 1912; SALZMANN, *The Anatomy and Histology of the Human Eyeball in the Normal State. Its Development and Senescence.* Annotated Translation by Dr. E.V. L. Brown. Chicago University Press 1912.

817 Peter C. Kronfeld (1900–1980). Originally from Vienna. Son of Adolf Kronfeld (see below). Studied in Vienna (Dr. med. univ. 1923). 1921–1924 Demonstrator at the Inst. of Physiology. Until 1927 ophthalmol. specialis. at the 1st Univ. Eye Clinic under Meller. 1927–1933 Assist. Prof., then Assoc. Prof. under E. V. L. Brown at the Univ. Eye Clinic of Chicago. 1933–1939 Prof. and Dir. of Department at the Peking Union Medical College, where, at the initiative of the Rockefeller Foundation, he was following in the footsteps of Ernst Fuchs, Adalbert Fuchs, Arnold Pillat and Ludwig v. Sallmann. (See Ch. 11). In Beijing he continued his research on glaucoma and on retinal detachment. After his return to the United States, from 1941 Assist. Prof. at Northwestern University. 1947 Prof. at the Illinois Eye and Ear Infirmary of the College of Med. of the Univ. of Illinois., 1959–1969 Dir. of the Eye Clinic of that Univ. The honours and awards that were heaped on him include the prize of the Wien. Ophthalmol. Gesellsch. Cf.: IBBO (as in FN 18); Obituary, in: *Transact. Am. Ophthalmol. Soc.* 78 (1980), p. 11–12 (William F. Hughes); T. M. LI, "Report of the Department of Ophthalmology", in: *Sixteenth Annual Report of the Medical Superintendent of the Peking Union Medical College Hospital. For the Year Ending June 30, 1924.* Peking 1924, pp. 64–67.

818 Adolf Kronfeld (1861–1938). Originally from Lemberg (in the Habsburg Empire the capital of the Crownland of Galicia and Lodomeria, today Lviv/Ukraine). Studied medicine, art history and classics at Vienna Univ. (Dr. med. 1887). 1887–1892 Medical training at the Wr. Allg. Krankenhaus, which included a spell as junior doc-

tor under Fuchs at the Hospital Department at the Allg. Krankenhaus Fuchs was in charge of in addition to the 2nd Univ. Clinic. 1899 Joined the editorial staff of the *Wien. Med. Wochenschr*, 1909–1938 Editor-in-chief. Honorary organiser/editor at medical conferences, the Naturforscherversammlung and the Hygieneausstellung in Vienna, co-founder and secretary of the Wiener Aerzteorchester. 1922–1938 Honorary secretary of the International Advanced Training Courses at the Med. Fac. of Vienna Univ. Cf.: EISENBERG 2 (as in FN 13); FISCHER (as in FN 28); ÖBL (as in FN 11).

819 Cf. FUCHS, *Diseases of the Eye*. Tenth English edition 1933 (as in FN 812), p. VI.

820 Cf. the review by S. R. Gifford, in: *Arch. Ophthalmol.* 9 (1933), pp. 1019–21 and by John N. Evans, in: *The Sight-Saving Review* III/4, Dec. 1933, pp. 307–308. The latter took exception to some of Brown's cuts.

821 Camille Lacompte (life data not retrievable). 1883–1889 Assist. at the Eye Clinic under Fuchs and under Fuchs's successor, Jean-Pierre Nuel. Fuchs's call to Vienna in 1885 did not interrupt his contact with Lacompte. Co-founder of the Sociéte Belge d'Ophtalmologie (1896). Established the private Institut ophtalmique in Ghent. Cf. van DUYSE (as in FN 282), p. 60 and 180.

822 Cf. FN 430.

823 Ernst FUCHS, *Manuel d'Ophtalmologie.* Traduit sur la deuxième édition allemande par le Docteur C. Lacompte et le Docteur L. Leplat. Georges Carré, Paris 1892; FUCHS, *Manuel d'Ophtalmologie.* Seconde édition française, traduite sur la cinquième édition allemande par C. Lacompte et L. Leplat, G. Carré & C. Naud, Paris 1897; FUCHS, *Manuel d'Ophtalmologie*. Troisième édition française traduite sur la dixième édition allemande par le Dr. L. Leplat et le Dr. C. Lacompte, Steinheil, Paris 1906.

824 Manuel Márquez Rodríguez (1872–1962). Studied in Madrid (graduation in 1896). Participated in a state sponsored post-doc programme in Germany and Austria. Collaborator of the renowned histologist and Nobel Prize winner (1906) Santiago Ramón y Cajal (1852–1934). 1898 Ophthalmol. special. in Paris (Antonelli), Freiburg (Axenfeld) u. Vienna (Fuchs, Wintersteiner). 1908–1936 Dir. of the Univ. Eye Clinic Madrid. 1916 Member of the Real Academia Nacional de Medicina. 1934 Dean of the Med. Fac. Fled from the Civil War by emigrating to Mexico. President of the Mexican Ateneo Ramón y Cajal. 1943 Prof. at Mexico Univ.; honorary member of the Ophthalmol. Societies of France, Austria, Belgium, the United States and Mexico. Went blind in the last years of his life. Cf. Francisco GIBRAL, *Ciencia española en el exilio (1939–1949). El exilio de los científicos españoles.* Editorial Anthropos, Barcelona 1994, pp. 278–281.

825 Cf. Ernst FUCHS, "Tiefe Keratitis, hervorgerufen durch eine pathologische Zusammensetzung des Humor aqueus". (Lecture delivered to the Ophthalmol. Society. Madrid, 19 Feb. 1920), in: *Archivos de Oftalmología Hispano-Americanos* [*Arch. Oftalmol. Hisp.-Americ.*] 20 (1920), pp. 49–53 and *España oftalmol.* 5 (1920) pp. 121–128 and *Zentralbl. ges. Ophthalmol.* 4 (1920), pp. 522ff.; Ernst FUCHS, "Relaciones entre el ojo y la tabes". Conferencia dada en esta corporación el día 24 de Febrero de 1920, por el Profesor Fuchs (de Viena) in: *Anales de la Real Academia Nacional de Medicina [= Anal. R. Acad. Nac. Med.]* 40 (1920), pp. 531–547.

[826] Cf. W. A. FISHER, *Catarata senil: métodos operatorios*. Con la colaboración de E. FUCHS, I. BARRAQUER, Enrique SMITH, H. T. HOLLAND, John Westley WRIGHT. Traducción por Melchor Parrizas Torres 1924. Engl. original: W. A. FISHER, *Senile Cataract*. Methods of Operating. With the collaboration of Prof. E. FUCHS, Vienna, Austria; Prof. L. I. BARAQUER, Barcelona, Spain; Lt. Col. Henry SMITH, London, England; Dr. H. T. HOLLAND, Shikarpur, Sindh, India; Dr. John Westley WRIGHT, Columbus, O[hio]. Published by the Chicago Eye, Ear, Nose and Throat College. Chicago 1923. With the assistance of a competent translator, Fuchs published in 1927 the lectures he had delivered to the Med. Faculty of Madrid Univ. on topics such as glaucoma, sympath. ophthalmia, interior secretion in ophthalmol., ocular tuberculosis and ocular syphilis: Profesor E. FUCHS (de Viena), *Cuestiones Oftalmologicas (Cinco lecciones dadas en la facultad de medicina de Madrid)*. Traducción de la Dra. T. Arroyo de Márquez. Editorial Paracelso, Madrid 1927. For the appreciation of Ernst Fuchs, cf. Manuel MÁRQUEZ, Hans LAUBER, "El Profesor Fuchs", in: *Arch. Oftalmol. Hisp.-Americ.* 31 (1931). On the multiple relations between Fuchs and Spanish ophthalmologists, cf. Carlos LÓPEZ DE LETONA, "El Profesor Ernesto Fuchs y España" (1931), in: *Arch. Soc. Esp. Oftalmol.* 78/9 (2003), pp. 517–518.

[827] See Ch. 9.

[828] Ernst FUCHS, *Tratado de enfermedades de los ojos por el Dr. E. Fuchs catedrâtico ordinario de oftalmología en la Universidad de Viena traducido por Don Víctor Cebrián y Díez medico de número del Hospital de Madrid. Con un prologo del Doctor Osío y 74 figuras intercaladas en el texto*. Tomo I + II. Biblioteca escogida del Siglo Médico, Madrid 1893.

[829] Víctor CEBRIÁN y DÍEZ, *Patogenia de la glucosuria en sus relaciones con la terapéutica*. Madrid Imp. de Segundo Martínez 1881.

[830] Ernst FUCHS, *Tratado de oftalmología por el Prof. Dr. Ernst Fuchs† completado por el Maximilian Salzmann Profesor de Oftalmología en la Universidad de Graz. Traducción de la 15.ª Edición Alemana por el Dr. M. Renedo Jefe del Servicio de Oftalmologiá del Hospital Militar de Madrid-Carabanchel con un Apéndice a las Operaciones oculares por el Dr. Salvador Viusá*. Editorial Labor, Barcelona/Madrid/Buenos Aires/Rio de Janeiro 1935.

[831] Agustín Albarracín TEULÓN, *Die Stipendiaten des spanischen Rates für die wissenschaftliche Fortbildung und die Wiener Medizin des 20. Jahrhunderts*, in: LESKY, *Wien und die Weltmedizin* (as in FN 130), pp. 219–224.

[832] Ernst FUCHS, *Lehrbuch der Augenheilkunde*. 15. Auflage. Herausgegeben von Maximilian Salzmann. Maudrich, Leipzig/Vienna 1926.

[833] Ernst FUCHS †, *Oftalmología actualizada por el Dr. Adalbert Fuchs Profesor de Oftalmología en la Universidad de Viena. Tercera Edición Española. Traducción de la 18.ª edición alemana revisada y ampliada por el Dr. Santiago Vilahur Pedrals Jefe de Clinica Oftalmolólogica de Hospital Provincial M. de la Real Academia de Medicina*. Tomo I+II. Editorial Labor, S. A. Barcelona/Madrid/Buenos Aires/Rio de Janeiro/México/Montevideo 1958.

[834] Ernst FUCHS, *Lehrbuch der Augenheilkunde*. Japanese Translation by Tatsushichiro Inouye and Y. Morosumi. (Parts 1 and 2). Asakaya. Tokyo 1895.

835 Joseph Jakob Plenck (Plenk) (1739–1807). Originally from Vienna. 1770 Prof. of Anat., Theor. and Pract. Surgery and Obstetrics at the then Hungarian Univ. of Tyrnau (today Trnava/Slovakia); in the same capacity at the Univ. of Ofen from 1777, where he added ophththalmology to his remit. 1785–1806 Prof. of Botany and Chemistry at the Med.-Chir. Josephs-Akademie in Vienna, Inspector General of the system of Military Pharmacy. Extremely versatile author with a great number of textbooks to his credit, covering a wide range of specialties and translated into several languages. Cf. GORIN (as in FN 38), p. 267; HIRSCHBERG, *Geschichte der Augenheilkunde* (as in FN 18), vol. 14/I (= Reprint vol. II), §427, pp. 244–245 and §480, pp. 588–589; IBBO (as in FN 18); WYKLICKY, *Josephinum* (as in FN 165), pp. 39–40.

836 Joseph Jakob PLENCK, *Doctrina de morbis oculorum*. Apud Rudolphum Graeffer, Viennæ 1777.

837 (Joseph Jacob PLENCK), *Verhandeling over de Oogziekten door den Heer Joseph Jakob Plenck door Martinus Pruys*. Pols & Knap, Rotterdam 1787.

838 Cf. GORIN (as in FN 38), p. 112; Saiichi MISHIMA, *The History of Ophthalmology in Japan*. G. Schmidt, Oostende 2004, pp. 167–169.

839 (Joseph Jakob PLENCK), *Ganka Shinso* (New work on ophthalmology). Edo, Osaka, Kyoto 1815.

840 Ernst FUCHS, *Lehrbuch der Augenheilkunde*. Japanese translation by Tatsushichiro Inouye and Y. Morosumi. (Parts 1 and 2). Asakaya, Tokyo 1895.

841 Tatsushichiro Inouye (1869–1902). Adoptive son of the outstanding ophthalmologist Tatsuya Inouye (1848–1895, see below.). Studied medicine at a private university in Tokyo. Ophthalmol. specialis. under his adoptive father, who had established his own eye hospital and research institute in 1881. Publication of his translation of the *Lehrbuch* in 1895, the year the elder Inouye died. 1895–1897 Advanced training at Leipzig Univ. Eye Clinic (Sattler) and Breslau (Uhthoff). After his return, Director of the Inouye Eye Hospital. 1898 Co-founder of the Japan. Ophthalmological Society. Developed an ophthalmoscope named after him. Monographs on eye hygiene, diseases of the ocular fundus and trachoma. Delivered lectures to the annual meetings of the Dt. Ophthalmol. Gesellsch. in Heidelberg; many original papers in German published in prestigious ophthalmol. journals, e.g. Tatsushichiro INOUYE, "Ueber die eigenthümliche Farbe des Augenhintergrundes der mongolischen Race", in: *Centralbl. f. Augenheilk.* 20 (1896), pp. 200–205; INOUYE, "Bericht über einen neuen Netzhautreflex", in: *25. Versamml. d. ophthalmol. Gesellsch. Heidelberg*. J. F. Bergmann, Wiesbaden 1897, pp. 297–299; INOUYE, "Ein Fall von Veränderungen des Augenhintergrundes durch Filixvergiftung", in: ibid., pp. 300–301; INOUYE, "Ueber einen Fall von Augenverletzung durch stumpfe Gewalt und insbesondere ueber Linsenkapsel-Abhebung", in: *Centralbl. Augenheilk.* 21 (1897), pp. 147–149; INOUYE, "Ueber einen Fall von Retinitis albuminurica ohne ausgesprochene Nephritis bei einem Neger". Aus der Augenklinik Leipzig, in: *Klin. Monatsbl. Augenheilk.* 36 (1898), pp. 297–309. Cf. IBBO (as in FN 18); MISHIMA (as in FN 838), pp. 276–277 and pp. 294–295. – Unfortunately, no particulars of the career of Inouye's partner for this translation, Y. Morosumi, have come to light yet.

842 Tatsuya Inouye (1848–1895). Studied medicine in his native country under German professors, which made him fluent in German. 1885/86 Travels in Europe to

visit eye clinics in Vienna, Berlin (Hirschberg), Leipzig (Sattler), Snellen (Utrecht) u. Paris. Cf. HIRSCHBERG, *Geschichte der Augenheilkunde* (as in FN 18), vol. 14/VII [= Reprint vol. V], §997, pp. 390–392; IBBO (as in FN 18); MISHIMA (as in FN 838), Reg.; Obituary, in: *Centralbl. Augenheilk.*, pp. 286–287 (J. Hirschberg).

843 Cf. FN 304.

844 See Julius HIRSCHBERG, *Um die Erde. Eine Reisebeschreibung.* Georg Thieme, Leipzig 1894.

845 Cf. FN 220.

846 Cf. FN 292.

847 Cf. FN 253.

848 This is borne out by two postcards Tatsuya Inouye sent Ferdinand v. Arlt in 1886, one from Paris (stamped Boulevard St. Germain) and one from Berlin (Artilleriestraße 8). Cf. Sammlungen d. Med. Univ. Wien, Handschriftenarchiv No. 2088.

849 Ferdinand ARLT, "Operationslehre", in: Alfred GRAEFE, Theodor SAEMISCH (eds.), *Handbuch der gesammten Augenheilkunde.* Vol. 3. Pathologie und Therapie. Part 1. Wilhelm Engelmann, Leipzig 1874, pp. 249–500.

850 Cf. FN 848. On the postcard from Paris (1886) Inouye told Arlt, in somewhat idiosyncratic German, that *"ich bin jetzt Ihr Operationsbuch nach Japan übersetzt."*

851 Cf. FN 840.

852 Josef MELLER, Prof. Ernst Fuchs †, in: *Wien. klin. Wochenschr.* 42 (1931), pp. 1493–1495.

853 Giuseppe Cirincione (1863–1929). Originally from Sicily. Studied medicine in Naples (graduation 1889). Early special. in histopathol. and ophthalmology under Carlo de Vincentiis (1849–1904). Further training in Berlin (Hertwig, Hirschberg, Virchow), Leipzig (Wilhelm His sen., Sattler, Hess, Spateholz). 1894 Habilitation in Ophthalmology at Naples Univ., until1896 assist. under de Vincentiis. 1896 Dir. of the Department of Ophthalm. at the Italian Hospital in Tunis. 1898 Foundation of an ophthalm. and research institute in Palermo. 1902 Appointment to the Chair at the Univ. Eye Clinic Siena, and 1903–1908 at Genoa Univ. Genua; 1894–1908 at Palermo Univ.; from 1909 Dir. of the Univ. Eye Clinic Rome, which he reorganised to meet modern standards. Main areas of interest: embryol. and histopathol. of the eye. Cf. FISCHER (as in FN 28); HIRSCHBERG, *Geschichte der Augenheilkunde* (as in FN 18), vol. 14/V (= reprint vol. IV), §734, pp. 84–85; IBBO (as in FN 18); Obituary, in: *Am. J. Ophthalmol.* 13 (1930), pp. 707–709 (F. Park Lewis).

854 Ernst FUCHS, *Trattato di oftalmiatria, ad uso degli studenti e di medici pratici.* Traduzione italiana eseguita sull'ultima edizione tedesca dal dott. Gius. Cirincione, con prefazione del prof. Carlo de Vincentiis, Casa Edit. Dott. V. Pasquale, Napoli 1897.

855 Carlo de Vincentiis (1849–1904). Studied in Naples (graduation 1871). Early special. in the histopathol. of the eye. 1876 Habilitation in Pathol. and Clinic of Ophthalmology. 1877 Assoc. Prof. at the Univ. Eye Clinic in Palermo (Full Prof. 1884), 1887 Full Prof. at Naples Univ., where he initiated a scientifically oriented school of ophthalmology. One of the pioneers of ophthalmol. pathol. in Italy. Teacher of Giuseppe Cirincione (cf. FN 853). Cf. FISCHER (as in FN 28); HIRSCHBERG, *Geschichte der Augenheilkunde* (as in FN 18), vol. 14/V (= reprint vol. IV), §736, pp. 99–101; IBBO (as in FN 18); *Dizionario biografico degli Italiani*, vol. 39.

856 Ernst FUCHS, *Trattato di oftalmologia del Prof. Dott. Ernst Fuchs*. Traduzione italiana sulla 15ª edizione tedesca aumentata ed elaborata dal Dott. Massimiliano Salzmann, Professore di Oculistica nell' Università di Graz eseguita dal Prof. Mario Pagani libero docente. Edizione S.A.V.I.T, Vercelli 1932.

857 Mario Pagani (1898–1972). Ophthalm. specialis. at the Univ. of Modena and Genoa. 1930 Habilitation. Head physician at the Eye Department of the hospital at Vercelli, and 1954–1967 in Novara. Cf. Obituary, in: *Boll. oculist.* 52 (1973), p. 170.

858 "Fuchs used to say with justifiable pride that none of his other works had contributed as much to his fame [as the *Lehrbuch*]. This is evidenced by the impatience with which Italy's ophthalmological community has been looking forward to the [publication of the translation]." – Cf. FN 856, Preface del traduttore. Vercelli, aprile 1932.

859 Ernst FUCHS, *Rukovodstwo k glasnym bolsnjam*. (Lehrbuch der Augenheilkunde). Russian translation by A. V. Natanson and L. E. Vorontsova, based on the 5th German edition. St. Petersburg 1897, and FUCHS, *Rukovodstwo k glasnym bolsnjam* (Textbook of Ophthalmology). Russian translation by E. P. Eberman and S. A. Kaplan, based on the 11th German edition. A. A. Karzeva, Moskau 1910.

860 Alexander Natanson (1862–1909). Dr. med. 1888, Dorpat Univ. (then Russian Tsarist Empire. 1893 renamed Yuryev, since 1918 Tartu/Estonia). Ophthalmol. specialis. at the St. Petersburg Eye Clinic, 1896 Relocation to Moscow and Habilitation (because of his Jewish descent he had a delay of ten years imposed on his venia legendi). Director of the Alexeyev Eye Hospital. Cf. GORIN (as in FN 38), p. 284–285; HIRSCHBERG, *Geschichte der Augenheilkunde* (as in FN 18), vol. XIV/7 (= reprint vol. V), § 903, pp. 224–225.

861 Ernst FUCHS, *Lehrbuch*. 5th ed., Maudrich, Vienna/Leipzig 1895.

862 Cf. *Liste Général des Membres du Congrès*, in: *Comptes-rendues du XII Congrès International de Médecine, Moscou, 7 (19)–14 (26) août 1897*. Publiés par le Comité Exécutif sous la rédaction du Sécretaire Général W. Roth. Volume I. Partie générale. Typ.-lith. Soc. I. N. Kouchnérev & Cie, Moscou 1900, Appendix XVIII (Fuchs, Ernst. Prof. Vienne) and pp. XLIV (Natanson, Alexandre V. Dr. Moscou).

863 E. PFLÜGER, "Moskau. Internationaler medicinischer Congress", in: *Klin. Monatsbl. Augenheilk.* 35 (1897), pp. 391–397 (Rev.); *Wien. klin. Wochenschr.* 10 (1897), pp. 1044ff., pp. 1091ff. u. pp. 1115ff. (Ed.).

864 Cf. FN 303.

865 Jan (Johann) Deyl, disciple of the Arlt successor Joseph Hasner R.v. Artha (cf. FN 473) at the Eye Clinic of the German Univ. of Prague. 1902–1924 Dir. of the Eye Clinic of the Czech Univ. of Prague. Cf. GORIN (as in FN 8), p. 265ff.; HIRSCHBERG, *Geschichte der Augenheilkunde* (as in FN 18), vol. XV/2, §1223, p. 350.

866 Cf. FN 862 (Comptes-rendues), Section XI. Ophtalmologie. vol. VI (1898), p. 3.

867 Ibid., p. 76.

868 Ibid., p. 4.

869 Ibid., pp. 284–287.

870 Ernst FUCHS, *Rukovodstwo k glasnym bolsnjam*. (Textbook of Ophthalmology). Russian translation by E. P. Eberman and S. A. Kaplan, based on the 11th German edition. A. A. Karzeva, Moscow 1910.

871 FUCHS, *Lehrbuch der Augenheilkunde*. 11th ed. 1907.

872 Cf. FN 862, Appendix, p. XXIX ("Kaplan, Samouil Dr. Oufa")

873 In 1911, a revolution took place in China: Sun Yat-sen toppled the Manchu dynasty.

874 Ernst FUCHS, *Text-Book of Ophthalmology by Ernst Fuchs Vienna*. Eleventh edition. Translated from the Third American edition by James Boyd Neal, M. A., M. D., Union Medical College, Tsinan. China Medical Missionary Association, Shanghai 1911.

875 The objective of this association with Protestant roots was the teaching and promotion of Western medical expertise and the practice and promotion of Christianity in China. High priority was given to the translation of Western textbooks into Chinese and an interdisciplinary specialist journal, the *China Medical Missionary Journal*, was called to life. Cf. James Boyd NEAL, *Report of the Chinanfu Medical Work. In Charge of the American Presbyterian Mission, Chinanfu, China for Six Years 1891–1896*. American Presbyterian Mission Press 1897; NEAL, "Medical Training in China", in: *China Med. Miss. J.* [= *CMMJ*] 11/2 (1897), pp. 89–91; C. S. F. LINCOLN, "Medical Missionary Association of China", in: *J. Am. Med. Assoc.* [*JAMA*] 44/12 (1905), p. 970; James Boyd NEAL, "The Medical Missionary Association of China, in: *CMMJ* 19 (1905), p. 62; "The China Medical Missionary Association", in: *The Lancet* 183 (1914), p. 1412; Harold BALME, *China and Modern Medicine. A Study in Medical Missionary Development*. United Council for Missionary Education, London 1921; J. H. LIU, Wu-Lien TEH, Yui C. VOONPING, "Western Ophthalmology in China", in: *Nat. Med. J. of China* 17 (1931), pp. 120–121; Peter BUCK, *American Science and Modern China*. Cambridge University Press, Cambridge et al. 1980; G. H. CHOA, *"Heal the Sick" Was Their Motto. The Protestant Medical Missionaries in China*. The Chinese University Press, Hong Kong 1990.

876 James Boyd Neal (1855–1925). Originally from Pennsylvania. Graduated from Yale (M. A. 1877) and the School of Medicine of the Univ. of Pennsylvania (M. D. 1883). 1883 Marriage and relocation to China as a member of the Am. Presbyt. Mission, where he remained until 1921. First Prof. of Ophthalmol. and Dean and later President of the School of Medicine at Shantung Christian Univ., Tsinan. Editor-in-chief of the *China Med. Miss. J.* A great number of translations of med. works into Chinese. Cf. Obituaries: "Dr. J. B. Neal Dies in the United States", in: *Nat. Med. J. of China* 11 (1925), p. 147; "Dr. James Boyd Neal" in: *The Chinese Recorder* 56 (1925), pp. 255–256; Peter BUCK, *American Science and Modern China, 1876–1936*. Cambridge University Press, Cambridge et al. 1980, pp. 12–13 and Reg.

877 1. Chorioiditis, 2. Retinitis albuminurica, 3. Ophthalmoscopic appearances in retinitis syphilitica, 4. Glaucoma, 5. Normal eye-ground (average tint), 6. Ophthalmoscopic appearances in early stage of papillitis, 7. Ophthalmoscopic appearances in regressive neuritis.

878 Examination of Anterior Chamber and Iris, Examination of Tension of Eyeball, Examination with Ophthalmoscope (2x).

879 See Ch. 11.

880 Cf. FN 808.

881 Hua-Teh Pi.

882 Wen-Ping Ling.

883 Shih-Pu Chang.

884 Cf. Arnold PILLAT, *Report of the Ophthalmological Service*, in: *Twenty-Fourth Annual Report of the Medical Superintendent June 30, 1932*. Peiping Union Medical College Hospital. Formerly the Peking Union Medical College Hospital. P. U. M. C. Press 1932, pp. 45–47 (here: p. 46).

7. Fuchs's Description of Newly Discovered Anatomical Structures and Pathologies and Their Histological Substantiation

Ernst Fuchs had at his command a remarkable gift of clinical observation, which enabled him to quickly identify and differentiate any given phenomenon and, aided by his thorough familiarity with the literature, to assess whether it had already been described or whether it was indeed a new pathology. About his working method and the innovative results it generated Fuchs had this to say:

I myself have published individual cases only when they added up to a specific new pathology [...]. *The wish to establish new disease entities was greatest when I had the opportunity to observe several similar cases and put them together, a task for which I relied on my record of rare cases.*[885] *This is how the papers on keratitis punctata superficialis, ring abscess, epithelial dystrophy, etc. came into being.* [...] *Several previously unknown pathologies were described for the first time in my textbook, such as keratitis marginalis superficialis profunda*[886] *and, initially, keratitis punctata superficialis and heterochromic iridocyclitis. Often I was left with only little time for scientific work.*

I did histological work when I was inspired by special preparations or when I wanted to get to the bottom of some question that had arisen, such as the difference between common endophthalmitis and ophthalmitis sympathica or the nature of chronic endogenous uveitis. When I had reached a certain point and saw that no further progress was in sight, I closed the case and did not as a rule take up the same topic again at a later stage, as many others do. This I did only when I realised that I had made some mistake in my first attempt, as was the case for example in my research on the postoperative detachment of the choroid.

I have always steered clear of polemics and priority debates.[887]

While Fuchs did not believe in hiding his light under a bushel, he always spoke about his work with characteristic openness and modesty:

If my works have met with recognition, it is because they were done with diligence and attention to detail and because I have never proposed any daring hypotheses; I preferred to admit that I did not know for sure.[888]

Fuchs's painstaking histological studies of pathologically altered eyes – he had privately accumulated a unique collection of some 40,000 tissue sections – made him the founder of ophthalmic pathology:

Ophthalmic pathology came into being along the lines of the cellular pathology of Virchow of which one principal proponent was Ernst Fuchs.[889]

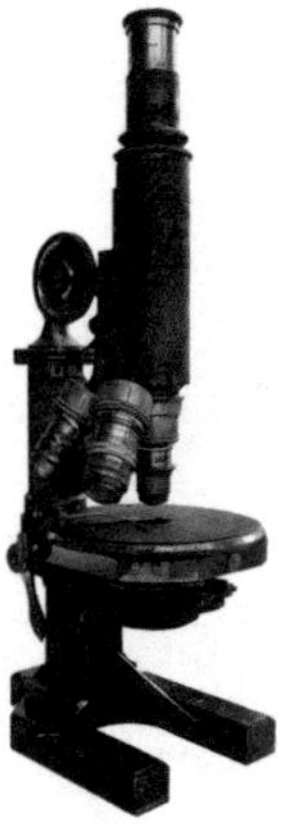

Fig. 73 Microscope formerly owned by Ernst Fuchs

For his histological studies Fuchs acquired in his early years as professor in Vienna a microscope made in Jena in 1889 by Carl Zeiss[890], at that time the leading manufacturer of optical instruments, a model called Stativ II^{a},[891] serial number 13733. (Figs. 73, 74) It is still part of the family's collection, alongside a caricature of Ernst Fuchs, which was made in Buenos Aires in 1927, depicting him with microscope, histological preparation and a bottle of atropine as his attributes. (Fig. 75)

What follows below are those anatomical structures and pathologies that are associated eponymously with Fuchs in ophthalmologic nomenclature, together with details of their historical emergence. They are listed in chronological order in subgroups organised according to the different regions of the eye.

Eye Lids

PTOSIS AMYOTROPHICA

In a meeting of the Gesellschaft der Ärzte in Vienna on December 22, 1889, Ernst Fuchs showcased the case histories of "Zwei Fälle von doppelseitiger Ptosis".[892] Two months later, in February 1890, Hungarian ophthalmologist Wilhelm Goldzieher (1849–1916)[893] presented his paper on a tissue pathology affecting the musculus levator palpebrae for which he proposed the term ptosis amyotrophica in February 1890.[894] In both cases these were purely clinical descriptions. Persevering in his research, Fuchs succeeded in the course of a routine Panas[895] operation on one of these two female patients in excising a small sample of the elevator muscle of the upper eyelid. He went on to publish in detail the results of the histological analysis in the following year alongside three new cases.[896]

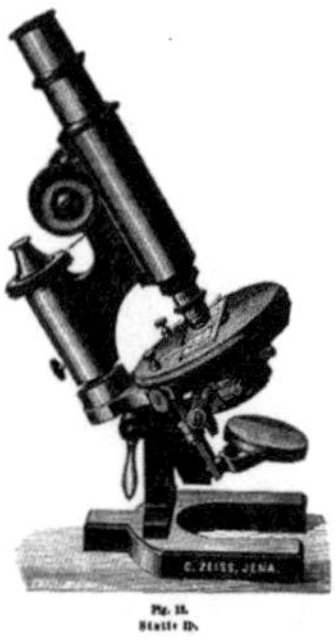

Fig. 74 Zeiss microscope Stativ II

All five patients exclusively presented the clinical picture of a more or less strongly pronounced ptosis. With some, the weakness of the elevator muscle was congenital, others developed ptosis later in life. Progress of the condition was always slow. What was common to all the patients was that the malfunction was confined bilaterally to the elevator muscle, which led Fuchs to classify the pathology as an "isolated, bilateral" ptosis. This meant there was no systemic degradation of the muscular or the nervous systems, which might have led to peripheral or central paralysis. This discovery and the histological analysis of the excised sample of the elevator muscle made Fuchs conclude that the cause underlying this clinical picture must be the atrophy of the elevator muscle of the upper eyelid. His conclusions were accepted by his colleagues and later came to be referred to as ptosis myopathica, a term that was to become established. In the 13th edition of the Lehrbuch, the entry on diseases of the elevator muscles reads as follows:

There is a sort of ptosis that develops without known cause in women (very rarely in men) of middle age. It is always bilateral, and sets in so gradually that not until after a series of years is it pronounced enough to cause any considerable interference with vision. In these cases it is not paralysis of the nerve, but a primary atrophy of muscle itself that is present (ptosis myopathica).[897]

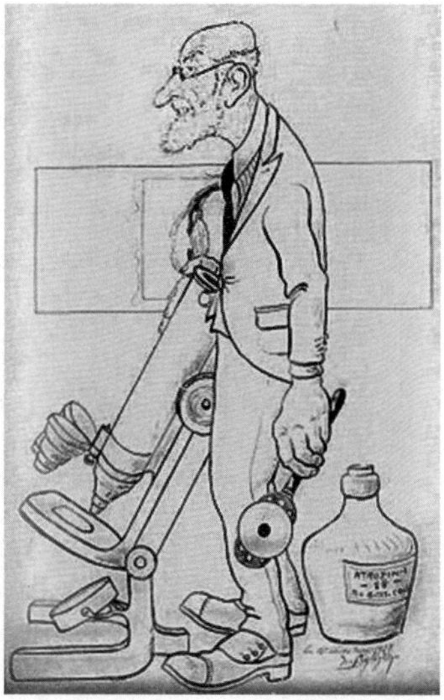

Fig. 75
Ernst Fuchs, cartoon, Buenos Aires 1927

BLEPHAROCHALASIS

The disease exclusively affects the upper eyelids and only ever occurs bilaterally. It involves primarily the skin of the eyelids. The skin is exceedingly thin, as one can ascertain by grasping it between the fingers. This is compounded by an almost complete loss of elasticity, and by consequence of these two changes the skin is folded into countless fine wrinkles crossing and recrossing one another in all directions, of the sort familiar to us from advanced senile atrophy and relaxation of the skin. The comparison with crumpled cigarette paper (Pospelow)[898] *is very apt. Thinning of the skin is combined with a genuine increase in the surface of the skin. If one determines the expansion of the skin of the upper eyelid by taking hold of the eyelid at the cilia and gently pulling it downward and stretching it, and then measures the distance between the margin of the eyelid and the eyebrow, one will arrive at far larger figures than in people of the same age and same size with normal eyelid skin.*

In addition to the senile, wilted aspect of the eyelid skin the patients are disfigured by the reddish appearance of the eyelid. The eyelid skin is crossed by a great number of small superficial veins, especially where the curvature of the eyelid is most pronounced, veins comparable in their widening to those one sees in the skin of elderly people's red cheeks. The eyelid skin does not display abnormal pigmentation. The skin's sensitivity for touch and temperature is normal.

[…]

The nature of this disease is to be found in the atrophy of the eyelid skin, leading to its thinning and loss of elasticity and, by consequence, to its distention. It also involves atrophy, or at least relaxation, of the subcutaneous tissue. I believe that the widening of the fine superficial veins is a secondary phenomenon and this may well apply also to what ptosis there is. I am therefore opposed to referring to this affection as ptosis atonica*, as this term is in use already for the aforementioned cases where an enlarged fold droops over the lid edge. I am even against calling it ptosis at all, as there is in fact no such thing in the strict sense of the word. Instead, I would like to propose the term blepharochalasis, relaxation of the skin of the upper eyelid (*χάλαρις *= relaxation).*[899]

Ernst Fuchs presented this newly defined disease entity for the first time in the Gesellschaft der Ärzte on December 6, 1895, referring to several cases in his care.[900]

The thoroughness and accuracy of differentiation Fuchs applied to the observation of what was in fact a small number of patients and the specific nature of his talent led him to the perception of this pathology. This is how he accounted for his discovery in the paper which first reported it in 1896:

There can be no doubt that this highly conspicuous pathology was noted by researchers in the past without being singled out for comment. Instead, it was grouped together with that condition where a longer-than-usual covering fold droops over the lid edge like a curtain, especially at is outer half; however, in these cases the skin is normal.[901]

Fuchs then cited examples from the ophthalmic specialist literature of the generation before him, without making any claim as to the completeness of his list.

In addition to Fuchs and his generally recognised achievements in delimiting, defining and aptly naming blepharochalasis, a survey of the more recent literature on blepharochalasis mentions the founder of the Vienna School of Ophthalmology, Georg Joseph Beer,[902] as the first known describer of this pathology,[903] and cites Beer's *Nosologie des Augenliedvorfalles* [Nosology of Blepharoptosis], a paragraph in his seminal 1817 textbook. As is to be expected in a book dating from the dawn of scientific ophthalmology, the description is still heavily indebted to the philosophy of nature:

While it does not often occur in isolation, this disease is sometimes one of the consequences of an inflammation of the eye. It is characterised by the conspicuous relaxation and distention of the cover of the upper eyelid, which takes the form of a more or less extensive skin fold protruding over the closed palpebral fissure. The same cause that has brought about the relaxation of the skin leads to the musculus levator palpebrae superioris being more or less deprived of energy so that the weight becomes too heavy for it to properly lift the eyelid. One can quite clearly see the effort being made the moment the patient attempts to open the palpebral fissure in earnest, but he will only ever succeed in opening it a little or most often not at all. – Apart from his inability to lift the upper eyelid the patient does not feel the least discomfort, the eye is not reddened but, shielded as it normally is from light, it is sensitive to light when the upper eyelid is lifted. There is no epiphora. The lid edge with all its dry cilia becomes visible the moment one lifts the upper lid with the thumb, and if one takes hold of the limp skin fold with thumb and index without pulling, let alone stretching it, but with a view to lifting the superfluous skin to make the task easier for the m. levator palpebrae superioris, the patient can open the palpebral fissure without further ado, the only drawback being that the moment one lets go of the fold, the upper eyelid slowly starts on its way down again. Occasionally such a limp skin fold forms not only in the middle of the palpebral fissure but rather towards the temporal corner, and the upper eye lid can then be lifted at least slightly in the corner of the nose. By consequence, the eyeball directs the cornea towards the nose to see, which produces a misalignment of the eyes and strabismus, if this blepharoptosis is not treated without further delay. There are even cases where the upper eyelid is shaped in a way that seems to constitute a kind of predisposition for such lengthening of the skin in the temporal angle.[904]

Fuchs's delimitation of this rare clinical picture and his description of its pathomechanism were quickly disseminated through ophthalmological circles and welcomed for their precision. This led to blepharochalasis frequently being linked to the eponym 'Fuchs', as can be seen from two papers in Fuchs's collection which he incorporated as a whole into the library of his clinic.[905] Both date to the early twentieth century. They were written by the renowned Italian ophthalmologists Gaetano Lodato (d. 1936)[906] and Erasmo Scimemi.[907] The well-known American ophthalmologist Casey A. Wood (1856–1942),[908] the editor of the *American Encyclopedia and Directory of Ophthalmology*, a multi-volume work that became a standard textbook in the United States, singled out Fuchs in 1913 for praise for his apt coinage.[909]

Two decades after Fuchs's initial description of blepharochalasis (1896), W. B. Laffer[910] (1909) and Karl Wolfgang Ascher (1887–1971)[911] (1920) defined a syndrome to which blepharochalasis contributes a characteristic share. Ophthalmologic terminology often refers to this condition alternatively as Fuchs syndrome III or Laffer-Ascher syndrome.[912]

Ernst Fuchs's pathohistological collection comprises several histological preparations illustrating blepharochalasis.[913]

Conjunctiva
HERPES IRIS CONJUNCTIVAE

The pioneer of scientific dermatology Thomas Bateman (1778–1821)[914] first described the characteristic skin changes associated with herpes iris in 1817. Another milestone in the study of this clinical picture was reached several decades later with the description of the related eczema marginatum[915] by Ferdinand Ritter von Hebra,[916] who laid the scientific foundations for dermatology in the German-speaking world around the middle of the nineteenth century. In his standard work, *Atlas der Hautkrankheiten*,[917] he provides a graphic illustration of herpes iris.

Hebra's student and son-in-law Moriz Kaposi (1837–1902) had succeeded, under his original name Kohn, in establishing the aetiological connection between the erythema (exsudativum) multiforme group of disorders and herpes iris in a manner that is considered valid to this day. He had done so only a few years after the latter disease had been instructively documented by his father-in-law.[918]

In 1876, when Ernst Fuchs, 25 at the time, was still an assistant at Arlt's clinic, the very first paper he published described herpes iris in conjunction with conjunctivitis caused by herpes efflorescens, as he had observed it in a single patient.[919] This is why he coined the term *herpes iris conjunctivae* for the newly defined pathology, placing it in the group of conjunctivitides exanthematicae. It is noteworthy that even at the beginning of his training Fuchs showed himself capable of delimiting newly observed phenomena from already known ones and of describing them with great accuracy. What is so impressive in Fuchs's first scientific publication is the detailed, painstaking microscopic analysis of the exudate found in equal measure on the conjunctiva, the affected parts of the lips, oral mucosa, hands, fingers, elbows and soles of the feet.

Even though the era of bacteriology was only beginning to dawn at that stage, Fuchs stated explicitly as the upshot of his microscopic analysis that *"it should be noted by way of conclusion that, apart from coccus and coccus chains in varying amounts, no fungi or algae of any kind were found either in the membranes of the conjunctiva and the oral mucosa or in the serum of skin efflorescences".*[920]

In 1881, Ferdinand von Arlt drew attention to the initial description of herpes iris conjunctivae by his disciple Ernst Fuchs by citing from his paper, providing a brief summary of the original case study and noting that *"up until now, the sole description of herpes iris conjunctivae has been published by my clinic".*[921]

Arlt's disciple Otto Bergmeister,[922] Fuchs's senior by six years, published another case study of herpes iris conjunctivae in 1883.[923] This was followed in 1901 by a paper written by one of Fuchs's assistants, Viktor Hanke (1871–1945),[924] with the author providing a detailed histological description of the clinical picture.[925]

It is worth pointing out here that Fuchs saw to it that his students from abroad, predominantly from the United States, were closely involved in everyday day life at the Clinic and in clinical research. In 1912, to quote only one example, Fuchs singled out volunteer assistant Hans Barkan (1882–1960)[926] from San Francisco, the son of his one-time private pupil Adolph Barkan,[927] for the treatment of an especially dramatic case of herpes iris conjunctivae and for the publication of the case history in the prestigious *Archives of Ophthalmology.*[928]

In the first edition of his textbook (1889), Fuchs only mentions herpes iris conjunctivae in a brief note on the formation of membranes in conjunctivitis crouposa (sive membranacea):

In herpes iris conjunctivae, which is very rare, these membranes constitute what is considered to be a characteristic symptom.[929]

In this context Fuchs forbore to mention his initial description of the condition.

In later editions of the textbook the relevant text was amplified by a series of small addenda. The third edition adds the characteristic membranes on oral mucosa.[930] The fifth edition features a brief description of the characteristic efflorescences:

The cases of membrane formation upon the conjunctiva that pursue a more chronic *course include the very rare instances of* herpes iris *of the conjunctiva. The cornea is not affected in these instances. These latter cases can easily be diagnosed, provided the characteristic exanthem of herpes iris (a central reddened or pigmented area of skin surrounded by a wall of vesicles) is to be found upon the skin. Sometimes, too, a formation of membrane like that upon the conjunctiva occurs upon the mucous membrane of the mouth. In some cases the disease recurs frequently.*[931]

German editions of the *Lehrbuch* from the eighth edition onward point out that the characteristic exanthem is not necessarily seen on the skin.[932]

Herpes iris conjunctivae has entered ophthalmological terminology as Fuchs syndrome I (Syndroma cutaneo-muco-oculoepitheliale erythematicum Fuchs)[933] and is considered to belong to the erythema multiforme exsudativum[934] group of diseases, for which the name Stevens-Johnson syndrome was coined later.

Cornea

Ernst Fuchs devoted special attention in his pathohistological research to diseases of the cornea. This was to bear fruit in the initial description and mutual delimitation of different types of inflammations, dystrophies and other pathological changes.[935]

ANNULAR ABSCESS OF THE CORNEA

In 1880, when Fuchs was still an assistant at Arlt's Clinic, he first recorded his observation of a ring-shaped infiltration after cataract surgery enclosing the entire cornea, describing it in anatomical terms.[936] Twenty-three years later, in 1903, helped by the study of additional cases, Fuchs understood this insidious disease[937] (Fig. 76) sufficiently clearly to provide a detailed description of the pathological changes it causes:

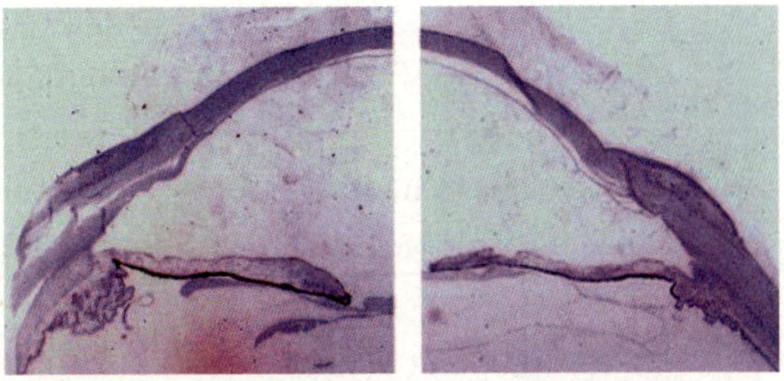

Fig. 76
Annular abscess. Histological preparation from Ernst Fuchs's collection

The term annular abscess of the cornea refers to a rapidly evolving infiltration, which forms in the shape of a ring along the rim of the cornea, usually leading within a very few days to suppuration of the cornea and to panophthalmitis. The annular abscess of the cornea usually occurs after perforating injuries, which includes operations, followed by wound sepsis. Suppuration of the cornea after a cataract operation often assumes the form of an annular abscess. In the days before the antiseptic era this was a common occurrence, as I remember very well from my time as an assistant.[938]

[…]

The ring is initially grey before turning yellow within a very short time. Its average width is 1.5 mm. Its peripheral margin is sometimes located on the limbus itself but more commonly between 1 and 1.5 mm away from it. It is more sharply delineated than the central rim, which is clouded by the portion of the cornea enclosed by the ring uniformly turning grey. As long as this clouding is not predominant, the exudate in the pupil and at the floor of the chamber and the inflamed iris are clearly visible. Within the next few days the centre of the cornea clouds over more and more and the disintegration of the cornea sets in, usually starting at the yellow ring.

Not only is qualitative vision suspended early on, but the perception of light decreases as a symptom of suppurative retinitis. An increase in intraocular pressure is proof of abundant exudation into the vitreous body. Shortly afterwards the other symptoms of panophthalmitis appear.[939]

[…]

What can be observed first is the agglomeration of pus cells between the lamellae of the cornea. Where the concentration of cells is greatest, the nuclei lose their contour before disappearing altogether. The perished cells are replaced by a granular mass which is located between the lamellae of the cornea, marked by their lighter colour. Very soon these, too, disintegrate and what ensues is the destruction of the entire cornea, proceeding from the surface of the eye to its depth.[940]

At that time Fuchs asked his assistant Viktor Hanke[941] to carry out aetiological-bacteriological investigations on those cases of the ring abscess of the cornea for which he himself had provided a pathological-anatomical description.

This soon led to first pathogenic agents being identified. Hanke reported in a meeting of Vienna's Ophthalmologische Gesellschaft on November 11, 1903 on the bacillus proteus fluorescens,[942] which he had discovered. This was followed in quick succession by the discovery of other pathogens, such as bacillus pyocyaneus and bacillus subtilis.[943]

Fuchs's contribution to the clarification of the pathogenesis and pathomorphology of this disease was emphatically acknowledged by the ophthalmological community:

Even though various authors in the past had mentioned the annular abscess of the cornea, it was left to Fuchs to describe it in 1903 as a disease in its own right and to provide an explanation of its genesis: microorganisms invade the eye in the wake of its perforation by a foreign body, causing iridocyclitis and a necrosis of the hindmost lamellae of the cornea. The ring abscess then forms as a demarcation zone around the necrotic tissue. The ring is frequently composed of an anterior and a posterior part. The cells of the anterior part derive from the margin of the cornea's lower vascular network, while those of the posterior part come from the anterior chamber and penetrate the cornea around the Descemet membrane. This penetration only happens once "en masse". According to Fuchs, *this accounts for the fact that, in clinical observation of the abscess, the periphery of the cornea is found to have cleared up again. The only lamellae of the cornea that are found to have remained undamaged are the stationary ones at the periphery. The microorganisms do not penetrate the cornea. The abscess forms both after perforating wounds in the cornea and the sclera and in ophthalmia metastatica. Whether it occurs in the latter case or not depends on a sufficiently large number of microorganisms penetrating the anterior chamber.*[944]

As his father's disciple, Adalbert Fuchs illustrated this description with a highly instructive drawing in his *Atlas der Histopathologie des Auges* (1923) and documented it with a case history.[945]

KERATITIS PUNCTATA SUPERFICIALIS

In the first edition of his 1889 *Lehrbuch* Fuchs gave the first detailed description of this condition, specifying its clinical symptoms and the histological changes it induces:

A type of superficial keratitis, which is related to herpes febrilis corneae, but not associated with the formation of vesicles, is characterised as follows: The disease begins with the symptoms of an acute conjunctivitis. While this resembles an acute catarrh, it differs from the latter in that the ciliary injection comes very much to the fore compared with a not very pronounced conjunctival infection; in addition, the secretion is not mucous or suppurative; there is, however, abundant lacrimation. Symptoms include photophobia and pain. Either at the same time or not until some days or weeks afterwards extremely minute, grey dots can be observed which, as in herpes febrilis, are arranged in groups or in short chains. These are sometimes only ten or twenty in number, sometimes very abundant, as many as 100. Either they are irregularly dispersed across the cornea or they cluster together, especially in the central portions of the cornea. In all cases the marginal portions of the cornea are the region least covered by the spots. Seen through a magnifying glass, the spots appear quite clearly circumscribed and comprise minute dots; similar dots, if less densely congregated, mark the rest of the cornea, which looks clear to the unaided eye. The spots lie in the most superficial layers of the cornea, which look dull because the epithelium above the spots bulges out in the form of a nodule. – The irritative symptoms soon vanish but the spots, together with the mottled appearance of the corneal surface, generally remain almost unchanged for months and then disappear very gradually. If the spots are not numerous, sight remains undisturbed; if, however, many spots are present, particularly in the centre, acuity of vision is reduced considerably.

This disease, for which I have proposed the name keratitis punctata superficialis, *is found most frequently in young people. Its occurrence after the 30th year of life is rare. In a quarter to a third of the (more than thirty) cases I have seen, both eyes were affected at the same time and generally to a comparable degree. With regard to aetiology I have observed that the onset of the disease often coincides with a cold, a cough or a catarrhal fever; only in one case have I noted the eruption of a few herpes vesicles in the face. – The onset of the disease as coincidental with a catarrh of the respiratory airways and the arrangement and superficial location of the foci may suggest herpes febrilis corneae but it is distinguished from the latter by the absence of vesicles in the face, its frequent occurrence in both eyes, the shorter duration of the inflammatory symptoms and the frequently great number of spots. It is especially noteworthy that there is a total absence of vesicles on the cornea, of losses of epithelium, of ulcers, hypopyon and iritis.*[946]

Six months later, in October 1889, Fuchs returned to this disease to give it a more detailed treatment.[947] In both the material Fuchs published in this paper and the first depiction in the form of a drawing of the changes described in it, it is remarkable how the author draws attention to work done by his Viennese colleagues Stellwag, Reuss and Adler,[948] who had presented their own ideas about this disease in the same *Wiener klinische Wochenschrift* only shortly before; the incidence of this type of keratitis had recently been on the increase in Vienna.[949] Since these three descriptions seemed to diverge considerably from each other, Fuchs, pursuing his passion for precise observation and documentation, summed up his own data to establish clarity:

I observed the form of keratitis described above for the first time in the academic year 1885–86, at least I found the first exact notes on it, complete with drawings, in my books dating to that time. I made notes on one case in December 1885 and on two cases in January 1886. The next cases did not occur until January and March 1887. Nor did 1888 yield more than a few isolated cases. However, this changed in the winter months, when the disease suddenly became much more common. Given that I observed the first cases almost four years ago, I believe that this disease is by no means a new development; it has probably always been around, though it used to be much less common. Its recent vogue may be attributed to its current near epidemic incidence.[950]

[…]

Of the cases I have seen myself I have made detailed notes on thirty-six, including drawings of almost all of them, representing the various stages of the disease. This means there is no need for me to rely only on my memory. In addition, I have had the opportunity to check up on roughly half the number of cases after some time, sometimes after several years, so that I am in a position to report on their final outcomes.

[…]

I believe I was the first to describe this disease in writing, in April of this year in my Lehrbuch der Augenheilkunde, *which was published by Deuticke in Vienna this summer.*[951]

Here Fuchs added verbatim the passage cited above from the *Lehrbuch*, which did not contain an illustration, with the description of the disease, noting that he "*did not see the need to change anything, apart from the last remark on the formation of ulcers*".[952]

Having documented the clinical symptoms and his findings regarding the cornea in great detail, Fuchs raised the question of what kind of lesion caused the disease:

What anatomical precondition *causes the visible changes in the cornea? Since it has not been possible to date to subject such cases to a histological examination, we are forced to resort to conjecture. The tiny grey dots the cornea displays in fresh cases across its entire surface are likely to correspond to the corneal corpuscles. I am led to infer this from the observation of human corneas whose corneal corpuscles had been dyed.* […]

I therefore believe that the visible changes in the affected cornea are caused by the presence in the lymphatics in the cornea's superficial layers of an opaque substance or of a substance that refracts light differently. The precise nature of this substance is unclear. It is, however, highly probable that it is not, by and large, made up of distinct elements such as wandering cells, as the dots develop so quickly, and the entire process unfolds so easily, hardly ever leading to the formation of ulcers. It seems safe to assume that what we have here is an extremely cell-depleted, largely amorphous liquid or semi-liquid exudate. In those places where this substance is present most markedly, i.e. where the dots are, it makes its way, even across Bowman's membrane, to under the epithelium, pushing it up to form small lumps. It is noteworthy that the opacity caused by a liquid exudate should remain nearly unchanged for months. Are we to suppose that the exudate itself remains in the cornea that long? There is no reason to come to this supposition. The exudate washing over the corneal tissue in its vicinity could possibly cause changes in the latter that affect its transparency. This secondary change could well persist even after the exudate itself has withdrawn from the cornea. This is consistent with the fact that the irritative symptoms only last for a short time as a rule whereas the opacity persists in the completely irritation free eye for a long time.[953]

In his efforts to distinguish "his" keratitis punctata superficialis both from the familiar keratitis with exudate lumps at the posterior wall of the cornea and keratitis punctata syphilitica, Fuchs summed up the matter as follows:

To avoid any confusion of these two diseases, I called the one I had described keratitis punctata superficialis, *on account of the consistently superficial location of the clouding.*[954]

[…]

Opposed as I am to superfluous terminology, I would have loved to adopt either of the two other names,[955] *if I had not described the disease already as keratitis punctata superficialis in my* Lehrbuch *before those two papers were published.*[956]

In 1902, when Fuchs received the honour of being asked to deliver the Bowman Lecture[957] to the Ophthalmological Society of the United Kingdom in London, he described the examination of the cornea and its specific changes in line with his delineation of the disease:

I take it for granted that for the minute examination the aid of a strong magnifying glass or a corneal microscope is necessary. With this aid it is, for instance, often possible to recognise a diffuse opacity of the cornea as consisting of an infinite number of minute grey points, which correspond to swollen corneal corpuscles or to lymph cells lying at the side of the corneal corpuscles in the lymph spaces. You may easily convince yourself of the visibility of the corneal corpuscles by examining, with the help of a good magnifying glass, a stained lamella of a human cornea.[958]

Until the 12th edition of the *Lehrbuch* (1910), the last to be revised by Fuchs himself, the description of keratitis punctata superficialis remained substantially unchanged. Rather than being assigned a separate chapter, the disease was treated as an appendix to keratitis vesiculosa and bullosa. Even the drawing of the punctiform changes always remained the same.[959]

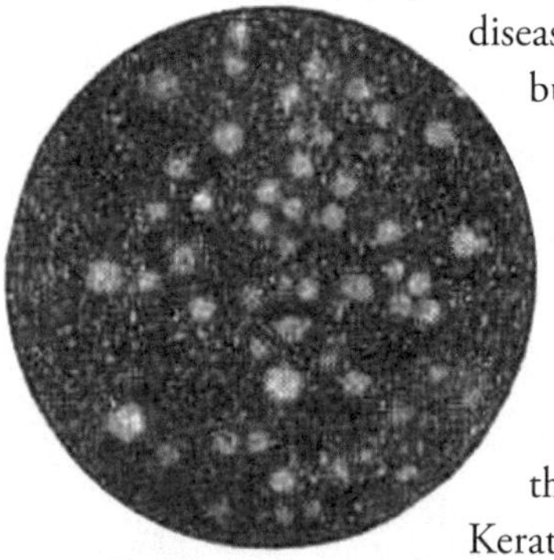

Fig. 77 Keratitis punctata superficialis. Fluorescein staining

When after an interval of 11 years, attributable in the main to World War I, the 13th edition of the *Lehrbuch*, no longer overseen by Fuchs himself but by his disciple Maximilian Salzmann,[960] appeared in 1921, the keratitides were rearranged and partly re-described. Keratitis punctata superficialis was for the first time given the eponym "Fuchs".[961] In the 15th edition published five years later, again under the aegis of Salzmann, the drawing of the characteristic sharply delineated dots was replaced by a magnified image of the changes, thrown into sharp relief by a fluorescein dye.[962] (Fig. 77) The same image remained in use until the last edition of the *Lehrbuch* in 1945, which was revised by Fuchs's son, Adalbert.[963]

KERATITIS PUNCTATA PROFUNDA

In the first edition of the *Lehrbuch* (1889), Fuchs adds to his discussion of keratitis parenchymatosa the following excursus:

The opacities in the cornea are initially composed of isolated grey specks, which are only discernible with a magnifying glass. Soon these specks flow together. It sometimes happens that the opacity achieves only a low intensity so that it appears as a number of isolated grey specks in the deeper and deepest layers of the cornea. This form of keratitis, which occurs mainly as a consequence of lues acquisita concurrently with syphilitic iritis, has been described by Hock,[964] *Mauthner,*[965] *Purtscher*[966] *and others as keratitis punctata syphilitica. This is distinguished from keratitis punctata superficialis* [...] *not only by the aetiology, but also by the situation of the specks in the deep layers of the cornea, and might therefore be appropriately be characterised as* keratitis punctata profunda.[967]

In the 13th edition, revised by Salzmann and published in 1921, keratitis punctata profunda is given a short section by itself – this time without mentioning Fuchs as the author of the name.[968] It is interesting to note that the disease is no longer mentioned in the last three editions of the *Lehrbuch*,[969] all of which were overseen by Adalbert Fuchs.

KERATITIS MARGINALIS (SUPERFICIALIS)

This disease is described as one of the varieties of keratitis non suppurativa by Fuchs in the first edition of the *Lehrbuch* (1889):

Up until now I have observed this rare disease seven times. It is mostly found in persons in middle age and usually affects only one side, only once both. Causing only moderate symptoms of irritation, a grey or grey-yellow opacity forms at the margin of the cornea, which directly adjoins the sclera and extends into the transparent cornea by roughly 2 mm. This marginal opaque zone usually covers between ⅓ and ½ of the cornea, most often at the top. Only in rare cases does it cover the entire cornea. The surface of the cornea above the opacity is slightly dull but does not exhibit any loss of substance, not even rejection of the epithelium. Soon the limbus advances and covers the opacity with its vessels. Over several weeks the irritative symptoms gradually disappear, while the infiltrate in the margin is transformed into a permanent grey cloudiness of the cornea.

This closely resembles the arcus senilis, the main difference being that it is not separated from the margin of the sclera by a transparent zone but shades into the latter without a distinct border. This disease of the cornea neither leads to iritis nor, as a rule, to the formation of ulcers on the cornea. I have only ever seen a single ulcer form on the cornea, which was entirely superficial. Given the marginal location of the residual opacity, it does not endanger vision. I have looked in vain for a description in the textbooks, the only exception being Arlt's,[970] *which describes the disease in connection with sclerosing keratitis. However, I have never seen symptoms of scleritis in conjunction with this inflammation of the cornea.*[971]

This rare disease continued to claim Fuchs's attention over the following years, with the result that keratitis marginalis – now with the added qualification "superficialis" – was dealt with in the 3rd edition of the *Lehrbuch* (1893) on three occasions. First, Fuchs pointed out what distinguished this form of keratitis:

A different type of pseudopterygium appears after a chronic superficial ulceration of the marginal zone (keratitis marginalis superficialis) [...]. *For these pseudopterygia to be distinguished from genuine pterygia it is necessary to diagnose the ulcerating process or its consequences (superficial corneal opacities) in those marginal regions of the cornea that are free from pterygium.*[972]

[...]

Keratitis marginalis superficialis *is* [...] *a rare disease, found in persons in middle life. A quite superficial ulceration spreads over the cornea, starting from its margin. It does not, however, start from all parts of the margin at the same time, nor does it advance uniformly. Consequently, the ulcerated marginal zone of the cornea is demarcated from the transparent central portion by a sinuous border formed by a fine gray line. This variety of keratitis drags on for a long time (sometimes for years),* [*with*] *periods of intermission alternating with relapses, which are associated with moderate symptoms of irritation. It is distinguished from ulcus rodens in that the ulcer is extremely shallow. Moreover, the edge of the ulcer is not undermined. The ulceration never reaches the center of the cornea so that the extremely faint opacities that remain do not interfere with sight. Keratitis marginalis superior often gives rise to a drawing of the conjunctive up over the cornea in the form of pseudopterygium* [...].

The vascular fasciculus, keratitis dendritica, ulcus rodens, and keratitis marginalis superficialis have the common trait of creeping slowly in the cornea, for which reason they are also designated by the name of serpiginous ulcers of the cornea.[973]

The passage dealing in the 3rd edition of the *Lehrbuch* with Keratitis marginalis superficialis differs only marginally from the initial description in 1889.[974] The 7th edition (1898) was the first to feature a drawing to illustrate this pathology.[975]

The consistency with which Fuchs's name is associated in the international specialist literature with keratitis marginalis superficialis more than a hundred years after his initial description testifies to the accuracy with which he observed, examined, and defined newly discovered pathologies.[976]

KERATITIS MARGINALIS PROFUNDA

Fuchs mentioned deeper located forms of marginal keratitis for the first time in the second edition of the Lehrbuch (1891).[977] In the following year he returned to this newly identified pathology in his comprehensive treatment of pterygium.[978]

Salzmann summarised Fuchs's findings in the 13th edition of the *Lehrbuch* (1921) as follows:

A narrow, yellowish-gray to almost pus-yellow clouding, extending scarcely 1 mm beyond the limbus, develops at the margin of the cornea (most often in the topmost region), along with moderate symptoms of irritation mostly in older people and in only one eye. Its central margin is sharp; toward the periphery it loses itself in the limbus, whose vessels are plainly seen to be in front of the clouding. [...] *The surface is not notably changed. The opacity has no tendency to extend further or to ulcerate but is soon resorbed without leaving opacities behind. According to* Fuchs *it leaves an opacity similar to the that of arcus senilis which is of no significance for vision because of its location at the border of the cornea. Etiology and anatomical findings are unknown. The prognosis is favorable, the treatment symptomatic.*[979]

CLEARING LINES OF THE CORNEA

In the first edition of the *Lehrbuch* Fuchs described a process he called "clearing up of corneal cicatrices" as follows:

After a long time has elapsed – months or years, that is – the cicatrix left by an ulcer appears less large and less opaque than it was directly after the healing of the ulcer was completed; the cicatrix has partially "cleared up". In this way quite small cicatrices may become altogether invisible. The extent to which clearing takes place depends principally on two circumstances: upon the thickness of the cicatricial tissue and upon the age of the individual. The deeper the cicatrix penetrates into the cornea, the less it clears up; perforating cicatrices of the cornea, if they are ever so small, remain permanently opaque. (A fine example of this is afforded by the punctures which the discission needle makes, and which remain visible as gray points upon the cornea all during life.) The age of the individual influences the process of clearing, in that the latter makes greater advances the younger the patient is. For this reason cicatrices after ophthalmia neonatorum often clear up in a wonderful way.[980]

Not content with the exclusively morphological description of newly observed pathological changes, Fuchs always prioritised research on the mechanism of their genesis. His interest in the clearing lines of the cornea, which continued unabated over the next years, led to a paper in 1893.[981]

What explanation can be found for light, line-shaped stripes, arranged in a distinct order, appearing in opaque cicatricial tissue? We find lines arranged in that same order in fresh keratitis, where the stripes stand out as clouded grey lines against the transparent – or at least less clouded – background. These line-shaped opacities were first observed after the extraction of cataracts, with parallel opaque lines protruding from the wound into the transparent cornea.

[…]

These parallel lines are found much more frequently after non-suppurative corneal ulcers, i.e. mainly after keratitis parenchymatosa and keratitis profunda (central parenchymatous ulcer of the cornea).

The opaque lines associated with keratitis display the same arrangement as the light lines in old cicatrices to such an extent that there is no doubt that both are caused by the same anatomical substrate. No anatomical findings are available as yet regarding the light lines in the cicatrice.[982]

[…]

As the light lines in old cicatrices display the same characteristics as the grey lines associated with keratitis, the question needs to be asked whether a connection may be established between them and the minuscule corneal tubes. Could it be the case that the latter grow over time from the healthy cornea into the cicatrice and that this is followed by the clearing of the cicatrice? An answer to this question depends on knowing the histological properties of the corneal cicatrices and their relationship with the neighbouring healthy tissue of the cornea.[983]

The cases Fuchs had observed and documented meticulously, making several of the drawings himself, made him come to the following conclusions:

The transformation of the cicatrices, shot through with lymphatic spaces, into a more compact and more homogeneous tissue results in reducing cicatricial opacity; the opacity has been 'cleared up' to a certain extent.[984]

[…]

Over time, the aqueous humour pressing against the cicatrice will be aiming to open up incrementally better channels into the cicatricial tissue. It is not probable that the passage of time will allow the establishment of a regular lymphatic system with anastomosing lymphatic spaces within the cicatrix. What is easily conceivable, however, is for the extended crevices, the corneal tubes, which can so easily be filled and expanded with injection fluid, to protrude into the cicatrices more and more, which is effected by lymph inserting itself between the lamellae of the cornea in the direction of their fibrillation. Furthermore, it is equally conceivable for the fibres in the vicinity of the crevices to become more homogeneous, more like normal corneal fibres in places where such lymph-filled crevices are created in the cicatrices. This would put us in a position to understand why over time transparent lines form within opacities whose direction corresponds to the grain of the fibres in individual lamellae and to the direction of the corneal tubes. It could be said that the opacity is gradually being washed out by the penetrating lymph.[985]

Further studies on corneal cicatrices continued to modify Fuchs's understanding of this phenomenon:

Corneal scars frequently undergo subsequent metamorphoses. *Delicate scars arising in childhood frequently do not appear any longer in adults as an uninterrupted opacity but are permeated by transparent lines which cross in various directions and thereby divide the opacity into little fields.*[986]

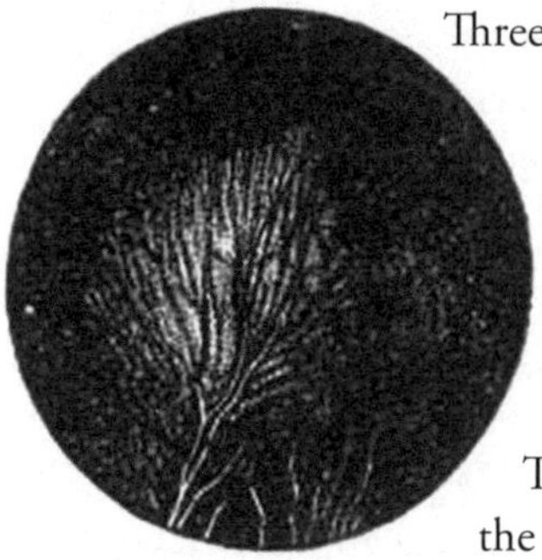

Fig. 78
Clearing lines

Three years later Fuchs added this comment in his *Lehrbuch*:

> *This makeup therefore always indicates its very long existence and may be explained by the fact that young transparent fibers arise among the old ones due to the interstitial growth of the cornea.*[987]

Twelve years later Fuchs had this to say on the aetiology of the changes he had described:

> *In other cases the transparent stripes follow the ramification of vessels that had existed in the cicatrice when it was still young* […].[988]

This passage comes with an illustration whose caption for the first time explicitly includes the term "clearing lines". (Fig. 78)

ISLANDS ON THE CORNEA ASSOCIATED WITH PTERYGIUM

The first description of these grey-whitish, intraepithelial small specks on the cornea near the head of the pterygium is to be found in Fuchs's 90-page paper published in 1892.[989] Having first dealt in detail with the macroscopic evidence, Fuchs presents the documentation of the histological examination of this pathological change, a survey of hypotheses on its genesis and his own clinical observations. He then adds a description of the pseudopterygium.[990] In accordance with Fuchs's research practice, the main part of the paper is devoted to histology.

Given that it was Fuchs who first noticed certain changes in the relationship between the pterygium and Bowman's membrane, it is only reasonable that these "islands of the cornea" should be associated with his name in the specialist literature.

Still further away from the border of the pterygium, beyond the point where the destruction of Bowman's membrane has taken place, island-shaped changes surrounded by healthy tissue are to be found. They correspond no doubt to those minute grey points mentioned in the clinical description of the pterygium […], *which one frequently finds outside the pterygium in the otherwise transparent cornea. Under the microscope these changes are revealed to belong to several different types. The simplest change consists in the absence of Bowman's membrane in a small, island-shaped spot. The membrane gives out at its border and disintegrates into lamellae [...]. Places marked by the absence of the membrane feature thin, irregularly curved lamellae below the epithelium, which encloses fairly large interstices housing isolated nuclei. The whole thing looks like decompressed corneal tissue. In places that have undergone this change the epithelium is also changed. Tissue sections show thin basal cells, like narrow platelets with a bulge where the nucleus is located. Furthermore, they display strange, twisted forms and are mostly positioned at an angle toward Bowman's membrane; the outermost cells are almost pushed over [...]. One gets the impression that these cells have been pushed to one side and flattened in the process. This change in the basal cells reduces the cohesion between the epithelial cells, as is shown by the fact that the superficial layers of epithelium have mostly been cast off in precisely those places in the histological sections. However, where they have been preserved, it is plain to see that they are much less changed than the layer of basal cells.*

Another change in the shape of an island in front of the pterygium is the superimposition of dense, fibrous connective tissue, quite abundantly equipped with elongated nuclei. This tissue may rest on the intact Bowman' s membrane, resulting only in an elevation of the epithelium; if the epithelium is thick enough, it can absorb this unevenness entirely so that the surface of the epithelium appears completely even. However, as a rule Bowman's membrane is found to have been eroded below the connective tissue so that it displays a trough like depression [...] or it has disintegrated into a network of fine lamellae or has disappeared altogether. –

Similar islands of newly formed connective tissue can be discovered to have formed directly under Bowman's membrane so that they push it up and erode it from below.

That such changes really occur in the form of islands can only be shown by having recourse to a series of histological sections. Given that the anterior border of the pterygium is often jagged and dispatches shorter or longer offshoots into healthy areas of the cornea, a section passing close to the anterior border of the pterygium might be cut off and subsequently be interpreted as an island shaped change [...].[991]

In 1916 Fuchs returned once more to the island shaped changes of the cornea.[992]

DIMPLES IN THE CORNEA

Ernst Fuchs mentioned the formation of dimples in the margin of the cornea for the first time in 1901 in his paper on marginal sclerosis and marginal atrophy of the cornea:

Finally, I would like to mention several noteworthy cases I have observed of the formation of dimples in the margin of the cornea. The patient becomes aware of a moderate burning sensation in his eye. The doctor then discovers a fairly deep depression, 2 to 3 mm in diameter, exactly adjacent to the margin of the cornea; compared with the rest of the cornea, its borders sometimes appear to be distinctly raised. Regardless of this, the cornea is almost entirely clear in the zone of the dimple, it is perfectly shiny and the eye is hardly injected at all. The next day, the dimple is less deep and on the third day it disappears altogether. In one case the dimple had formed at the head of a pterygium, in several of the other cases the eye was otherwise normal. In one case the dimple returned twice.[993]

Ten years later Fuchs again took up the subject of dimples in the cornea, dealing with it in greater depth. Interestingly enough, he does so without mentioning his own first description. Of the *"strange, dimple-like depressions in the cornea* [...]*, which have not yet been described comprehensively"*[994] he said:

A flat, saucer-shaped depression is located in the margin of the cornea, from where it slightly expands into the limbus. Its borders are clearly discernible, but they are rounded rather than sharp-edged. The border that is visible in the middle of the cornea is usually steep, while the one reaching out toward the limbus subsides gradually. The dimple is usually elliptical, with the long axis parallel to the margin of the cornea. If the dimple is located in the temporal margin of the cornea, as is most commonly the case, it takes the form of a vertically positioned ellipsis, 1–2 mm wide and 2.5–3.5 mm long. At times [the dimples] are also smaller or circular. Dimples located at some distance from the margin of the cornea are very rare [...]*. Their depth cannot be measured, only estimated. It is unlikely to ever exceed 0.5 mm. The floor shows a slight, somewhat silvery opacity and has a fine tubercular appearance; at its deepest point it looks somewhat desiccated, even xerotic. Only in exceptional cases is the della entirely clear and transparent. Tested by touching it with a thread, the sensitiveness of the cornea is lower than in the other marginal areas of the cornea, where it is generally* *found to be lower again than in the cornea's middle areas. There is usually only an insignificant injection of the sclera and the neighbouring conjunctival vessels at points adjacent to the peripheral border of the dimple.*[995]

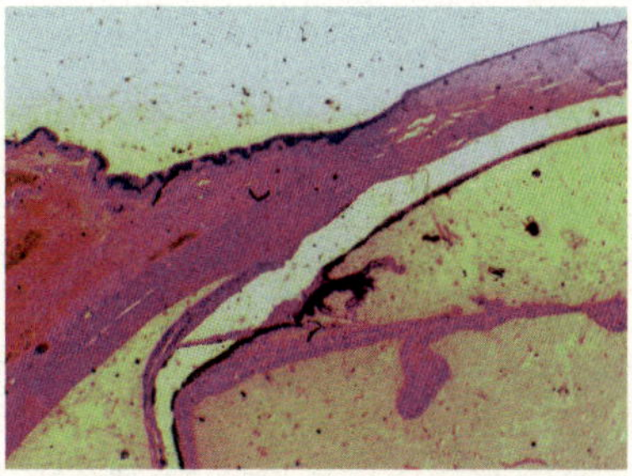

Fig. 79 Pathological dimple in the cornea (fovea). Histological collection Ernst Fuchs

Ernst Fuchs's collection of histological sections comprises a highly illustrative preparation of such a dimple. (Fig. 79)

Fuchs observed the formation of such corneal dimples in cases of inflammatory swelling of the conjunctiva and episcleral tissues, on the second or third day after cataract extractions, and in cases of day blindness and lagophthalmus paralyticus. It also occurred spontaneously without any recognisable connection to an underlying pathological condition. In all cases the dimples disappeared again after a few hours or days. Fuchs showed that dimples like the one illustrated in the figure could experimentally be made to form with subconjunctival injections of a saline solution or of cocaine. He attributed their formation to a dysfunction in the short, extremely fine and entirely superficial nerve trunks branching out to the marginal zones of the cornea from the conjunctiva. He realised that this phenomenon lacked clinical relevance and did not amount to a disease.

As was the case with several other previous eponyms, Maximilian Salzmann pointed out Fuchs's first description of the dimples in the 13th edition of the *Lehrbuch* (1921),[996] and Adalbert Fuchs followed suit in a paper he published in 1929 in a leading American ophthalmological journal.[997] In this way, Fuchs's discovery and painstaking description of these rare changes became more and more widely known.[998]

From today's point of view, the dimples are desiccation spots of the epithelium in the margin of the cornea next to demarcated swellings of the conjunctiva:

Fuchs's dimples [...] *are roundish areas of attenuated cornea, mostly in a horizontal position and located either at the nasal or the temporal side. The epithelium is intact, the cornea transparent. Fuchs's dimples are formed by a localised drying-out of the cornea.*[999]

KERATITIS DISCIFORMIS

In 1901, Fuchs delimited the clinical picture of keratitis disciformis from keratitis annularis, which had first been described by Adolf Vossius (1855–1925)[1000] in 1885.

The disease is mainly found in middle-aged people, being common especially in association with slight defects of the epithelium, caused either by injury or by herpes corneae. It is characterised by a faint grey disc in the region of the middle part of the cornea, sharply delimited from the transparent marginal parts by an intensely grey border. The surface of the cornea on top of this disc is clouded and insensitive. In the course of the disease, which usually lasts several months, small ulcerations are common, and the opacity that remains is usually rather marked.

As far as the surface *of the cornea in the affected part is concerned, it is mostly level with the rest of the cornea; in two cases (where there was no ulceration yet) I noticed a very slight depression, and in one case, where the infiltrate was located close to the surface, there was a slight bulge. The cornea has lost its lustre there and is dotted or grained. With a magnifying glass often minute vesicle-like protrusions come into view, rarely larger vesicles of the kind associated with keratitis vesiculosa.*

The disc shaped *opacity occupies most of the central parts of the cornea, as in ulcus serpens. As far as can be ascertained with a magnifying glass, it is located in the middle layers of the cornea, frequently even deeper, only rarely closer to the surface. A powerful magnifying glass or a corneal microscope will dissolve it into the most minute chalk-white dots. It is quite common for these dots to be arranged in a cluster in the central parts of the disc, resulting in a point- or disc-shaped zone that is intensely grey or whitish* […]. *It is in places such as these that small ulcerations frequently form later.*

The most striking characteristic of this disease is the saturated grey *border of the disc. If one follows with a magnifying glass the minute dots the disc is made up of to its border, they are seen to congregate ever more densely until they can no longer be identified individually in the grey border itself. On the far side of the border they mostly disappear very quickly in the transparent cornea. While the saturation of the grey border on the inside of the disc therefore decreases only gradually on its outside, the same process occurs abruptly in the direction of the transparent cornea, which is why the grey disc is always sharply demarcated on its periphery.*[1001]

The graphic quality of the illustration in the original publication is too poor to be reproduced here but Fuchs incorporated this pathology into the 9th edition of his *Lehrbuch* (1903) together with an instructive drawing.[1002]

Fuchs's first description was followed over time by a series of case histories of keratitis disciformis. In the same year, 1903, Eïsaburo Hadano,[1003] a Japanese ophthalmologist then active at the Eye Clinic of the University of Rostock, published his own observations on this disease.[1004] Albert Peters (1862–1938),[1005] Professor of Ophthalmology at Rostock, gave a presentation on the topic at the 31st Meeting of the Deutsche Ophthalmologische Gesellschaft in Heidelberg in 1903 and published a monograph in the following year on traumatic pathologies of the cornea, which at that time were understood to include keratitis disciformis.[1006] In his discussion of the aetiology of this pathology, Peters explicitly mentioned Fuchs's hypothesis of 1901 suspecting a bacterial infection:

We are well advised to make use of the research on bacteria for ophthalmology, and it is therefore understandable for Fuchs to attempt to make a bacterial causation plausible for keratitis disciformis; the comparison with ulcus serpens actually reveals quite a few clues.[1007]

Further investigations were undertaken by Otto Schirmer (1864–1917)[1008] in 1904[1009] and again by Peters[1010] in 1905.

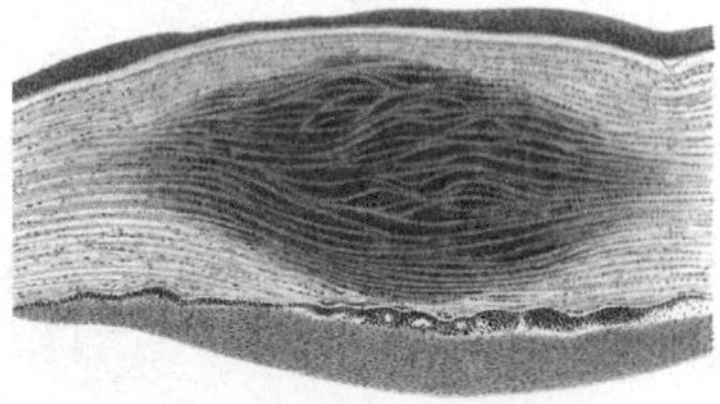

Fig. 80 Keratitis disciformis. Drawing by Joseph Meller

As Fuchs's assistant at the Second University Eye Clinic, Josef Meller published the first detailed histological description of the newly demarcated pathology in 1905 together with drawings of the pathological changes of the cornea. (Fig. 80) The patient in question had been under observation for several months at Fuchs's clinic.[1011] In 1907 a doctoral thesis on keratitis disciformis as a disease entity was commissioned by Rostock University.[1012]

In Salzmann's 13th edition of the *Lehrbuch* (1921), which has already been referred to repeatedly in these pages for its documentation of Fuchs's genuine contributions to ophthalmopathology, the eponym "Fuchs" is assigned to keratitis disciformis arguably for the first time.[1013] 1921 was the year of Fuchs's seventieth birthday, and *Albrecht von Græfes Archiv für Ophthalmologie*, which had already published many original papers by Fuchs and was co-edited by him, rose to the occasion with a *Festband.*[1014] It included a comprehensive paper by the Bonn ophthalmologist Paul Junius (1871–1948)[1015] dealing with keratitis disciformis. In it, Junius highlighted the contribution Fuchs had made to the identification of the crucial characteristics of this pathology:

In 1901 Fuchs was the first to describe the clinical disease entity k[eratitis] disciformis. The condition was known, if imperfectly, to an older generation of eye specialists as abscessus siccus. It was described under that name for example by Arlt. Th. Saemisch[1016] *referred to it as the* infiltratum corneae centrale profundum. *We are indebted to* Ernst Fuchs *for having identified the characteristics typical of k[eratitis] disciformis amid a welter of erroneous diagnoses and for having enshrined them in a description that has now become a classic. This included delimiting the new disease from* k[eratitis] annularis (Vossius) *and from* k[eratitis] profunda (Fuchs).

[...]

The definition of this disease as it appeared to Ernst Fuchs *at the beginning of the twentieth century has often been quoted, but every practising physician stands to gain from rereading this exemplar of the most refined art of observation. It is assumed here that everyone knows it. The description is largely identical with the clinical picture we still see today.*[1017]

Adalbert Fuchs included keratitis disciformis in his 1923 pathohistological atlas, for which he largely drew on his father's collection, together with a drawing, a case history and a detailed description.[1018]

MARGINAL SCLEROSIS AND MARGINAL ATROPHY OF THE CORNEA

In 1901, Ernst Fuchs published the following observation:

I have had the opportunity to study several patients whose corneas had developed a furrow-like depression in the margin. This change took place spontaneously and was not attended by any ulceration; one of these cases was subsequently subjected to anatomical examination. As such cases are exceedingly rare and have never been examined anatomically, it is justified in my view to describe them here.

The majority of these cases concern people of advanced age and must be seen as an especially pronounced senile change in connection with the arcus senilis. The latter consists of hyaline shoals deposited in the superficial layers of the cornea.

[…]

Arcus senilis has several characteristics in common with this band-form opacity of the cornea: both present in superficial layers, both are consequences of the presence of amorphous substances (in one case hyaline, in the other chalk), and both are caused by a dystrophy of the cornea, whose nature, however, cannot be the same in both cases. […] *It is, on the other hand, to be noted that the arcus senilis* in its common extension *is confined to the margin of the cornea, a region of the eye the band-form opacity strictly avoids; and that it initially starts at the upper margin of the cornea, which is permanently covered by the upper lid, again a region the band-form opacity shies away from.* Leber *proceeds from the assumption that the deposition of calcium salts in Bowman's membrane, which is the cause of the band-form opacity, is connected with evaporation in the area of the palpebral fissure. Conversely, the deposition of the hyaline shoals of the arcus senilis initially occurs in those parts of the cornea that are permanently covered. Is it not therefore tempting to assume that this is due to the suppression of evaporation? Evaporation at the surface of the cornea is undoubtedly a factor in the movement of fluid in the cornea, whether this takes place in a system of juice canals or, as Leber claims, through totally diffuse saturation of the cornea. When parts of the cornea are dehydrated due to evaporation, this sets in motion an influx of fluid from more abundantly supplied regions; the absence of evaporation may therefore cause a slowdown in the circulation of fluids and perhaps the precipitation of insoluble chemical substances such as hyaline.*

In cases where the arcus senilis has become unusually broad, it goes without saying that the transparent area of the cornea is reduced in size, but it is even smaller than follows from the broadening of the arcus senilis because the latter has at the same time contracted over all to a circle with a shorter radius. In such advanced cases the peripheral margin of the arcus senilis is located deeper in the cornea.[1019]

Fuchs subsequently went on to describe the formation of a marginal groove[1020] in the cornea:

It inserted itself in the arcus senilis, causing a broadening or bevelling of the latter. It did not display any clinically perceptible scarred opacities and microscopic findings did not provide any evidence of a recent or past inflammation.

The process leading to the formation of the groove involves the disappearance of Bowman's membrane and the transformation of the anterior corneal lamellae into a fibrous tissue of low volume. This is arguably best visualised along the lines of Bowman*'s membrane being dissolved alongside the glue-like substance between the corneal fibrils so that the corneal lamellae disintegrate into fibrillar bundles; in addition, this process of disintegration must also affect a number of these fibrillar bundles, as otherwise the result would be an increase in volume, not a reduction. While this process affects the deeper layers of the cornea below the groove, it confines itself to the most superficial layers in the middle. Are we to assume that this process starts in the middle and gradually works its way from the surface to the regions below? I do not think so because in that case the result would be a wide and shallow depression. What we get instead is the rather sudden absence of corneal lamellae at the steep central border of the groove. This suggests that the process, rather than working its way downward from the surface to the deeps, advances from the border towards the transparent cornea, penetrating to a certain depth as it does so.*[1021]

Roughly a decade and a half after this first description Fuchs returned once more to the topic of senile marginal atrophy of the cornea.[1022] His continued histological research work enabled him to cast more light on the presumed onset of the disease and to sum up its progress:

1. *The transformation always proceeds vertically, never horizontally.*
2. *The thinner lamellae resulting from the disintegration of corneal lamellae are reminiscent of connective tissue or are substituted by connective tissue invading the diseased zone together with vessels from the limbus. At the groove's central border the connective tissue even inserts itself between the ends of the corneal lamellae. Other cells than those replacing fixed corneal corpuscles appear alongside the connective tissue and the vessels, and sometimes a slightly inflamed infiltration is present, which is prone to inflammation, as has been reported by some researchers.* […].
3. *Complete disintegration of individual corneal lamellae at the central border of the groove. There is no such disintegration at the onset of the disease.* […].
4. *Ectasis of the floor of the furrow, causing the Descemet membrane to expand, with such attendant consequences as tearing, total destruction or, conversely, thickening due to the accumulation of deposits.*[1023]

ULCUS ATHEROMATOSUM CORNEAE

In 1901 Fuchs delimited a hitherto unknown type of ulceration in the cornea from the common ulcus corneae:

Atheromatose ulceration is accompanied by necrosis of dystrophied scar tissue, be it only in its superficial layers or, in more severe cases, in its entire thickness. Necrosis is triggered by the invasion of bacteria, which is boosted by the morbid quality of the epithelium. The necrotic parts are pushed off by sequestrating suppuration, which very often expands downward from here.

As far as anatomy is concerned, common ulceration differs from atheromatose ulceration in that the primary actor in the former is an infiltrate which disintegrates, causing a loss of substance, while in atheromatose ulceration the primary change is necrosis, followed by sequestrating suppuration. In anatomical terms, atheromatose ulceration resembles more closely ulcus serpens, in which the anterior layers of the cornea are destroyed by suppuration, while the posterior layers partly fall victim to necrosis without the involvement of suppuration. However, the process as a whole differs from atheromatose ulceration, where necrosis of a comparatively large piece of tissue is present from the first beginnings and suppuration only goes so far as is required for the sequestration of that piece of tissue.[1024]

NODULAR OPACITY OF THE CORNEA

The description of this change in the cornea by Ernst Fuchs is not a primary description in the strict sense. This, as Fuchs himself pointed out, had already been made a few years earlier by the Breslau ophthalmologist Arthur Groenouw (1862–1945).[1025] However, Fuchs had made notes on the first case as early as 1889 and had only seen seven more cases by the time of the publication of his paper devoted to the disease in 1902.[1026]

The total number of cases that have come to light to date warrant the opportunity to supplement the clinical picture of the nodular opacity of the cornea that Groenouw *has already outlined quite correctly, and to revise some of the details.*

[…]

In the majority of cases, the disease had been triggered by a usually short-lived inflammation; afterwards the eyes either remained permanently irritation-free or occasionally displayed mild inflammations or at least enhanced sensitiveness.

[…]

Let us now have a look at the individual symptoms of the disease. The surface of the cornea can hardly be called lustreless even though it is highly uneven. Displaying elevations above the spots, the unevenness is especially pronounced in the area of the pupil, and this constitutes no doubt the most important cause of the frequently significant impairment of vision.

[…]

The opacity of the cornea consists in circumscribed spots and a diffuse cloudiness. The spots mainly occupy the pupillary area of the cornea. They are grey-white or blueish-white and clearly circumscribed, as can be seen with the naked eye. Seen through the magnifying glass, they are usually less sharply defined. […] *The spots are quite superficial and push up the epithelium* […].

In most cases two types of spots can be distinguished: larger and smaller. The larger usually occupy the middle and are irregular in shape […]. *Their shape is caused by the coalescence of smaller spots.* […]

The number and size of the spots vary considerably, depending undoubtedly not only on individual cases as such but on the stage at which one gets to see them. The spots undergo changes over the years: they rearrange themselves, join up to form larger spots or disappear altogether, while new spots appear. The cornea meanwhile gradually becomes more and more cloudy and vision suffers accordingly; in the worst cases finger counting is reduced to a distance of 1 m.

[…]

In addition to the circumscribed spots a diffuse clouding prevails […] *in all cases in the rest of the cornea, sometimes evenly across the entire area, sometimes slightly more markedly in the area of the pupil. Under the magnifying glass this clouding dissolves into minute blurred grey dots.* […] *The deep layers of the cornea and the deeper parts of the eye are always normal.*[1027]

Using a trephine, Fuchs succeeded in obtaining a piece of the superficial layers of the cornea with a view to examining it histologically:

The superficial corneal lamellae […] *appear to be more saturated with fluid, causing the lamellae to appear more homogeneous and slightly bloated; the lymphatic crypts are expanded and the corneal corpuscles enlarged. – The layers that exhibit these changes are located directly below the epithelium. No traces of Bowman's membrane are visible.*

The evenly altered superficial layers are interspersed with elevations caused by fraying. These correspond to the macroscopically visible larger grey spots in the cornea, measuring at most 0.5 mm across. The bloated superficial lamellae disintegrate in this place into ever finer layers, which appear as fine fibres in histological preparations. They proceed along a curved path, coalesce, split up again and leave wide interstices, causing the surface to rise up above the level of the neighbouring tissue in these places.[1028]

[…]

Another change, likewise confined to isolated places, is the deposition of an amorphous substance in the cornea […]. *This occurs where the superficial light corneal lamellae border on the deeper normal ones. Here the corneal lamellae are forced apart in places by a substance whose colour contrasts sharply with the lamellae.* […] *While it appears homogeneous under weak magnification, powerful magnification reveals it to be extremely fine-grained and shot through with a diffuse network of lines. The impression one gets is of a substance that has coagulated under the effect of a hardening agent but has not done so evenly.*

[…]

The amorphous substance is most frequently found in places where the changes in the topmost corneal lamellae have progressed furthest, i.e. where fraying has led to the formation of nodules. In the larger specimens one finds the following sequence of layers […]*: at the top the attenuated epithelium, followed by the frayed lamellae* […]*, followed by the amorphous substance …, which is followed in turn by normal corneal lamellae further down.*[1029]

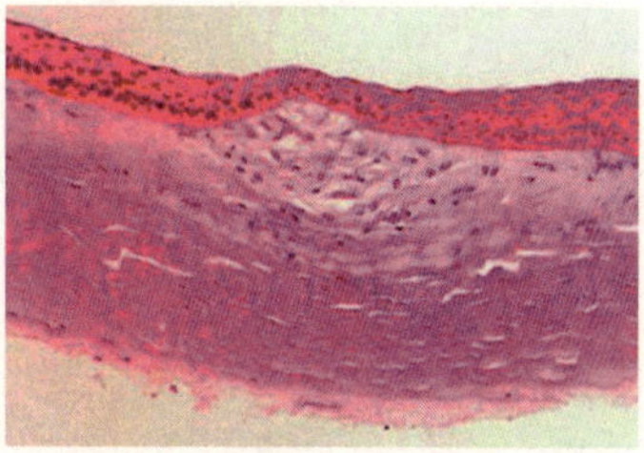

Fig. 81 Nodiform opacity of the cornea. Histological collection Ernst Fuchs

The cause Fuchs attributed to the deposition process described above was a change in the metabolism in the superficial corneal lamellae, leading to the formation of a liquid substance not normally present in the cornea. He saw the aetiology of this disease in a dystrophy caused by the deposition of a fluid leading to the degeneration of the cornea. In his view, the nodular opacity of the cornea and the metabolic deficiency as its underlying cause were more than a sporadically occurring disease of the eye, as he noticed that it ran in families.

Fuchs's collection of histological preparations comprises a highly instructive specimen that illustrates this condition. (Fig. 81)

In the Anglo-American world, Fuchs's achievement in delimiting this pathology from, say, keratitits punctata superficialis, was soon explicitly acknowledged:

Our knowledge of the condition was considerably extended by Fuchs on the basis of eight carefully observed cases.[1030]

In 1915 Fuchs published another paper on the nodular opacity of the cornea predicated on two new cases, where he attempted a precise localisation of the deposition process underlying the formation of the nodules. To achieve this, he used different dyes.[1031]

DYSTROPHIA EPITHELIALIS CORNEAE

In 1910, Fuchs summarised the observations on degenerative diseases of the cornea he had made over many years. In light of his clinical and pathological-anatomical findings he assigned them a position midway between inflammation and clouding. In keeping with his habitual way of thinking, he developed a new systematic order for these changes, which enabled him to define the new pathology of dystrophia epithelialis corneae:

I have observed and documented over many years a substantive number of cases characterised by odd changes in the cornea. They occurred mostly in both eyes, becoming more pronounced very gradually, with incrementally negative consequences for vision. Given the scarcity of cases, I was denied the opportunity of seeing a sufficiently great number to sketch appropriate clinical pictures; all I could have done was to give case-by-case accounts. However, for only one of these dystrophies, arguably the most common of all, I have been able to gather a total of 13 cases, a base on whose examination the shared – and therefore characteristic – changes can be deduced with a relatively high degree of accuracy. These changes concern the cornea, which displays a clouding as in serious cases of glaucoma. In some cases, the condition affected only one side, in others both; some cases involved an increase of intraocular pressure.[1032]

Fuchs's subtle style of investigation and his personal modesty are on full display in the following summary of characteristics shared by the cases under his observation:

In light of the clinical characteristics, the epithelium must be considered to be the first and main seat of the changes. I would therefore like to name this condition dystrophia epithelialis, a name that can be replaced by a better one later, when the true nature of the disease has been understood. Objections may be raised against this name on the grounds that this is certainly not a primary disease of the epithelium. [...] The primary disease of the cornea, which must be assumed to be present in dystrophia ep[ithelialis], appears to cause remarkably little change in the corneal parenchyma, as after the removal of the epithelium the latter is found transparent in some cases. Only occasionally a very fine-grained clouding is present. No changes in the cornea worth mentioning have been found in those cases that have been subjected to an anatomical examination. We are therefore reduced to speculation. Given the very substantial deposit present in the later stages of the disease, the fine-grained superficial clouding visible early on could perhaps be the first beginnings of the formation of this deposit.[1033]

Fuchs identified the following pathological-anatomical characteristics in the condition he had defined:

Dystrophia epithelialis corneae is a degenerative condition of the cornea, which exclusively affects people of advanced age, usually females. Sometimes both eyes are affected, sometimes only one. The condition first makes itself felt by a decrease in sensitivity to touch on the part of the cornea's surface. This is followed at a later stage by clouding of the cornea, sometimes accompanied by slight irritations. Where this is not the case, patients only become aware of the condition through defects in vision. The clouding of the cornea is superficial and appears diffuse to the naked eye. It is most pronounced in the pupillary zone of the cornea and it subsides without a sharp demarcation toward the transparent margin. As a rule, the opacity expands furthest downward, while the upper margin of the cornea remains most clear. The ephithelium bears the brunt of the changes. Its surface is lustreless or markedly uneven, it is clouded and looks bloated, displaying either easily discernible vesicles or fine dark spots, which are visible under the magnifying glass. The spots mark small cavities within the epithelium. Both the spots and the larger vesicles appear as black when seen against the backdrop of the pupil, which allows the conclusion that the clouding is mainly located in the epithelium. However, after its removal the cornea itself displays a very faint superficial fine-grained cloudiness. The surface of the cornea is totally insensitive to touch, and in those cases where only one eye is affected the seemingly normal cornea of the other eye likewise evinces a high degree of insensitivity. The deep parts of the eye are normal, with the exception of those cases that are complicated by an increase in pressure. In the majority of cases, however, intraocular pressure remains permanently normal. The cloudiness of the cornea increases over the years gradually, but steadily. In the end, a somewhat more clearly demarcated grey opacity forms in the area of the pupil, which rises above the level of the only faintly clouded marginal regions. This elevation corresponds to the deposition of newly formed connective tissue on the cornea between Bowman's membrane and the epithelium. Vision has been reduced in the meantime to finger counting at a very short distance. – The cause of the condition is unknown, as is an effective therapy.[1034]

Only one year later, in 1911, the clinical picture of dystrophia epithelialis corneae as described by Fuchs was presented to the 47th Annual Meeting of the American Ophthalmological Society by the New York ophthalmologist Arnold Knapp in a paper whose title eponymously linked the condition to Fuchs:

Professor Fuchs in his article, based on thirteen personal observations, gives us an unusually clear and complete picture of this interesting condition. He summarizes it as being a degenerative process of the cornea occurring in the aged, and usually in females. One or both eyes are involved. The first symptom is diminished sensibility of the cornea. The cornea then becomes opaque, generally in the superficial layers, and most marked in the pupillary zone. The corneal surface is opaque, uneven, with fine vesicles. In some of the cases glaucoma is present, though the opacity does not seem to be in any way the result of increased intraocular tension. The opacity slowly increases, and finally newly formed tissue is deposited on the cornea between Bowman's membrane and the epithelium. The cause is unknown and there is no treatment.[1035]

Fuchs witnessed Knapp's address as a guest of honour on his first visit to the United States. At this meeting[1036] he himself gave three lectures.[1037]

Ten years after Fuchs's first publication of dystrophia epithelialis corneae, in 1920, Ernst Kraupa (1884–1945)[1038] added the eponym "Fuchs" to this condition.[1039] One year later Salzmann followed suit in the 13th edition of the *Lehrbuch*.[1040]

The invention of the slit lamp[1041] in 1911, an instrument first presented one year after Fuchs's initial description of dystrophia epithelialis at the annual meeting of the Ophthalmologische Gesellschaft in Heidelberg by Allvar Gullstrand (1862–1930),[1042] made a significant advance possible in the histological examination of the different layers of the cornea. One of the consequences was the realisation that Fuchs's dystrophy originated in the corneal endothelium rather than in the epithelium:

The first description of the condition was made by ERNST FUCHS (1910), who also coined its name. Strictly speaking, dystrophia epithelialis is a misnomer in light of what we now know about the condition. Fuchs's view that it is caused by a primary degeneration of the top layer due to unknown causes needs to be adapted in light of the results provided by the slit lamp. Rather than the epithelium it is the posterior endothelium of the cornea that is the point of origin of this change. FUCHS himself had surmised as much but a close examination of DESCEMET's membrane was beyond the reach of the methods then in common use.[1043]

This fact was underscored by Kraupa in a presentation he gave in 1932 to the Gesellschaft der Ärzte in Vienna:

Secondary dystrophies of the epithelium include dystrophi[a] epithelii senilis, which was first described by E. Fuchs *in 1910. It was the introduction of the slit lamp that put the present speaker in a position to identify in 1919 far-reaching changes at the posterior endothelium of the cornea and other changes in the cornea.*[1044]

A doctoral thesis published in 1937 acknowledges Fuchs's pioneering role and this particular scientific achievement. In the introduction the author points out that while

Fuchs observed the most striking changes in the epithelium of the cornea, *he himself hypothesized* […] *that the primary changes were not confined to the epithelium and left it to future researchers to substitute for the name he had proposed for the condition one that actually captured the primary changes. It was the deployment of the slit lamp, a tool that was not yet available to Fuchs, that enabled the investigating eye to pry into the deeper layers of the cornea.*[1045]

This is why the most commonly used name for this condition now is either "Fuchs's endothelial dystrophy" or simply "Fuchs's dystrophy".[1046]

KERATITIS PUSTULIFORMIS PROFUNDA

This condition of the cornea is chronologically the last condition to be linked eponymically to Fuchs's name. He described this inflammation in 1915, the year he resigned from his chair.[1047] Characteristically, he had postponed the publication of the cases he had observed until he could supplement the clinical description with histological findings. All in all, Fuchs presented 16 case histories from first-hand observation in this very substantial paper.

Adding the eponym to the condition in 1921,[1048] Salzmann succinctly summarized its characteristic traits as follows:

The disease begins with the symptoms of an iritis; deeply placed gray stripes then form in the cornea as in keratitis parenchymatosa and later pus-yellow infiltrates, looking like pustules of varying size and varying location appear. At times there are several infiltrates; one large infiltrate alone is seldom present. These infiltrates are in part only clumps of exudate clinging on the back surface of the cornea, in other portions however they are actually located in the cornea because they cannot always be removed by puncture of the anterior chamber. Along with this there exists a delicate diffuse clouding of the cornea. The surface is dull but not ulcerated. Inflammatory symptoms and pain are severe.

The iris is markedly swollen and discolored; flakes of pus also often lie upon it; posterior synechiae and pupillary membrane are present; before all however a large hypopyon is at times united with the infiltrates by means of exudate striae. Moreover, the deeper structures are drawn into sympathy (vitreous opacities, marked disturbance of vision).

The course of the disease is very chronic. The infiltrations undergo transformation into dense gray, often vascularized, deep-lying opacities. At times anterior synechiae also form, even when no perforation has taken place. Elevations of pressure and staphyloma can also then develop. In very severe cases atrophia bulbi takes place.

Keratitis pustuliformis as a rule occurs only on one side, is seldom bilateral, affects older people, men by preference. According to Meller[1049] *the disease depends upon lues and Fuchs also now inclines to this view. The prognosis is unfavourable.*

On anatomic study one finds changes especially in the iris; in addition, there is massive exudate in the anterior chamber made up of polynuclear cells. The cornea shows severe injury to its endothelium, arrosion of Descemet's membrane and proliferation of the corneal corpuscles […]. *Later leucocytes also immigrate and in especially severe cases destruction of the posterior layers of the cornea also comes about.*

The treatment is quite of no avail. Puncture alleviates the pain and takes care of the exudate for a short time, yet these things soon recur. In general, the treatment can only be symptomatic.[1050]

Five years later, Adalbert Fuchs, who paid special attention to several rare luetic diseases of the eye, also concluded that keratitis pustuliformis most probably depended on lues.[1051] In the last edition of his father's epoch-making *Lehrbuch* (1945) he provided a brief outline of the frequently fulminant course this inflammation took, culminating in an aetiology for the majority of cases:

The disease mostly depends on lues and an antiluetic treatment often yields surprising results.[1052]

That Fuchs was on the right track, even though he did not yet have sufficient proof, was underscored as early as 1922:

While Fuchs was unwilling to make any pronouncements on the aetiology of the disease, he nevertheless considered syphilis in that light in some cases. We need to bear in mind that all of Fuchs*'s cases bar one* [...] *belonged to the era before the* Wassermann *test. In 1917* Meller *presented one case in Innsbruck whose aetiology was undoubtedly syphilitic.*[1053]

In a similar vein, Josef Igersheimer (1879–1965)[1054] pointed out explicitly in his reference work on the manifestations of syphilis in the eye, whose first edition was published in 1918, that Fuchs had already mooted a syphilitic aetiology in his first description of the disease.[1055]

The three decades following Fuchs's first description of the disease had not in the least diminished his authority:

The clinical picture of k[eratitis] p[ustuliformis] pr[ofunda] was described for the first time in 1915 by Fuchs *in an outline that left nothing significant to be added later. At a time when the Wassermann test was still unknown, Fuchs already mooted a luetic genesis.* Meller[1056] *und* R[udolf] Schneider [1886–1975, A/N] *successfully followed up this hypothesis.*[1057]

Sclera

EPISCLERITIS PERIODICA FUGAX

On July 31, at the 63rd Annual Meeting of the British Medical Association held between July 30 and August 1, 1895 in London, Fuchs presented to the Ophthalmological Section a description of the newly delimited disease of episcleritis periodica fugax based on twenty-three patients. It was so exhaustive that it has been associated with his name ever since. The paper was first published on August 22, 1895 in the *Wiener klinische Wochenschrift*,[1058] before appearing on October 19, 1895 in the *British Medical Journal* as part of the conference proceedings.[1059] A more detailed paper on this newly discovered disease was published in *Graefes Archiv* in the same year.[1060]

I mean by the name "episcleritis periodica fugax" a special form of frequently recurring inflammation of the eye which attacks pre-eminently the conjunctiva and the episcleral tissue, runs its course without extensive exudation and is of a very transitory nature. The symptoms of the disease are in many cases so characteristic that we can diagnose it from the history alone with a great probability of success.[1061]

The course the disease typically takes is described by Fuchs as follows:

The disease in question consists in a severe inflammation of the conjunctiva bulbi, but especially of the underlying episcleral tissue. From acute conjunctival catarrh it is distinguished by the absence of secretion and by limiting itself to the conjunctiva bulbi, of which at times only one quadrant is affected. From the usual episcleritis it is distinguished by the absence of any nodes and its very rapid disappearance, after which no traces of the disease are to be found. It consists chiefly in a severe inflammatory oedema of the episcleral tissue; the deeper structures often take part in the hyperaemia, as is shown sometimes by the presence of pain on accommodation or movement of the eyeball, a spasm of the sphincter of the pupil, which causes miosis, or a spasm of the ciliary muscle which produces transient myopia. The inflammation is frequently accompanied by severe photophobia, lachrymation, and pain; the latter often makes its appearance before the inflammation and denotes its imminent onset.[1062]

At the 47th Annual Meeting of the American Ophthalmological Society in 1911,[1063] where Fuchs was present in the course of his first trip to the United

States, Albert Conrad Snell (1871–1954), an ophthalmologist based in Rochester, NY, underscored in his presentation on episcleritis periodica fugax the significance of Fuchs's original publications sixteen years after Fuchs had first constituted this disease entity:

It was his articles which first brought these interesting and peculiar cases to the wider notice of ophthalmologists in general.[1064]

Two decades after the first description and naming of episcleritis periodica fugax Fuchs returned once more to this inflammation of the sclera and its differentiation from secondary scleritis.[1065]

SCLERITIS POSTERIOR

In 1902, Ernst Fuchs gave a report to the Deutsche Ophthalmologische Gesellschaft on this benign, short-lived form of scleritis:

A 16-year-old student, who had gone through an episode of pharyngeal diphtheria two weeks previously, fell ill with severe pain in the left eye, which was primarily located in the outermost corner of the eye, radiating to the left half of the head. A few days later, the vision of this eye began to deteriorate. The conjunctiva was found to be swollen and reddened in the outermost corner of the eye. Neuritis nervi optici, severe grey clouding of the retina at the posterior pole and proptosis of the entire area of the macula by 3–4 dptrs; S=6/12. Irregular restriction of the field of vision. Pushing back the bulbus into the orbita proved painful. The disease disappeared as quickly as it had developed so that findings were normal two weeks later and vision had regained its former strength. Roughly two months later the disease erupted in the other eye and ran the same course.[1066]

Fuchs's subsequent deliberations on the localisation, symptomatology and differential diagnosis of this rare disease led to scleritis posterior being diagnosed more effectively and more frequently in future. This is why it was eponymously linked to his name:

Severe clouding and the proptosis of the hindmost parts of the retina necessarily created the impression [of their being located, A/N] *either in the retina itself or in the underlying choroid, with secondary involvement of the retina. The argu-*

ments against this are, first, the relatively mild disturbance of vision; second, the quick disappearance of the clouding without any residual traces, not even the least changes in the retinal pigment epithelium; and, finally, the severe pain.[1067]

According to Fuchs, the criteria for a diagnosis of scleritis posterior were the following: infection of the conjunctiva, swelling of the episcleral tissue in the outermost corner of the eye and pressure sensitivity in this area. To account for these symptoms, Fuchs assumed the presence of an inflammatory focus in the posterior sector of the sclera, causing oedemas in the retina and choroid.

Even decades later, appreciation of Fuchs's achievement in the delimitation of this disease was not confined to the School of Ophthalmology established by Fuchs.[1068]

Uvea – Iris – Anatomical Structures
CRYPTS OF THE IRIS

In 1885, the year Fuchs was recalled from Liège to Vienna, he devoted a great deal of time to the study of the fine structures of the human iris and published two papers on this topic in close succession, one in Liège,[1069] the other in Vienna.[1070]

In his description of the anterior surface of the iris Fuchs discussed the following structures in his Liège paper:

The ridges departing from the lesser circle are interspersed in some places with larger triangular or rhombic depressions. These are the openings in the anterior surface of the iris that the authors refer to as crypts. *These crypts form a wreath whose location corresponds to the lesser circle around the pupil. Most of them are located in the ciliary margin of the lesser circle, a few also in its pupillary margin. Often they continue from the ciliary to the pupillary side so that one sees them straddled by both coarse and delicate trabeculae of the lesser circle. Lying clear of any substrate, the latter achieve a greater degree of autonomy in this way. Coarse or delicate cords extend downward from the margin of the crypts to their floor* […]. – *The small crypts appear to be black since their steep margins cast a shadow over their floor. With larger crypts, the floor is clearly visible. It displays the numerous parallel vessels of the stroma, spun about by the same delicate brown meshwork we have already observed in the pupillary zone.*[1071]

[…]

On the floor of the crypts one can see the vessels of the deeper layers.[1072]
[…]

Frequently the lesser circle is absent either in part or altogether. In this case it is common for the anterior surface of the iris to be divided by radial ridges into convex sectors, whose blunt points protrude as far as the margin of the pupil. Occasionally the radial ridges deepen near the margin of the pupil to become narrow crypts.

The crypts located close to the lesser circle are extraordinarily variable in number and size. Very often crypts are found in more peripheral locations in the ciliary zone […]. *Where they are numerous, the entire surface of the iris acquires an irregular, almost tattered look. It is by no means unusual to meet people whose blue irides bear a dark, usually triangular mark on their underside. These cases have been called the lightest variant of incomplete or superficial coloboma. In some of these cases, which I had the opportunity to examine recently, I found that the cause of the dark mark was a very large shallow crypt in the ciliary zone. Something similar also applies to brown eyes.*[1073]

In his detailed sketch tracing the anatomical foundations underlying the relief of the iris's anterior surface, Fuchs once again achieved the masterful plasticity that habitually characterized his observation of histological structures.[1074]

In the paper on the anatomical structure of the iris, which he published shortly after his return to Vienna, he gave a summary overview of the structure and significance of the crypts as revealed by his own research:

Special significance accrues to the crypts. *These are by no means the open pits or blind sacs they were previously taken for. Instead, they are openings in the anterior surface of the iris leading into the tissue of the iris itself. At the margin of the crypts the anterior endothelium stops; the anterior marginal layer folds back on itself, lining the entrance to the crypt for part of the way and becoming thinner along the way until it disappears completely. In this way, the crypt gradually transforms into a crevice-like space that is not clearly demarcated and merges into the stroma of the iris itself. That space is straddled by extremely delicate, acaryote fibres, extending from one wall of the space to the other. Tangential sections across several adjacent crypts reveal that the lateral walls of the crypts are undermined and that the crevices the crypts lead into are interconnected.*[1075]

In his comprehensive study of the structure of the human eyeball,[1076] Maximilian Salzmann had this to say about crypts as described by Fuchs, "*his revered teacher and thoroughly versed expert and authority on the normal and pathological anatomy of the eye*":[1077]

In general, the stroma of the iris is delimited from the anterior chamber by the anterior border membrane and the endothelium. In the crypts this delimitation is missing: crypts are places where the aqueous humour washes against the stroma of the vascular layer. Histological examination reveals peripheral crypts to be simple defects of the anterior border layer and the endothelium that open up a deeper layer of the stroma; these crypts are therefore shaped like pit-like depressions.

The larger pupillary crypts, on the other hand, are cavities in the tissue of the iris, often extending far toward the periphery so that the peripheral wall of the crypt appears to be undermined. Often the entrance to such a crypt is straddled by freely suspended trabeculae. […] *To the extent the floor of such crypts is visible from in front, it does not entirely lack a boundary layer, but the latter is much less solidly developed than at the anterior surface of the iris.* Fuchs, *who was the first to study the histology of crypts in detail, concluded that the crypts are not entirely covered with endothelium and that tissue crevices of the stroma of the iris communicate freely with the anterior chamber. It needs to be said, however, that it is impossible to inject the tissue crevices from the chamber.*[1078]

CREVICES OF THE IRIS / IRIS SLITS

Another result of his anatomical research on the vascular system of the iris in the context of the study and the description of the iris crypts is the following set of observations:

There is one capillary meshwork in the iris close to the anterior surface and another close to the posterior surface […]. *These meshworks are located in the two layers of tissue that owe their dense structure largely to the blood vessels with their adventitia and the superimposed cell networks.*

In its turn, the tissue located between the layers mentioned above is remarkable for its especially loose structure. It also contains a layer of radial vessels, such as the arteries and veins of the iris, in addition to numerous capillaries. Like the other vessels, those in the intermediate layer have a thick adventitia doubling as the basis for a meshwork of ramified cells. Apart from this, these vessels are surrounded by little or even no stroma tissue. By consequence, there are relatively large, almost empty spaces between their own surfaces and the anterior layers of denser tissue. In histological preparations these spaces appear as crevices or as relatively large, irregularly shaped apertures [...] *bridged by the same extremely delicate fibrils we have already encountered in the description of the crypts.* [...] *Looking at a radial cross-section of the iris at low magnification* [...], *one sees the middle part of the iris marked by light-coloured, crevice-shaped empty spaces, located sometimes at the anterior, sometimes at the posterior side of the intermediate vessels, and sometimes at both sides. All these spaces are actually interconnected, while at the ciliary margin of the iris they merge gradually into the system of spaces of the ligamentum pect[inatum]. What we find here are not clearly delimited lymphatic spaces, but a system of relatively large crevices directly linked to the more delicate lymphatic spaces of the stroma close to the anterior and posterior surfaces of the iris. Both the crypts close to the lesser circle and the openings of the peripheral iris zone directly give on to these crevices.*

The iris therefore contains a system of relatively large crevice-shaped empty spaces, which encases the vessels of the intermediate layer. For the sake of brevity, I will in future refer to this system as the iris slit. The iris slit is on one hand connected to the lymphatic spaces of the lig[amentum] pect[inatum] and on the other to the anterior chamber via its pupillary and ciliary outlets (crypts and openings in the marginal zone). [1079]

Fuchs describes the technique he applied in making pertinent histological preparations as follows:

In my attempts to make the iris slit visible by injection I was only partially successful. Applying a constant pressure of 40 mmHg, I injected Prussian blue into the anterior chamber. Even though I continued the experiment for hours, the injection fluid penetrated no further than to those parts of the iris slit that were adjacent to the outlets. This result was to have been anticipated since the pressure at which the injection fluid enters the iris is no higher than the pressure that prevails inside the chamber and is brought to bear on the iris from outside. [1080]

LAMELLA OF THE IRIS

Alongside the structures of the iris listed above, Fuchs examined in 1885 the anatomical foundations of the relief of the posterior surface of the iris in detail:

The anterior pigment layer is succeeded by the posterior limiting lamella *of the iris. The latter is made up of parallel, delicate, rigid fibrils held together by an intermediate, only faintly coloured substance* […]. *The width of the fibrils varies between 0,001 and 0,002 mm.* […] *Sections performed at a right angle to the radius of the iris reveal the limiting lamella to be a series of subsequent round cross-sections that correspond to the individual fibrils. The limiting lamella has no nuclei of its own. The nuclei that rest upon it belong to the anterior layer of pigment. They cling so closely to the fibrils of the limiting lamella that they can be removed only with difficulty.*

[…]

The nature of the limiting lamella in the pupillary zone of the iris is highly remarkable. In the ciliary zone the fibres of the limiting lamella form a single layer. In the region that marks the beginning of the short radial folds of the pupillary zone, that is at a short distance outside the peripheral margin of the sphincter, they start to form multiple layers. The individual layers branch out in different directions. The hindmost continue on their way along the posterior surface of the iris towards the margin of the pupil; however, they do not make it all the way because they dissolve before they do so. The fibres located in front of them extend forward at an angle to the sphincter, with which they achieve contact. This happens in the following manner: as has already been said above, the tissue behind the sphincter features deep grooves. The posterior limiting lamella, which follows these bumps, sprouts extensions *into the iris stroma from the floor of these grooves extending as far as the peripheral margin of the sphincter* […]. *These extensions follow the blood vessels, one or two of which lie in each of the grooves; they also extend forward at an angle toward the sphincter. In some cases, the vessels are regularly encased in the extensions of the limiting lamella* […]. *Elsewhere the extensions appear to be only rudimentary or to be lacking altogether. The latter are heading mainly for the peripheral margin of the sphincter, with which they become entangled. Occasionally they are accompanied by pigment cells and lumps of pigment, which stem from the foremost pigment layers and are identical in their makeup with the clot cells located in front of and behind the sphincter.*

Appropriately performed radial cross sections reveal how all this relates to the limiting lamella. What one gets to see is a strand that extends forward at an angle on the inside toward the peripheral margin of the sphincter […]. *Often this strand is encased in pigment and displays a fold in this place.*[1081]

Fuchs followed up this description with a reference to the contemporary discussion centring on the existence of an iris dilator muscle:

The controversy on whether or not there is such a structure as a dilator in the human iris boils down to the nature of the posterior limiting lamella.[1082]

On the basis of his research results at the time Fuchs reached a conclusion that is no longer valid today:

The question regarding the dilator needs to be answered as follows: There is in the human iris no structure which could be credited with the potential of enlarging the pupil apart from the posterior limiting lamella. Regardless of its physiological properties – whether it functions through its sheer elasticity or through active contraction – it needs to be borne in mind that it differs substantially from muscular tissue in its anatomical properties.[1083]

The structure of the m[usculus] dilatator pupillae and its embryonic development was described in 1912 by Fuchs's disciple Salzmann in the context of the ectodermal layers of the posterior surface of the iris:

Like the sphincter, the m[usculus] dilatator pupillae is an epithelial muscle, i.e. its fibres have developed from epithelial cells or, to be precise, from the external sheet of the eye cup. But while in the sphincter pupillae a complete transformation of the epithelium cells into muscle cells has taken place, this transformation has become effective only at the base of the dilatator pupillae cells, while the head of the cell has retained its epithelial character and pigmentation.

In its typical development, the dilator element is therefore seen to be a spindle-shaped cell with an oval nucleus and moderately pigmented protoplasm, which changes at either end into an unpigmented, fibre shaped spur. As these spurs correspond to the cell bases, they are located at a different level (further toward the front) than the nucleated heads of the cells, and a cursory inspection of a cross section leaves one with the impression that the dilatator pupillae is comprised of two layers: an acaryote, membrane like layer in front (posterior limiting lamella or border membrane [Fuchs, Bruch[1084] *or* Henle[1085] *membrane*]*) and another layer of nucleated, pigmented spindle cells (anterior pigment layer* [Fuchs], *anterior epithelium* Gruenhagen[1086] *et al.).*[1087]

PIGMENT LAYER OF THE IRIS

As part of his study of the posterior limiting lamella Fuchs went on to turn his attention to the pigment layer:

The concentric furrows and ridges of the posterior surface of the iris are located exclusively in the pigment layer (at its back, to be precise), while the radial folding involves not only the pigment layer but the tissue of the iris as such. I will start with the concentric folding that concerns only the pigment layer.

According to Schwalbe,[1088] *the pigment layer is the retinal part of the iris. He distinguishes between the two layers accordingly. The thin layer in front is made up of spindle-shaped, radially arranged cells and corresponds to the pigment epithelium of the retina. The thick layer at the back must be considered to be the continuation of the retina proper. The latter is covered on its posterior surface by the limitans iridis. I wholly agree with this view and will cite several facts in support below. – Radial cross sections of the iris reveal the posterior surface of the pigment layer to be marked with regular notches, which tally with the concentric ridges* […]. *Near the ciliary margin, where the pigment layer is generally thicker, the notches are deep, and it is not uncommon for the interspersed ridges to rise above the level of the iris like mushrooms. Toward the pupillary margin the pigment layer becomes thinner and its notches less deep. Notches only occur in the layer at the back of the pigment layer. From thin cross sections it can be seen that the pigment layer is divided by delicate, light-coloured lines into narrow ribbons that correspond to the concentric ridges* […]*; at considerable intervals, defects occur in these ribbons in a radial direction toward the iris* […]. *The latter are linked to the suture-like defects of the concentric ridges that a surface view of the iris reveals to be located deep down in the radial furrows. – Where the concentric demarcation lines of the ribbons are completely light and empty, they must be seen as optical cross sections of the furrows that keep the ridges apart. In cross sections located further down (and further to the front), the lines are coloured red by carmine and contain isolated grains of pigment. This would be the beginning of the segmentation of the cell protoplasm of the posterior pigment layer, which does not quite make it to the anterior surface of the layer. – In the dark ribbons the unpigmented nuclei appear as light dots. Similarly, contours of cells are occasionally visible inside the sheets. On this evidence, the cells in the posterior pigment layer are roughly hexagonal.*[1089]

SPUR OF THE IRIS

This is a small spur in the cross section of the iris protruding from the posterior pigment epithelium into the *m[usculus] sphincter pupillae*, which incorporates individual fibres of that muscle.[1090] The discovery of this structure and the assignation of the name "pigment spur" to it is in all likelihood to be credited to the ophthalmologist Fuchs mentions in this context, Julius von Michel (1843–1911).[1091] In his discussion of the histological examination of the irides of new-born children Fuchs says:

The posterior layer of the pigment coating [...] *is thicker than the anterior and one occasionally sees the light nuclei lying on top of each other so that one gets the impression that even in children there is already more than one layer of cells in place. At the pupillary margin the two layers turn toward each other. At the ciliary margin the anterior layer merges into the pigment epithelium of the ciliary body, the posterior into the pars ciliaris retinae. I have been able to observe this merger beyond all doubt, though Michel sought to call it into question. The two pigment layers at the posterior surface of the iris therefore correspond to the two sheets of the secondary optic vesicle. In the pupillary zone, the anterior pigment layer emits a series of extensions towards the sphincter, a structure Michel has called attention to. The largest among them, called* Pigmentsporn *by* Michel,[1092] *courses to the peripheral margin of the sphincter; it is still visible in grown-ups as a pigment sheath of the extensions of the limiting lamella, which run to the sphincter.*[1093]

At the beginning of the twentieth century it had already become common in ophthalmological literature to associate the name Ernst Fuchs with the pigment spur of the iris:

The fibres connecting the dilatator pupillae to the posterior surface of the sphincter pupillae are significantly weaker, if more numerous, than the ridge bundles and are mostly made up of one specimen or of only a few. A meridional cross section throughout reveals dilatator fibres rising from the underlying plane coursing to the sphincter across the rough connective tissue in a forward leaning, concave sweep [...]. *However, only rarely is it possible to follow them through to that point as they deviate from the meridional direction at the same time. A transversal cross section yields different images: both sphincter bundles coursing backward at an angle, and imperfectly formed dilatator fibres branching out in a forward direction, which on account of their perfect pigmentation are at times referred to as* Fuchs's *pigment spurs, are visible in the vicinity of the pupillary margin* [...].

Cross sections of dilatator elements are visible in the connective tissue at some distance from the pupillary margin, frequently arranged crosswise around the vessels, as graphically illustrated by Fuchs.[1094]

Pathological changes
HETEROCHROMIA-CYCLITIS

This aetio-pathologically still unaccounted for congenital disease is marked by a difference in the colour of the two irides or by a colour difference within the same iris. Other characteristics that may be found are uveitis in the lighter-coloured eye, iridocyclitis, keratitic deposits, characteristic clouding of the vitreous body and, frequently, cataract. Often secondary glaucoma develops at a later stage. The onset of the disease typically takes place in the third or fourth decade of life.

In the first edition of the *Lehrbuch* (1889) Fuchs described heterochromia iridis as follows:

As is universally known, the color of the iris *changes in the first years of life. Most children are born with a deep-blue iris. The stroma contains but little pigment and is still very thin, so that the posterior pigment layer is seen through it, having a bluish look. With increasing age the stroma becomes thicker and more dense. If, while this is taking place, the pigmentation does not increase, the iris simply becomes of a light blue or gray; but if, simultaneously, there is an increase of the pigment of the stroma, the iris takes on a brown color. The transformation of a blue iris into a brown one is sometimes confined to a part of the membrane, so that a brown sector is seen in an otherwise light-colored iris. Moreover, the iris of one eye may be blue and that of the other brown. The color of the iris is always proportioned to the pigmentation of the rest of the body. The dark races always have a dark iris.*[1095]

In the 8th edition of the *Lehrbuch* (1900 Fuchs) the description of the difference in the colour of the iris in the two eyes was augmented by a bracketed remark:

(In such cases the eye with the lighter iris often becomes affected with [...] *cataract.)*[1096]

In the section dealing with cataracta complicata in the next edition of the *Lehrbuch* three years later Fuchs added further details:

If the two eyes are of a different color, (e.g., one has a brown, the other a blue iris [heterochromia iridis] *it may happen that a cataract develops in one of them and in that case it always develops in the* lighter eye *of the two. In the absence of other causes, this must be regarded as something connected to the lack of pigmentation in the lighter eye; it being assumed that a disturbance of nutrition is at the bottom of both morbid conditions. It is true that nothing more definite than this is known regarding such a disturbance of nutrition; but that it is present is clear from the fact that in the lighter-colored eyes we always find the evidence of a chronic cyclitis in the form of very minute deposits. Accordingly, the cataract in these eyes is to be put under the category of complicated cataract.*[1097]

In the detailed description Georges Weill (1866–1952)[1098] provided in 1904 of seven cases of heterochromia,[1099] the disease was congenital in all patients; five had developed a cataract. Using the same journal as Weill, Fuchs published a wide-ranging survey of this disease in 1906.[1100] He added to Weill's patients another 38 cases he had observed in the course of the preceding ten to fifteen years plus a report on the histopathology of six eyes. In his view, the syndrome was caused by an as yet unidentified pathological process, whose onset was to be dated as early as the embryonic or early postnatal stage. This process developed concurrently with a disturbance in the development of uveal pigment, resulting in heterochromia iridis. This in turn made the eye react with a low-grade inflammation. In the absence of pain, this iridocyclitis continued to develop slowly over several years, steadily producing minute corneal deposits. This led to an atrophy of the iris, often accompanied by clouding of the vitreous body and the formation of a cataract. The latter, according to Fuchs, was arguably caused by pathological changes in the intraocular fluids, a secondary consequence of the disease affecting the iris and the ciliary body. In some cases, the situation deteriorated further by the formation of secondary glaucoma, which Fuchs suggested was caused by an obstruction of the drainage system.[1101]

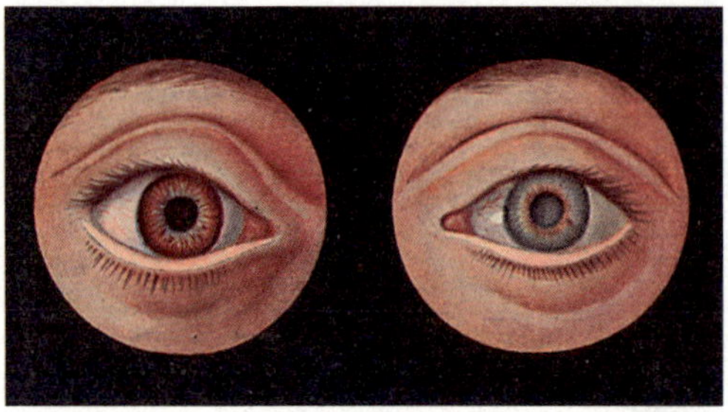

Fig. 82 Heterochromia according to a watercolour by Georg Joseph Beer

A few years later, Fuchs contributed another two papers on pigment anomalies of the iris,[1102] on heterochromia, and other congenital anomalies.[1103] To this day, the name Fuchs is generally associated with heterochromia in the ophthalmological specialist literature, while the precise terminology for this disease, whose nature was first elucidated by Fuchs on the basis of his histological studies, varied over the years: Fuchs's heterochromic iridocyclitis (FHI), Fuchs's uveitis syndrome (FUS), and Fuchs's heterochromic uveitis are the most common.[1104]

When Adalbert Fuchs published the 16th edition of his father's *Lehrbuch* in 1939, he added a historically highly significant illustration to the description of *Cataracta in oculo coeruleo, Heterochromiekatarakt*. The founder of Vienna's Ophthalmological School, Georg Joseph Beer,[1105] had painted the water colour himself. It had been kept as a treasure at the First University Eye Clinic, where Adalbert Fuchs used to work as assistant under Josef Meller.[1106] (Fig. 82)

In this way Ernst Fuchs, having identified and linked up the characteristic elements of this pathology, was paid homage for this achievement in the ophthalmological literature many decades after the event. From the wealth of testimonies, only two Anglo-American examples are quoted here. In 1929, one year before Fuchs's death, Ferdinand Herbert Haessler (1895–1965)[1107] from Milwaukee wrote:

Heterochromia as such was popularized first by Fuchs, who reported a large series of cases. That this paper made physicians conscious of the problem is emphasized by the fact that complicated heterochromia is frequently called the "Fuchs type", though the phenomenon had been reported earlier.[1108]

The pioneer of iris research, Irene Löwenfeld (1921–2009),[1109] succinctly noted in 1973:

His meticulous descriptions and lucid discussion left little to add for later authors, and the syndrome is rightfully called by Fuchs's name, even though others had reported such cases previously.[1110]

ENDOPHTHALMITIS SEPTICA

One of the preoccupations that took up a great deal of Fuchs's time in 1904 was the localisation and the spread of inflammation processes in the inner eye. Among other things, this resulted in the coinage of the term "endophthalmitis septica":

It is one of our chief concerns to consistently improve the accuracy of our diagnoses and to substitute anatomical for clinical diagnoses. – The inflammations at the centre of this investigation particularly affect the coats of the eye, because the inflammatory noxious agents are brought to bear first and foremost on their internal surfaces. In analogy to endocarditis, endometritis etc. it would appear most logical to me to assign to this disease with all its variants the name "endophthalmitis septica", a coinage where "septic", taken in its broader meaning, denotes only that the inflammation has been caused by infection.[1111]

[...]

In cases of common acute inflammation of the inner eye resulting from lesions (endophthalmitis septica) the phlogogenic germs penetrate into the space either within the chambers or within the vitreous body. In the former case, the germs – and therefore the inflammation – may continue to be confined to the chambers, but it remains possible for germs to enter the vitreous body from the chambers at a later stage. This depends on a number of different factors, such as, above all, the virulence of the germs, which determines their potential to multiply and spread, and the anatomical preconditions in the eyeball. The chambers are separated from the vitreous body by a diaphragm (lens and zonule of Zinn), which offers resistance to penetration by phlogogenic agents. If the diaphragm has been adversely affected, e.g. by a cataract operation, the spread of the inflammation to the vitreous body is facilitated once the space within the chambers has succumbed to infection. This is why, in the times before the advent of antisepsis, cataract operations led to the suppuration of the eyeball much more frequently than did iridectomy.

The fact that an infection initially confined to the space within the chambers has spread to the vitreous body makes itself known clinically through a sudden increase in inflammatory symptoms, a rapid decrease in sensitivity to light and a slight exophthalmus.

The infection of the vitreous body may also proceed from the choroid or the retina, if, as is the case with metastatic ophthalmy, these membranes are invaded by phlogogenic agents via the bloodstream. And, finally, it happens, if only rarely, that germs penetrate to the inner eye from the rear through the intact sclera in cases of an inflammation of the orbita.

Once the internal spaces of the eye are infected, the phlogogenic agents get to work on the surfaces of the inner coats, i. e., iris, ciliary body, and retina.[1112]

Detailed histological investigation enabled Fuchs to understand how inflammation spread step by step in the inner eye:

Once the vitreous body has been infiltrated, the inflammation spreads to the inner lining of the vitreous cavity, especially to the pars ciliaris retinae and to the retina proper. These membranes are the first to become inflamed, a process that results in very extensive purulent retinitis. The effect projects to the deeps only in places where this innermost membrane is in contact with the uvea, the membrane that comes next. The ciliary body is therefore regularly affected in its superficial layers, while the choroid is affected to a significant extent only when the inflamed retina remains in contact. In the numerous cases where the retina becomes detached early on, the choroid displays only slight inflammation. The spread of the inflammation in the continuity of the membranes does not extend to any great distance. In the case of the ciliary body the anterior margin is affected, in the case of the optic disc it is the posterior margin of the uvea that is affected. The suprachorioideal cavity is an outlier in that it participates very extensively in the inflammation once it has been penetrated by inflammatory pathogens in a place located in the flat part of the ciliary body; its stroma is intensely afflicted by the inflammation of the pars ciliaris retinae, with which it has inseparable links.[1113]

In his description of the histological evidence of iridocyclitis Fuchs summarized the results of his own investigation at length[1114] and, having further specified the newly coined term endophthalmitis septica, he included it in the 10th edition of the *Lehrbuch* (1905):

The clinical designations for the types of inflammation described above, which moreover present all possible combinations and transition forms, are as follows:

The cases in which the main clinical feature is the inflammation of the anterior division of the eye and which terminate in organization of the exudate are known as plastic iridocyclitis. When the exudate is purulent, we speak of a purulent iridocyclitis or, if the suppuration is in the vitreous body, of a purulent iridochorioiditis. If the suppuration in the vitreous becomes encapsulated, we call it an abscess of the vitreous or a hyalitis; if pus breaks through, we call the condition panophthalmitis. These terms are not quite proper if we have regard to the anatomical findings, and it would accord best with the latter if we were to call the inflammation of the inner coats of the eyes that is produced by an infection an endophthalmitis septica.[1115]

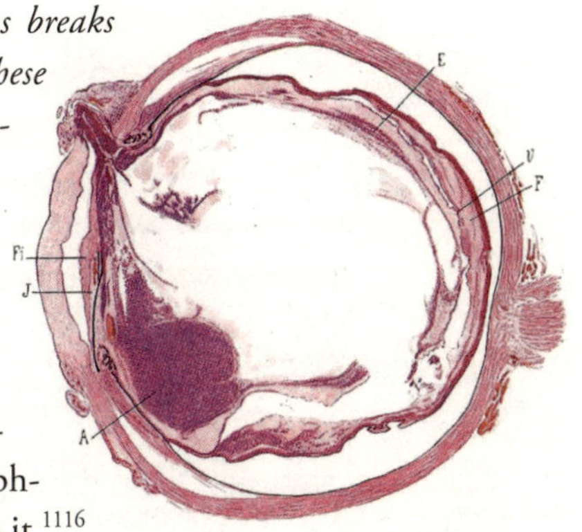

Fig. 83 Endophthalmitis septica

In the 13th edition of the *Lehrbuch* (1921), Maximilian Salzmann devoted an entire chapter to endophthalmitis septica and attached the eponym Fuchs to it.[1116]

Largely based on his father's collection, Adalbert Fuchs's *Atlas der Histopathologie des Auges* (1923) features the detailed description and illustration of an eye that became infected long after a cataract operation *(Endophthalmitis septica)*:

Case history: A 60-year-old woman had the lacrimal sac removed on account of chronic dacryocystitis; ten days later, a mature cataract was extracted with iridectomy. After the operation astigmatism against the rule of 12 diopters.

Nine months later an abrupt and very severe inflammation developed, accompanied by pain. Severe chemosis. A suppurative focus at the surgical site. The cornea is slightly clouded, the chamber shallow, the iris indistinct. The coloboma is filled with pus. After six days sensitivity to light had decreased to 1 m[etre]; projection wrong. Enucleation.

The conjunctiva on top of the extraction wound is oedematous and bulges. In the wound itself there is pus, which, filling the coloboma, runs from there to behind the iris and an abscess (A) located on the ciliary body. The Iris (J) is topped by a red-coloured fibrin coagulum (Fi), coagulated aqueous fluid. While in the anterior chamber significant suppuration is absent, all membranes encompassing the vitreous body are severely inflamed and covered with suppurative exudate: endophthalmitis septica. The exudate is deposited on the retina (next to E) and even more so on the ciliary body below, where an abscess (A) has formed. The inflamed retina has also excreted a fluid rich in protein (F) and has lifted the vitreous body (V) at the posterior pole of the eye from the retina.[1117] (Fig. 83)

In 1925, Fuchs summed up the great number of his histological investigations into this clinical picture:

I tried to show twenty years ago that the inflammation of the inner eye that was formerly referred to as suppurative iridochorioiditis is the consequence of the impact toxins have on the inner surfaces of the membranes lining the inner eye. It would therefore be better to refer to this condition as endophthalmitis, a designation that has gained widespread acceptance.[1118]

Fuchs's histological collection[1119] still contains a great number of preparations that graphically document the different stages of this disease and the range of different trajectories it may take.

COMMON ENDOPHTHALMITIS VS. OPHTHALMIA SYMPATHICA

The meticulous histological investigations into endophthalmitis outlined above, for which Fuchs relied on bulbi enucleated after trauma, enabled him to unambiguously delimit the common inflammation of the inner eye from the long-familiar – and much feared – ophthalmia, which in the wake of a perforating injury or an operation on one eye very often affects and destroys the other.[1120] On the evidence of the composition of the exudate, Fuchs declared endophthalmitis septica to be a fibrinous-plastic or purulent iridocyclitis or iridochorioiditis, while sympathetic inflammation was found to lead to the formation of granulation tissue.

For the description of these nodules, Fuchs cited research carried out one year previously by Swedish ophthalmologist Johan Albin Dalén (1886–1940).[1121] [1122] The pigmented zones consisting of epithelium cells between Bruch's membrane and the retinal pigment epithelium soon came to be referred to as Dalén-Fuchs nodules, a designation they have retained to this day.

Four years later Fuchs added other typical cases of sympathetic ophthalmia he had observed himself to his earlier comprehensive description.[1123]

The main differences between septic endophthalmitis and sympathetic ophthalmia as defined by Fuchs are the following:

Sympathetic inflammation, the disease that spreads to the other, uninjured eye where it causes sympathetic ophthalmia, differs fundamentally, as Ernst Fuchs [...] *has shown, from suppurative posttraumatic inflammation. While suppurative inflammation may affect all coats of the eye and depends for its gravity on the number and virulence of germs and the location of the focus of the infection in the inner eye, sympathetic inflammation is a selective disease affecting the uvea. It develops as a primarily chronic inflammation, in which the uvea is densely permeated predominantly by lymphocytes, forming nodules in many places, in whose centre agglomerations of epitheloid cells are found, interspersed with giant cells of the* Langhans *type. Right from the beginning of the outbreak of what is called serous traumatic iritis, the tissue of the retina, as* Ernst Fuchs *has shown, is permeated by lymphocytes. Gradually chronic granulation tissue is formed, which affects only the uvea. Even in the walls of the retinal vessels analogous infiltrates are found. As the disease subsides, it leaves behind fibrous scars. In the second, uninjured eye the sympathetic inflammation runs the same course.*

With these two studies, Ernst Fuchs *has clearly delimited the two forms of posttraumatic inflammation of the inner eye and has shown them to be completely different processes. He has demonstrated that they are independent of each other and can even exist side by side, provided suppurative inflammation, as is the rule in endophthalmitis septica, has not destroyed all parts of the uvea. This accounts for the experience of the old eye specialists which told them that in exceptional cases sympathetic ophthalmia may occur even after panophthalmitis, if parts of uveal tissue have remained untouched by suppuration. Endophthalmitis, however, is not, as* Fuchs *has explicitly emphasized, a precondition for the development of sympathetic inflammation. The latter disease develops independently of suppuration. It is, as he has pointed out, a disease in its own right, whose occurrence presupposes a specific infection and the presence of uveal tissue.*[1124]

At the time when Fuchs was working on a definition of the symptoms of sympathetic ophthalmia, no therapy for this insidious disease was yet in sight. As there was the very real possibility for this trauma induced inflammation to repeat itself in the other, uninjured eye within the first weeks after the lesion, Fuchs, together with a large number of fellow ophthalmologists, recommended enucleation of the initially affected eye in cases where the latter was severely damaged and had only vestigial vision left. This drastic measure was designed to prevent sympathetic ophthalmia from breaking out in

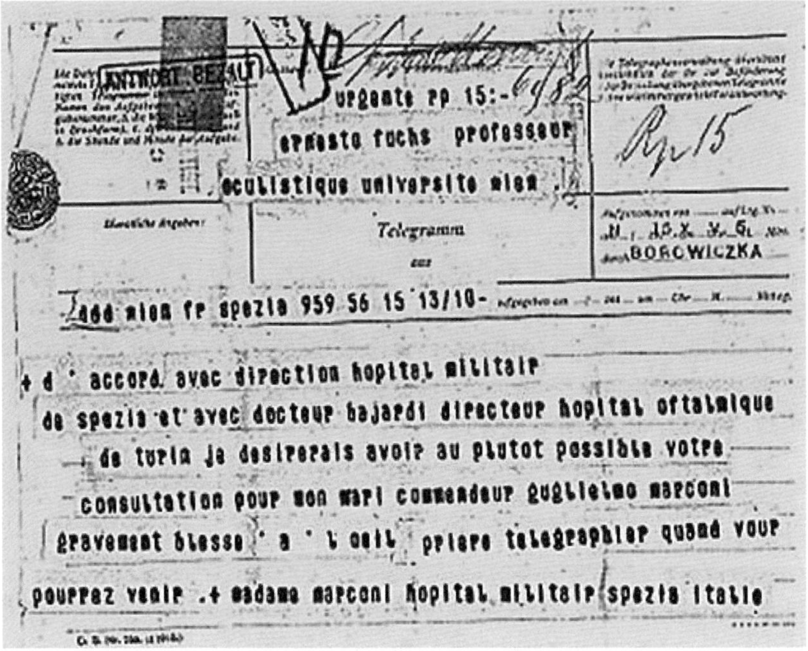
ANTWORT BEZAHLT

urgente pp 15:-

ernesto fuchs professeur

oculistique universite wien

Telegramm

aus

BORCWICZKA

Zadd wien fr spezia 959 56 15 13/10-

+ d ' accord avec direction hopital militair

de spezia et avec docteur bajardi directeur hopital oftalmique

de turin je desirerais avoir au plutot possible votre

consultation pour mon mari commendeur guglielmo marconi

gravement blesse ' a ' l oeil priere telegraphier quand vour

pourrez venir .+ madame marconi hopital militair spezia italie

Fig. 84 Madame Marconi's telegram

the uninjured eye, since the extremely stormy course the disease was prone to take had in many cases led to severe visual impairment or the total loss of vision in the formerly healthy eye.

A case in point is the medical history of Guglielmo Marconi (1874–1937),[1125] the inventor of wireless telegraphy and the radio.

On September 25, 1912, Marconi was involved in a car accident; a glass fragment from the broken windscreen penetrated into his right eye. As the status of the injured eye deteriorated very rapidly, the doctors in charge at the military hospital in La Spezia feared that sympathetic ophthalmia might develop in the uninjured left eye. To prevent this from happening they advised the enucleation of the injured and inflamed eye which was no longer functionable. In October, they decided to ask Pietro Bajardi (1862–1922),[1126] then Director of the University Eye Clinic in Torino, and Ernst Fuchs as an internationally recognized expert in this field to act as consultants. Marconi's wife sent Fuchs an express telegram (Fig. 84), asking him to come to Torino for a consultation. Published here for the first time, the telegram reads as follows:

d'accord avec direction hopital militair de spezia et avec docteur bajardi directeur hospital oftalmique de turin je desirerais avoir au plutot possible votre consultation pour mon mari commandeur Guglielmo Marconi gravement blesse a l'oeil priere telegraphier quand vous pourrez venir. Madame Marconi hospital militair spezia italie[1127]

Fuchs complied with this request without delay. After jointly examining the patient on October 17, Bajardi and Fuchs agreed that it was imperative to remove Marconi's right eye. The enucleation was performed on the same day by Fuchs in Bajardi's presence. The healing process proved straightforward and took place without any complications. The left, uninjured eye was spared sympathetic ophthalmia, in all probability thanks to the measures adopted.[1128]

Ciliary body
DICTYOMA

In 1908, Fuchs had first described in detail and named a very rare tumour of the ciliary body. With most cases occurring in young children, this tumour is characterised by a network of strands of epithelial cells.[1129]

In 1892 Badal[1130] *and Lagrange*[1131] *were the first to describe a tumour which, originating in the epithelium of the pars ciliaris retinae, develops in the region of the corpus ciliare from amorphous masses of cells and from strands of cells reminiscent of tubular glands.*[1132] *By 1908 Fuchs had found three similar cases in the literature*[1133] *and provided a first comprehensive overview of these rare eye tumours. He called them dictyomata because of their morphological behaviour.*[1134] *In the early stages of their development they spread as a two-dimensional, mesh-like growth across the surface of the ciliary body and the walls of the anterior chamber. Later they form compact tumourous masses which destructively penetrate the adjacent tissue* […].[1135]

Fuchs mentions dictyoma in the 13th edition of the *Lehrbuch* (1921) among the tumours of the retina:

In addition to glioma, only sarcoma *has been observed in the retina proper. The remaining segment of the internal coat of the eye, the pigment epithelium, the ciliary and the iris portion of the retina give rise to the formation of epithelial tumours, which sometimes consist of simple cell tubes (adenomata), sometimes show the structure of the embryonal retina (dict[y]oma), sometimes solid heaps of cells. They are referred to as* carcinoma, glioma *or* neurinema. *All these tumours are great rarities. The majority occur in eyes that have previously been destroyed by inflammation so that in general they could not have been diagnosed clinically. They are of anatomical interest only and have no clinical significance.*[1136]

To this day, Fuchs's name is associated in the specialist literature with the description of this rare tumour.[1137]

Chorioidea
FUCHS' COLOBOMA and CONUS INFERIOR

In 1882, in his second year in Liège, Fuchs made a comprehensive study of crescent formation in the chorioid,[1138] which included the delimitation of this condition from congenital coloboma of the chorioid, which spreads downward from the papilla nervi optici. Basing his remarks on 45 cases he had observed himself, Fuchs underscored the following characteristics:

1. *Special attention is to be paid to the occurrence of downward pointing crescents, especially those of the narrow, inconspicuous and therefore often overlooked type.*
2. *This crescent is congenital and analogous to the coloboma of the inner coats of the eye. It needs to be clearly distinguished from the common, outward pointing crescent-shaped atrophies of the chorioid. The extent to which the latter are congenital remains outside of consideration in this study.*
3. *The downward pointing crescent is nearly always associated with a refraction deficiency, most commonly with (congenital) myopia. It would, however, be a mistake to conclude from this that a great number of myopia cases are congenital. This view could only be taken by those who group downward pointing crescents together with those that point outwards and also regard the latter as congenital in many cases (*Schnabel*).*[1139] *Instead, the quota of cases of metropia is relatively high among individuals with a downward pointing crescent.*
4. *The downward pointing crescent is nearly always associated with deficient acuity of vision and is therefore an important symptom of congenital amblyopia.*[1140]

Fuchs mentioned the formation of colomboma outlined above in the first edition of the *Lehrbuch* (1889). He did so without mentioning his own contribution to the clarification of this phenomenon and even without so much as quoting from his own relevant earlier publication:

White crescents are also observed at the lower *border of the papilla* [...]. *These resemble in their appearance the acquired crescents due to myopia, but have an altogether different significance. They are congenital (presumably linked to the fetal ocular fissure which is also located on the nether side of the bulbus) and are associated frequently with astigmatism and almost always with incomplete acuity of vision.*[1141]

More than three decades later Fuchs returned to the topic of the congenital anomalies of the retina and the optic nerve, subjecting them to further extensive treatment.[1142] On the basis of the description of several new cases he had observed himself, he examined the nature and the causes of the "*crescent pointing downward at the papilla*":[1143]

The anatomical finding in uncomplicated cases of crescent pointing downward is the same as in those of temporal crescent. It is therefore not possible to refer to these cases as colobomata. It would, however, be equally mistaken to assume that the downward distortion of the papilla corresponds exactly to the outward distortion in every respect apart from the direction. Both are the results of a strain on the coats of the eye, but even though the result may be the same morphologically in both cases, it does not follow that the strain that precedes it is identical. That the downward pointing crescent occupies a special place follows from a number of clinical and anatomical facts. I had pointed this out when I had been the first to show[1144] *that such eyes display a host of other abnormalities, such as the abnormal form of the papilla, astigmatism and poor acuity of vision.*[1145]

[...]

The developmental disorder affecting the ocular fissure that causes the formation of the downward pointing crescent therefore leads, rather than to the formation of a coloboma, to a certain degree of hyperplasia of the inner coats of the eye, most notably of the sclera, causing in turn ectasia of the latter and, subsequently, distortion of the scleral canal.[1146]

The form of the downward pointing crescent as described by Fuchs was soon accepted as part of ophthalmological terminology, especially in the Anglo-American world:

In 1882 Fuchs emphasised the difference between the acquired atrophic crescents and congenital crescents due to a defect in the development of the choroid which usually occurs at the lower margin of the optic disc and which is small and oval horizontally – a condition now often referred to as ***Fuchs coloboma****.*[1147]

ATROPHIA GYRATA CHORIOIDEAE ET RETINAE

In his quest for clear definitions and delimitations of the ophthalmo-pathological changes he observed, Fuchs's clinical and histological investigations led him in 1896 to the constitution of a new clinical picture within the range of congenital degenerations of the chorioid, which he proposed to call *atrophia gyrata chorioideae et retinae.*

Fuchs had had the opportunity to observe the condition in three sisters, who were his private patients. He presented the findings and conclusions he had arrived at in this context on 5 August 1895 at the 24th Annual Meeting of the Ophthalmologische Gesellschaft in Heidelberg as retinitis gyrata, delimiting it from retinitis pigmentosa. Fuchs handed these case histories for publication to a member of his clinical staff, New York ophthalmologist Colman W. Cutler (1862–1935).[1148, 1149] Cutler had done research at Fuchs's clinic on congenital night blindness and pigment degeneration.[1150]

As the presentation of his paper, in Fuchs's own words, *"had left no trace in the proceedings of that conference"*, he published a detailed original paper in the following year, in which he described a fourth case:

Another type of chronic retinal degeneration is that to which I would like to give the name of atrophia gyrata chorioideae et retinae.[1151]

[...]

The disease is apt to occur in several members of the same family, either handed down or in the same generation, and at times in children whose parents are related by blood. It begins in childhood with night-blindness. The ophthalmoscope shows signs of atrophy of the papilla, retina and choroid. The papilla has the same appearance as in retinitis pigmentosa, and the atrophy of the retina is shown by the narrowing of its vessels. The characteristic feature of the disease

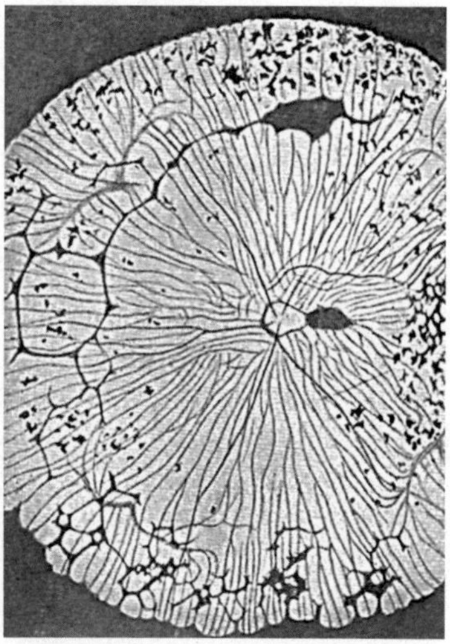

Fig. 85
Atrophia gyrata chorioideae et retinae

is the peculiar form of choroidal atrophy. This occurs first discreetly, in the form of round, sharply margined bright dots, which increase in size until they become confluent. They now melt completely into one another or remain divided by small strips of normally coloured fundus. Over the atrophic areas a few choroidal vessels and pigment flecks are to be seen. The atrophy then involves both the pigment epithelium and the stroma of the choroid; that of the first is complete; the latter has vanished to a great extent. The atrophic spots lie in a zone having the papilla for centre and extend from the equator nearly to this point. Thus the papilla is surrounded by a broad white girdle, from which it is separated by a band of normally coloured fundus. The edge of the girdle which lies towards the papilla is scalloped, because the separate, rounded parts of which it is composed extend backwards varying distances, while the remains of the normal fundus project forwards between them in sharp processes. This lobulated edge of the white zone is sharp, and in places is brought into greater relief by a narrow pigment margin. The longer the disease lasts the nearer this zone approaches the papilla, thus narrowing more and more the area of normal fundus, until finally only a slender ring remains around the papilla; in addition to this, an island of normal fundus, somewhat larger, may be preserved in the region of the macula.

The normal zone will sometimes be farther diminished still by the occurrence of atrophy around the papilla, either in the form of the familiar staphyloma or like the lobulated white areas, which finally unite with the broad white zone. While the atrophic zone is sharply limited posteriorly, anteriorly the pigment flecks become more and more numerous, until the fundus in the extreme periphery may appear almost black. In my last case there appeared to be normal fundus still farther towards the periphery. The opacity of the posterior cortical layers of the lens is to be mentioned as existing in all cases so far observed; it is the same kind of star-shaped, posterior cortical cataract that occurs in retinitis pigmentosa.[1152] (Fig. 85)

When he described this disease for the first time, Fuchs conceived of the mechanism of its genesis in purely morphological terms and hypothesised that it was caused by pathological changes in the local vascular supply:

Atrophia gyrata chorioideae et retinae *is differentiated from retinitis pigmentosa by the prominence of the choroidal atrophy, which dominates the ophthalmoscopic picture. The appearance of the atrophy in the shape of round spots, constantly increasing in size, suggests that it starts in middle of an area supplied by a single vessel, and advances towards the periphery. It is known that the smallest arteries of the choroid, which pass from the middle vessels (Sattler) to the capillary layer divide here into numerous radiating capillaries. It is possible that these groups of capillaries may have a part to play in this disease. In any case, this disease seems to demonstrate that chronic degeneration of the retina in general, the different forms of which I have just dealt with, is preceded by a primary disease of the choroid.*[1153]

In the 13th edition of the *Lehrbuch* (1921), Salzmann added the eponym "Fuchs" to atrophia gyrata chorioideae et retinae and summed up the typical characteristics and distinguishing features of this disease, whose progressive destruction of tissue may lead to blindness:

Atrophia gyrata chorioideae et retinae (Fuchs) is a peculiar atrophy of the chorioid related to typical pigment degeneration. It has the atrophy and pigmentation of the retina, the course and subjective disturbances in common with pigmentary degeneration [...], *is however distinguished from it by the addition of a complete atrophy of the chorioid which is extended over the greater part of the fundus, so that only a narrow girdle about the papilla or only the macular region is exempt. The atrophy arises in foci but the foci are so numerous and large that they coalesce into an apparently diffused atrophy. The border of the atrophic zone only shows the manner of origin by the crenated outline. Small portions of the normal fundus also remain here and there as uninvolved dark brown crenated serrated flecks.*[1154]

Fuchs's new coinage soon established itself in international ophthalmological terminology and atrophia gyrata chorioideae et retinae was frequently associated with the name of the man who first delimited it.[1155] Even more frequent were references to Ernst Fuchs's first description by the authors of ophthalmological papers in one form or another.[1156]

Several decades passed before the cause of this condition, a congenital disturbance in the metabolism of ornithine aminotransferase, was identified on the basis of insights provided by genetic research.[1157]

DETACHMENT OF THE CHORIOID AFTER CATARACT OPERATIONS

Several pathologies are eponymously associated with Fuchs even though he had no claim to their first description in the strict sense. What he did deserve credit for was the meticulous histological research that frequently made him the first to identify specific tissue changes and to unravel and describe the pathomechanism of the condition in question. A case in point is the detachment of the chorioid after operations, which had only rarely been diagnosed correctly before.

Having kept a watch on this complication for more than quarter of a century, Fuchs gave a presentation on it at the 28th Annual Meeting of the Ophthalmologische Gesellschaft in Heidelberg on 14 September 1900.[1158] He then proceeded to publish the case histories of the patients in question and the results of his histological research in two detailed papers.[1159]

An important factor Fuchs isolated first of all was advanced age and the consequent increase in the rigidity of the sclera. Incisions with Graefe's knife during iridectomies could result in a tear in the base of the iris and the ciliary body. In iridectomy necessitated by glaucoma, the pre-existing increase in pressure would act as a facilitating factor. The finding Fuchs considered to be typical was the continued shallowness or the shrinkage of the anterior chamber due to a decrease in pressure. Both symptoms were prone to subside spontaneously, with a tendency to reappear later. In 1902, Fuchs distinguished between four types of detachment of the choroid:

Detachment can be due to a tear in the base of the ciliary body, to pull applied to the choroid, to the bursting of choroidal vessels, or to an inflammatory effusion.

In the first case the fluid under the choroid is aqueous humour; in the second, transudative serum; in the third, blood; in the fourth, exudate. The extension of the detachment depends on the amount of liquid seeping out, on the strength of the pull that is being applied, or on the resistance put up by the vortex veins, which attach the choroid to the sclera. The subchorioideal liquid can either sate the subchorioideal [lamellae] *evenly – oedema of the suprachorioidea – or cause a genuine anatomic detachment of the choroid. Distention of the suprachorioideal lamellae may lead to the formation of relatively large circumscribed cavities; these cavities may be lined by a coarse wall, or else fibrous scar tissue may form in the suprachorioideal space. – A complete restitutio ad integrum is only possible with detachments of the first type. Detachments of the second type (caused by pull) will remain for ever. With detachments caused by the influx of blood or of exudation under the choroid, the choroid may in isolated cases come close again to the sclera later, but never so as to completely re-establish normal conditions in the suprachorioideal space.*[1160]

More than a decade and a half after this classification Fuchs revisited the complex topic of the detachment of the choroid in another two papers.[1161]

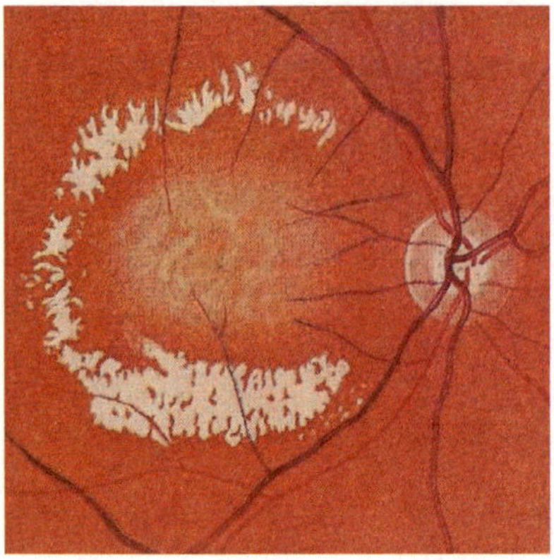

Fig. 86
Retinitis circinata

Retina

RETINITIS CIRCINATA

I have over the years observed a number of cases of a peculiar retinitis, some of them over a longer period of time, in some cases as long as seven years. As this disease, which I would like to call retinitis circinata, has never been described adequately and in sufficient detail, the cases I have observed myself will be described at some length.[1162]

Fuchs described this clinical picture he had established in 1893 on the basis of twelve cases as

a disease of unknown aetiology, appearing by preference in older women and characterized by a corona of clear white confluent sharply-delimited little flecks, which encircle the delicately grayishly clouded macular region.

[…]

The papilla and the retinal vessels are normal. The macula lutea and its surroundings have been transformed into a yellowish-grayish area, which is not sharply delimited and is encircled by a girdle composed of white flecks. The flecks coalesce to form map-like shapes, but they are absent in the vicinity of the papilla, leaving the ring open.[1163] (Fig. 86)

As was the case with several other clinical pictures eponymously linked to his name, Fuchs felt called upon to delimit retinitis circinata from other types of inflammation of the retina, as previous descriptions of similar changes by other authors were not in his view sufficiently unambiguous. In

1874, renowned English ophthalmologist Sir Jonathan Hutchinson,[1164] for instance, had assigned inflammatory changes he had seen predominantly to the choroidea, *"speckled with minute dots of yellowish white deposits"* and had called it a symmetrical central choroido-retinal disease.[1165] Hutchinson's terminology was subsequently accepted by the Hungarian ophthalmologist Wilhelm Goldzieher (1849–1916).[1166] However, after the publication of Fuchs's paper Goldzieher equated Hutchinson's choroidoretinal disease with retinitis circinata.[1167]

Fuchs documented the pathohistological changes he had observed in only a relatively small number of patients in his characteristically painstaking manner so comprehensively that he paved the way for further research. A veritable flood of research papers appeared over time devoted to the substrate and cause of this degenerative change in the retina, based on the typical central spot surrounded by a circle of dots and flecks, causing incremental loss of central visual acuity.[1168]

It became gradually more and more accepted that retinitis circinata, rather than being a disease in its own right, is one of the variants of age-related macula degeneration.[1169]

FUCHS SPOT

In current ophthalmologic terminology, a black spot in the macula, the result of the proliferation of pigment epithelium associated with choroidal haemorrhage due to powerful myopia-related strain, is still widely referred to as Fuchs spot. This phenomenon, whose first description Fuchs traced to a paper Wrocław ophthalmologist Carl Friedrich Richard Förster[1170] had published in 1862,[1171] he sought to elucidate further in a paper in 1901.[1172] In his description, Fuchs was at pains to stress

that [the black spot] *is radically different from other, more common macular changes. I have come to this conclusion because it occurs entirely independently of other changes in the fundus and follows its course independently of the latter.*[1173]

His new insights were based on the observation of more than 50 cases in his private practice:

The disease initially makes itself felt through the sudden onset of impaired vision. In the majority of cases patients say that objects appear distorted to them, in the form of metamorphopsia Förster *described in a classic text; often it is a dark spot at the centre of the field of vision that veils the objects the eyes focus on. This spot is sometimes described as dark, sometimes as greenish or reddish. In some cases, distinct scintillation is seen in the area of the spot, which is also perceived with eyes closed and in the dark. When this symptom occurs, it is usually very persistent and causes patients great distress.*

A test always reveals reduced vision, in most cases to between 1/4 and 1/10 of normal visual acuity. In particularly serious and in inveterate cases vision is even more reduced, to finger counting over a short distance. The cause of the reduction of visual acuity is a central scotoma, which in recent cases is still small and can often only be demonstrated to exist with reference to colours, which means that small print can still be read with an effort; later the scotoma always becomes absolute and in consequence reading is no longer possible.

In recent cases, where impaired vision has only existed for a few weeks or months, the ophthalmoscope allows us to see the characteristic black spot in the macula. Its size is at that stage still considerably smaller than the papilla […]*; it was only in exceptional cases that I found larger spots in recent cases (even as large as three times the size of the papilla). The spot is usually circular and well-defined. Only rarely is it evenly pitch black throughout; usually a grey or whitish hue is faintly perceptible in its central parts.*[1174]

Fuchs's real achievement, which subsequently caused his name to be eponymously linked to the black spot in specialist literature, lies in the explanation he provided of what caused the black spot to form in cases of high myopia. The explanation that had previously held sway was haemorrhage in the macula. His observations enabled Fuchs to refute conclusively this hypothesis that even Förster had supported in his first description of the condition:

Personally I believe […] *the haemorrhages that one occasionally sees at the margin of the black spot to be something that is merely accidental, caused presumably by disturbances in circulation in the vicinity of the focus of the disease.*[1175]

It was the close study of the autopsy findings presented in a Zurich dissertation written a quarter of a century earlier[1176] that gave Fuchs the breakthrough to understand the aetiology of the black spot:

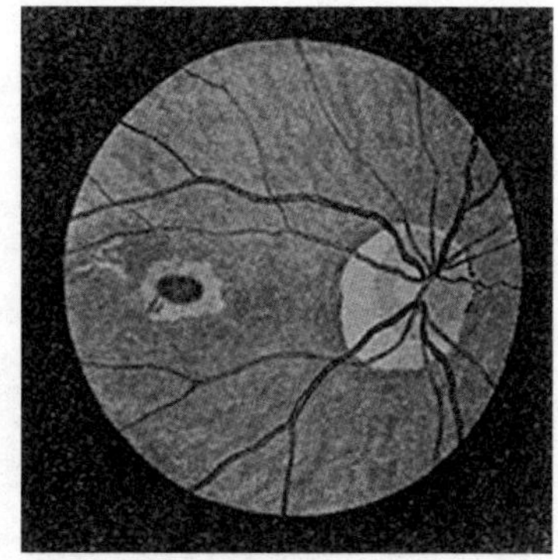

Fig. 87
Fuchs spot

[The findings] concerned a 52-year-old man the macula of whose left eye featured a longitudinal-oval black spot almost the size of the papilla. At the site of the spot the choroid displayed no significant changes and the glass membrane was also normal. However, the pigment epithelium lying on the glass membrane had proliferated so vigorously that it had grown to two thirds of the thickness of the choroid in the middle of the focus. At the periphery of this growth the pigment epithelium was paler or completely devoid of pigment, taking on its normal quality by contrast at a greater distance from the focus. Where the pigment epithelium had proliferated, it was covered by an ostensibly gelatinous, acellular exudate (clotted fibrine?), which likewise reached its greatest thickness of two thirds of the thickness of the choroid in the middle of the focus. The proliferating pigment layer and the exudate formed a hill which subsided evenly towards one side. The retina had grown together with its surface. No specifications are given as to its nature.

The findings in question correspond closely with the clinically observed facts. The proliferating pigment accounts for the black spot. The gelatinous exudate deposited on the pigment is possibly the reason why the black spot appears to be a lighter grey in the middle. The zone of paler or pigmentless epithelium cells in the vicinity of the growth arguably corresponds to the lighter red zone surrounding the black spot. When the exudate organises and shrinks, which spells the end for the proliferating pigment epithelium, the spot assumes a lighter colour and is replaced by grey or blueish-white tissue, the exudate callus. The fact that in the autopsy findings there is no mention either of extravasated blood nor of pigment arising from it (which is easily distinguishable from the pigment of the proliferating epithelium cells) accords with my experience that haemorrhage plays no significant part in this disease.[1177]

The 12th edition of the *Lehrbuch* (1910), the last to be overseen by Ernst Fuchs himself, includes a first illustration of the central black spot.[1178] (Fig. 87) Having mentioned the occurrence of haemorrhages in his description of the changes of the choroid in the area of the macula lutea, Fuchs noted:

Another, rare change in myopic eyes consists in the formation of a pitch black, circular spot in the macula itself, which expands until it is roughly the size of the papilla […]; over time, the centre of the spot becomes progressively lighter.[1179]

It was again Maximilian Salzmann who established an eponymous connection between the description of the central black spot and the name of Ernst Fuchs. In the 13th edition of the *Lehrbuch* he wrote:

The central black spot (Fuchs) […] *is a transverse oval, pitch black or at least dark grey spot in the area of the fovea, which causes severe impairment of vision (absolute scotoma). Over time, it may become lighter in the centre.*[1180]

The passage remained unchanged in the next two editions.[1181] The last three editions of Fuchs's classic work were overseen by his son, Adalbert, who retained the original illustration and the legend, but changed the text. In the first of these editions, published in 1939, nine years after Ernst Fuchs's death, Adalbert's text failed to mention his father in this context:

Two rare changes in the macula are distinct from central chorioiditis. First, the often ambilateral lacquer cracks, whitish yellow, reasonably straight stripes that branch out and may even form networks […]. *Visual acuity is not impaired by them. Second, the central black spot* […], *a pigment focus the size of between 1/2 and 1/4 of a p[apilla] d[diameter] that occurs spontaneously and is accompanied by severely impaired vision (metamorphopsia and central scotoma); it becomes lighter in the middle later and may even turn entirely grey or greenish. The black spot due to myopia can occur in the other eye years later; over time distorted vision disappears, but the scotoma does not. It seems that the lacquer cracks are caused by tears in the lamina vitrea and the pigment epithelium, while the black spot is caused by proliferations of the pigment epithelium.*[1182]

In the 17th edition (1944) and in the last edition (1945) of the *Lehrbuch*, the legend of the illustration in question included the eponym, "Fuchs spot", in brackets.[1183]

Nervus opticus

ATROPHY OF THE OPTIC NERVE (FUCHS)

Ernst Fuchs's description of the (senile) atrophy of the peripheral fibres of the optic nerve dates to his last year as Chair of Ophthalmology at Liège University (1885).[1184] Meticulous examination of the kind typical of him, involving 60 optic nerves of individuals of all age groups,[1185] allowed him to reach the following conclusions:

The physiological strengthening of the septa system in the vicinity of the apple of the eye must not be confused with the sclerotic thickening of the latter, which constitutes a pathological change. It is not only a constant companion of many diseases of the optic nerve, but is often encountered even in otherwise normal optic nerves, which are most likely to belong to elderly persons […] *The* sclerotic thickening *of the connective-tissue septa is much more pronounced in the vicinity of the bulbus than further toward the back and is frequently present only in front. Even the walls of the smaller blood vessels, sometimes even those of the central vessels, are sclerotic* […]. *Furthermore, this is often accompanied by a thickening of the pial sheath, especially of the longitudinal fibres, which are so prominent in cross sections* […]. *In these cases of sclerosis among old people I have never found a multiplication of nuclei in the septa, so that in my view they are not due to inflammation.*[1186]

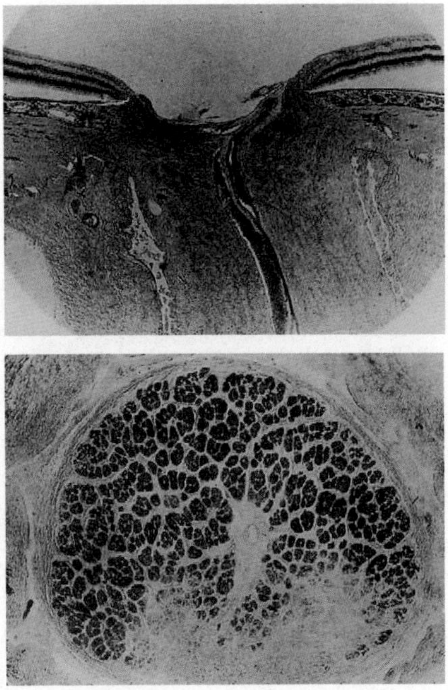

Fig. 88 Senile optic atrophy

Fuchs commented on the histological structure of the changes he had observed as follows:

The nerve bundles enclosed between the peripheral septa and the pial sheath are precisely those peripheral atrophied bundles *already mentioned. The nerve fibres have gone missing and what remains is an empty network of delicate fibres – grey atrophy.*[1187] (Fig. 88)

Fuchs reached the following conclusions in the interpretation of his research results:

Fairly long series of cross sections were made with a microtome from the majority of the optic nerves under consideration. Among all these optic nerves I did not come across a single one *that did not show peripheral and central atrophy, be it in its beginning, be it further advanced. I cannot believe that this is the result of coincidence which happened to hand me exclusively pathological optic nerves. I believe instead that the atrophy I have described, which by its nature is a pathological change, occurs* as a rule in all human beings. *One could group it together with the other age-related changes if its first traces were not already apparent in newborn babies.*[1188]

Going beyond a morphological description, Fuchs already raised the following question – and provided at least tentative answers:

What are the functional consequences *of these atrophic changes in the human optic nerve that are invariably present? Thanks to a series of investigations undertaken only recently we are now in a position to say at least with a high degree of probability what parts of the retina the affected nerve bundles are allocated to. The most peripheral bundles located immediately under the pial sheath supply those parts of the retina that border on the papilla (Bunge).*[1189] *This is true at least of the anterior, vascular part of the optic nerve, which is the one that chiefly matters. At the same time, it is in the forefront as far as peripheral atrophy is concerned. Accordingly, the loss of the peripheral bundles would cause an enlargement of the blind spot. This, too, would make itself felt only at an advanced age, when the atrophy of the peripheral bundles had become absolute. As long as at least part of the fibres remains conductive, those parts of the retina that surround the papilla would register a decrease in visual acuity rather than a complete loss of the sensitivity to light. – Further research is needed to show whether an enlargement of the blind spot is in fact attendant on advanced age.*[1190]

More than thirty-five years later, Fuchs took advantage of new methods of preparation and of dyeing to revisit the senile degeneration of the optic nerve.[1191] He summed up his findings as follows:

Most foci were located at the periphery of the nerves, far fewer in the parts in the middle and only isolated cases spread for part of their course from the periphery to the middle or the other way round. The peripheral foci were located most frequently on the upper side. They occupied parts of varying size of the nerve periphery, sometimes as much as one half. They varied in the extent they stretched from the margin to the inside, sometimes only a short way, sometimes further, even as far as the middle, so that some foci were seen to be very extensive, taking up as much as one third of the entire cross section.[1192]

On the evidence of the optic nerves he had examined himself, Fuchs identified a common cause for these atrophic foci: the advanced age of the patients. It was the same cause he had already proposed last time round thirty-five years earlier. However, he now added an important distinction:

The only factor that is common to all these cases is advanced age, and the cause of the disease affecting the optic nerve will have to be sought in age-related degeneration. Among these degenerative changes, senile vascular changes are prime candidates, as has indeed been confirmed by section in all cases under consideration, sometimes to a greater and sometimes to a lesser degree and reconfirmed by the microscopic examination of the vessels supplying the optic nerve. In all likelihood the atrophic foci are caused by local disturbances of circulation in the small vessels entering the optic nerve with the septa from the pia. These vessels may be affected by stenosis or blockage due to vascular walls thickening or due to thrombosis, or by both factors at the same time. The vessels in the septa are, after all, few in number, they are narrow, have deposits of rough tissue stored in them and some of them are perhaps end arteries.

[...] *A deficient blood supply would be detrimental to nerve substance and would cause it to shrink, while the tougher tissue of the septa would be able to put up resistance and even grow at the expense of the nerve substance.*[1193]

Orbita
MYXOMA ORBITAE

On 15 June 1914 Ernst Fuchs presented to the Wiener Ophthalmologische Gesellschaft the case history of a patient suffering from a tumour located in the orbital cavity. Given its histological structure, Fuchs referred to this tumour as myxoma orbitae:

A 40-year-old woman suffered, when she was seven, from a continually growing exophthalmus, which finally measured almost 2 cm. After the removal of the lacrimal gland, which had been dislocated from its niche, and after the transection of the rectus lateralis, which allowed dislocating the bulbus as far as the nose, it was easy to remove the well encapsulated tumour. 1½ times bigger than the bulbus, the tumour was nowhere attached to any of the neighbouring organs of the orbita. Healing occurred per primam with complete restitution of visual acuity. The round tumour is enclosed in a delicate fibrous capsule and shows an unadulterated myxoma structure without any admixture. As far as I could make out,

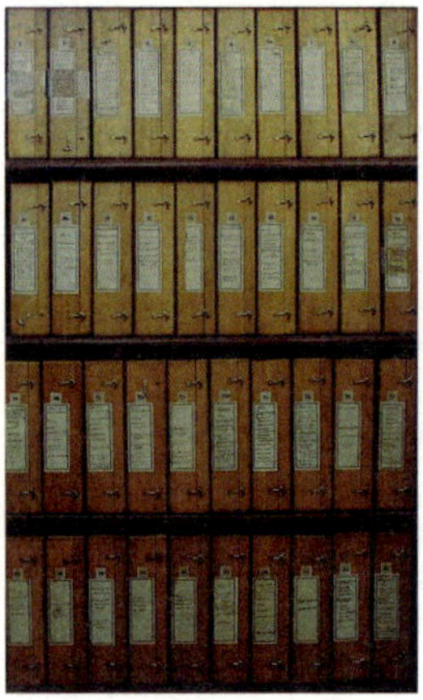

only myxofibromata or myxosarcomata have been described to this day. Myxomatous tumours often proceed from the sheaths of optic nerves; in addition, mixed tumours of the lacrimal gland contain myxomatous tissue. In the present case the point of departure of the tumour could not be ascertained.[1194]

Ernst Fuchs's first description of this extremely rare tumour is still mentioned in specialist literature a century after the event:

Ocular myxomas were first described by Fuchs in 1914; only a few cases have been reported since.[1195]

Fig. 89
Cupboard for Ernst Fuchs's histological preparations (detail)

Ernst Fuchs's Collection of Histological Preparations

According to his son Adalbert, Ernst Fuchs's legendary collection of histological preparations comprised roughly 40,000 items.[1196] It is highly likely that it is the most comprehensive historical collection of histological ocular preparations in the world. What is more, it has survived almost completely intact. It is three times the size of the collection assembled by Viennese ophthalmologist Hugo Wintersteiner (1865–1918),[1197] which at his death is said to have amounted to 13,000 tissue sections of pathologically altered eyes.[1198]

Ernst Fuchs, again according to his son, used the following system to help him navigate his collection:

The preparations are stored in 74 upright boxes of 1,000 items each.[1199] *The boxes are inscribed on the outside with the groups and sections of the preparations. Each group is arranged according to the bulbus numbers. Of each bulbus sliced into a series of tissue sections, one section per series, equipped with two labels, was consigned to the collection. The sections of the different series were sorted into different groups reflecting pathological criteria. One of the labels contained a shorthand note stating the group where the other sections of that series were to be found; the other label contained the diagnosis and a condensed case history.*[1200] (Fig. 89)

The collection began to take shape during Fuchs's assistantship under Ferdinand von Arlt at the First University Eye Clinic. Fuchs compiled notes, predominantly in shorthand, on patients' pathologies in special logbooks. The

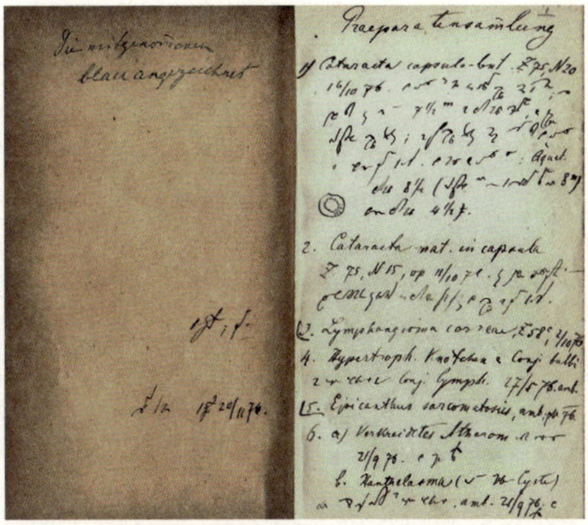

Fig. 90 Protokollbuch I. Ernst Fuchs's handwritten catalogue of his preparations

numbers he assigned to these notes reflected the chronological order of their histological processing. The first of these notes in Fuchs's own handwriting date to October 16, 1876.[1201] Initially, the chronological order was not strictly adhered to; later entries refer all the way back to 1869.[1202] It may therefore be assumed that these are in fact the dates of the operation originally performed on patients. As in 1869 and in the immediately ensuing years Fuchs was not yet an ophthalmologist, these old preparations frequently state the names of the surgeons who had carried out the operation. In later years, the notes made by Fuchs or his assistants and other staff members always included such information as whether a patient had been referred to the Eye Clinic from some other department or clinic of the Allgemeines Krankenhaus; whether the operation had been performed at the outpatient clinic; and whether a patient had been referred to the Eye Clinic from Fuchs's own private practice or the private practice of one of the other clinical professors. In addition, Fuchs had initially concerned himself with questions of comparative anatomy so his notes include references to histological preparations made from the eyes of pigs and their embryos; of an owl and a frog; of rabbits, monkeys, birds, cephalopods, pikes and carps; of a goose; of dogs, cats and calves; of an elephant, a partridge and a duck.

Eleven logbooks in black binding have survived, with the last entry dating to December 30, 1937. By 17 December 1927, 8,248 entries had been made. From the beginning of 1928 entries were numbered chronologically, starting from scratch at the beginning of every year.[1203] In the first volume[1204] Fuchs had made all the entries himself, supplementing them occasionally with his own drawings. Later on, most of the log entries were made by his assistants or other staff members. The preparations served Fuchs not only for documentation but as material for classes in microscopy. To facilitate the return to their proper place of preparations that had been removed Fuchs added a note on the flyleaf of the first volume: *"Removed [preparations] marked blue"*.[1205] (Fig. 90) His students, both those from Austria and from abroad, had free access to their teacher's unique collection. All they were required to do was to put their names against the number of any preparations they wished to borrow.

Other data recorded alongside the consecutive numbering of the histological preparations include the patients' names, the number of the surgical operative log, the date of the operation, salient details of the case history, and the number of the hospital room. A concerted effort involving the Wiener Stadt- und Landesarchiv, where the case histories of female patients of the Second University Eye Clinic from 1905 to 1914[1206] are stored, would make it possible to identify those original files that correspond to the histological preparations in Fuchs's collection. In these cases, the entire trajectory of individual case histories could be laid bare. When Fuchs performed the operation himself, this fact was documented in the case history with the remark "fecit Hofrath".[1207] This peculiarity actually creates the possibility of selecting from the mass of existing preparations those that are directly linked to Ernst Fuchs's activities as a surgeon.

The histological processing of the preparations was not necessarily done by Fuchs himself, and occasionally a considerable length of time elapsed after the operation before it was done. This, too, is meticulously documented in the logbooks of the collection. The last time Ernst Fuchs is mentioned by name in the logbooks – he had successfully requested to be allowed to retire in 1915[1208] – is four years after that date, together with Ludwig J. K. von Sallmann (1892–1975),[1209] on October 20, 1919.[1210] On that day Fuchs worked on altogether eleven histological preparations together with assistants and other staff members in what was now the clinic of his successor (and brother-in-law) Friedrich Dimmer.[1211, 1212] His retirement made no difference to the high esteem accorded to Fuchs's collaboration.

Fuchs used a custom made portable wooden case to facilitate the transport of any greater number of histological preparations whenever he needed them for work during vacations or for lectures he gave during his many trips abroad.

1	Development
1a	Congenital anomalies
2	Normal eyes
3	Conjunctiva
4	(missing)
5	Conjunctiva
6	Sclera

6a	Traumatic and secondary scleritis
7	Sclera
8	Sclera
9	Normal cornea
10	Foremost layers of the cornea
10a	Pannus

11	Corneal ulcers
12	Corneal ulcers
13	Ulcus corneae serpens
14	Corneal ulcers
15	Keratitis
16	Corneal wounds fresh
17	Corneal scars after injury
18	Corneal scars without iridencleisis
19	Corneal scars after ulceration with iridencleisis
20	Abnormal corneal scars
21	Abnormal corneal scars
22	Posterior layers of the cornea
23	Staphyloma corneae
23a	Myopia
24	Iris
25	Chamber
26	Iridocyclitis
27	Iridocyclitis
28	Endophthalmitis recens
29	Endophthalmitis recens
29a	Iridocyclitis traumatica
30	Exitus iridocyclitidis
31	Exitus iridocyclitidis
32	Phthisis b[ulbi]
33	Iridocyclitis
34	Ophthalmia sympathica
35	O[phthalmia] sympathica
36	Traumata

37	Iris surgery
38	Proliferation of the ciliar[y] epithelium
39	Epithelium lining of the chamber
40	(Missing)
41	Normal chorioidea
41a	Tissue on chorioidea
42	Chorioiditis recens
43	Chorioiditis obsoleta
44	Detachment
45	Detachment
45a	Chorioidea
46	Sarcoma chorioideae
47	Sarcoma chorioideae
48	Sarcoma chorioideae
49	Glaucoma
50	Glaucoma secundarium
51	Vitreous body
52	Lens
53	Cataracta traumatica
54	Extraction
55	Retina normal
55a	Anterior margin of the retina
56	Retina
57	Retinitis
58	Atrophia ret[inae] without pigment
59	Retina
60	Ablatio retinae

61	Retina	67	Eyelids
62	Opticus	68	Eyelids
63	Neuritis in […]	69	Lacrimal gland
64	Neuritis	70	(Missing)
65	Atrophia n[ervi] o[ptici] after […]	71	Orbita
66	Opticus	72	Orbita

Table 4: Ernst Fuchs's collection of histological preparations. Authentic arrangement according to Ernst Fuchs's own labelling on the outside of the wooden boxes and the order and sequence he gave to the collection.

Notes

885 See FUCHS, *Augenarzt* (as in FN 2), p. 101. – In his 1946 edition of his father's autobiography, Adalbert Fuchs noted that *"my father left behind 15 volumes of these records"*. As is the case with many others of Ernst Fuchs's scientific papers, the whereabouts of these volumes are now unknown. CF. FN 1683.

886 In Ernst Fuchs's original typescript, the passage read quite correctly *"Keratitis marginalis superficialis und profunda"*. Cf. Typoskript, Family archive, p. 50.

887 FUCHS, as in FN 885.

888 Ibid.

889 George E. ARRINGTON, *A History of Ophthalmology*. MD Publications, Inc., New York 1959, p. 100.

890 Carl Zeiss (1816–1888). Originally from Weimar. 1834–1838 Apprenticed to a mechanic; studied at Jena Univ. His interest in mechanical engineering led him to lead a journeyman's life until 1845 [Stuttgart, Darmstadt, Vienna (1843), Berlin)]. Guest student at Vienna's Polytechn. Institut in mechanics with diploma. Back in Jena, his friendship with Jena botanist Matthias Jacob Schleiden (1804–1881) resulted in the construction of his first opt. instruments and microscopes. 1846 Established his own workshop in Jena. 1860 Appointed mechanic to Jena Univ. and awarded the venia legendi. Collaboration with physician Ernst Abbe (1840–1905) led to the improvement of simple microscopes and the manufacture of more complex models using a new production technique based on the mathematical calculation of objectives. 1880 Dr. phil. h. c. (Univ. Jena). See Rüdiger STOLZ, Joachim WITTIG, Günter SCHMIDT, *Carl Zeiss und Ernst Abbe: Leben, Wirken und Bedeutung*. Universitätsverlag, Jena 1993.

891 See S. CZAPSKI, "Mittheilungen aus der Werkstatt von Carl Zeiss in Jena", in: *Zeitschr. f. wissenschaftl. Mikroskopie u. mikroskop. Technik* 4 (1887), pp. 289–292; Carl ZEISS Optische Werkstätte Jena. *Mikroskope und mikroskopische Hilfsapparate.*

No. 28, Jena 1889, p. 35, Fig. 12. – The 1902 Zeiss sales catalogue comprises a detailed description of this model: *Medium-size* Stative [= microscopes, T/N]. *Medium-size* Stative [...] *feature the ABBE illumination apparatus. The upper part can be tilted until the lens barrel is in a horizontal position; only available with the older form of fine adjustment. Rough adjustment is achieved by rack and pinion. The draw-tube moves inside a sleeve. The distance between the object table and the sleeve-like foot is somewhat shorter than in the larger* Stativen *so that some of the* [...] *illumination apparatuses can only be used when the upper part is in a tilted or horizontal position.*
Stativ II^{a}. *This* Stativ *features a revolvable hard rubber table with a centring device. The table's diameter is 100 mm.* [...] *This is the only medium-size* Stativ *suitable for observation under polarised light as it features a revolvable object table.* See Carl ZEISS Optische Werkstätte Jena, *Mikroskope und mikroskopische Hilfsapparate*. 32nd issue, Jena 1902, pp. 58–59.

892 Ernst FUCHS, "Zwei Fälle von doppelseitiger Ptosis", in: *Wien. med. Wochenschr.* 39 (1889), Nr. 52; *Wien. klin. Wochenschr.* 2 (1890), p. 13; *Centralbl. prakt. Augenheilk.* 14 (1890), pp. 63–64. (Reports).

893 Wilhelm (Vilmos) Goldzieher (1849–1916). Originally from Kittsee, Burgenland (then in the Hungarian half of the Austro-Hungarian Empire, today Republic of Austria). Studied at the Univ. of Vienna and Heidelberg (Dr. med. 1871, Wien). Ophthalmol. specialis. as assist. under Otto Becker (cf. FN 178) at the Univ. Eye Clinics Heidelberg, Berlin, Prague and Leipzig. 1875 Set up an ophthalmolog. practice in Budapest. 1878 Habilitation (Assoc. Prof. 1895). 1883 Leading eye specialist of the newly established Red Cross Hospital in Pest. 1895 Head physician at the Eye Dept. of the Allg. Krankenh. in Ofen, from 1901 in the same capacity in Pest. See HIRSCHBERG, *Geschichte der Augenheilkunde* (as in FN 18), vol. 15/2 [= Reprint vol. VII), §1260, pp. 459–468; PAGEL (as in FN 13).

894 Wilhelm GOLDZIEHER, "Einfachstes Verfahren gegen Ptosis und Entropium spasticum senile", in: *Centralbl. prakt. Augenheilk.* 14 (1890), pp. 34–36.

895 Photinos Panas (1832–1903). Cf. FN 258.

896 Ernst FUCHS, "Ueber isolirte doppelseitige Ptosis", in: *Graefes Archiv* 36/Abtheil. I (1890), pp. 234–259.

897 FUCHS, *Lehrbuch*. 13. Auflage, 1921, p. 180. Cf. FUCHS, *Text-Book* (as in FN 810), p. 656. Cf. *"Fuchs presented a report (1890) on typical 'myopathic' changes in the biopsy of a patient with a circumscribed form of disease (Ptosis myopathica)* [...]", in: J. Michael SCHRÖDER, "Pathologie der Muskulatur", in: W. DOERR, G. SEIFERT, E. UEHLINGER, *Spezielle pathologische Anatomie*. vol. 15. Springer, Berlin/Heidelberg/New York 1982, p. 219.

898 Alexei Ivanovich Pospelow (1846–1921). Studied in Moscow (Dr. med. 1874). 1884 Habil. in Dermatol. (1887 Assoc. Prof.). 1893–1909 Dir. of the new Moscow Clinic for Dermatology and Venereology (1898 Full Prof.). Founder of the Moscow Dermato-Venerol. School. See FISCHER (as in FN 28).

899 Ernst FUCHS, "Ueber Blepharochalasis (Erschlaffung der Lidhaut)", in: *Wien. klin. Wochenschr.* 9 (1896), pp. 109–110.

900 Ibid., p. 110.

901 Ibid.

902 Cf. FN 525.

903 See e.g.: J. R. O. COLLIN, C. BEARD, W. H. STERN, D. SCHOENGARTH, "Blepharochalasis", in: *Brit. J. Ophthalmol.* 63 (1979), pp. 542–546.

904 Georg Joseph BEER, *Lehre von den Augenkrankheiten, als Leitfaden zu seinen öffentlichen Vorlesungen entworfen.* Zweyter Band. Heubner und Volke, Vienna 1817, § 94, pp. 109–111.

905 See Ch. 8.

906 Gaetano Lodato (d.1936). 1893 Graduation from Palermo Univ.; assistant at the city's Eye Clinic. 1906 Prof. of Ophthalmol. at Siena. 1909 Return to Palermo as Dir. of the Univ. Eye Clinic. See Obituary, in: *Am. J. Ophthalmol.* 20 (1937), p. 205 (Melchiore Lombardo); Gaetano LODATO, "Blefarocalasi. Contribuito clinico ed anatomico-patologico", in: *Archivio d'ottalmologia* [*Arch. Ottalmol.*] (1903), offprint.

907 Erasmo Scimemi (1852–1935). Prof. of Ophthalm. at the Univ. of Cagliari (1880–1890) and Messina (1890–1908). See HIRSCHBERG, *Geschichte der Augenheilkunde* (as in FN 18), vol. 14/5 [= Reprint, vol. IV, Georg Olms, Hildesheim/New York 1977, § 735, p. 85 and § 738, p. 104; Erasmo SCIMEMI, "Dermatolisia palpebrale (Blefarocalasi di Fuchs)", in: *Bollettino della Società tra i Cultori delle Scienze Mediche e Naturali* [= *Boll. Soc. Cult. Sci, Med. Nat.*], Cagliari, No. 4 (1907), offprint.

908 Casey Albert Wood (1856–1942). Originally from Canada. Graduate of Bishop's College, Montreal (Master of Surgery, M. D. 1877). From 1886 special. in ophthalmol. and otol. in New York and at various eye clinics in Europe. 1889 Set up a practice in Chicago. Prof. of Ophthalm. at the Chicago Post-Graduate Med. School and at Northwestern Univ. After WW I he concerned himself with the comparative study of the visual apparatus of animals. He then took up residence in the Vatican, where he translated Latin works on ophthalm. See: Obituaries, in: *Arch. Ophthalmol.* 27/4 (1942), pp. 779–781 (Frank Brawley); *Brit. J. Ophthalmol.* 26/6 (1942), p. 287.

909 See (Ed.), Casey A. WOOD, "Blepharochalasis", in: *The American Encyclopedia and Directory of Ophthalmology*. Vol. II – B to Cataract, Incipient. Cleveland Press, Chicago 1913, pp. 1033–38.

910 W. B. LAFFER, "Blepharochalasis. Report of a case of this trophoneurosis, involving also the upper lip", in: *Cleveland Med. J.* 8 (1909), pp. 131–135.

911 Karl Wolfgang Ascher (1887–1971). Originally from Prague. 1911 Graduation from Prague Univ. (Dr. med.) Ophthalmolog. special. at the Univ. of Strasbourg and Prague (Elschnig). 1922 Habilitation in Prague (1937 Assoc. Prof.). Active at the Prague hospital of the Barmherz. Brüder. After the establishment of the Protectorate of Bohemia and Moravia by the Nazis in March 1939, emigration first to Great Britain and in August 1939 to the United States. Research associate at the Eye Clinic of the Univ. of Cincinnati until 1947. Teacher at the university's College of Medicine (1949 Assist. Prof., 1952 Assoc. Prof.) until 1962. See IBBO (as in FN 18); Obituaries: *Transact. Am. Ophthalmol. Soc.* 69 (1971), pp. 5–9; *Am. J. Ophthalmol.* 73 (1972), p. 140; *Klin. Monatsbl. Augenheilk.* 101 (1972), pp. 126–128; K. W. ASCHER, "Blepharochalasis mit Struma und Doppellippe", in: *Klin. Monatsbl. Augenheilk.* 65 (1920), pp. 86–97.

912 See www.whonamedit.com (last accessed: 6 Sept. 2022). See also: H. MÜHLENDYCK, M. HUNDEIKER, "Blepharochalasis (Fuchs) und Laffer-Ascher-Syndrom", in: *Hautarzt* 29 (1978), p. 474.

913 On permanent loan to the Sammlungen d. Med. Univ. Wien, cassette 67.

914 Thomas Bateman (1778–1821). First apprenticed to an apothecary, from 1797 med. studies in London under renowned pathologist Matthew Baillie (1761–1823) and others. Pract. training at St. George's Hospital, studied at Edinburgh Univ. from 1798 (Graduation 1801). After his return to London a student of Robert Willan (1757–1812), who did pioneering research on skin diseases. Bateman perfected and expanded Willan's dermatolog. system by introducing eight genera: *A Practical Synopsis of Cutaneous Diseases according to the Arrangement of Dr. Willan, Exhibiting a Concise View of the Diagnostic Symptoms and the Method of Treatment* (1813). He completed the series of water colours begun by Willan. French, German and Italian translations made his doctrines internationally well-known and established him as an authority: Thomas BATEMAN, *Delineations of Cutaneous Diseases: Exhibiting the Characteristic Appearances of the Principal Genera and Species, Comprised in the Classification of Willan, and Completing the Series of Engravings Begun by that Author* (1817). The book also provides a description of herpes iris. See GARRISON/MORTON (as in FN 124); Nick J. NIVELL, "Thomas Bateman (1778–1821)", in: LÖSER/PLEWIG, *Pantheon der Dermatologie* (as in FN 162), pp. 57–66.

915 Ferdinand HEBRA, "Das umschriebene Eczem. Eczema marginatum", in: Rudolf VIRCHOW, *Handbuch der speciellen Pathologie und Therapie*. Abth. I. Ferdinand Enke, Erlangen 1860, pp. 361–363.

916 Cf. FN 163.

917 Ferdinand HEBRA, *Atlas der Hautkrankheiten*. Nach der Natur gemalt von Anton Elfinger. Lithographiert von Carl Heitzmann. 2. Lfg., 6. Tafel. Hof- u. Staatsdruckerei, Vienna 1866, pp. 43–58.

918 Moriz KOHN, "Zur Aetiologie des Erythema multiforme und des Herpes iris sowie zur Frage über die Identität der die Mykosen bedingenden Pilze", in: *Archiv für Dermatologie und Syphilis* [*Arch. Dermatol. Syphilis*] 3 (1871), pp. 381–396. For continuing research on erythema exudativum multiforme, see: a) R. RENDU, "Sur un syndrome caractérisé par l'inflammation simultanée de toutes les muqueuses externes (conjunctivale, nasale, linguale, buccopharyngée, orale et balanopréputiale) coexistant avec une éruption varicelliforme puis purpurique des quatre membres", in: *Revue Générale de Clinique et de Thérapeutique* [= *Rev. Gen. Clin. Ther.*] 30 (1916), pp. 351ff.; b) Noël FIESSINGER, R. RENDU, "Sur un syndrome caractérisé par l'inflammation simultanée de toutes les muqueuses externes coexistant avec une éruption vésiculeuse des quatre membres, non douloureuse et non récidivante", in: *Paris médicale* 25 (1917), pp. 54–58; c) Albert M. STEVENS, Frank C. JOHNSON, "A new eruptive fever associated with stomatitis and ophthalmia: report of two cases in children", in: *American Journal of Diseases of Children* [= *Am. J. Dis. Children*] 24 (1922), pp. 526–533; d) E. BAADER, "Dermatostomatitis", in: *Arch. Dermatol. Syphilis* 149 (1925), pp. 261–268.

919 Ernst FUCHS, "Herpes iris conjunctivae", in: *Klin. Monatsbl. Augenheilk.* 14 (1876), pp. 333–351.

[920] Ibid., p. 348.

[921] Ferdinand Ritter von ARLT, *Klinische Darstellung der Krankheiten des Auges zunächst der Binde-, Horn- und Lederhaut dann der Iris und des Ciliarkörpers*. Wilhelm Braumüller, Vienna 1881, p. 81.

[922] Cf. FN 223.

[923] Otto BERGMEISTER, "Ueber Herpes iris der Conjunctiva", in: *Anzeiger d. k. k. Gesellsch. d. Ärzte* (1883), p. 223; BERGMEISTER, "*Über Konjunktivitis bei Erythema multiforme*", in: *Zeitschr. Augenheilk*. 41, pp. 106ff.

[924] Viktor Hanke (1871–1945). Studied at Vienna Univ. (Dr. med. 1894), 1895–1906 Assist. under Ernst Fuchs at the 2nd Univ. Eye Clinic of the Allgem. Krankenhaus (1904 Habil., 1914 tit. Assoc. Prof, 1920 Assoc. Prof.). 1906–1914 Dir. of the Eye Dept. of the Krankenh. d. Barmherz. Brüder in Vienna. 1911 Dir. of the newly established Eye Dept. at the Kaiser-Franz-Joseph-Spital. 1917–1940 Head physician of the Eye Dept. of the Krankenanstalt Rudolfstiftung. Main areas of interest: bacteriol. of the eye, lesions of the eye. See CZEIKE (as in FN 13); FISCHER (as in FN 28); ÖBL (as in FN 11).

[925] Viktor HANKE, "Der Herpes iris des Auges", in: *Graefes Archiv* 52 (1901), pp. 263–284.

[926] Hans Barkan (1882–1960). Ophthalmol. special. at Harvard Med. School, in Munich and under Fuchs in Vienna (1912/13). Practised in San Francisco in 1914–1954. 1925–1950 Dir. of the Eye Clinic at Stanford Univ. in Francisco. See IBBO (as in FN 18); Obituaries, in: *Am. J. Ophthalmol.* 50 (1960), pp. 185–186 (Frederick Cordes); *Transactions of the American Ophthalmological Society* [*Trans. Am. Ophthalmol. Soc.*] 58 (1960), pp. 7–8 (F. Cordes).

[927] Cf. FN 349.

[928] Hans BARKAN, "Herpes iris of the conjunctiva, with report of a case", in: *Arch. Ophthalmol.* 42 (1913), pp. 236–240.

[929] Ernst FUCHS, *Lehrbuch* (as in FN 787). 1st edition 1889, p. 57.
The simultaneous occurrence on the palms of the hands and the soles of the feet, which Fuchs described in his initial publication, is not mentioned explicitly in the *Lehrbuch*.

[930] Ernst FUCHS, *Lehrbuch* (as in FN 787). 3rd ed.,1893, p. 63.

[931] Ernst FUCHS, *Lehrbuch* (as in FN 787). 5th ed. 1895, p. 100. Cf. FUCHS, Text-Book (as in FN 810), p. 177.

[932] Ernst FUCHS, *Lehrbuch* (as in FN 787). 8th ed. 1900, p. 104. This was to remain the definitive state of affairs in the *Lehrbuch* concerning the exanthem.

[933] Bernfried LEIBER, *Die klinischen Syndrome. Syndrome, Sequenzen und Symptomenkomplexe*. Ed. by G. ADLER, G. BURG, J. KUNZE, D. PONGRATZ, A. SCHINZEL, J. SPRANGER, 8th ed. Urban & Schwarzenberg, Munich/Vienna 1996.

[934] See E. CRAMER, H. KÖLLNER, W. REIS, F. SCHIECK, R.THIEL, *Kurzes Handbuch der Ophthalmologie*. Vol. 4. Julius Springer, Berlin 1931, pp. 153–156.

[935] See F. PHINIZY CALHOUN, "A Classification of Corneal Affections", in: *Am. J. Ophthalmol.* 3/5 (1922), pp. 8–13.

[936] Ernst FUCHS, "Vollständige Sequestration der Cornea nach einfacher Linearextraktion", in: *Klin. Monatsbl. f. Augenheilk.* 18 (1880), pp. 134–139.

937 Ernst FUCHS, "Über Ringabscess der Hornhaut", in: *Graefes Archiv 61* (1903), pp. 1–31.

938 Ibid., p. 1.

939 Ibid., p. 3.

940 Ibid., pp. 22–23.

941 Cf. FN 924.

942 Viktor HANKE, "Zur Aetiologie des Ringabszesses der Kornea", in: *Klin. Monatsbl. Augenheilk.* 42 (1904), pp. 172–173. (Ophthalmol. Gesellsch. in Wien. Bericht v. Doz. Dr. Wintersteiner. 2. Sitzung v. 11. November 1903). See original paper: Viktor HANKE, "Ein bisher unbekannter Bacillus, der Erreger des typischen Ringabszesses der Cornea", in: *Zeitschr. Augenheilk.* 10 (1904), pp. 373ff.

943 For more details, see e.g.: Viktor HANKE, Rudolf TERTSCH, "Einige seltene Infektionen des Auges", in: *Klin. Monatsbl. Augenheilk.* 45 (1907), pp. 545–560; Rudolf TERTSCH, "*Über den Ringabscess der Cornea*", in: *Graefes Archiv* 73/2 (1910), pp. 314–334; Philipp VERDERAME, "*Über Infektionen des Auges durch den Bacillus pyocyaneus*", in: *Centralblatt f. Bakteriologie, Parasitenkunde und Infektionskrankheiten* [= *Centralbl. Bakteriol. Parasitenk. Infektionskrankh.*] 58 (1911), pp. 302–317; Rudolf SCHNEIDER, "Klinisches und Experimentelles zur Infektion mit Pyocyaneus und Bact. fluorescens liq. und zur Ringabszessbildung", in: *Klin. Monatsbl. Augenheilk.* 77/2 (1926), pp. 103–115.

944 H. J. FLIERINGA, "Der Ringabszess in der Hornhaut," in: *Klin. Monatsbl. Augenheilk.* 69/2 (1922), pp. 241–248.

945 Adalbert FUCHS, *Atlas der Histopathologie des Auges.* Franz Deuticke, Leipzig/Vienna 1923, Table 4, Fig. 3 and pp. 7–8.

946 Ernst FUCHS, *Lehrbuch.* 1st ed. 1889, pp. 189–190. See also FUCHS, *Text-Book* (as in FN 810), p. 271.

947 Ernst FUCHS, "Keratitis punctata superficialis", in: *Wien. klin. Wochenschr.* 2 (1889), pp. 837–841.

948 Hans Adler (1843–1923). Studied in Vienna (Dr. med. 1867). Disciple of Ferdinand v. Arlt and Eduard Jaeger v. Jaxtthal. 1872 Eye specialist at the Wiedener Krankenhaus, 1894–1923 Head physician of that hospital's Eye Department, eye specialist at the St. Josephs-Kinderspital and at the K. K. Theresian. Akademie in Vienna (1891–1897). Founder of the Pensionsinstitut and President of the Witwen- u. Waisen-Societät of the Wien. med. Doct.-Coll. See EISENBERG 2 (as in FN 13); HIRSCHBERG, *Geschichte der Augenheilk.* (as in FN 18) (as in FN 18), vol. 15/2, § 1235, pp. 378–379; *Wien. med. Wochenschr.* 44 (1894), col. 1365 (Notiz); Karl Heinz TRAGL, *Chronik der Wiener Krankenanstalten.* Böhlau, Vienna/Cologne/Weimar 2007, p. 230.

949 a) Carl STELLWAG v. CARION, "Ueber eine eigenthümliche Form der Hornhautentzündung", in: *Wien. klin. Wochenschr.* 2 (1889), pp. 613–614; b) August R. v. REUSS, "Keratitis maculosa," in: Ibid., pp. 665 –666; c) Hans ADLER, "Ueber Keratitis subepithelialis centralis", in: Ibid., pp. 713–714, and *Centralbl. prakt. Augenheilk.* 1889, p. 289 and 321. See L. ROSENZWEIG, "Zwei Fälle von Keratitis punctata nach Influenza", in: *Centralbl. prakt. Augenheilk.* May 1890; Jean-Pierre NUEL, "De la kératide punctuée superficielle", in: *Arch. d'Ophtalm.* 14 (1894), pp. 145ff.;

Toshima KURAWA, "Ueber eine eigenthümliche Art von Keratitis superficialis punctata nach Influenza", in: *Centralbl. prakt. Augenheilk.* Sept. 1902; Eugen WEHRLI, "Zur Histologie der Keratitis punctata superficialis (FUCHS), Keratitis subepithelialis (ADLER)", in: *Klin. Monatsbl. Augenheilk.* 44, II (1906), pp. 224ff.; Leonard KOEPPE, "Keratitis epithelialis punctata", in: *Graefes Archiv* 95 (1917), pp. 250ff.
Stellwag's description deviated so much from Fuchs's own that the latter expressed doubts whether the two descriptions referred to the same disease. (cf. FN 947, p. 841).

950 Ernst FUCHS, "Keratitis punctata superficialis" (as in FN 947), p. 840.

951 Ibid., p. 837.

952 Ibid.

953 Ibid., p. 840.

954 Ibid.

955 This is a reference to the terminology proposed by Reuss and Adler. Cf. FN 949b and 949c.

956 Ernst FUCHS, "Keratitis punctata superficialis" (as in FN 947), p. 841. For a change, and as an exception to the rule stated earlier, Fuchs does make a priority claim here.

957 To honour the first President of the Ophthalmol. Society of the United Kingdom, the renowned ophthalmologist William Bowman (cf. FN 299), the Society, which was founded in 1880, instituted in 1883 the *Bowman Lecture*. See (Ed.), "Ophthalmological Society of the United Kingdom. Brief History of the Society", in: *Annals of the Royal College of Surgeons of England* [*Ann. R. Coll. Surg. Engl.*] 56 (1975), pp. 52–53.

958 Ernst FUCHS, "On Keratitis. Being the Bowman Lecture". Delivered on June 13, 1902, in: *Transactions of the Ophthalmological Society of the United Kingdom* [*Transact. Ophthalmol. Soc. United Kingdom*] 22 (1902), pp. 15–34. (here: pp. 16–17).

959 FUCHS, *Lehrbuch* (as in FN 787). 12th ed. 1910, pp. 284–285.

960 Cf. FN 45.

961 FUCHS, *Lehrbuch* (as in FN 787). 13th ed. 1921, p. 354.

962 FUCHS, *Lehrbuch* (as in FN 787). 15th ed. 1926, p. 354.

963 FUCHS, *Lehrbuch* (as in FN 787). 18th ed. 1945, p. 232.

964 For Jakob Hock, cf. FN 446. Fuchs is referring to keratitis interstitialis punctiformis specifica as described by Hock (Cf. Wiener Klinik 1876).

965 For Ludwig Mauthner, cf. FN 200. Fuchs is referring to the inflammation of the cornea described by Mauthner under the name *keratitis punctata*. See the section on the manifestations of syphilis in the eye Mauthner contributed to Hermann ZEISSL, *Grundriss der Pathologie und Therapie der Syphilis und der mit dieser verwandten venerischen Krankheiten.* Ferdinand Enke, Stuttgart 1876. On syphil. keratitis parenchymatosa, Mauthner writes: *"A genuine keratitis punctata, which is characterised by the formation of inconspicuous specks the size of a pinhead in various layers of the substantia propria corneae, is possibly linked more intimately to syphilis, but it is so phenomenally rare that it is enough to have mentioned it."* (p. 258). This has led to the disease being referred to in the literature as keratitis punctata profunda (syphilitica) MAUTHNER. See e.g.: CRAMER et al: *Kurzes Handbuch der Ophthalmologie*, as in FN 934, pp. 337–338; Josef IGERSHEIMER, *Syphilis u. Auge.* Springer, Berlin/Heidelberg 1918, p. 183 and p. 227; O. H. BAUMERT, "Zur Kenntnis der Keratitis punctata profunda Mauthner", in: *Klin. Monatsbl. Augenheilk.* 79 (1927), pp. 782ff.

966 Fuchs seems to be referring to a paper by Purtscher in: *Bolletino di Oculistica* [*Boll. Ocul.*] 7 (1884), p. 237. The efforts of the author of the present work to get hold of this paper have been to no avail. – Othmar Purtscher (1852–1927). Assist. under Ferdinand v. Arlt, disciple of Mauthner. 1887 Establishment of a prov. Eye Dept. in Klagenfurt (1897 tenure), Head physician until 1922, followed by his son Adolf Purtscher (1882–1976). Contributed significantly to lowering the number of people going blind in Carinthia. He coined the term *angiopathia retinae traumatica* (Othmar PURTSCHER, "Angiopathia retinae traumatica, Lymphorrhagien des Augengrundes", in: *Graefes Archiv* 82 (1912), pp. 347–371). See FISCHER (as in FN 28); HIRSCHBERG, *Geschichte der Augenheilkunde* (as in FN 18), vol. 15/2 [= Reprint vol. VI, §1258, pp. 443–445; LESKY, *Wien. Med. Schule* (as in FN 12), p. 226, FN 30 and pp. 485–486.; Othmar PURTSCHER, *Erinnerungen aus meinem Berufsleben*. Artur Kollitsch, Klagenfurt 1926; Obituaries: *Wien. med. Wochenschr.* 77 (1927), col. 1760; *Zeitschr. Augenheilk.* 64 (1928), pp. 346–347 (Josef Meller); *Klin. Monatsbl. Augenheilk.* 80 (1928), pp. 99–100 (Richard Krämer); Karl LISCH, "Beziehungen von Othmar Purtscher zu Julius Hirschberg und zur Reform der Augenheilkunde", in: *Spektrum Augenheilk.* 1 (1988), pp. 157–159.

967 FUCHS, *Lehrbuch* (as in FN 787). 1st ed. 1889, pp. 196–197. See also FUCHS, *Text-Book* (as in FN 810), p. 271.

968 FUCHS, *Lehrbuch* (as in FN 787). 13th ed. 1921, p. 369.

969 FUCHS, *Lehrbuch* (as in FN 787). 16th ed. 1939; 17th ed. 1944; 18th ed. 1945.

970 Ferdinand R. v. ARLT, *Klinische Darstellung der Krankheiten des Auges zunächst der Binde-, Horn-, und Lederhaut, dann der Iris und des Ciliarkörpers*. Wilhelm Braumüller, Vienna 1881.

971 FUCHS, *Lehrbuch* (as in FN 787). 1st ed. 1889, p. 204.

972 FUCHS, *Lehrbuch*. 3rd ed. 1893, p. 127.

973 Ibid., pp 174–175. See also FUCHS, *Text-Book* (as in FN 810), pp. 248–249.

974 FUCHS, *Lehrbuch*. 3rd ed. 1893, p. 211. The frequent mention of Keratitis marginalis (superficialis) in the 3rd edition of the *Lehrbuch* may be the reason why 1893 is sometimes cited in the literature as the year of Fuchs's initial description of the disease. See www.whonamedit.com (last accessed: 6 Sept. 2022).

975 FUCHS, *Lehrbuch*. 7th ed. 1898, p. 178.

976 See e.g.: J. R. BIERLY, J. P. DUNN, C. R. DAWSON, H. B. OSTLER, I. G. WONG, "Fuchs's superficial marginal keratitis", in: *Am. J. Ophthalmol.* 113/5 (1992), pp. 541–545; Harilaos S. BRILAKIS, Michael L. NORDLUND, Edward J. HOLLAND, "Recurrence of Fuchs's Marginal Keratitis Within a Graft", in: *Cornea* 23/6 (2004), pp. 639–640.

977 FUCHS, *Lehrbuch*, 2nd ed. 1891, pp. 205–206.

978 Ernst FUCHS, "Ueber das Pterygium", in: *Graefes Archiv* 38/II (1892), pp. 1–90.

979 FUCHS, *Lehrbuch*. 13th ed. 1921, p. 355. Cf. FUCHS, *Diseases of the Eye* (as in FN 812), p. 186.

980 FUCHS, *Lehrbuch*. 1st ed. 1889, p. 160. Cf. FUCHS, *Text-Book* (as in FN 810), p. 241.

981 Ernst FUCHS, "*Über Aufhellung von Hornhautnarben*", in: Richard DEUTSCHMANN (Ed.), *Beiträge zur Augenheilkunde*. IX. Heft, Leopold Voss, Hamburg/Leipzig 1893, pp. 1–11.

[982] Ibid., pp. 3–4.
[983] Ibid., p. 8.
[984] Ibid., p. 10.
[985] Ibid., p. 11.
[986] FUCHS, *Lehrbuch*. 5th ed. 1895, p. 225. Cf. FUCHS, *Diseases of the Eye* (as in FN 812), p. 216.
[987] FUCHS, *Lehrbuch*. 7th ed. 1898, p. 229. Cf. FUCHS, *Diseases of the Eye* (as in FN 812), p. 216.
[988] FUCHS, *Lehrbuch*. 12th ed. 1910, p. 320. The same illustration was retained in all subsequent German editions, including the last one, see: FUCHS, *Lehrbuch*. 18th ed. 1945, p. 263, Fig. 95: *Hornhautnarbe mit Aufhellungsstreifen*.
[989] FUCHS, "Ueber das Pterygium", cf. FN 978.
[990] See the section on keratitis marginalis superficialis.
[991] Cf. FN 978, pp. 70–72.
[992] Ernst FUCHS, "Erkrankung der Hornhaut durch Schädigung von hinten", in: *Graefes Archiv* 92 (1916), pp. 145–236.
[993] Ernst FUCHS, "Ueber Randsklerose und Randatrophie der Hornhaut," in: *Graefes Archiv* 52 (1901), pp. 317– 329 (here: p. 329).
[994] Ernst FUCHS, "Über Dellen in der Hornhaut", in: *Graefes Archiv* 78 (1911), pp. 82–92.
[995] Ibid., p. 82.
[996] FUCHS, *Lehrbuch* (as in FN 787), 13th ed., p. 389.
[997] Adalbert FUCHS, "Pathological Dimples ('Dellen') of the Cornea", in: *Americ. J. Ophthalmol.* 12 (1929), pp. 877–883.
[998] See e.g.: J. G. LINDBERG, "Zwei Fälle von sogenannten 'Dellen' in der Hornhaut," in: *Acta Ophthalmol.* 9 (1931), pp. 88–93.
[999] Peter WALTER, Niklas PLANGE, *Basiswissen Augenheilkunde*. Springer, Berlin/Heidelberg 2017, p. 183.
[1000] Adolf Vossius (1855–1925). Originally from West Prussia. Studied at the Univ. of Königsberg (today Kaliningrad/Russian Federation). Dr. med. 1878. 1879–1881 Assist. at the Eye Clinic of Gießen Univ.; 1882 Habilitation at the Univ. Eye Clinic in Königsberg (1887 Assoc. Prof.). After the death of Julius Jacobson (1828–1889) Deputy Dir. of the Clinic in the winter semester of 1889/90. 1890–1923 Full Prof. and Dir. of the Univ. Eye Clinic Gießen, which was rebuilt from scratch at his instigation and inaugurated in 1907. He is credited with the first description of keratitis interstitialis centralis annularis and the Vossius ring (1906). See EULNER (as in FN 13); FISCHER (as in FN 28); HIRSCHBERG, *Geschichte der Augenheilkunde* (as in FN 18), vol. 15/2 [= Reprint vol. VI], § 1200, pp. 295–296; IBBO (as in FN 18); PAGEL (as in FN 13).
[1001] Ernst FUCHS, "Ueber ringförmige und scheibenförmige Keratitis (Keratitis annularis et disciformis)", in: *Klin. Monatsbl. Augenheilk.* 39 (1901), pp. 513–523 (here: pp. 515–516).
[1002] Ernst FUCHS, *Lehrbuch* (as in FN 787), 9th ed. 1903, p. 199.
[1003] Eïsaburo Hadano (a.k.a Eizaburo Hatano), originally from Kazusa in Japan, graduated in 1903 from Rostock Univ. Rostock with his thesis "*Über die Behandlung von Hornhauterkrankungen mit dem scharfen Löffel*". Later Dir. of the Eye Dept. of the

Military Hospital in Hiroshima. See http://matrikel.uni-rostock.de/periode/1902WS (last accessed: 6 Sept. 2022); *Jahresverzeichnis der an den deutschen Universitäten erschienenen Schriften XVIII. 15. August 1902 bis 14. August 1903*. A. Asher & Co., Berlin 1903, p. 353; MISHIMA, *History of Ophthalmology in Japan* (as in FN 838), pp. 296–297.

1004 Eïsaburo HADANO, "Beitrag zur Kenntnis der Keratitis disciformis", in: *Zeitschr. Augenheilk.* 10 (1903), pp. 500–504.

1005 Albert Peters (1862–1938). Studied at the Univ. of Bonn, Berlin, Tübingen. Dr. med. 1885. 1886–1888 Junior doctor at the University Eye Clinic in Bonn. Set up his own practice. 1882 Habilitation, 1898 tit. Assoc Prof. at Bonn Univ.; 1901–1933 Full Prof. and Dir. of the University Eye Clinic Rostock. 1906/07 and 1914/15 Dean of the Med. Fac, 1915/16 Rector. See EULNER (as in FN 13); FISCHER (as in FN 28); HIRSCHBERG, *Geschichte der Augenheilkunde* (as in FN 18), vol. 15/2 [= Reprint vol. VI], § 1132, p. 143; PAGEL (as in FN 13).

1006 Albert PETERS, "Über traumatische Hornhauterkrankungen (Erosionen, Keratitis disciformis und Ulcus serpens) und ihre Beziehungen zum Herpes corneae", in: *Graefes Archiv* 57 (1904), pp. 93–137.

1007 Ibid., p. 94.

1008 Otto Schirmer (1864–1917). Son of ophthalmol. Rudolf Schirmer (1831–1896). Studied at the Univ. of Munich, Freiburg and Greifswald (Dr. med. 1886). 1889 Habilitation in Ophthalmology at Göttingen Univ. 1896–1907 Successor of his father at Greifswald Univ., then Full Prof. and Dir. of the Clinic at the Univ. of Kiel (1907) and Strasbourg (1907–1909). Developed the eponymous Schirmer test, a method used to measure the eye's lacrimal secretion with absorbent paper. 1909 Emigration to New York. See EULNER (as in FN 13); FISCHER (as in FN 28); HIRSCHBERG, *Geschichte der Augenheilkunde* (as in FN 18), vol. 15/2 [= Reprint vol. VI], § 1130, p. 139.

1009 Otto SCHIRMER, "Keratitis disciformis und Keratitis postvaccinolosa", in: *Graefes Archiv* 59 (1904), pp. 133ff.

1010 Albert PETERS, "Zur Frage der Keratitis disciformis", in: *Klin. Monatsbl. Augenheilk.* 43/II (1905), pp. 535ff.

1011 Josef MELLER, "Die histologischen Veränderungen des Auges bei der Keratitis disciformis", in: *Klin. Monatsbl. Augenheilk.* 43 (1905), pp. 335–352.

1012 Martin BARTELS, *Beiträge zur pathologischen Anatomie der Keratitis disciformis.* Inaugural-Diss., Univ. Rostock 1907.

1013 FUCHS, *Lehrbuch* (as in FN 787), 13th ed. 1921, p. 342.

1014 See Ch. 9.

1015 Paul Junius (1871–1948). Studied at Königsberg Univ. (Dr. med. 1895). 1913 Habilitation in Ophthalmol. at Bonn Univ. (Assoc. Prof. 1921). Collaborated with Dir. of Clinic Hermann Kuhnt (1850–1937) in innovative research on congenital macula degeneration. See FISCHER (as in FN 28); Suzan HUNT, "Leben und Werk von Hermann Kuhnt (1850–1937) und Paul Junius (1871–1948)", in: *Klin. Monatsbl. Augenheilk.* 224/8 (2007), pp. 678–682.

1016 Edwin Theodor Saemisch (1833–1909). Studied at Berlin Univ. (Dr. med. 1858), then assistant under Albrecht v. Graefe in Berlin and Alexander Pagenstecher (1828–1879) in Wiesbaden. 1862 Habilitation at Bonn Univ. (1867 Assoc. Prof.,

Dir. of the Univ. Eye Clinic. 1873 Full Prof.). The first edition of his epoch-making *Handbuch der gesammten Augenheilkunde* was published in seven volumes in 1874–1880, co-edited by Alfred Graefe (1830–1899). The second edition (from 1899) ran to 15 vols, incl. *Die Geschichte der Augenheilkunde* (vols. 12–15) by Julius Hirschberg. See EULNER (as in FN 28); HIRSCHBERG, *Geschichte der Augenheilkunde* (as in FN 18), vol. 15/2 [= Reprint vol. VI], § 1203, pp. 301–302; IBBO (as in FN 18); PAGEL (as in FN 13); Obituaries: *Centralbl. f. Augenheilk.*; Jan. 1910 (J. Hirschberg); *Klin. Monatsbl. Augenheilk.* 48 (1910), p. 86 (Zur Nedden); *Archiv Augenheilk.* 45 (1910), p. 268; *Zeitschr. Augenheilk.* 23 (1910), p. 90.

1017 Paul JUNIUS, "Über Keratitis disciformis. Ein Beitrag zur Klinik und zur Entstehungsweise der Krankheit", in: Graefes *Archiv* 105 (1921), pp. 177–204. (= Festschrift zur Feier des siebzigsten Geburtstages Herrn Hofrat Prof. Dr. Ernst Fuchs in Wien gewidmet von Freunden und dankbaren Schülern). See the paper Junius presented at the 39th Versammlung d. Rheinisch-Westfälischen Augenärzte on 5 June 1921 in Bonn: Paul JUNIUS, "Zur Frage der Keratitis disciformis", in: *Klin. Monatsbl. Augenheilk.* 67 (1921/2), pp. 110–112 (Minutes).

1018 Adalbert FUCHS, *Atlas der Histopathologie des Auges* (as in FN 945). Pl. 8, Fig. 1 and p. 13.

1019 Ernst FUCHS, "Ueber Randsklerose und Randatrophie der Hornhaut"; in: *Graefes Archiv* 52 (1901), pp. 317– 329 (here: pp. 317–320).

1020 A preliminary phase of the Fuchs furrow is a shallow dimple in the corneal epithelium near the limbus, which is described as a *"mostly senile change or the consequence of a dystrophy in the sclera (e.g. after episcleritis or a cataract operation)".* See *Reallexikon der Medizin und ihrer Grenzgebiete.* 3rd vol., Urban & Schwarzenberg, Munich/Berlin/Vienna 1969, F 210.

1021 See FUCHS, as in FN 993, pp. 325–326.

1022 Ernst FUCHS, "Über senile Randatrophie der Hornhaut", in: *Graefes Archiv* 89 (1915), pp. 386–392.

1023 Ibid., pp. 391–392.

1024 Ernst FUCHS, "Das Ulcus atheromatosum corneae (sequestrirende Narbenkeratitis)", in: *Graefes Archiv* 53 (1901), pp. 61–73 (here: pp. 71–72).

1025 Arthur Groenouw (1862–1945). Originally from a place near Ratibor (today Razibórz/Poland). Studied at the Univ. of Breslau/Wroclaw (Dr. med. 1886), 1887–1896 Assist. at the Breslau Eye Clinic under Carl Friedrich Richard Förster (cf. FN 263) and his successor Wilhelm Uhthoff (1853–1927). 1892 Habilitation, 1899 tit. Assoc. Prof. See FISCHER (as in FN 28); HIRSCHBERG, *Geschichte der Augenheilkunde* (as in FN 18), vol. 15/2 [= Reprint vol. VI], § 1144, p. 176; IBBO (as in FN 18); PAGEL (as in FN 13); Arthur GROENOW, "Knötchenförmige Hornhauttrübungen (Noduli corneae)", in: *Graefes Archiv* 21 (1890), pp. 281–289, GROENOW., "Knötchenförmige Hornhauttrübungen", in: *Graefes Archiv* 46 (1898), pp. 85–102.

1026 Ernst FUCHS, "Ueber knötchenförmige Hornhauttrübung", in: *Graefes Archiv* 53 (1902), pp. 423–438.

1027 Ibid., pp. 428–430.

1028 Ibid., pp. 432–433.

1029 Ibid., p. 434.

[1030] John GREEN, "Nodular Opacity of the Cornea with Special Reference to Its Etiology", in: *J. Am. Med. Assoc.* 53 (1909), pp. 151ff.

[1031] Ernst FUCHS, "Über knötchenförmige Hornhauttrübung", in: *Graefes Archiv* 89 (1915), p. 337–349.

[1032] Ernst FUCHS, "Dystrophia epithelialis corneae", in: *Graefes Archiv* 76 (1910), pp. 478–508 (here: p. 479).

[1033] Ibid., p. 505.

[1034] Ibid., pp. 507–508.

[1035] Arnold KNAPP, "Dystrophia epithelialis corneae (Fuchs), with report of a case", in: *Transact. Am. Ophthalmol. Soc.* 12 (1911), pp. 745–747. (Here: pp. 746–747).

[1036] (Ed.), "Minutes of the Proceedings". Forty-Seventh Annual Meeting. American Ophthalmological Society 1911, in: *Transact. Am. Ophthalmol. Soc.* 12/3 (1911), pp. 708–717.

[1037] See Ch. 11.

[1038] Ernst Kraupa (1884–1945). Studied at the German Univ. of Prague (Dr. med. univ. 1908). 1911–1914 Assist. at the Eye Clinic of the German Univ. of Prague, 1914–1940 Ophthalmologist in Brno. 1945 Murdered in the Terezín concentration camp. See Kal MENŠ, *MUDr. (Arnošt) Ernst Kraupa*, in: Encyklopedie dějin města Brna (Internet version, last accessed: 12 Aug. 2020).

[1039] Ernst KRAUPA, "Pigmentierungen der Hornhauthinterfläche bei 'Dystrophia epithelialis' (Fuchs)", in: *Zeitschr. Augenheilk.* 44 (1920), pp. 247–250.

[1040] FUCHS, *Lehrbuch* (as in FN 787), 13th ed. 1921, p. 383.

[1041] Allvar GULLSTRAND, "Demonstration der Nernst-Spaltlampe", in: *Bericht über die Siebenunddreissigste Versammlung der Ophthalmologischen Gesellschaft Heidelberg*, Bergmann, Wiesbaden 1911, pp. 374–376.

[1042] Allvar Gullstrand (1862–1930). 1891 Habil. in Ophthalmol. at the Karolinska Institutet in Stockholm, 1894 Prof. at the Univ. Uppsala; 1903 Establishment of the Univ. Eye Clinic. Pioneering research on ophthalmol. dioptics, numerous opto-technological innovations; 1911 Nobel Prize. See FISCHER (as in FN 28); GARRISON/MORTON (as in FN 124); GERABEK et al. (as in FN 13); IBBO (as in FN 18); Obituaries, in: *Deutsche Optische Wochenschrift* [*Dt. Opt. Wochenschr.*] 16 (1930), pp. 546–548 (Shozo Hashimoto); *Zeitschrift für ophthalmologische Optik* [= *Zeitschr. ophthalmol. Optik*] 18 (1930), pp. 129–134 (Moritz v. Rohr); *Zeitschr. Augenheilk.* 73 (1931), pp. 326–330 (Heinrich Erggelet); Appreciation: Richard KEELER, "Allvar Gullstrand: Dioptrics of the Eye and the Slit Lamp", in: Michael F. MARMOR, Daniel ALBERT (eds.), *Foundations of Ophthalmology. Great Insights that Established the Discipline*. Springer Internat. Publ. 2017, pp. 129–144.

[1043] CRAMER et al., *Kurzes Handbuch der Ophthalmologie* (as in FN 934), p. 391.

[1044] Presentation at a meeting at the Gesellschaft d. Ärzte in Vienna on 15 April 1932: "E. Kraupa (Brno) reports on dystrophies of the corneal epithelium and illustrates this with slides," in: *Med. Klinik*, 20 April 1932, p. 567.

[1045] Otto BRUCHHÄUSER, *Betrachtungen über Dystrophia epithelialis Corneä.* Med. Diss. Univ. Gießen 1937, p. 3.

[1046] The disease and its identification with the name of Fuchs, who had been the first to describe it, have become so firmly established in the Anglo-American world that in popular discussions and patient forums they are simply referred to as "Fuchs' dystrophy". The publication of information material to facilitate an early diagnosis and to alert patients suffering from the condition is an ongoing process. The eponym ensures that the memory of Ernst Fuchs's achievement is kept alive. See e.g.: James N. PARKER, Philip M. PARKER (eds.), *The Official Patient's Sourcebook on FUCHS'S DYSTROPHY. A Reference Manual for Self-Directed Patient Research*. ICON Group International, Inc., San Diego 2002.

[1047] Ernst FUCHS, "Über Keratitis pustuliformis profunda", in: *Graefes Archiv* 90 (1915), pp. 13–75.

[1048] FUCHS, *Lehrbuch* (as in FN 787), 13th ed. 1921, p. 370.

[1049] Cf. FN 45.

[1050] FUCHS, *Lehrbuch* (as in FN 787), 13th ed. 1921, pp. 370–371. Cf. FUCHS, *Diseases of the Eye* (as in FN 812), pp. 198–199.

[1051] Adalbert FUCHS, "Über einige seltene luetische Erkrankungen des Auges", in: *Zeitschr. Augenheilk.* 8 (1926), pp. 315–342.

[1052] FUCHS, *Lehrbuch*, 18th ed. 1945, p. 246.

[1053] Rudolf SCHNEIDER, "Zur Keratitis pustuliformis profunda", in: *Klin. Monatsbl.* Augenheilk. 69 (1922), pp. 238–241.

[1054] Josef Igersheimer (1879–1965). Originally from Frankfurt/Main. Studied at the Univ. of Heidelberg, Munich, Berlin, Strasbourg and Tübingen (Dr. med. 1904). 1906 1st Assist. at the University Eye Clinic at Heidelberg. Moved on together with the Dir. of the Clinic, Eugen v. Hippel (1867–1939) to the University Eye Clinic at Halle/Saale (1910 Habilitation). 1914 Followed Hippel to Göttingen Univ. (1915 tit. Assoc. Prof., 1920 Assoc. Prof.). 1925 Dir. of the Dept. of Ophthalm. at the Univ. Hospital (later Univ. Clinic) of his hometown Frankfurt. 1933 Deprived by the Nazis of his venia legendi on account of his Jewish descent, he emigrated first to Turkey (Dir. of the University Eye Clinic Istanbul) and, in 1939, to the United States (Assoc. Prof. at the Tufts Med. School/Boston). 1945 US citizenship. Main areas of interest: research on infectious diseases and their manifestations in the eye, such a tuberculosis and syphilis, a disease to which he devoted a comprehensive monograph in 1918 (cf. FN 965). He was the first ophthalmologist to use Salvarsan (E 606) for the therapy of syphilis, an antiluetic first prescribed by Paul Ehrlich (1854–1915). He was also the first German ophthalmolog. to use the method developed by Jules Gonin (1870–1935) for the treatment of retinal detachment by transfixing the break by cauterization. See Obituary, in: *Trans. Am. Ophthalmol. Soc.* 64 (1966), pp. 7–8 (Albert E. Sloane); Appreciation: Arin NAMAL, Arnold REISMAN, "Joseph Igersheimer (1879–1965): a visionary ophthalmologist and his contributions before and after exile", in: *Journal of Medical Biography* [*J. Med. Biogr.*] 15/4 (2007), pp. 227–234.

[1055] See IGERSHEIMER, *Syphilis und Auge* (as in FN 965), p. 175.

[1056] Josef MELLER, "Zur Ätiologie der Keratitis pustuliformis profunda", in: *Centralbl. prakt. Augenheilk.* 42 (1918), pp. 1–8.

[1057] Rudolf SCHNEIDER, "Zur Keratitis pustuliformis profunda", in: *Wien. klin. Wochenschr.* 64 (1952), p. 949.

[1058] Ernst FUCHS, "Ueber Episcleritis periodica fugax", in: *Wien. klin. Wochenschr.* 8 (1895), pp. 601–603.

[1059] Ernst FUCHS, "Episcleritis periodica fugax", in: Brit. Med. J., Oct. 19, 1895, pp. 951–953.

[1060] Ernst FUCHS, "Ueber Episcleritis periodica fugax", in: *Graefes Archiv* 41/Abtheil. I (1895), pp. 229–273.

[1061] Ernst FUCHS, "Episcleritis periodica fugax", as in FN 1058, p. 601.

[1062] Ibid., p. 602.

[1063] *Minutes of the Proceedings*. Forty-Seventh Annual Meeting. American Ophthalmological Society 1911, in: *Transact. Am. Ophthalmol. Soc.* 12/3 (1911), pp. 708–717.

[1064] Albert C. SNELL, "Episcleritis periodica fugax", in: *Transact. Am. Ophthalmol. Soc.* 12/3 (1911), pp. 736–745.

[1065] Ernst FUCHS, "Sekundäre Skleritis und Episkleritis", in: *Bericht ueber die vierzigste Versammlung der Ophthalmologischen Gesellschaft Heidelberg 1916*. Bergmann, Wiesbaden 1916, p. 365.

[1066] Ernst FUCHS, "Scleritis posterior", in: *Bericht ueber die dreissigste Versammlung der Ophthalmologischen Gesellschaft Heidelberg 1902*. Bergmann, Wiesbaden 1903, pp. 71–77. (Cited in: CRAMER, KÖLLNER, REIS, SCHIECK, THIEL, *Kurzes Handbuch der Ophthalmologie*. Vol. 4 (as in FN 934), pp. 429–430.

[1067] Ibid.

[1068] See e.g.: Ernst PURTSCHER, "Zur Aetiologie der 'spontanen' Choroidabhebung und der 'serösen Tenonitis'", in: *Zeitschr. Augenheilk.* 94 (1938), pp. 141–151; Peter WATSON, Sohan SINGH HAYREH, "Scleritis and episcleritis", in: *Brit. J. Ophthalmol.* 60 (1976), pp. 163–191.

[1069] Ernst FUCHS, "Beiträge zur normalen Anatomie der menschlichen Iris", in: *Graefes Archiv* 31 (1885) Abtheil. III, pp. 39–86.

[1070] Ernst FUCHS, "Zur Anatomie der Iris", in: *Klin. Monatsbl. Augenheilk.* 23 (1885), pp. 467–478.

[1071] Cf. FN 1069, pp. 41–42.

[1072] Ibid., p. 45.

[1073] Ibid., p. 47.

[1074] Ibid., pp. 52–60.

[1075] Cf. FN 1070, pp. 470–471.

[1076] SALZMANN, *Anatomie und Histologie des menschlichen Augapfels* (as in FN 816).

[1077] Ibid., Dedication.

[1078] Ibid., pp. 147–148.

[1079] Cf. FN 1069, pp. 57–59. A paragraph very similar to the last paragraph in its wording is to be found in Fuchs's article on the anatomy of the iris. Cf. FN 1070, p. 472.

[1080] Cf. FN 1069, p. 59.

[1081] Ibid., pp. 66–67.

[1082] Ibid., pp. 67–68.

[1083] Ibid., p. 69.

[1084] Karl Wilhelm Ludwig Bruch (1819–1884). Originally from Mainz. Studied at the Univ. of Berlin and Gießen (Dr. med. 1842). 1845 Habilitation in Anat. at Heidelberg Univ. Heidelberg under Jakob Henle (cf. FN 1085). 1850 Full Prof. of Anat. and Physiol. at Basel Univ., 1855–1860 in the same function at the Univ. of Gießen. Bruch's membrane is the name given to the lamina basalis of the chorioidea which separates the chorioidea from the retina (first description in 1844). See EULNER (as in FN 28); Claudia ZRENNER, "The Discovery of the Lamina Basalis Choroideae by Carl Wilhelm Ludwig Bruch (1819–1884)", in: *Hist. Ophthal. Intern.* 3 (1984), pp. 213–260.

[1085] Jakob (Jacob) Henle (1809–1885). Studied at the universities of Bonn (disciple of renowned anat. and physiol. Johannes Müller, cf. FN 135) and Heidelberg (Dr. med. 1831). 1834 Prosector under Müller, after the latter had moved from Bonn to Berlin. 1837 Habilitation. 1840–1844 Prof. of Anat. at Zürich Univ.; 1844–1851 Prof. at Heidelberg Univ.; 1852–1885 Full Prof. of Anatomy at Göttingen Univ.; first describer of the goblet cells in the small intestines, of the loop shape of the renal tubules (Henle's loop) and of the fine structure of the cornea. He was the first to realize that the fovea centralis and the macula lutea contained exclusively cone photoreceptors. Pioneering work also in the fields of pathology and microbiology. See EULNER (as in FN 28); GERABEK et al. (as in FN 13); HIRSCH (as in FN 13); IBBO (as in FN 18); NDB (as in FN 15); PAGEL (as in FN 13); DHOM, *Histopathologie* (as in FN 40), pp. 73–80; Friedrich MERKEL, *Jacob Henle: Ein deutsches Gelehrtenleben, nach Aufzeichnungen und Erinnerungen*. Friedrich Vieweg, Braunschweig 1891; Victor ROBINSON, *The Life of Jacob Henle*. Medical Life Company, New York 1921.

[1086] Probably a reference to Alfred Wilhelm Gruenhagen (1842–1912): 1842 Dr. med. Univ. Königsberg, 1868 Habilitation. 1872–1894 Assoc. Prof. of Physics and Dir. of the Med.-Physical. Collection. Cf. PAGEL (as in FN 13).

[1087] Cf. SALZMANN, *Anatomie und Histologie des menschlichen Augapfels* (as in FN 816), p. 149.

[1088] Gustav Schwalbe (1844–1916). Studied at the Univ. of Berlin, Zürich and Bonn (Dr. med. 1866). Histol. studies under Max Schultze (1825–1874) in Bonn. 1870 Habilitation in Anat. at the Univ. of Halle/Saale. 1871 Private lecturer at the Univ. of Freiburg im Breisgau. 1871–1873 Assoc. Prof. at Leipzig Univ. 1873–1881 Full Prof. and Dir. of the Anat. Institute of Jena Univ. 1881–1883 Full Prof. at Königsberg Univ. and 1883–1914 Full Prof. at Strasbourg Univ. (Rector 1893/94). Main areas of interest: microscop. anat. of the sensory organs, anthropolog. studies. See EULNER (as in FN 13); PAGEL (as in FN 13).

[1089] Cf. FN 1069, pp. 62–63. From the vantage point of the present, this refers to the anterior part of the pigment layer of the iris, which comprises the pigmented myoepithel. components of the *m. dilatator pupillae*. Cf. *Reallexikon* (as in FN 1020), F 211.

[1090] Ibid.

[1091] Julius von Michel (1843–1911). Studied at the Univ. of Würzburg and Zürich (Dr. med. Würzburg 1866). 1868–1870 Ophthalmol. training as assist. under Johann Friedrich Horner (1831–1886) at the University Eye Clinic in Zürich. Ophthalmol. and histol. training at Leipzig Univ.; 1872 Habilitation. 1873 Assoc Prof. and founder of the University Eye Clinic in Erlangen (Full Prof. 1874). 1879–1900 Full Prof. at the Würzburg Univ. and in 1900–1911 at Berlin Univ. See EULNER (as in FN 13); HIRSCHBERG, *Geschichte der Augenheilkunde* (as in FN 18), vol. 15/2 [= Reprint vol. VI], §§ 1174–1177, pp. 225–239; IBBO (as in FN 18); PAGEL (as in FN 13).

[1092] While Michel was in Erlangen, he published the monograph *Die histologische Struktur des Irisstromas* (Erlangen 1875), to which Fuchs is presumably referring here. Furthermore, Michel published a comprehensive paper in 1881, "Ueber Iris und Iritis", in: *Graefes Archiv* 27, Abth. II (1881), pp. 171–282.

1093 Cf. FN 1069, p. 71.

1094 SALZMANN, *Anatomie und Histologie des menschlichen Augapfels* (as in FN 816), p. 153.

1095 FUCHS, *Lehrbuch*. 1st ed. 1889, p. 263. Cf. FUCHS, *Text-Book* (as in FN 810), p. 354.

1096 FUCHS, *Lehrbuch*. 8th ed. 1900, p. 289. Cf. FUCHS, *Text-Book* (as in FN 810), p. 354.

1097 FUCHS, *Lehrbuch*. 9th ed. 1903, p. 494. Cf. FUCHS, *Text-Book* (as in FN 810), p. 523.

1098 Georges Weill (1866–1952). Originally from Alsace-Lorraine, which in the wake of the French defeat in the Franco-German war (1870/71) was part of the German Reich between 1871 and 1918. Ophthalmol. special. under Jakob Stilling (1842–1915) at Strasbourg Univ, whose eye clinic Weill headed later on. He and Tyrolean Oswald Marchesani (1900–1952) provided the eponym for a rare genetically determined disease, the Weill-Marchesani syndrome (1932/39), which, in addition to other symptoms, presents in close association with the ocular symptoms of microspherophakia, ectopia lentis, severe myopia and glaucoma. See GORIN (as in FN 38), p. 409; IBBO (as in FN 18); H. V. NEMA, *Ophthalmic Syndromes*. Butterworth & Co., London et al. 1973, p. 271.

1099 Georges WEILL, "Über Heterophthalmus", in: *Zeitschr. Augenheilk*. 11 (1904), pp. 165–176.

1100 Ernst FUCHS, "Über Komplikationen der Heterochromie", in: *Zeitschr. Augenheilk*. 15 (1906), pp. 191–212.

1101 Irene E. LOEWENFELD and H. Stanley THOMPSON, "Fuchs's Heterochromic Cyclitis: A Critical Review of the Literature. II. Etiology and Mechanisms", in: *Survey of Ophthalmology* [*Surv. Ophthalmol]* 18 (1973), pp. 2–61.

1102 Ernst FUCHS, "Normal pigmentierte und albinotische Iris", in: *Graefes Archiv* 84 (1913), pp. 521–529.

1103 Ernst FUCHS, "Über Heterochromie nebst Bemerkungen über angeborene Anomalien", in: *Graefes Archiv* 93 (1917), pp. 381–398.

1104 See Ronald E. SMITH, Robert A. NOZIK, *Uveitis*. Translated from American English and revised by Günther Grabner. Springer, Berlin/Heidelberg/New York/Tokyo 1986, pp. 267–281; Carl P. HERBORT, Moncef KHAIRALLAH, "Editorial: Fuchs's uveitis: from Imperial Vienna to global appraisal", in: *Internat. Ophthalmol.* 30 (2010), pp. 449–452; Neerav Neel LAMBA, *Fuchs Heterochromic Iridocyclitis (Fuchs Heterochromic Uveitis)*, available online at: https://emedicine.medscape.com/article/1208706-overview (last accessed: 6 Sept. 2022).

1105 Cf. FN 525.

1106 FUCHS, *Lehrbuch* (as in FN 787). 16th ed. 1939, p. 486. The original is signed *"Beer ad nat. pinx. 1791"*. The legend reads "*Ambo oculi puellae, irides diverse coloratas exhibentes"*. See Karl HOLUBAR, Stella FATOVIĆ-FERENČIĆ, Gerd PLEWIG, *Looking at Eyes and Faces.* Ophthalmologic water-colours drawn largely by physician-artists Vienna late 18th and 19th centuries. Austrian Academy of Sciences Press, Vienna 2006, pp. 52–53, fig. 13.

1107 Ferdinand Herbert Haessler (1895–1965). Originally from Milwaukee. Studied at the Univ. of Milwaukee and at Johns Hopkins Univ. in Baltimore (M. D. 1916). Having trained as a GP, he specialised in ophthalmol. and returned to this native city. 1922–1949 Private practice. 1949–1959 First full-time Prof. of his specialty at the private Cathol. Marquette Univ. in Milwaukee. Since 1929 on the staff of *Am. J. Ophthalmol.* (1945–1964 Chief editor of the Abstract Departm.). See IBBO (as in FN 18); Obituaries: *Transact. Am. Ophthalmol. Soc.* 64 (1966), pp. 5–6; *Am. J. Ophthalmol.* 61 (1966), pp. 357–358.

1108 F. Herbert HAESSLER, *Heterochromia Irides*, in: Arch. Ophthalmol. 2/3 (1929), pp. 333–347.

1109 Irene E. Löwenfeld (Loewenfeld) (1922–2009). Originally from Munich. Forced to flee on account of her Jewish descent with her family to Zurich in 1933/34 and on to New York in 1938. From 1940 lab assistant under neuropsychiatrist Otto Löwenstein (1889–1965). Joint specialisation in research on pupillary phenomena. 1955 Rehabilitation and graduation from Bonn Univ. Started in the following year on their monumental work on the human pupil, which Loewenfeld completed on her own in 1993: *The Pupil: Anatomy, Physiology, and Clinical Applications*. 1973 Prof. of Ophthalmology at the Kresge Eye Institute of Wayne State Univ. Detroit/Michigan (Research documentation archived in the Irene E. Loewenfeld Neuro-Ophthalmology Collection). 1999 Endowment of the Loewenfeld Lecture at the biannual meetings of the Internat. Pupil Conference. See H. Stanley THOMPSON, Randy H. J. KARDON, "Irene E. Loewenfeld, PhD Physiologist of the pupil", in: *Neuroophthalmol.* 26/2 (2006), pp. 139–148; Neil R. MILLER, "Remembrance: Dr. Irene Loewenfeld", in: *Neuro-Ophthalmol.* 34 (2010), p. 78.

1110 Irene LOEWENFELD, H. Stanley THOMPSON, "Fuchs's Heterochromic Cyclitis. I. Clinical Characteristics of the Syndrome." *Surv. Ophthalmol.* 17 (1973), pp. 394–414. (Here: p. 401). Cf. the following surveys: S. J. KIMURA, M. J. HOGAN, P. THYGESON, "Fuchs' syndrome of heterochromic cyclitis", in: *Arch. Ophthalmol.* 54 (1955), pp. 179–186; F. HOLLWICH, "Zur Differentialdiagnose der Heterochromiezyklitis", in: *Klin. Monatsbl. Augenheilk.* 142 (1963), pp. 129–139 and K.-H. SCHMAUTZ, "Status dysrrhaphicus und Heterochromiezyklitis", in: *Dt. Gesundh.-Wesen* 25 (1970), pp. 991–993.

1111 Ernst FUCHS, "Anatomische Veränderungen bei Entzündung der Aderhaut", in: *Graefes Archiv* 58 (1904), pp. 391–428 (here: p. 392, FN 1).

1112 Ibid., pp. 395–396.

1113 Ibid., pp. 416–417.

1114 Ernst FUCHS, "*Über sympathisierende Entzündung (nebst Bemerkungen über seröse traumatische Iritis)*", in: *Graefes Archiv* 61 (1905), pp. 365–456.

1115 FUCHS, *Lehrbuch*. 10th ed. 1905, p. 367. Cf. FUCHS, *Text-Book* (as in FN 810), pp. 403–404.

1116 FUCHS, *Lehrbuch*. 13th ed. 1921, pp. 476–486. Cf. FUCHS, *Diseases of the Eye* (as in FN 812), p. 290.

1117 Adalbert FUCHS, *Atlas der Histopathologie des Auges* [as in FN 945], pp. 26–27 and Plate 15/Fig. 1.

1118 Ernst FUCHS, "Zur Anatomie der Endophthalmitis", in: *Graefes Archiv* 115 (1925), pp. 387–398. (Here: p. 398).

1119 On permanent loan to the Collections of the Medical University Vienna.

1120 FUCHS, *Sympath. Entzündung* (as in FN 1114).

1121 Johan Albin Dalén (1866–1940). Studied medicine at Stockholm Univ. (1895 Graduation). Ophthalmol. specialisation, 1897 Habilitation in Ophthalmology at Stockholm Univ.; August 1898–June 1899 study visits to Vienna (2nd Univ. Eye Clinic under Fuchs), Switzerland and Paris in the autumn of 1899. 1897–1902 Lecturer at Stockholm's Karolinska Institutet. 1904–1906 Lecturer, from 1906 Assoc Prof. of Ophthalmol. at Lund Univ.; 1910–1931 Dir. of the Eye Clinic at the Karolinska Institutet. See Obituary, in: *Acta Ophthalmol.* 18 (1940), pp. 221–223 (Fredrik Berg).

1122 Albin DALÉN, "Zur Kenntnis der sogenannten Chorioiditis sympathica", in: *Mitteil. Carol. medico.–chir. Inst. zu Stockholm* 6 (1904), pp. 6–21.

1123 Ernst FUCHS, "*Über Ophthalmia sympathica*", in: *Graefes Archiv* 70 (1909), pp. 465–485.

1124 Josef BÖCK, "Ernst Fuchs' Lehre von der posttraumatischen Entzündung des Augeninneren", *Wien. med. Wochenschr.* 106 (1956), Special edition (offprint). See also: Josef MELLER, "Ueber die Entwicklung der Lehre von der sympathischen Ophthalmie in der Wiener Ophthalmologischen Schule", in: *Wien. klin. Wochenschr.* 48 (1935), pp. 622–629.

1125 Guglielmo Marconi (1874–1937). Privately educated, he began to experiment aged 20 or so with electromagnet. waves for the wireless transmission of signals over great distances. In 1895 he succeeded in transmitting signals from his self-built devices over a distance of 1.5 km in the Alps. 1896 British patent for his transmitter and receiver for "Improvement in the Transmission of Electrical Impulses and Signals and Apparatus therefor". 1897 Established the Wireless Telegraph and Signal Co. in London (later Marconi's Wireless Telegraph Co. Ltd.). 1899 First wireless transmission of radio signals across the Atlantic, foundation of the Am. Marconi Wireless Corporation. 1900 Foundation of the Marconi Internat. Marine Co., which installed radio equipment on ocean liners such as the Atlantic. 1901 First transatlant. wireless communication. Inventor of the radio. 1909 Nobel Prize in physics. 1930 Co-founder of Radio Vatican. See *Nobel Lectures, Physics 1901–1921*. Elsevier Publishing Company, Amsterdam 1967.

1126 Pietro Bajardi (also Baiardi, Bayardi) (1862–1921). Studied medicine at Turin Univ. and specialised in ophthalmol. there under Carlo Reymond (cf. FN 479). 1911 Full Prof. and Dir. of the University Eye Clinic at Genoa, shortly afterwards in the same function at Torino Univ. as the successor of Reymond. See Obituaries: *Archivio di ottalmologia giornale mensile* 1922, pp. 89–96; *Am. J. Ophthalmol.* 5 (1922), p. 416, p. 842.

1127 *In agreement with the directorate of the military hospital in La Spezia and Dr. Bajardi, Director of the Eye Hospital in Torino, I entreat you to make yourself available as soon as possible for a consultation concerning my husband, Commander Guglielmo Marconi, who has a serious eye injury. Telegraph when you reckon you will arrive. Madame Marconi Military Hospital La Spezia Italy.* – Original telegram in the Family archive.

1128 (Ed.), "L'estirpazione dell'occhio offeso a Guglielmo Marconi per salvargli l'occhio sano", in: *Corriere della Sera*, 17 Oct. 1912, evening ed., p. 4; *Marconi ha perduto l'occhio* (unidentifiable newspaper cutting, 17 Oct. 1912, evening ed., in the Family archive; *L'incidente d'auto di Marconi*; *The Accident to Mr. Marconi*, available at: http://radiomarconi.com/marconi/incidente.html (last accessed: 19 July 2020).

1129 Ernst FUCHS, "Wucherungen und Geschwülste des Ciliarepithels", in: *Graefes Archiv* 68/ Abth. II (1908), pp. 534–587.

1130 Jules Badal (1840–1929). Cf. FN 302.

1131 Pierre-Félix Lagrange (1857–1928). Studied at Bordeaux Univ.; initially Assoc. Prof. of Surgery, then ophthalmol. specialisation. 1910 Full Prof. of Ophthalm. at Bordeaux Univ.; special fields of interest: strabismus, refraction anomalies, eye tumours, glaucoma surgery. See FISCHER (as in FN 28), GARRISON/MORTON (as in FN 124).

1132 Jules BADAL, Félix LAGRANGE, "Carcinome primitif des procès et du corps ciliaire", in: *Arch. d'opht.* 12 (1892), p. 143. (Classification as adenocarcinoma).

1133 Carl EMANUEL, "Ein Fall von Gliom der Pars ciliaris retinae nebst Bemerkungen zur Lehre von den Retina-Tumoren", in: *Graefes Archiv* 161/II (1900), pp. 338–364; F. H. VERHOEFF, "A rare tumour arising from the pars ciliaris retinæ (terato-neuroma) of a nature hitherto unrecognized, and its relation to the so-called glioma retinæ", in: *Transact. Am. Ophthalmol. Soc.* 10/2 (1904), pp. 351–377; Siegmund GINSBERG, *Grundriss der pathologischen Histologie des Auges*. Karger, Berlin 1903, p. 186 (Classification as adenocarcinoma or as destructrive adenoma of the ciliary body); R. KUHTE, S. GINSBERG, "Malignes Epitheliom d. Ziliarkörpers bei einem fünfjährigen Kinde", in: *Beiträge zur Augenheilkunde*. Festschrift Julius Hirschberg von Schülern und Freunden aus Anlass seiner fünfundzwanzigjährigen Wirksamkeit als Professor an der Universität Berlin in Verehrung überreicht. Veit & Comp., Leipzig 1905, pp. 127–160. See also e.g.: L. LEVY-WOLFF, "Zur Genese der ‚gutartigen Epitheliumwucherung des Ziliarkoerpers' nach Fuchs", in: *Klin. Monatsbl. Augenh.* 89 (1932), pp. 593ff.; I. CZUKRÁSZ, "*Über das Diktyom des Strahlenkörpers*", in: *Graefes Archiv* 142 (1941), pp. 619–626; Bertha A. KLIEN, "Diktyoma retinae", in: *Arch. Ophthalmol.* 22/3 (1939), pp. 432–438; J. HILLEMANN, G. NAUMANN, "Beitrag zum benignen Epitheliom (Fuchs) des Ziliarkörpers", in: *Ophthalmologica* 164 (1972), pp. 321–335.

1134 τὸ δίκτυον (to diktyon) = net.

1135 René BERNOULLI, "*Über das sogenannte Diktyom – Neuroepithelioma teratoides ciliare*", in: *Ophthalmologica* 141 (1961), pp. 386–397.

1136 FUCHS, *Lehrbuch* (as in FN 787). 13th ed. 1921, p. 593. Cf. FUCHS, *Diseases of the Eye* (as in FN 812), p. 390. In the German 1921 *Lehrbuch* as edited by Salzmann, this is the only mention Ernst Fuchs makes of dictyoma. In the last three editions (1939, 1944 and 1945) overseen by Adalbert Fuchs, dictyoma was again mentioned only once and not described in any detail.

1137 See e.g.: L. RAZZAQ, M. MARINKOVIC, W. SWART, G. P. M. LUYTEN, S. G. van DUINEN, J. E. E. KEUNEN, "Fuchs' adenoma of the choroid simulating a choroidal hemangioma", in: *Case Rep. in Ophthalmol.* 3/1 (2012), pp. 83–86.

1138 Ernst FUCHS, "Beitrag zu den angeborenen Anomalien des Sehnerven", in: *Graefes Archiv* 28/Abth. I (1882), pp. 139–169.

[1139] For Schnabel, cf. FN 602. Fuchs refers here to the following two papers: Isidor SCHNABEL, "Ueber die Disposition zum erworbenen Staphyloma posticum Scarpae", in: *Wien. med. Wochenschr.* 26 (1876), Cols. 888–891; Isidor SCHNABEL, in: *Graefes Archiv* 20/Abth. II, pp. 43ff. Schnabel continued to uphold his point of view which differed from Fuchs's. See Isidor SCHNABEL, "Ueber Maculakolobom, physiologische Exkavation und angeborenen Conus", in: *Wien. med. Bl.* 7 (1884), cols. 161–166, 197–201, 229–232, and 259–261.

[1140] Cf. FN 1138, p. 159.

[1141] FUCHS, *Lehrbuch* (as in FN 787). 1st ed. 1889, p. 345. Cf. FUCHS, Text-Book (as in FN 810), p. 444.

[1142] Ernst FUCHS, "*Über den anatomischen Befund einiger angeborener Anomalien der Retina und des Sehnerven",* in: *Graefes Archiv* 93 (1917), pp. 1–48.

[1143] Ibid., pp. 20–21.

[1144] Here Fuchs is quoting from his paper on congenital anomalies of the optic nerve (1882), cf. FN 1138.

[1145] FUCHS (as in FN 1142), p. 26.

[1146] Ibid., p. 28.

[1147] Cited in.: http://www.whonamedit.com (Ernst Fuchs), entry author: Daniel Enerson (last accessed: 6 Sept. 2022). See Ch. 3 of this monograph on Fuchs's time in Liège.

[1148] Colman Ward Cutler (1862–1935). Originally from New Haven/New York. Studied at the College of Physicians and Surgeons of Columbia Univ. (M. D. 1889). Assistant at St. Luke's Hosp. for two years, ophthalmol. specialisation for three years at the 2nd Univ. Eye Clinic under Ernst Fuchs (studies on congenital night blindness and pigment degeneration). Dir. of the Eye Dept. of St. Luke's Hospital, consultant at several New York hospitals. Active support of measures for the prevention of blindness. See Obituary, in: *Transact. Am. Ophthalmol. Soc.* 33 (1935), pp. 24–25 (Conrad Berens).

[1149] Colman W. CUTLER, "Drei ungewöhnliche Fälle von Retino-Chorioideal-Degeneration", in: *Archiv Augenheilk.* 30 (1895), pp. 117–122.

[1150] Colman W. CUTLER, "Ueber angeborene Nachtblindheit und Pigmentdegeneration", in: *Arch. Augenheilk.* 30 (1895), pp. 92–116.

[1151] Ernst FUCHS, "Ueber zwei der Retinitis pigmentosa verwandte Krankheiten (Retinitis punctata albescens und Atrophia gyrata chorioideae et retinae)", in: *Archiv Augenheilk.* 32 (1896), pp. 111–116 (here: p. 113). Two years later this paper was published in English: Ernst FUCHS, "Two diseases related to retinitis pigmentosa; retinitis punctata albescens and atrophia gyrata choroideae et retinae", in: *Arch. Ophth.* 27 (1898), pp. 484–489, (here: p. 486).

[1152] Ibid., p. 114–116. Cf. "Two diseases", etc., as in FN 1151, pp. 488–489.

[1153] Ibid., p. 116. Cf. "Two diseases", etc., as in FN 1151, p. 489.

[1154] FUCHS, *Lehrbuch* (as in FN 787). 13th ed. 1921 (Maximilian Salzmann), p. 509. Cf. FUCHS, *Diseases of the Eye* (as in FN 812), pp. 318–319.

[1155] See e.g.: Hunter McGUIRE, "Gyrate Atrophy of the Choroid and Retina (FUCHS)", in: *Arch. Ophthalmol.* 8/3 (1932), pp. 372–379.

[1156] See e.g.: Johan SÆBØ, "Atrophia gyrata choroideae et retinae", in: *Brit. J. Ophthalmol.* 1948, pp. 824–847; Hellmut NEUBAUER, "Progressive Aderhautatrophie", in: *Graefes Archiv* 156 (1955), pp. 577–589.

1157 See e.g.: James J. O'DONNELL, "Gyrate atrophy of the retina and choroid is an inborn error of metabolism of ornithine aminotransferase", in: *Neurochemistry International* 1 (1980), pp. 459–463; Alireza JAVADZADEH, Davood GHARABAGHI, "Gyrate atrophy of the choroid and retina with hyper-ornithinemia responsive to vitamin B6: a case report," in: *J. Med. Case Reports* 1 (2007), p. 27; Andreas SCHULZE, Tyler REIMSCHISEL, "Hyperornithinemia", in: *Neurology MedLink*, available online at: https://www.medlink.com/articles/hyperornithinemia (last accessed: 6 Sept. 2022); Julio César GONZÁLEZ GÓMEZ, Eliecer PÉREZ GARCÍA, Odelaisys HERNÁNDEZ ECHEVARRÍA, Daniel LÓPEZ FELIPE, Yanelys LEAL DELGADO, Hiperornitinemia con atrofia gyrata de coroides y retina, in: *Revista Cubana de Oftalmología* [= *Rev. Cub. Oftalmol.*]. 30/3 (jul.–set. 2017), available online at: www.sciELO.org (last accessed: 19 July 2020).

1158 Ernst FUCHS, "Ablösung der Aderhaut nach Staaroperation", in: *Bericht über die 28. Versammlung d. Ophthalmol. Gesellsch. Heidelberg 1900*. Bergmann, Wiesbaden 1901, pp. 84–87.

1159 Ernst FUCHS, "Ablösung der Aderhaut nach Staaroperation", in: *Graefes Archiv* 51 (1900), pp. 199–224; FUCHS, "Ablösung der Aderhaut nach Operation", in: *Graefes Archiv* 53 (1902), pp. 375– 400.

1160 FUCHS, ibid., p. 400.

1161 Ernst FUCHS, "*Über eine angeborene Abnormität der Retina nebst Bemerkungen über Scleraleinbuchtung und Aderhautabhebung*", in: *Graefes Archiv* 94 (1917), pp. 107–116, and FUCHS, Über seröse Choroidabhebung, in: *Graefes Archiv* 104 (1921), pp. 247–263.

1162 Ernst FUCHS, "Retinitis circinata", in: *Graefes Archiv* 39 /Abth. III (1893), pp. 229–279.

1163 FUCHS, *Lehrbuch* (as in FN 787). 13th ed. 1921, p. 575, Fig. 196 (caption). Cf. FUCHS, *Diseases of the Eye* (as in FN 812), p. 375.

1164 Cf. FN 275.

1165 Jonathan HUTCHINSON, "Symmetrical central choroidoretinal disease occurring in senile persons", in: *R. London Ophthalmic Hosp. Rep.* 8 (1875), pp. 231–244.

1166 Cf. FN 893.

1167 Wilhelm GOLDZIEHER, "Ueber die Hutchinson'sche Veränderung des Augenhintergrundes", in: *Wien. med. Wochenschr.* 37 (1887), cols. 861–865; GOLDZIEHER, "Die Hutchinsonsche Veränderung des Augenhintergrundes. (Retinitis circinata Fuchs)", in: *Arch. Augenheilk.* 34 (1897), pp. 112–134.

1168 For the first four decades after Fuchs's description and terminological coinage, see e.g.: Louis de WECKER, "Faut-il différencier la rétinite circinée, ou dégénérescence blanche, de la rétinite apoplectiforme", in: *Arch. d'opht.* 14 (1894), special print; Joseph WELTERT, "Ein Fall von 'Retinitis circinata'", in: *Archiv Augenheilk.* 32 (1896), pp. 187–193; E. AMMANN, "Ein Fall von Retinitis circinata mit anatomischer Untersuchung", in: *Archiv Augenheilk.* 35 (1897), pp. 123–136; Edward FRIDENBERG, "A Case of Retinitis Circinata", in: *Transact. Am. Ophthalmol. Soc.* 8 (1897), pp. 181–185; Karl HOOR, "Eine eigenartige Veränderung der Retina um die Macula lutea und die Retinitis circinata Fuchs", in: *Zeitschr. Augenheilk.* 3 (1900), pp. 26–31; George Edmund de SCHWEINITZ, "A Case of Retinitis circinata", in: *Ophthal. Rec.* 1900, p. 1; SCHWEINITZ, Circinate Retinitis, in: *Ophthal.*

Rec. 1901, p. 160; SCHWEINITZ., "Disappearance of the lesions in circinate retinitis", in: *Ophthal. Rec.* 1902; LASKER, *Ein Beitrag zur Retinitis circinata.* Med. Diss. Univ. Leipzig 1904; Otto HEINRICY, *Klinische Beiträge zur Degeneratio circinata retinae [Retinitis circinata (Fuchs)] mit besonderer Berücksichtigung der atypischen Formen dieses Krankheitsbildes.* Med. Diss. Univ. Tübingen, Wilhelm Engelmann 1913; Eugene BLAKE, "The Etiology of Retinitis Circinata", in: *Transact. Am. Ophthalmol. Soc.* 14/2 (1916), pp. 753–762; Paul JUNIUS, Hermann KUHNT, *Die scheibenförmige Entartung der Retinamitte: Degeneratio maculae luteae disciformis.* S. Karger, Berlin 1925; Leo POLLNOW, "Beiträge zur Retinitis circinata und zur Lochbildung in der Makula", in: *Zeitschr. Augenheilk.* 70 (1930), pp. 257–264, F. SCHIECK, A. BRÜCKNER (eds.), *Kurzes Handbuch der Ophthalmologie.* Vol. 5. Julius Springer, Berlin 1930, pp. 578ff.; Ambrose Earl EDGERTON, "Circinate Retinitis", in: *Am. J. Ophthalmol.* 19 (1936), pp. 463–469.

1169 For the gradual growth of the understanding of age-related macula degeneration, see: Paulus T. V. M. de JONG, "A Historical Analysis of the Quest for the Origins of Aging Macula Disorder, the Tissues Involved, and Its Terminology", in: *Ophthalmology and Eye Diseases [= Ophthalmol. Eye Dis.*] 8/Suppl. 1 (2016), pp. 5–14 and de JONG, "Elusive drusen and changing terminology of AMD", in: *Eye* 32 (2018), pp. 904–914.

1170 Cf. FN 263.

1171 Carl F. R. FÖRSTER, *Ophthalmologische Beiträge.* Enslin, Berlin 1862, pp. 52–68.

1172 Ernst FUCHS, "Der centrale schwarze Fleck bei Myopie", in: *Zeitschr. Augenheilk.* 5 (1901), pp. 171–178.

1173 Ibid., p. 171.

1174 Ibid., p. 172.

1175 Ibid., p. 177.

1176 Emilie LEHMUS, *Die Erkrankungen der Macula lutea bei progressiver Myopie.* Inaug. Diss. Univ. Zürich 1875, p. 26.

1177 Cf. FN 1172, pp. 177–178.

1178 FUCHS, *Lehrbuch* (as in FN 787). 12th ed. 1910, Fig. 188, p. 482.

1179 Ibid., p. 483.

1180 FUCHS, *Lehrbuch*, 13th ed. 1921, p. 901 and Fig. 313, p. 902 (The figure is the same as the original in the previous edition).

1181 FUCHS, *Lehrbuch.* 14th ed. 1922, p. 896 and 15th ed. 1926, p. 891.

1182 FUCHS, *Lehrbuch.* 16th ed. 1939, p. 40.

1183 FUCHS, *Lehrbuch.* 17th ed. 1944; FUCHS, *Lehrbuch*, 18th ed. 1945, p. 410, Fig. 179.

1184 Ernst FUCHS, "Die periphere Atrophie des Sehnerven", *Graefes Archiv* 31/Abth. I (1885), pp. 177–200.

1185 Ibid., p. 192.

1186 Ibid., pp. 179–180.

1187 Ibid., p. 183.

1188 Ibid., p. 193.

1189 Paul Bunge (1853–1926). Studied at the Univ. of Jena, Kiel, Leipzig and Halle (Graduation 1877). 1878–1892 Assist. at the University Eye Clinic in Halle/Saale (Habilitation 1884, Assoc. Prof. 1889). Here Fuchs quotes Bunge's habilitation dissertation: Paul BUNGE, *Ueber Gesichtsfeld und Faserverlauf im optischen Leitungsapparate*. Halle 1884. See FISCHER (as in FN 28); HIRSCHBERG, *Geschichte der Augenheilkunde* (as in FN 18), vol. 15/2 [= Reprint vol. VI], § 1104, pp. 43–44; PAGEL (as in FN 13).

1190 Cf. FN 1184, pp. 197–198.

1191 Ernst FUCHS, "Über senile Veränderungen am Sehnerven", in: *Graefes Archiv* 103 (1920), pp. 304–330.

1192 Ibid., pp. 328–329.

1193 Ibid., p. 329.

1194 Ernst FUCHS, "Myxoma orbitae", in: *Zeitschr. Augenheilk.* 32 (1914), p. 192. (Pres.). Cf.the report on the meeting in: *Klin. Monatsbl. Augenheilk.* 53 (1914), p. 244, and *Wien. med. Wochenschr.* 65 (1915), col. 214.

1195 Cf. e.g.: Aaron FAY, Peter J. DOLMAN, *Diseases and Disorders of the Orbit and Ocular Adnexa*. Elsevier, Edinburgh etc. 2017, pp. 365–367 (here: p. 365).

1196 FUCHS, *Augenarzt* (as in FN 2), p. 10, FN 6.

1197 Hugo Wintersteiner (1865–1918). Studied at Vienna Univ. (Dr. med. univ. 1890). Ophthalmol. specialis. at the First University Eye Clinic at Vienna's Allg. Krankenhaus under Carl Stellwag v. Carion (cf. FN 165). 1897 Habilitation in Ophthalmol. at Vienna Univ.; 1911 Dir. of the Eye Dept. of Vienna's Wilhelminenspital. Cf. HIRSCHBERG, *Geschichte d. Augenheilkunde* (as in FN 18). Reprint vol. VII, §1252, p. 429; Obituary, in: *Centralbl. prakt. Augenheilk.* 43 (1919), p. 188.

1198 In the United States, the "Wintersteiner collection" was nevertheless touted as the largest collection of its kind in Europe and in the world. In 1916 there were first rumours of wholesale liquor magnate Charles Rebstock (1846–1928) purchasing the collection from Vienna Univ., but, on the evidence of contemporary reports, it took until 1922 for the collection to reach the Univ. of St. Louis, where it was to serve the purpose of "graduate instruction in ophthalmology". See "Newsletter", in: *National Society for the Prevention of Blindness 1916*, p. 302; "News Items", in: *Am. J. Ophthalmol.* 3/5 (1922), p. 851; *Southern Med. J.* 15 (1922), p. 864; *Bull. Chicago School Med. Instruct.*, Chicago (III) Dept. of Health 1922, p. 190; *Eighth Annual Report of the National Committee for the Prevention of Blindness*. December 31, 1922, New York 1922, p. 22. Housed in the R. L. Thomson Pathological Laboratory of St. Louis Univ., the Wintersteiner Collection was made accessible to the public on 18 February 1924 during the Convention of the American Congress of Internal Medicine and College of Physicians. See J. *Missouri State Med. Assoc.* 21 (1924), p. 117.
Rebstock generously donated to several other university and humanitarian institutions. He gave, to name only one example, $1,000,000 for an Institute of Zoology and Botany at Washington Univ. in St. Louis (1926), on the understanding that the institute and the endowed chair that went with it was to bear his name. At the time of the purchase of the Wintersteiner Collection, Rebstock was Director of the Missouri Assoc. for the Blind.

1199 The histol. preparations were stored in an apparently purpose-made wooden box with a capacity of 2 times 4 compartments for 10 cassettes each. Not all cassettes are completely full and some are missing altogether. On the occasion of the 150th anniversary of the foundation of the First University Eye Clinic in Vienna in 1962, the descendants of Ernst Fuchs gave the collection on permanent loan to what was then the

Institut für Geschichte d. Medizin d. Univ. Wien (today: Sammlungen d. Med. Univ. Wien). See Jutta LAUBER, Helmut WYKLICKY, *150 Jahre Wiener Augenheilkunde* (In 1812, the world's first University Eye Clinic was established in Vienna). Das Institut für Geschichte der Medizin in Wien (Leitung: Doz. E. Lesky) in Verbindung mit I. Univ.-Augenklinik Wien (Vorstand: Prof. A. Pillat), II. Univ. Augenklinik Wien (Vorstand: J. Böck), Univ.- Augenklinik Graz (Vorstand: K. Hruby) stellt Dokumente, Handschriften, Publikationen, Bilder und Instrumente aus. Ausstellungskatalog 1.–30. Juni 1962. Eigenverlag der Wiener medizinischen Akademie für ärztliche Fortbildung, Vienna 1962, p. 15; Gabriela SCHMIDT-WYKLICKY, "Ein ophthalmohistorischer Schatz: Die pathohistologische Sammlung von Ernst Fuchs in Wien", in: *Mitteilungen der Julius-Hirschberg-Gesellschaft* 16–2014 (2018), pp. 181–196.

1200 FUCHS, *Augenarzt* (as in FN 2), p. 10, FN 6.

1201 "Praeparatesammlung" I. 1–582.

1202 Ibid., Logbook no. 135 (Sarcoma chorioideae).

1203 The following consecutive numbers are printed in gold on the side of the binding: II. 583–1117, III. 1118–1605, IV. 1606–2240, V. 2241–3031, VI. 3032–3799, VII. 3800–4523, VIII. 4524–6005, IX. 6006–7471, X. 7472–8106, XI. 8107–8246 and, after the introduction of a new counting system, 1/28–58/37. In 1915, Fuchs resigned from his post at the Clinic, which means that all entries from roughly the middle of volume VIII belong to a time when he was no longer an active member of the University. All eleven volumes are now part of a private collection.

1204 Cf. FN 1201. It comprises as an attachment the complete case history of a 19-year-old female patient afflicted with meningitis tuberculosa, from 18 April 1878 (d. 29 May 1878), which belongs to Preparation No. 446.

1205 Ibid. The numbers of the preparations and the pertinent pathology are underscored in blue.

1206 Wiener Stadt- u. Landesarchiv. Krankenprotokolle Augenklinik Frauen Saal Nr. 43, Signatur M. Abt. 209.1 B 50. The period 1905–1914 is covered in 18 volumes.

1207 Ernst Fuchs was awarded the title Hofrat in 1896. See the decree signed by the then Minister f. Cultus u. Unterricht, Paul Gautsch v. Frankenthurn, now in the Family archive:

Seine Kaiserliche und Königliche Apostolische Majestät haben mit Allerhöchster Entschließung vom 6. April l. J. Ihnen den Titel eines Hofrathes mit Nachsicht der Taxen allergnädigst zu verleihen geruht.

Es gereicht mir zum Vergnügen, Eure Hochwohlgeboren von dieser Allerhöchsten Schlußfassung in Kenntnis zu setzen. Wien, am 7. April 1896. Der Minister für Cultus und Unterricht

[His Imperial and Royal Apostolic Majesty has graciously deigned to award to you the title of Hofrat [Aulic Councillor], exempt from fees. It is with great pleasure that I herewith inform your honour of His Majesty's resolution. Vienna, etc.]

Hofrat was awarded as a title from the 16th century to members of the highest collegial government bodies. On the pattern of the Aulic Council in Vienna these bodies were tasked with the discharge of governmental and administrative duties and doubled as regional appeal courts. Until the end of the Austro-Hungarian Monarchy in 1918, *Hofrat* was a honorific title that came in different flavours – *Hofrat, Geheimer Hofrat*, etc. – and was awarded to senior civil servants, professors and medical doctors. Until 1921 *Hofrat* was associated with the 5th tier of civil servants (between *Regierungsrat* and *Sektionschef*). Since 1926 *Hofrat* has been awarded as an official title (*Wirkl. Hofrat*) and as a mark of distinction. See Meyers Lexikon. 7. ed., vol. 5. Bibliographisches Institut, Leipzig 1926, col. 1664. – Another Imperial resolution of March 24, 1902 topped up the title by awarding Fuchs what was known as the "character of Hofrat". See Family archive. – The distinction between titular and actual Aulic Councillor – even though in the sunset of the Empire the latter qualification remained largely fictive – goes back at least to the days of Maria Theresa (1717–1780).

1208 See Ch. 5.

1209 Ludwig J. K. von Sallmann (1892–1975). Studied at Vienna Univ. (Dr. med. univ. 1919). Ophthalmol. specialis. under Fuchs's successor Friedrich Dimmer (1856–1926, Cf. FN 44), Dir. of the 2nd Univ. Eye Clinic (Assistant 1923, habilitation 1931). 1930 Dir. of the Dept. of Ophthalmology at Peking Union Med. College as successor of Arnold Pillat (cf. FN 808). 1931–1937 Senior consultant at the 2nd Univ. Eye Clinic under Karl David Lindner (cf. FN 751). 1939 Head physician at Vienna's Kaiserin-Elisabeth-Spital. As an outspoken critic of the Nazi regime he left Austria. 1939 Dir. of the laboratories of the Hermann Knapp Memorial Hospital in New York. 1940 Relocation of this institution to Columbia University (1946 Prof., in charge of research). 1955–1970 National Institutes of Health (initially Visiting Professor, then Dir. of the Ophthalmol. Dept. of the National Institute of Neurological Diseases and Blindness). Continued his ophthalmol. basic research on such topics as the lens (e.g. experim. cataract) and the influence of the central nervous system on the control of intraocular pressure at the Lab. of the National Institute of Neurological and Communicative Disorders and Stroke. Himself the recipient of numerous awards and prizes, he and his wife founded the Ludwig u. Henrietta v. Sallmann Stiftung, which awards a research prize every other year. In 2011 the ARVO Foundation of Eye Research established the Ludwig von Sallmann Clinician-Scientist Award, an annual prize associated with the Ludwig von Sallmann Lecture. See Herbert E. KAUFMAN, "Ludwig von Sallmann", in: *Investigative Ophthalmology and Visual Science* [= *Invest. Ophthalmol. Vis. Sc.*] 9 (1970), pp. 1–2; Obituaries: *Trans. Am. Ophthalmol. Soc.* 74 (1976), pp. 8–11 (Peter C. Kronfeld); *Arch. Ophthalmol.* 94/4 (1976), p. 685 (G. Richard O'Connor).

1210 Cf. FN 1203, Protokollbuch [= Logbook] IX, no. 7364.

1211 Cf. FN 44.

1212 Cf. FN 1203. Nos. 7214, 7221, 7230 with Dr. Philipovitsch; nos 7217, 7240, 7274 and 7352 with Arnold Pillat; nos 7252, 7284 and 7285 with Ludwig J. K. von Sallmann; nos. 7280 and 7330 with Dr. Teichner; and 7328 (Ernst Fuchs solo).

8. The "Fuchs Library"

As an assistant at Vienna's First University Eye Clinic headed by Arlt Ernst Fuchs had made the specialist library of this institution, the oldest of its kind, his home from home. The library owed its core holdings of monographs, some of which date to the eighteenth century, to its founder, Georg Josef Beer. Fuchs's remit as a clinical assistant included administrative work at the library, which he used to excellent effect: as he himself said later, he read the bulk of the library in those years,[1213] acquiring a profound knowledge of the literature of his specialty as part of his training.

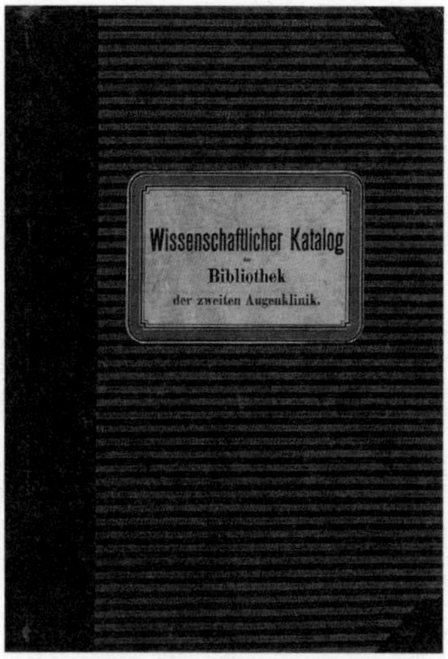

Fig. 91
Library catalogue of the 2nd University Eye Clinic

Having been recalled from Liège to Vienna in 1885 to take charge of the Second University Eye Clinic, Fuchs focused his energy on the establishment of this newly founded clinic, stocking its library with the pertinent scientific literature. Over the thirty years between 1885 and 1915 he spent in charge of this clinic, the library held subscriptions to all relevant international ophthalmological journals and steadily increased its collection of the most important textbooks and ophthalmological monographs both in German and in all the major foreign languages.

The monographs were listed – just when is now impossible to say – under Fuchs's auspices in a two-volume, hand-written, bound catalogue[1214] (Fig. 91) under two times eighteen headings:

1. General Ophthalmological Literature – Textbooks, Atlantes
2. General Pathology, Clinical Diagnostics and Therapy
3. Anatomy and Embryonic Development
4. Physiology
5. Examination Methods
6. Malformations – Congenital Diseases
7. Lids
8. Lacrimal organs
9. Conjunctiva
10. Blennorrhea –Trachoma
11. Cornea
12. Sclera – Anterior Chamber
13. Iris Corpus ciliare
14. Pupil – Adaptation
15. Lens
16. Vitreous Body
17. Glaucoma – Hydrophthalmus – Hypotension
18. Chorioidea
19. Sympathetic and Metastatic Ophthalmia
20. Retina
21. Nervus opticus – Brain and Visual Pathway
22. Visual Field – Functional Disturbances – Simulation – Colours
23. Orbita – Sinuses
24. Tumours of the Eye and the Adnexa
25. Ocular Muscles and Their Disorders
26. Injuries – Poisonings
27. Links to Other Diseases
28. Optics – Refraction and Accommodation
29. Bacteriology and Serology
30. Non-Operative Therapy
31. Operations for Cataract and Glaucoma
32. Other Operations
33. Hygiene – Welfare of the Blind
34. Writing – Book Printing
35. History – Speeches and Biographies
36. Statistics –Varia

Table 5: The thematic fields in the handwritten catalogue of monographs in the library of the 2nd University Eye Clinic, initiated by Ernst Fuchs

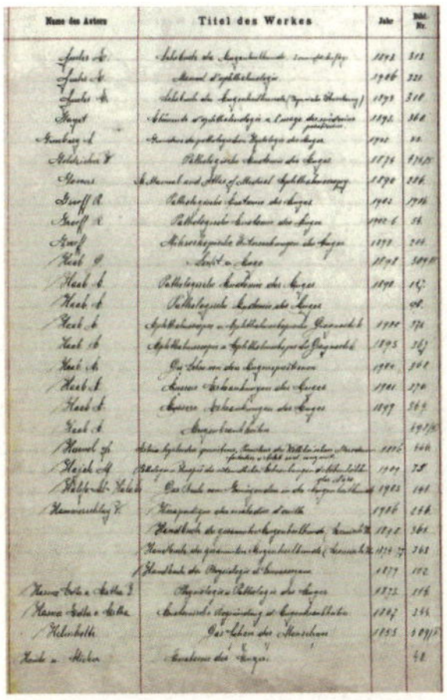

Fig. 92
Page 10 of the Library catalogue of the 2nd University Eye Clinic

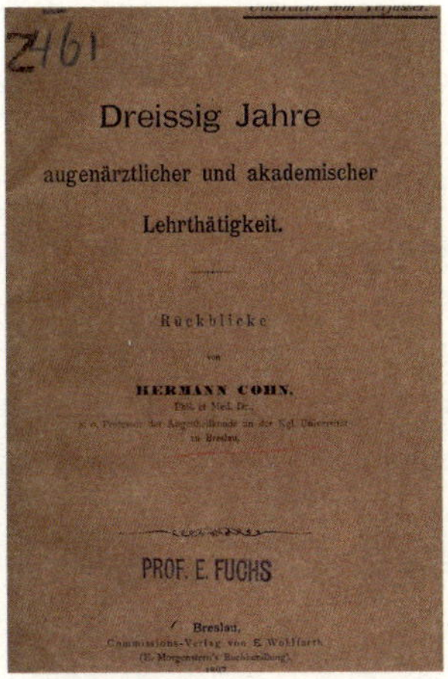

Fig. 93
Ernst Fuchs's private rubber stamp

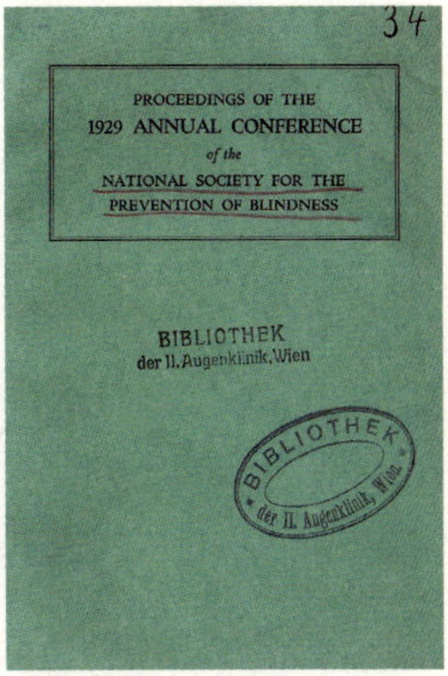

Fig. 94
Library stamp of the 2nd University Eye Clinic

Books were listed under their specific headings in laterally arranged columns stating the author's name – in alphabetical order in the cataloguing of the core collection, later in chronological order reflecting the date of a book's arrival in the library – title, the year of publication, and the shelf number, which in the case of books from the core collection was retained, while new arrivals were assigned numbers that picked up where the old collection had left off. (Fig. 92) Each of the 36 headings had 10 double sided sheets at two times 31 lines assigned for the cataloguing of monographs or bound offprints. This catalogue was added to for more than a decade after Fuchs's retirement in 1915, when he had thirty years of service to his record.

An important role among the latest specialist publications was played by special prints of the most recently published papers both by up-and-coming novices and internationally established authors. Fuchs was in direct scientific contact with many of them. Papers they had sent him personally, often inscribed with a personal dedication, did not, in Fuchs's view, belong to him alone. Marked with his special rubber-stamp (Fig. 93), they were incorporated into the library of the Clinic. (Fig. 94)

Special prints, of which there are a great number, are arranged according to the part of the bulbus they dealt with. Kept in cardboard boxes of uniform size and appearance and either remaining in their original state or bound in book form at a later stage, they have largely survived intact, apart from the loss of several entire boxes or of their cardboard exterior.[1215] The user-friendliness of this system was probably the reason why special prints were not subjected to the same handwritten cataloguing as the monographs. Offprints were in any case disposed of according to this system until well into the 1970s. Then the system was given up – presumably because modern developments in ophthalmology could no longer be fitted into the pre-existing thematic categories of Ernst Fuchs's time. Special prints were now stored in bundles by author name and assigned consecutive numbers per publication. No inventory that could be called a catalogue for the many hundreds of special prints has been found.

The original labels on the cardboard boxes containing special prints cover the following subjects:

1	Normal and Comparative Anatomy, Embryonic Development A–K
1	Normal and Comparative Anatomy, Embryonic Development L–Z
1/III	Congenital Anomalies
2	Spatial Perception, Binocul[ar] Vision
3	Sense of Colour and Disorders A–L
3	Sense of Colour and Disorders M–Z
4	4 Physiology of the Retina, the Impact of Light, General Remarks on Sensual Perception A–M
4	The Eye and General Disorders
5	5 Brain, Simulation, Functional Disturbances
5/III	Brain, Simulation, Functional Disturbances
5/IV	Brain, Simulation, Functional Disturbances

6	Aetiology, Correlation with Other Diseases, Occupational Diseases A–G
6	Aetiology, Correlation with Other Diseases, Occupational Diseases H–O
6	6 Aetiology, Correlation with Other Diseases, Occupational Diseases P–Z
6/I	The Eye in Its Correlation with Other Diseases
6/II	The Eye in Its Correlation with Other Diseases
6/III	Aetiology of Ocular Diseases in their Correlation with other Diseases
7	General and Experimental Pathology, Methods of Examination M–Z
7/II	General and Experimental Pathology, Methods of Examination
8	Methods of Examination, Instruments A–H
8	Methods of Examination, Instruments J–Z (empty)
9	Retina – Opticus – Visual Pathway
10	Eyes – Injuries A–L
11	Exchange of Fluids, Glaucoma, Elevation of Pressure H–L
11	Exchange of Fluids, Glaucoma, Elevation of Pressure SCH–Z
11/I	Glaucomata, Hydrophthalmus
11/II	Metabolism, Glaucoma, Hypotony
11/III	Primary Juvenile Glaucoma Exchange of Fluids
12	Heredity
13	Lids
13/I	Lids
14	Lacrimal organs (empty)
14/I	Lacrimal Tools

15	Conjunctiva A–O
15	Conjunctiva P–Z
15/I	Conjunctiva
15/II	Conjunctiva
16	Trachoma, Blennorrhea J–R
16	Trachoma, Blennorrhea S–Z
16/II	Blennorrhea, Trachoma
16/III	Trachoma – Blennorrhea
17	Cornea, Sclera A–F
17	Cornea, Sclera O–Z
18	Iris, Corpus ciliare A–K
18	Iris, Corpus ciliare L–Z
19	Pupil
20	Lens, Cataract Cataract operations A–J
20	Lens, Cataract Cataract operations K–Q
20	Lens, Cataract Cataract operations R–Z
20/II	Cataracts
20/IV	Operation of Cataracts
21/I	Vitreous Body
22	Chorioidea, Metastatic and symp[athetic] Ophthalmia

23	Retina C–F
23	Retina G–J
23	Retina K–L
23	Retina M–R
23	Retina S–Z
23/I	Retina
23/II	Retina
23/III	RETINA
23/IV	Retina Normal and Pathological
24	Nervus opticus A–L
24	Nervus opticus M–Z
24/III	OPTIC NERVE
25	Tumours
26	Orbita Sinuses
27	Amblyopia Strabismus Eye Muscles A–G
27	Amblyopia Eye Muscles Strabismus G–N
27	Amblyopia Eye Muscles Strabismus O–Z
27/IV	Latent and Manifest Strabismus
28	Ultrasound A–Z (old box, original labelling overstickered)
28	Field of Vision

29	Refraction A–L
29	Refraction M–R
29	Refraction S–Z
29/I	Anomalies of Refraction
30/I	Accommodation
31	Radio- and Physical Therapy A–Z (old box, original labelling overstickered)
31/III	Therapy
31/IV	Therapy
32	Non-Operative Therapy A–H
32	Non-Operative Therapy J–M
32	Non-Operative Therapy N–Z
33	Ocular Operations excl[uding] Cataract Operations A–B
33	Ocular Operations excl[uding] Cataract operations C–J
33	Ocular operations excl[uding] Cataract Operations K–R
33	Ocular Operations excl[uding] Cataract Operations S–Z
33/I	Ocular Operations
33/II	OCULAR OPERATIONS
34	Hygiene, Blindness, Geography A–F
34	Hygiene, Blindness, Geography G–M
34	Hygiene, Blindness, Geography N–Z

35	History, Speeches, Lectures A–L
36	Offprints on historical and biographical topics
37	(Without thematic focus, recent issues) A–F
37	(Without thematic focus, recent issues) G–L
37	(Without thematic focus, recent issues) M–Z
Unnumbered box: A selection of old ophthalmological papers, mostly pre-1850 dissertations	
Box A (modern contents)	
Box DA (modern contents)	

Table 6: Thematic catalogue of the offprint collection in the library of the 2nd University Eye Clinic, initiated by Ernst Fuchs; comprising the extant boxes.

Among other relics of the Second University Eye Clinic library there is a cardboard portfolio with ripped off ribbons, bearing the inscription "Eigene Arbeiten" [Own works] in Ernst Fuchs's handwriting. (Fig. 95) It was obviously designed to house one specimen copy of each of his hundreds of original publications. The portfolio was found to be empty.

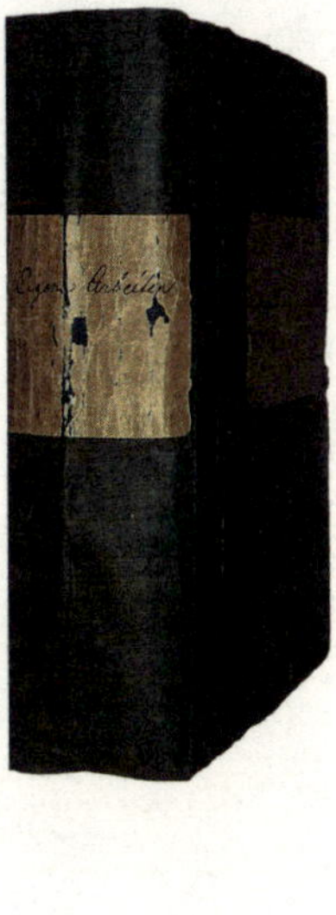

Fig. 95
File for offprints
by Ernst Fuchs

Notes

1213 FUCHS, *Augenarzt* (as in FN 2), p. 57.

1214 *Wissenschaftlicher Katalog der zweiten Augenklinik*. Private collection.

1215 See the bracketed notes in the list below.

9. Ernst Fuchs at 70: Academic Ceremonies, Honours, Homage

Six years after Ernst Fuchs had taken voluntary retirement from his position as Director of the Second University Eye Clinic, an institution he had single-handedly put at the top of the world of ophthalmology, the German-speaking ophthalmological establishment pooled its efforts to celebrate his 70th birthday on 14 June 1921.

Academic Birthday Celebration

The birthday celebration the University of Vienna[1216] put on in honour of Ernst Fuchs on June 14, 1921 rallied a great number of alumni, friends, representatives of the Republic of Austria, students, guests and family members so that the time-honoured auditorium of the First University Eye Clinic was filled to capacity. Ernst Fuchs's outstanding lifetime achievement was acknowledged by the presence of Federal President Michael Hainisch (1858–1940)[1217] at the festivity, all but raising the occasion to an official act of state. Other high-ranking guests included the Federal Minister of Education, Vice Chancellor Walter Breisky (1871–1944),[1218] the Director of the Office of Public Health, Carl von Helly (1865–1932),[1219] the Executive City Councillor for Welfare and Health and outstanding anatomist Julius Tandler (1869–1936),[1220] renowned historian and Rector of Vienna University Alfons Dopsch (1868–1953),[1221] the Fuchs disciple and representative of the Medical Faculty of Graz University Maximilian Salzmann,[1222] Professor of Pharmacology and Pharmacognosy Josef Nevinny (1853–1923)[1223] as the representative of the Medical Faculty of Innsbruck University; the deans of all the four faculties of Vienna University and many of its professors; the doyens of Vienna University, Viktor Ebner[1224] und Sigmund Exner;[1225] the Director of the Wiener Allgemeine Poliklinik Julius Mannaberg (1860–1941);[1226] the surgeon Anton Freiherr von Eiselsberg (1860–1939);[1227] pathological anatomist Richard Paltauf (1858–1924)[1228] and psychiatrist Julius Wagner Ritter von Jauregg[1229] as the representatives of the Gesellschaft der Ärzte; the members of the Ophthalmologische Gesellschaft in Vienna, led by their doyen, August Ritter von Reuss;[1230] and the sculptor Josef Müllner (1879–1968),[1231] who had created the marble relief which was unveiled on that occasion.

As the jubilarian was escorted into the auditorium, the "Weihelied" – "Brüder, reicht die Hand zum Bunde" [Brothers, join hands to pledge union] – rang out, music that was at that time still thought to have been written by Mozart,[1232] sung by the Vienna Academic Choir, the Ghibellinen. One of Fuchs's former students, Moriz Sachs,[1233] then opened the proceedings with a welcoming speech, whose beginning deserves to be cited here in full for the sake of the sentiments it expresses:

Ernst Fuchs, our teacher and mentor, is today turning 70. For us, who have served under him, who have been his assistants, it is a matter both of duty and heart's delight to celebrate this day with pomp and circumstance. – When we set about preparing today's festivity, we were acutely aware that what our jubilarian would like best was for any homage to be part – if you will pardon the expression – of a clinical family celebration.

However, we all of us agreed that this time we would put his wishes aside for once and focus instead on the unique position he holds as a teacher, scientist and doctor and turn the celebration of his seventieth birthday into an occasion that will ring down the ages.[1234]

Friedrich Dimmer[1235] – Fuchs's oldest student, assistant, brother in law,[1236] and his successor as Director of the Second University Eye Clinic between 1916 and 1926 – was assigned a task that was by no means easy: naming and describing those aspects of Fuchs's character that had enabled him to be so outstandingly successful as a doctor, teacher, and scientist:

No big words, no grand phrases are needed to pay homage to Fuchs. All that is needed is the unvarnished truth. Even an unskilled orator cannot fail to awaken an echo in the hearts of his listeners that owes its resonance to all of us knowing full well what Fuchs means to us.

[…]

If I am to draw up a picture of his career and dwell even briefly on its internal and external characteristics and effects, Fuchs will have to be prepared to hear a great deal of praise. As truth is my only guide in what I am going to say, he has only himself to blame if he is in for a great deal of praise and I only hope that he can muster the spirit his mentor Billroth once showed on a similar occasion, when he said: "You have no idea, gentlemen, how much praise I can bring myself to put up with."[1237]

Dimmer then quoted comments he had overheard other people make about Fuchs. Commenting on the test lecture Fuchs had delivered as part of his habilitation in 1881, Arlt, the teacher and mentor Fuchs thought of so highly, said: *"Fuchs has a knack of dealing with each topic exhaustively"*. An American doctor commended Fuchs with the words that *"he is remarkable for what is crucial in medicine – objectivity".* Shortly after World War I, an English ophthalmologist, reporting in a specialist journal on a tour of the most important eye clinics on the Continent, distilled what had struck him most about the way operations were carried out at the Fuchs Clinic into *"in this, the overriding rule is simplicity".*[1238]

Dimmer went on to name other characteristic traits, which in his view were preconditions for Fuchs's eminent success:

Cool, objective practicality; absolute reliability; unfailing thoroughness; implacable self-criticism; straight, targeted natural thinking, simplicity and matter-of-factness of action.[1239]

He then resoundingly appraised Ernst Fuchs's activities as a physician:

The way Fuchs examines his patients may serve as a pointer to how he has always proceeded in his work. This approach is all the more justified as Fuchs, in spite of the great deal of anatomical-histological work we have to thank him for has always remained a clinician at heart. Unlike many ophthalmologists whose works could equally well be done by anatomists, histologists or physiologists, Fuchs's work has always remained linked to the clinic. Even purely anatomical trains of thought have mostly been occasioned and sparked by clinical considerations.

When Fuchs examines a patient he never allows himself to be swayed by a prominent symptom, which may lead the examiner so easily astray that one might almost speak of seduction. Instead, a stock taking of symptoms is made, unhurriedly, methodically, and in systematic order. The symptoms are then combined to form an overall picture, which is then related to the wealth of images stored in the examiner's memory and to his comprehensive knowledge of the literature. This thoroughness and objective methodology made Fuchs a model for his students. These qualities impressed themselves upon his students and left their stamp on the work done at his clinic.[1240]

The same style, according to Dimmer, distinguished Fuchs's work at the microscope,[1241] assuring it in many cases of lasting significance and of making valuable contributions to scientific progress. Due to his inexorable self-criticism and the exacting standards Fuchs had set for himself, quite a few papers had never been put forward for publication. This highlights Fuchs's objectivity and the total lack of excessive ambition he had shown in all situations.

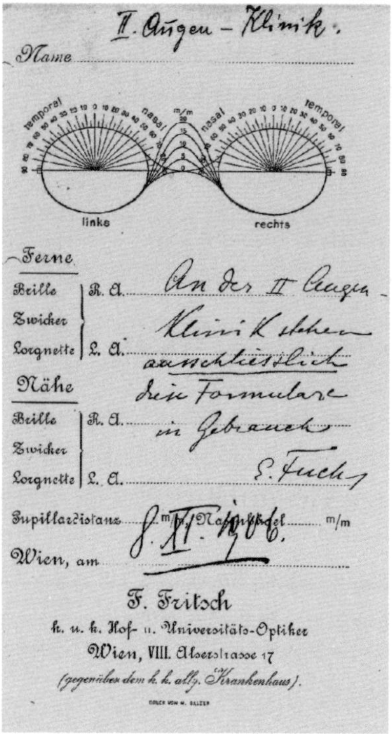
II. Augen-Klinik.
Name
temporal nasal m/m nasal temporal
linke rechts
Ferne
Brille R. A. An der II Augen-
Zwicker Klinik stehen
Lorgnette L. A. ausschliesslich
Nähe drei Formulare
Brille R. A. in Gebrauch
Zwicker
Lorgnette L. A. E. Fuchs
Pupillardistanz m/m
Wien, am 8. XI. 1906.
F. Fritsch
k. u. k. Hof- u. Universitäts-Optiker
Wien, VIII. Alserstrasse 17
(gegenüber dem k. k. allg. Krankenhaus).

Fig. 96
Prescription for glasses with handwritten commentary by Ernst Fuchs for the Directorate of the Allgemeines Krankenhaus, 8 November 1906

Next Dimmer expressed his appreciation of Fuchs's outstanding talents as a teacher, which had also manifested themselves in his world famous *Lehrbuch*.[1242] Due to World War I and the economic downturn it had caused, no new edition had been forthcoming for more than a decade. Now, on the occasion of his 70th birthday, the 13th edition was published, overseen by his former student Maximilian Salzmann.

While extremely popular as a teacher, Fuchs, according to Dimmer, tended to be feared as an examiner. This was down to his uncompromising sense of justice and integrity, which characterised him as an academic teacher. This is borne out by the orthopaedist Albert Lorenz (1885–1970),[1243] the elder brother of zoologist, ethologist and Nobel Prize winner Konrad Lorenz (1903–1989),[1244] in the memoir he dedicated in 1952 to his father, the pioneer of orthopaedics in Austria, Adolf Lorenz (1854–1946).[1245] Fuchs, according to Albert Lorenz, used to maintain stoic calm during doctoral viva voce exams, showing no outward reaction whatever. He provided no help whatever that would have enabled the candidate, once he had taken a wrong turning, to get back on course again. What Albert Lorenz says about this cannot be described as flattering:

You might as well have expected a sign of life from a marble statue. When it was all over, the marble statue moved and handed down its verdict: fail or pass; very often – too often – the former.[1246]

Yet in Dimmer's view it was precisely Fuchs's understanding of the office he held at the university, his integrity, and his highly developed sense of responsibility for the students he trained and examined that accounted for the enthusiasm he inspired among students who worked with him and the great number of doctors from abroad, who *"flocked to Vienna and the Second Eye Clinic as the Mecca of Ophthalmology"*.[1247]

His medical expertise and skills had made Fuchs *"a blessing for an untold number of patients"*.[1248] Only a few years after he had taken office, more than 20,000 new outpatients a year were attending his clinic[1249] (Fig. 96), where the number of cataract operations exceeded 500.

This made Fuchs the clinician who single-handedly coped with the greatest number of patients in the world. The higher patient volume of some eye clinics such as Moorfields Hospital in London needs to be put into perspective in that they have several executive medical directors.[1250]

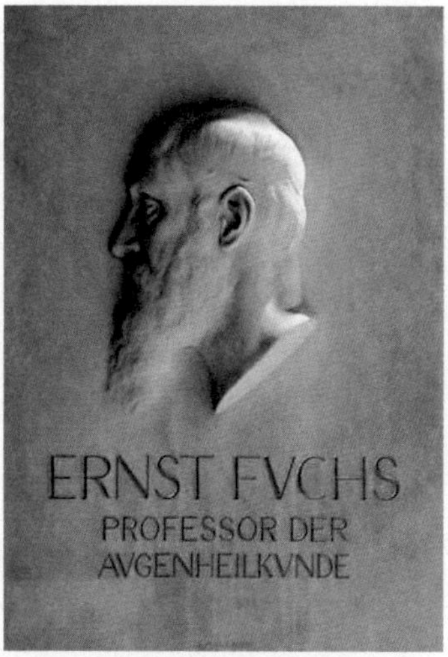

Fig. 97 Marble relief of Ernst Fuchs

Turning his attention to general human characteristics, Dimmer singled out the wide range of Fuchs's interests, his energy, his apparently unending zest for work and his strict work discipline, characteristics that needed to be taken into account if one was to understand how he had achieved so much in one lifetime. He never went on holiday without taking with him a great number of books, his microscope and histological preparations so as to be able to continue working wherever he happened to be. By way of compensation for his concentrated scientific work, Fuchs, who had a great love for nature, challenged himself with ambitious mountaineering and climbing exploits[1251] and travelled extensively.

Unveiling the Marble Relief Depicting Ernst Fuchs

Having decided to honour their teacher on his 70th birthday by adding his likeness to the portraits of the medical celebrities that adorned the walls of the First University Eye Clinic auditorium, former students from Ernst Fuchs's inner circle had commissioned the renowned sculptor and professor at Vienna's Academy of Fine Arts Josef Müllner (1879–1968)[1252] to create a marble relief. It depicts Fuchs in profile looking to the left. The rectangular slab of marble bears an engraved inscription in golden lettering at the bottom, stating the name and profession of the subject, the name of the artist, and the year of origin. (Fig. 97) The plaster model of the relief provided by Müllner beforehand today forms part of the Müllner bequest in the Rollett Museum in Baden near Vienna.[1253]

The relief having been unveiled by Dimmer in the presence of the artist, the gift was acknowledged by Meller in an acceptance speech,[1254] whose closing words were a fitting expression of the wishes, expectations, and hopes animating the Vienna Ophthalmological School in its faithful succession to Fuchs in spite of the unfavourable external conditions confronting it:

Thanks to the artist, Prof. Müllner, [Fuchs's] *eyes are permanently directed at us, as we engage in the serious work of passing on his teachings to the disciples of science in homage to his example. From the walls the pictures of his famous predecessors extend their greetings and welcome him joyfully to their company. Where they have laid the foundations, he has continued to build, working tirelessly, the very model of an honest steward of the legacy they have left him. He has endowed the Vienna Ophthalmological School with a renown that now spans the entire globe, and if it is the case today that physicians from all over the world again flock to our clinics to be trained for life in this profession, it is, as we know, thanks to the outstanding contribution Fuchs has made to our specialty. It has enabled our specialty to shine forth undiminished, even though he himself left the clinic years ago.*

And to those among us who are students of this University let me say: Gentlemen, may this portrait be an admonition to shape your lives along the lines the man at the centre of this festivity followed for seventy years, leading a life calmly engrossed in work.[1255]

[...]

Let the marble then reflect all the love we offer up to our mentor today, allowing it to settle in the young hearts of a generation who will, we hope, be more fortunate than us.[1256]

An option for the placement of the relief the festival committee would have preferred in view of Ernst Fuchs's worldwide renown was the *Arkadenhof* of Vienna University, where he would have been surrounded by a host of other eminent scholars. However, the legal situation at the time allowed the erection of monuments in this location to honour a scholar only several years after their death. The marble relief therefore remained in the auditorium of the First University Eye Clinic until Fuchs's centenary and was then transferred to the University's *Arkadenhof*, where its unveiling was marked by a festive ceremony on 21 June 1951.[1257]

Festschrift

As a token of the gratitude friends, colleagues, and students felt for the jubilarian, whom they venerated to a point where many were almost in awe of him, the most prestigious and longest established ophthalmological journal of the German-speaking world, Albrecht von Graefe's *Archiv für Ophthalmologie*, whose editorial committee counted Fuchs among its long-standing members, published a monumental *Festschrift* as its issue No. 105.[1258] Its date of publication, 14 June 1921, coincided with Fuchs's seventieth birthday. Priced at 458 marks, it featured a portrait of the jubilarian (Figs. 98a, b). After the unveiling of the portrait relief Maximilian Salzmann presented Fuchs with "his" *Festschrift*, wrapped as it were in words expressive of personal appreciation and gratitude.[1259]

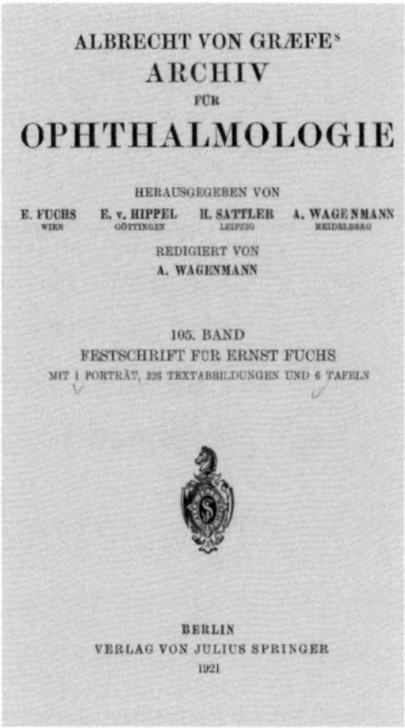
ALBRECHT VON GRÆFE'S
ARCHIV
FÜR
OPHTHALMOLOGIE
HERAUSGEGEBEN VON
E. FUCHS WIEN | E. v. HIPPEL GÖTTINGEN | H. SATTLER LEIPZIG | A. WAGENMANN HEIDELBERG
REDIGIERT VON
A. WAGENMANN
105. BAND
FESTSCHRIFT FÜR ERNST FUCHS
MIT 1 PORTRÄT, 326 TEXTABBILDUNGEN UND 6 TAFELN
BERLIN
VERLAG VON JULIUS SPRINGER
1921

Fig. 98a
Fuchs *Festschrift*
1921

The Festschrift contained seventy-three papers in German, all of which appeared there for the first time.[1260] Seventy-six authors from eleven nations contributed to the 1232-page tome: Germany (31), Austria (20), Sweden (5), Netherlands (3), Switzerland (3), Czechoslovakia (3), Hungary (3), Italy (2), Denmark (1), Finland (1) and Norway (1).

Two of the papers by Austrian authors were written by non-ophthalmologists: syphilidologist Josef Kyrle (1880–1924)[1261] reported on tabes and negative liquor[1262] in a paper whose ophthalmoscopic findings had been provided by Meller of the 1st Univ. Eye Clinic. The former Fuchs student Otto Marburg (1874–1948),[1263] then Director of the Institute of Neurology of Vienna University, in turn dealt with the phenomenon of papilloedema.[1264]

Special Issue of the Wiener Medizinische Wochenschrift

As a sign of their appreciation of Ernst Fuchs, the *Wiener Medizinische Wochenschrift*, Vienna's oldest medical weekly periodical in German (year of foundation: 1851) published a special issue[1265] in his honour. It was handed to Fuchs immediately after the presentation of the Graefe Archiv's *Festschrift* by the editor in charge, Adolf Kronfeld (1861–1938),[1266] who had received his medical training at Vienna's Allgemeines Krankenhaus under Ernst Fuchs, among others. The title page[1267] featured the reproduction of a portrait photograph of Fuchs as a young man, alongside a portrait of him in his old age, drawn by the well-known Viennese artist Olga Prager (1872–1930).[1268]

The introduction to this special issue, which Meller used to express his and the ophthalmological establishment's thanks to Fuchs,[1269] was followed by 19 original papers by Ernst Bachstez (1888–1954),[1270] Rudolf Bergmeister,[1271] Friedrich Dimmer,[1272] Adalbert Fuchs,[1273] Emil von Grósz (1865–1941),[1274] Gustav Guist (1892–1967),[1275] Viktor Hanke,[1276] Paul Kafka,[1277] Richard Krämer (1878–1937),[1278] Hans Lauber,[1279] Karl Lindner,[1280] Josef Meller,[1281] Marie Procksch,[1282] Adolf Purtscher,[1283] Moriz Sachs,[1284] Maximilian Salzmann,[1285] Hubert Sattler,[1286] Richard Seefelder, (1875–1949)[1287] and Eduard Konrad Zirm (1863–1944).[1288]

Award of the title "Freeman of the City of Vienna"

In his capacity as representative of the City of Vienna, Councillor Julius Tandler[1289] then extended the city's congratulations to Fuchs, announcing at the same time the award of the honorific title of Freeman of the City of Vienna.[1290] The pertinent resolution was passed at the meeting of the City Council on the very next day, June 22, and was followed a day later by the official presentation of the honorific title. The reason that was cited for the award was simply *"Professor at the University of Vienna, on the occasion of his seventieth birthday"*.[1291]

Honorary Member of the Wiener Ophthalmologische Gesellschaft

The oldest representative of the Vienna Ophthalmological School, August Leopold Ritter v. Reuss,[1292] presented Fuchs with the diploma attesting his honorary membership in the Wiener Ophthalmologische Gesellschaft (WOG),[1293] which had already elected him chairman in its meeting on April 19, 1920.[1294] The foundation of the WOG in 1903 was due to an initiative taken by one of Fuchs's students, Moriz Sachs.[1295]

Visibly moved by so many tokens of appreciation, Fuchs thanked the officials in the audience, the representatives of university and medical institutions, Josef Müllner and, last but not least, his former students, who had spared no effort to make the occasion truly festive. Fuchs found special words of gratitude for Dimmer, who had dedicated to him the third edition of his textbook of ophthalmoscopy,[1296] which was nearing completion, and for the heartfelt dedication[1297] of the new edition of Meller's textbook on ophthalmic surgery.[1298] He expressed his appreciation of Meller generously donating ten copies of Salzmann's 13th edition of the *Lehrbuch* to indigent students.

He showed himself delighted with the contributions to his *Festschrift* in *Graefes Archiv* and thanked the authors.[1299]

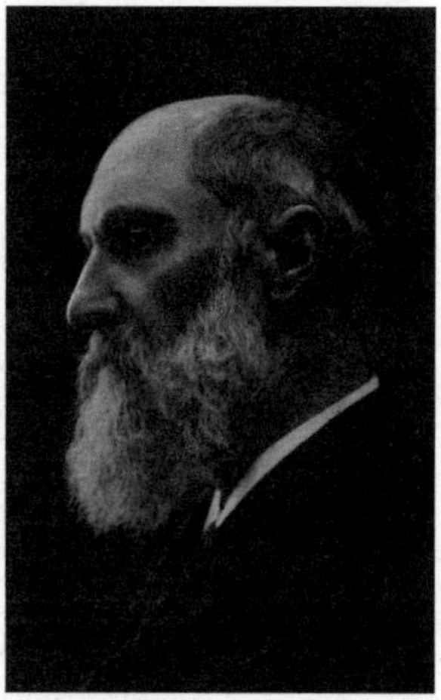

Fig. 98b Portrait of Ernst Fuchs in the 1921 *Festschrift*

At the end of this truly memorable occasion Fuchs briefly sketched the roadmap of his career in his acceptance speech.[1300] Downplaying in the way people had come to expect of him anything that might make his success look special in the eyes of others, he revealed that the "secret" behind his many achievements was sheer persistence:

My research work depended, rather than on strokes of genius, on steady, systematic work, which I value higher than anything else. Whenever I found myself in a situation where I could make neither head nor tail of a case, I took stock of the entire status and then often the breakthrough came in the shape of symptoms that had previously been overlooked. The same is true of scientific research. I believe that in this way everyone with no more than middling talent can achieve what I have achieved, given sufficient perseverance. It seems doubtful to me, however, whether this can be achieved in the modern eight-hour day.

I retired from teaching sooner than the law provides because I wanted to use what time remained to me to work through the great mass of material I had collected during the long time I worked at the clinic, a task for which I could not possibly have found the requisite time as director of the clinic. I am profoundly grateful to Professors Dimmer and Meller, who have supported me in this by putting the facilities of their clinics at my disposal right up to this very day.[1301]

The Ghibellinen then intoned the traditional academic commercium song, *Gaudeamus igitur*.

Birthday Lecture

As the great number of guests of honour had left very few seats for students in the relatively small lecture hall of the 1st Univ. Eye Clinic, Meller had suggested to Fuchs's delight that the students be recompensed for what they had missed. Moriz Sachs therefore announced in his opening speech that Fuchs was going to deliver a lecture to all comers at the same venue in two days' time.[1302] In this lecture Fuchs briefly cast light on the achievements and the significance of the world's oldest University Eye Clinic and went on to discuss the relationship between lighting and the eye.[1303]

Extraordinary Meeting of the Wiener Ophthalmologische Gesellschaft (WOG)

On 7 January 1921 Meller had announced that the WOG would meet for three days on 4–6 August for a four-session conference in honour of Ernst Fuchs.[1304] The venue for the conference, the time-honoured lecture hall of the First University Eye Clinic headed by Meller, was presumably chosen for its association with the development of ophthalmology as an academic specialty.[1305] On the same occasion, Meller set a deadline for the registration of presentations and demonstrations, June 15, the day after Fuchs's 70th birthday. In July, the detailed conference programme and the discussion topic – the efficacy of recently developed glaucoma operation techniques compared with classic iridectomy according to Graefe[1306] – were announced.[1307]

Opening the first session of the conference, Fuchs pointed out the achievements and significance of the world's oldest university eye clinic from an historical point of view:

E[rnst] Fuchs, speaking on behalf of the Wiener Ophthalmologische Gesellschaft, gave a cordial welcome to the numerous participants, reminding them that the conference's sessions were due to take place in the oldest university eye clinic in the world. The rise of the clinic, Fuchs said, dated to the eighteenth century, to the time of Empress Maria Theresa, who had appointed one of Wenzel*'s*[1308] *former students, Professor Barth,*[1309] *Full Professor of Ophthalmology. Under his successor Beer the chair of ophthalmology became an autonomous institution in 1812 and was soon followed by other such chairs established at other Austrian universities, including those of Padova and Pavia. It was not until much later, in 1866, that Berlin followed suit and established an autonomous chair; other countries took even longer and there were still some where ophthalmology was not on a par with the other specialties.*

Beer*'s clinic was then passed on to Rosas, Arlt, Schnabel, Dimmer and, most recently, to Meller. It is home to many historical-ophthalmological objects and from their serene portraits on the walls the old masters of our specialty extended their greeting. This conference was the first for which a great number of ophthalmologists, friends of ours, have accepted our invitation and have come to Vienna, many of them from Germany and from other countries, some of them from very far afield. This said, this meeting is not an "international conference". It goes without saying that we were unable to extend our invitation to those* *countries and colleagues who have imposed a boycott on German and Austrian ophthalmologists, who have refused to admit them to their own societies and conferences and who have even banned the German language (!) from Washington in 1922.*[1310] *But anyone who is friendly and fair minded, no matter where they are from, is welcome to join in our endeavours.*[1311]

These last words of Fuchs's introductory speech allude to the controversial, conflict-laden situation after World War I, which had pitted the Central Powers (the Austro-Hungarian Monarchy and Germany, later also the Ottoman Empire and Bulgaria) against the Entente (France, Great Britain and Russia, later also Italy and the United States). The victory of the Entente in 1918 led, as is well known, to the demise of the Austro-Hungarian Monarchy and the German *Kaiserreich*. War had also resulted in the rupture of diplomatic relations between the former enemies, which continued for several years after 1918. This was the reason why the US State Department extended invitations to the International Ophthalmological Conference scheduled for 1922 in Washington exclusively to the embassies and legations of countries with which it maintained diplomatic relations.[1312] It was against this backdrop that in 1919 the decision was taken by the organisers of the conference to substitute Spanish for German in the list of officially approved languages at the conference. To justify this decision it was claimed that the majority of participants, in addition to those from the United States itself, were in any case likely to come from England, France and Spain.[1313] German-speaking ophthalmologists naturally took offence at being thus excluded.[1314] Having been the vanguard of their specialty in science, research, teaching and therapy before the Great War, they now found themselves officially blacklisted and their achievements downplayed.

The Heidelberg-based Deutsche Ophthalmologische Gesellschaft having decided to forgo their own prestigious annual meeting in 1921 in favour of the conference in Vienna,[1315] the meeting of the Wiener Ophthalmologische Gesellschaft arranged in honour of Ernst Fuchs proved a resounding success and was attended not only by German and Austrian eye specialists but by a great number of colleagues from Spain, Scandinavia, the Netherlands, Switzerland, Hungary, Italy and even from Latin America.[1316]

Demonstrations and Lectures

Fourteen demonstrations were presented to the conference audience by researchers from eight countries, with Austria contributing five, Germany three, and Bulgaria, Denmark, Italy, Romania, Spain and Hungary one each.[1317]

Of the fifty-one lectures in German announced in the provisional programme forty-seven were in fact delivered in the conference's four sessions.[1318] The lecturers came from ten nations: seventeen from Germany, the same number from Austria, four from Hungary, two from Switzerland, another two from Spain, and one each from Italy, Norway, Romania, Sweden and Czechoslovakia.

It is worth pointing out that the lecturers included two women, E. Kleinsasser[1319] and Budapest-based Olga Palich-Szántó (1890–1971).[1320] This was still a rarity at conferences in the German-speaking world.

On August 6, during the fourth session of "his" conference, Ernst Fuchs delivered a lecture on chorioretinitis.[1321] In it, he discussed two possibilities for the localisation of the primary focus – choroid or retina – and the possibilities each of these possible points of origin opened up for the inflammation to spread. Based on his own clinical observations and the histological research he had carried out, Fuchs proposed that the majority of cases of chorioretinitis originated in the choroid. There were, however, isolated cases where the disease had originated in the retina and had only subsequently spread to the choroid. In the final phase, these latter cases displayed an appearance that often closely resembled the former.

Notes

1216 "Feier des 70. Geburtstages Ernst Fuchs's am 14. Juni 1921 in Wien", in: *Zeitschr. Augenheilk.* 47 (1922), pp. 47–63.

1217 Michael Hainisch (1858–1940). Studied law at the Univ. of Leipzig and Vienna (Dr. iur. 1882). Court internship, several years' service as a civil servant. 1920–1924 and 1924–1928 Federal President (independent) as the successor of Karl Seitz [(1869–1950), President of the Sozialdemokrat. Arbeiterpartei Deutschösterreichs – SDAPDÖ]. 1929/30 Federal Minister for Trade and Transport. Cf. CZEIKE (as in FN 13); ÖBL (as in FN 11); NDB (as in FN 15).

[1218] Walter Breisky (1871–1944). Studied law at Vienna Univ. 1895 Entered the civil service. 1905 In charge of the Protestant Desk at the Ministry of Education, from 1907 seconded to the press department of the Presidium of the Council of Ministers. 1919 Dir. of Department 1920 State Secretary for Domestic Affairs and Education. 1920–1922 Vice Chancellor and Federal Minister for Domestic Affairs and Education. 26/27 January 1922 Federal Chancellor for one day. 1923–1931 President of the Federal Office of Statistics. Cf. CZEIKE (as in FN 13); ÖBL (as in FN 11).

[1219] Carl von Helly (1865–1932). Studied at Graz Univ. (Dr. med. 1888). Assist. at the Patholog.-Anatom. Inst. in Graz, later junior doctor at the local Allg. Krankenhaus, 1890 Qualified as district physician, joined the state first-aid service (district physician), later in the First-Aid Department of Graz prefecture. 1896 Call to the Public Health Department of the Ministry of Domestic Affairs. 1911 In charge of public health in Lower Austria. 1920–25 Dir. of Department and Dir. of Public Health in the Federal Ministry of Social Affairs. Member of the Austrian National Institute of Health (OSR) and Vice President of the Austrian Society of the Red Cross. Great merits across almost all fields of public health, esp. in the war years and the difficult postwar years. Cf. *Mitt. d. Volksgesundheitsamtes Vienna* VI, 1932, p. 51; ÖBL (as in FN 11).

[1220] Cf. FN 769.

[1221] Alfons Dopsch (1868–1953). Studied at Vienna Univ., graduate of the Inst. f. österr. Geschichtsforschung (Dr. phil. 1890). 1892–1900 Member of the staff working on the *Monumenta Germaniae Historica* ("Diplomas of the Carolingians"). 1894 Habilitation. 1898 Assoc. Prof. 1900–1937 Full Prof. of General History and the History of Austria at Vienna Univ.; 1920/21 Rector of Vienna Univ.; 1929–1932 Senator. Main areas of interest: Economic, financial, social, constitutional and cultural history of the Middle Ages. Cf. CZEIKE (as in FN 13); NDB (as in FN 15); ÖBL (as in FN 11).

[1222] Cf. FN 45.

[1223] Josef Nevinny (1853–1923). 1878 Certified drug dispenser (Prague), 1879 Dr. med. univ. (Prague Univ.). From 1884 Assist. under Professor of Pharmacology and Pharmacognosy August Emil Vogl (cf. FN 604) in Vienna. 1888 Habilitation in Pharmacognosy at Vienna Univ.; 1893–1923 Prof. of Pharmacology and Pharmacognosy at Innsbruck Univ. (1893 Assoc. Prof., 1896 Full Prof.). His achievements include the construction and appointment of a new Pharmacolog. Institute (library, collection of drugs, stables). Cf. EULNER (as in FN 13); FISCHER (as in FN 28); ÖBL (as in FN 11); PAGEL (as in FN 13); HUTER, *100 Jahre Med. Fak. Innsbruck* (as in FN 177), pp. 291ff.

[1224] Cf. FN 686.

[1225] Cf. FN 137.

[1226] Julius Mannaberg (1860–1941). Studied at Vienna Univ. (Dr. med. univ. 1884). 1887 Assist. at the 1st Med. Univ. Clinic under Hermann Nothnagel (1841–1905) at the Allg. Krankenhaus. 1895 Habilitation in Internal Medicine at Vienna Univ.; 1895 (tit. Prof. 1902). 1898–1930 Dir. of the Department of Internal Medicine at the Wiener Allgem. Poliklinik (1917–1930 also Hospital Director). Main areas of interest: bacteriol., malaria, kidney diseases. Cf. CZEIKE (as in FN 13); EISENBERG 2 (as in FN 13); FISCHER (as in FN 28); DEIMER *Poliklinik* (as in FN 200), pp. 53ff.; Appreciations, in: *Wien. klin. Wochenschr.* 42 (1930), pp. 601–602 and 75 (1963), pp. 665ff.

1227 Cf. FN 745.

1228 Richard Paltauf (1858–1924). Studied at Graz Univ. (Dr. med. univ. 1880), 1881–1883 Ass. at the local Pathol.-Anatom. Inst. under Hans Eppinger sen. (1848–1916) and Hans Kundrat (cf. FN 597), whom he followed to Vienna in 1883. 1888 Habilitation in Pathol. Anatomy at Vienna Univ. (1892 tit. Assoc. Prof.). Establishment of the Patholog.-Anatom. Inst. of the Wr. Allgem. Poliklinik jointly with a Histol.-Bacteriol. Inst. 1893 Prosector of Krankenanstalt Rudolfstiftung, at the same time Dir. of the Inst. of Pathol. Histol. and Bacteriol. of Vienna Univ.; 1894 Foundation of a vaccination institute to protect humans from glanders, a contagious zoonotic disease, and of the State Serotherapeut. Inst. to produce an antiserum against diphtheria. 1898 Ad pers. Full Prof. of Histol. and General Pathol. 1900 Full Prof. of General and Experim. Pathol.; identification of what was known as rag pickers' disease as anthrax. Malign lymphogranuloma is now generally referred to as morbus Hodgkin-Paltauf-Sternberg: 1832 First description by Thomas Hodgkin (1798–1866), 1897 Paltauf and his disciple Carl Sternberg (1872–1935) succeeded in throwing light on the pathol. morphology of this blood disease. Cf. CZEIKE (as in FN 13); EISENBERG 2 (as in FN 13); FISCHER (as in FN 28); ÖBL (as in FN 11); PAGEL (as in FN 13); LESKY, *Wien. Med. Schule* (as in FN 12), cf. Ind.; Obituaries, in: *Wien. klin. Wochenschr.* 37 (1924), pp. 487ff., *Feierl. Inauguration* [...] *für das Studienjahr 1924/25* (with bibliography).

1229 Cf. FN 689.

1230 Cf. FN 589.

1231 Cf. FN 1252.

1232 A member of the Masonic lodge Zur Wohltätigkeit, Mozart composed a Masonic cantata (KV 623) 19 days before his death on 5 December 1791, the last work he was able to complete. Roughly a year later, a Viennese printer, one Joseph Hraschansky, published the score, adding the so-called *Kettenlied* (or *Bundeslied* or *Weihelied*) to part of the cantata's print run. Assigned the number 623a by Köchl, the *Kettenlied* received its name and its significance from the fact that freemasons used to end their meetings with that song while joining hands. New lyrics, beginning with "Brüder, reicht die Hand zum Bunde" were substituted in 1824 by Johann Gottfried Hientzsch (1787–1856), Director of the Royal Institutes of the Blind in Berlin. Austria's Council of Ministers passed a resolution on 22 October 1946 to adopt the tune of the *Weihelied/Bundeslied* for the new national anthem. Another government resolution passed on 25 February 1947 settled the question of the lyrics. A poem by Austrian poet Paula von Preradović (1887–1951), the wife of the diplomat, publicist, historian and resistance fighter against the Nazi regime Ernst Molden (1886–1953), was chosen and became the new anthem, after having been subjected to minor alterations agreed on by von Preradović. Musicologists began voicing doubts in the mid-1960s about Mozart's authorship of the *Bundeslied*, of which no autograph has yet come to light. Having initially been ascribed to the composer Johann Baptist Holzer (or Holtzer, 1753–1818), a member of the Viennese lodge "Zur wahren Eintracht", it is now increasingly being considered to be the work of another lodge brother, the Moravian-Austrian composer, conductor, violinist, and Mozart disciple Anton Wrani(t) zky (Antonín Vranický, 1761–1820); see: Richard BAMBERGER, Franz MAIER-BRUCK (eds), *Österreich Lexikon in zwei Bänden*. Österr. Bundesverlag für Unterricht, Wissenschaft u. Kunst/Verlag Jugend u. Volk, Volume 1 A–K, Vienna/Munich 1966, p. 161 (Bundeshymne); Joachim DIEDERICHS, "Von wem stammt die Melodie der österreichischen Bundeshymne?", in: *Österr. Musikzeitschr.* 73, (2018), Issue 1, pp. 79–82.

1233 Moriz Sachs (1865–1948). Studied at the Univ. of Vienna, Strasbourg and Heidelberg (Dr. med. univ. 1889, Vienna). 1891 Assist. under physiol. Carl Ewald Hering (see: FN 296) at the German Univ. in Prague. Hering encouraged Sachs's interest in the physiol. of the senses. 1894 Assist. at the 2nd Univ. Eye Clinic in Vienna under Fuchs (1899 Habilitation, 1911 tit. Assoc. Prof., 1917 Assoc. Prof.). 1904/05 Relaunch of the Eye Dept. of the Spital d. Barmherz. Brüder in Vienna, 1914–1934 Dir. of the Eye Dept. of the Krankenhaus Wieden, where he had modern facilities installed. 1903 Invention of the Sachs lamp for the transillumination of the eye, designed to find non-magnetic alien bodies in the vitreous. Other fields of work: detachment of the retina, physiology and pathology of eye movements (notably astigmatism and paralysis of the ocular muscles) and colour blindness. Cf. ÖBL (as in FN 11).

1234 Cf. FN 1216, p. 47.

1235 Cf. FN 44.

1236 Dimmer was the husband of the sister of Ernst Fuchs's wife Julie, née Mayr. Cf. Family archive.

1237 Cf. FN 1216, p. 48.

1238 Ibid., p. 49.

1239 Ibid., p. 50.

1240 Ibid.

1241 See Ch. 7.

1242 See Ch. 6.

1243 Albert Lorenz (1885–1970). Studied at Vienna Univ. (Dr. med. univ. 1910). Joined the 2nd Surg. Univ. Clinic at the Allgem. Krankenhaus, which was headed by Julius v. Hochenegg (cf. FN 744); Hochenegg entrusted him with the installation of an orthopaed. ward. After the end of World War I, this ward was discontinued for financial reasons, so that Albert Lorenz joined the practice of his father, Adolf Lorenz (cf. FN 1245), as private assist.; 1943 Habilitation in Surgery at Vienna Univ.; 1945–1951 Dir. of the orthopaed. ward of the 1st Surg. Univ. Clinic headed by Leopold Schönbauer (1888–1963). Continued to work at the orthopaed. outpatient clinic of the Wr. Gebietskrankenkasse in 1953–1959 after his official retirement. Main fields of work: amputation and prosthesis management, femoral neck fracture, high arch deformity, and acetabular bone grafting. Cf. CZEIKE (as in FN 13); https://austria-forum.org (last accessed: 6 Sept. 2022).

1244 Konrad Lorenz (1903–1989). Studied at Columbia Univ./New York and Vienna Univ. (Dr. med. univ. 1928). Studied zoology at Vienna Univ. (Dr. phil. 1933). During this time, he worked as assist. at the Anat. Instit. 1937 Habilitation in Comparative Animal Psychology and Anat.; a pioneer of comparative ethology of humans and animals. Advocate of the Nazi racist ideology. 1940 Appointed Prof. of Psychol., Dir. of the Psychol. Inst. at Königsberg Univ. and a staff member of the Office of Racial Policy of the NSDAP. 1941–1948 Active service and Russian prisoner of war.

1949–1951 Established a private research station of comparative ethology at his estate in Altenberg nr. Vienna. 1951 Dir. of the Forschungsstelle für Vergleichende Verhaltensforschung of the Max-Planck-Inst. in Buldern/ Westphalia. 1961–1973 Dir. of the Max-Planck-Inst. f. Verhaltenspsychol. in Seewiesen/Bavaria (trailblazing ethological research on greylag geese). Established the specialty ethology in the German-speaking world. 1953 Honorary Prof. at Münster Univ.; 1957 Honorary Prof. of Zoology at Munich Univ.; 1973 Nobel Prize for Medicine and Psychol. together with Nikolaas Tinbergen (1907–1988) and Karl Ritter von Frisch (1886–1982). Return to Austria; Dir. of the Inst. f. Tierpsychol. of the Academy of Sciences in Grünau/Almtal. From 1982 at the Konrad-Lorenz-Instit. in his native Altenberg. In old age activist for the protection of the environment and against nuclear power. Cf. CZEIKE (as in FN 13); Benedikt FÖGER, Klaus TASCHWER, *Die andere Seite des Spiegels. Konrad Lorenz und der Nationalsozialismus*. Czernin Verlag 2001; Gerhard KLUMBIES, "Konrad Lorenz 1903–1989. Verhaltensforscher – Professor in Königsberg (1940–45) – Nobelpreis 1973". In: Dietrich RAUSCHNING, Donata v. NERÉE (eds.): *Die Albertus-Universität zu Königsberg und ihre Professoren. Aus Anlaß der Gründung der Albertus-Universität vor 450 Jahren*. Duncker & Humblot, Berlin 1995.

1245 Adolf Lorenz (1854–1946). Originally from Austrian Silesia. Studied at Vienna Univ. (Dr. med. univ. 1880). Surg. specialisation under Eduard Albert (cf. FN 609) at the 1st Surg. Univ. Clinic at Vienna's Allgem. Krankenhaus. 1884 Habilitation. Prevented from pursuing surgery by chron. carbolic acid induced excema, he special. in orthopaedics ("dry surgery"), which he established as an autonomous specialty: 1886–1924 Founder-Director of the Universitätsambulatorium für orthopädische Chirurgie at the Allgem. Krankenhaus. 1889 Assoc. Professor of Orthopaedics. Worldwide recognition of his pioneering development of non-invasive orthopaed. treatment methods. Main fields of work: Pathol. and therapy of congen. dysplasia of the hip (trail-blazing cures), flat foot and clubfoot, curvature of the spine, tubercul. bone and joint diseases. 1924–1936 active in New York in the winter months. Honorary citizen of Newark/New York. Cf. CZEIKE (as in FN 13); FISCHER (as in FN 28); NDB (as in FN 15); ÖBL (as in FN 11); PAGEL (as in FN 13); Obituary: *Wien. klin. Wochenschr.* 58 (1946), pp. 96–97; LESKY, *Wiener Med. Schule* (as in FN 12), pp. 454ff; Adolf LORENZ, *Ich durfte helfen. Mein Leben und Wirken*. Albrecht, Vienna 1949; Manfred SKOPEC, "Adolf Lorenz und das Ringen um die Verselbständigung der Orthopädie", in: Rainer KOTZ (ed.), *100 Jahre Orthopädie an der Universität Wien*. Verlag d. Wiener Med. Akad. 1987, pp. 1ff.

1246 Albert LORENZ, *Wenn der Vater mit dem Sohne* [...] *Erinnerungen an Adolf Lorenz*. Franz Deuticke, Vienna 1952, p. 238.

1247 Cf. FN 1216, p. 52, and Ernst FUCHS, "Wien, das Mekka der amerikanischen Aerzte. Die Weltbedeutung der Wiener Schule", in: *Neue Freie Presse* Nr. 22963, 19 August 1928, and the reprint of the corresponding diary entry, in: FUCHS, *Augenarzt* (as in FN 2); pp. 335–341.

1248 Ibid.

1249 Cf. Outpatient clinic statistics of the 2nd Univ. Eye Clinic, headed by Ernst Fuchs for 1903:

Men: 12,905 Women: 7,334. Sum total: 20,239. Number of children: 6,264. How often outpatients frequent the outpatient clinic [...] *cannot be ascertained, as no records are kept on this. This said, some patients, e.g. patients suffering from trachoma or scrofulous inflammation of the eye, frequent the outpatient clinic often every day for months. E. Fuchs.* Printed form with handwritten notes, signed by Ernst Fuchs. Private collection.

1250 Cf. FN 1216, p. 52.

1251 According to his son Adalbert, Ernst Fuchs had climbed more than 70 mountains higher than 3,000 m, including six over 4,000 m. Cf. FUCHS, *Augenarzt* (as in FN 2), p. 11, FN 9.

1252 Josef Müllner (1879–1968). 1896–1902 Studied at the Academy of Fine Arts in Vienna under Edmund Ritter von Hellmer (1850–1935) and Kaspar Ritter von Zumbusch (1830–1915). 1903 Rome Prize, followed by a one-year study trip to Italy. 1906–1911 Member of the Viennese Secession, from 1912 member of the Künstlerhaus. 1910–1948 Prof. at the Vienna Academy of Fine Arts (Rector 1926–1928, then Vice Rector for eight years. 1949 Honorary citizen of the Stadt Baden, 1964 Awarded Baden's Culture Prize. Honorary citizen of Vienna.
Cf. CZEIKE (as in FN 13, with a work list); Walter PERKO, "Der akademische Bildhauer Josef Müllner (1879–1968)". Catalogue of the Rollett Museum Baden, No. 16, 2nd ed. revised by Rudolf Maurer 2004.

1253 Prof. Ernst Fuchs, plaster model of a medal, 100 x 80 mm (Collections of the Rollett Museum Baden, M 1078). Cf. PERKO, "Josef Müllner", p. 19.

1254 Josef MELLER, "Rede bei der Übernahme des Marmorbildnisses von E. Fuchs am 14. 6. 1921", in: *Bericht aus d. Versammlungen d. Ophthalmol. Gesellschaft in Wien. Feier d. 70. Geburtstages v. Ernst Fuchs am 14. Juni 1921 in Wien*, p. VIII, and in: Josef MELLER, *Ausgewählte Schriften und Reden*. Wilhelm Maudrich, Vienna 1935, pp. 75–78.

1255 Cf. FN 1216, p. 55.

1256 Ibid., p. 56. – This expression of the hope that the new generation will be more fortunate must be seen against the grim background of life in Austria in the postwar years.

1257 See Ch. 12. Cf. MAISEL, *Gelehrte in Stein und Bronze* (as in FN 740), p. 94. It is worth noting that on the occasion of Ernst Fuchs's 100th birthday in 1951 a postcard with a photo of Müllner's portrait relief was issued. It bears the inscription on its reverse, *"Aus der Fuchs-Festschrift / 5.* Österreichische Ärztetagung Salzburg (Wiener klinische Wochenschrift, 63. Jahrgang/1951, Nummer 35/36)". Original in a private collection.

1258 *Festschrift zur Feier des siebzigsten Geburtstages. Herrn Hofrat Prof. Dr. Ernst Fuchs gewidmet von Freunden und dankbaren Schülern.* See the announcement: "Festschrift für E. Fuchs, Wien", in: *Klin. Monatsbl. Augenheilk.* 67/2 (1921), p. 105, and the review by. Edward JACKSON, in: *Am. J. Ophthalmol.* 4 (1921), pp. 875–876.

1259 Cf. FN 1216, pp. 56–57.

1260 The Fuchs *Festschrift* comprises the following papers: 1. Rudolf BERGMEISTER (AT), "*Über gliöse Wucherungen im Auge bei Mikrophthalmus congenitus und deren Beziehungen zur Angiomatosis retinae"*, pp. 1–38; 2. Otmar PURTSCHER (AT), "Angeborene Mißbildung bei einem Brüderpaar", pp. 39–47; 3. Fritz RÖSSLER (IT), "Der blinde Fleck in schielenden Augen", pp. 48–103; 4. E. HORNIKER (IT),

"Augenspiegelstudien bei Kriegsnephritis", pp. 104–128; 5. Julius HIRSCHBERG (DE), "Alkmaion's Verdienst um die Augenheilkunde", pp. 129–133; 6. Richard GREEF (DE), "Flocculi am Pigmentsaum der Iris", pp. 134–136; 7. Carl v. HESS (DE), "Die relative Rotsichtigkeit und Grünsichtigkeit", pp. 137–153; 8. Albert PETERS (DE), "Zur Kenntnis des Kapselstares", pp. 154–158; 9. W. GILBERT (DE), "Zur Histologie des Aderhautsarkoms", pp. 159–176; 10. Paul JUNIUS (DE), "*Über Keratitis disciformis*", pp. 177–204; 11. Wilhelm UHTHOFF (DE), "Beiträge zur Klinik und Anatomie der degenerativen Veränderungen der Hornhaut und der Bindehaut", pp. 205–220; 12. Harald G. A. GJESSING (NO), "*Über Tonometrie*", pp. 221–242; 13. Sigurd HAGEN (SE), "Zur Ätiologie der transitorischen Hypermetropie bei Diabetes mellitus", pp. 243–250; 14. Heinrich SCHOEPPE (AT), "Das biologische Verhalten des Serums Altersstarkranker zum Linseneiweiß refraktometrisch untersucht in Anlehnung an die Mikro-Abderhalden-Reaktion", pp. 251–256; 15. F. SCHIECK (DE), "Die Abhängigkeit des Verlaufs der tuberkulösen Prozesse am Auge von dem Stadium der Allergie des Gesamtorganismus", pp. 257–270; 16. Richard SEEFELDER (AT), "Ein Beitrag zu den Geschwulstbildungen des retinalen Epithels der Regenbogenhaut", pp. 271–278; 17. Richard DEUTSCHMANN (DE), "Seltene Bindehauterkrankungen", pp. 279–285; 18. E. LINDGREN (DK), "Neuroretinitis eclamtica", pp. 286–298; 19. Josef MELLER (AT), "Chronische Iridocyclitis und Neuritis retrobulbaris", pp. 299–332; 20. Adalbert FUCHS (AT), "Zur Pathogenese und Anatomie der Netzhautcysten", pp. 333–375; 21. Moriz SACHS (AT), "*Über die transpalpebrale Eröffnung der vorderen Kammer*", pp. 376–383; 22. Paul KAFKA (AT), "*Über einen eigenartigen Pupillenbefund*", pp. 384–389; 23. Josef KYRLE (AT), "Tabes und negativer Liquor", pp. 390–400; 24. August WAGENMANN (DE), "*Über cystische Ektasie des Tränensacks durch Luft*", pp. 401–407; 25. L. HEINE (DE), "Beitrag zur 'chronischen, endogenen Uveitis'", pp. 408–420; 26. Ernst HERTEL (DE), "*Über die Bestimmung der Wasserstoffionenkonzentration im Kammerwasser*", pp. 421–427; 27. A. JESS (DE), "Die moderne Eiweißchemie im Dienste der Starforschung (1. Teil)", pp. 428–455; 28. M. GOLDSCHMIDT (DE), "Beitrag zur Pharmakologie des Optochins", pp. 456–464; 29. Henning RÖNNE (SE), "Pseudoglaukomatöse Exkavation der Papille", pp. 465–468; 30. Fritz SALZER (DE), "Beiträge zur Keratoplastik IV". (Schlußbetrachtungen), pp. 469–490; 31. Karl WESSELY (DE), "Beiträge zu den Wachstumsbeziehungen zwischen dem Augapfel und seinen Nachbarorganen", pp. 491–501; 32. C. H. SATTLER (DE), "Hornhautfistel, herbeigeführt anscheinend durch Perforation einer zum Teil verkalkten Linse", pp. 502–506; 33. Alfred VOGT (CH), "Fehldiagnosen am Spaltlampenmikroskop, mit besonderer Berücksichtigung von Trugbildern", pp. 507–527; 34. Karl STARGARDT (DE), "*Über Phlyktänen der Lidbindehaut des Auges*", pp. 528–537; 35. W. KOSTER (NL), "Schädigung des Auges durch Wasserstoffperoxyd (H_2O_2)", pp. 538–541; 36. L. v. LIEBERMANN (HU), "Kaustische Resektion der trachomatösen Tarsalbindehaut", pp. 542–550; 37. Maximilian SALZMANN (AT), "Die traumatische Cyclodialyse und ihre Diagnose am Lebenden", pp. 551–566; 38. Hans LAUBER (AT), "Klinische und anatomische Untersuchungen im Sehnervenkopf", pp. 567–589; 39. Otto MARBURG (AT), "Einiges über Grundlagen, Komplikationen und Erfolge der Sehnervenscheiden-Trepanation nach Müller", pp. 590–598; 40. Anton ELSCHNIG (CZ), "Die Grundlage der Spätinfektion nach Trepanation und der Wagenmannschen Infektion", pp. 599–604; 41. Henning RÖNNE (SE), "*Über Stauungspapille mit doppelseitiger plötzlicher Erblindung und deren eventuelle Behandlung mit Palliativtrepanation*", pp. 605–613; 42. G. F. ROCHAT (NL), "Sympathische Ophthalmie ohne Iridocyclitis auf dem verletzten Auge", pp. 614–616; 43. W. REIS (DE), "*Über Ophthalmomalacie*", pp. 617–639; 44. Josef IGERSHD, Walter PRINZ (DE), "Gedanken und Untersuchungen zur Pathogenese der phlyktänulären Augenentzündungen und zum Schicksal skrofulöser Augenpatienten", pp. 640–649; 45. Arthur BIRCH-HIRSCHFELD (DE), "Ein Fall von expulsiver Blutung nach Elliotscher Trepanation mit anatomischem Befund", pp. 650–655; 46. Alfred BIELSCHOWSKY (DE), "Beitrag zur operativen Behandlung der Vertikalablenkungen der Augen", pp. 656–687; 47. Albert v. PFLUGK (DE), "*Über Brillenmünzen und Medaillen*", pp. 688–707; 48. M. WOLFRUM, A. BÖHMIG (DE), "Zum Problem der Hornhautregeneration nebst Bemerkungen über den Keratokonus (II.Teil)", pp. 708–720; 49. J. W. NORDENSEN (SE), "*Über die Größe der Doppelbrechung der Hornhautsubstanz*", pp. 721–725; 50. Karl LINDNER (AT), "*Über die Topographie der parasitären Bindehautkeime*", pp. 726–777; 51. Arnold PILLAT (AT), "Zur Topographie der saprophytären Bindehautkeime des menschlichen Auges", pp. 778–793; 52. Friedrich DIMMER (AT), "*Über die Lichtempfindung bei geschlossenen Lidern*", pp. 794–798; 53. Alfred KESTENBAUM (AT), "Der Mechanismus des Nystagmus", pp. 799–843; 54. Arnold LÖWENSTEIN (CZ), "*Über den Einfluß einseitiger Beschränkung des Lichteinfalles auf die Sehschärfe*", pp. 844–850; 55. Viktor HANKE (AT), "Septische Metastasen in der Chorioidea", 851–864; 56. Ernst KRAUPA (CZ), "Beiträge zur Morphologie des Augenhintergrundes II", pp. 865–879; 57. J. van der HOEVE (NL), "Augengeschwülste bei der tuberösen Hirnsklerose (Bourneville)", pp. 880–898; 58. V. GRÖNHOLM (FI), "*Über prä-äquatoriale Sklerektomie bei Netzhautablösung*", pp. 899–915; 59. Richard CORDS (DE), "Papillitis und Glaukom", pp. 916–963; 60. Aurel v. SZILY (HU/DE), "Stereoskopische Versuche mit Schattenrissen", pp. 964–972; 61. Andreas RADOS (CH), "*Über die Veränderungen im Frühstadium der Retinitis exsudativa externa*", pp. 973–996; 62. Ernst BACHSTEZ (AT), "*Über Verfettung in der Hornhaut*", pp. 997–1036; 63. Eugen v. HIPPEL (DE), "Beiträge zur pathologischen Anatomie seltener Augenerkrankungen", pp. 1037–1049; 64. Adolf VOSSIUS (DE), "*Über die Bestsche familiäre Maculadegeneration*", pp. 1050–1057; 65. E. FRANKE (DE), "Zur Kenntnis des Lymphangioms der Bindehaut", pp. 1058–1068; 66. August SIEGRIST (CH), "Atrophie der Sehnerven durch Gefäßdruck bei Hypophysistumor", pp. 1069–1074; 67. Emil v. GRÓSZ (HU), "*Über einige Operationsmethoden an der königlich-ungarischen Universitäts-Augen Klinik Nr 1 in Budapest*", pp. 1075–1083; 68. Adolf PURTSCHER (AT), "Scheinbare Spiegelung der Iris und Pupille in der Hornhaut, ein bisher unbekanntes Phänomen", pp. 1084–1090; 69. Richard KRÄMER (AT), "Die optischen Grundlagen der 'scheinbaren Spiegelung der Pupille in der Hornhaut' (nebst Bemerkungen über konstruktive Optik)"; pp. 1091–1108; 70. Leonhard KOEPPE (DE), "Untersuchungen über Kreisgitterwirkungen bzw. Brennpunkteigenschaften der mit der Gullstrandschen Spaltlampe in den lebenden Augenmedien unter normalen und pathologischen Bedingungen zu beobachtenden mikroskopischen Gitterstrukturen nebst Bemerkungen über die beugungstheoretische Deutung des Sehens von Nebenlichtern", pp. 1109–1156;

71. Fritz ASK (SE), J. van der HOEVE (NL), "Beiträge zur Kenntnis der Entwicklung der Tränenröhrchen unter normalen und abnormen Verhältnissen, letzteres an Fällen von offener schräger Gesichtsspalte", pp. 1157–1196; 72. Theodor AXENFELD (DE), "Kosmetische Immobilisierung des Auges und Tenotomie des Levator palpebrae superioris, nebst Bemerkungen über Operationen an den Obliqui", pp. 1197–1206; 73. Hubert SATTLER (DE), "Ein Beitrag zur Kenntnis der epibulbären Carcinome und ihrer Behandlung", pp. 1207–1230.

[1261] Josef Kyrle (1880–1924). Studied at Graz Univ. (Dr. med. univ. 1904). Pathohistol. training under pathol. anat. and bacteriol. Anton Weichselbaum (1845–1920) at Vienna Univ. 1906 Joined the Univ. Clinic for Dermatol. u. Syphilis at the Allgem. Krankenhaus (1913 Habilitation, 1918 tit. Assoc Prof.). From 1917 together with psychiatrist Julius Wagner R. v. Jauregg (cf. FN 689) research on the malaria therapy for progress. paralysis, for which the latter received the Nobel Prize in 1927. 1916 Description of hyperkeratosis follicullaris et parafollicularis in cutem penetrans (1916). Cf. CZEIKE (as in FN 13); FISCHER (as in FN 28); Karl HOLUBAR, "Hyperkeratosis follicullaris et parafollicularis in cutem penetrans. Josef Kyrle and 'his' disease", in: *Americ. J. Dermatopathol.* 7 (1985), pp. 261–264; Obituaries, in: Wien. klin. Wochenschr. 39 (1926), pp. 377–378.; *Wiener med. Wochenschr.* 76 (1926), pp. 48ff.; *Feierl. Inaug. d. Rektors* [...] *Studienjahr 1926/27*, pp. 54–55.

[1262] Josef KYRLE, "Tabes und negativer Liquor," in: *Graefes Archiv* 105 (1921), pp. 390–400.

[1263] Otto Marburg (1874–1948). Studied at Vienna Univ. (Dr. med. 1899). 1900–1903 Assist. at the Neurol. Institute of Vienna Univ. under Heinrich Obersteiner (cf. FN 145). 1903–1905 Active at the 2nd Univ. Eye Clinic of Vienna's Allgem. Krankenhaus under Ernst Fuchs and at the Psychiatr. Univ. Clinic under Julius Wagner R. v. Jauregg (cf. FN 689). 1905 Habilitation in Neurol., tit. Assoc. Prof. 1912, Assoc. Prof. 1917. 1919 Full Prof. and successor of his teacher, Heinrich Obersteiner, as Dir. of the internationally renowned Neurol. Institute of Vienna Univ. 1938 Austria's Anschluss with Germany. M. ousted from his post on account of his Jewish descent. Emigration to the USA, where he continued his work at Columbia Univ./New York. Cf. CZEIKE (as in FN 13); FISCHER (as in FN 28); ÖBL (as in FN 11); NDB (as in FN 15); LESKY, *Wien. Med. Schule* (as in FN 12), pp. 386ff.; Obituaries, in: *Wien. med. Wochenschr.* 98 (1948), pp. 461–462; *JAMA* 138 (1948), p. 375*; Feierl. Inaug. d. Rektors d. Univ. Wien* [...] *Studienjahr 1948/49*, pp. 43 ff.; *Journal of Neuropathology and Experimental Neurology* [*J. Neuropathol. Exp. Neurol.*] 8 (1949), pp. 247ff; *Wien. Zeitschr. Nervenheilk.* 2 (1949), pp. 1ff.

[1264] Otto MARBURG, "Einiges über Grundlagen, Komplikationen und Erfolge der Sehnervenscheiden-Trepanation nach Müller", in: *Graefes Archiv* 105 (1921), pp. 590–598.

[1265] *Wien. med. Wochenschr.* Yr. 71/No. 24, 11 June 1921, cols. 1041–1093.

[1266] Cf. FN 818.

[1267] Cf. *Wien. med. Wochenschr.* 71 (1921), cols. 1041–1042.

[1268] Olga Prager (1872–1930). Trained as an artist with Adalbert F. Seligmann (cf. FN 355) in Vienna. Excelled as a portrait painter and her lifelike rendition of individuals in her large-format paintings of the Wr. Med. Professorenkollegium (1908) and the members of the Austrian Academy of Sciences (1912) added to her reputation. To pave the way for women to training as artists without being forced to resort to expensive private tuition she and Seligmann proposed in 1897 to set up a state-sponsored academy for women, with classes in painting, graphics and sculpture (Wiener Kunstschule f. Frauen u. Mädchen, later Wiener Frauen-Akademie f. freie u. angewandte Kunst). Cf. ÖBL (as in FN 11); Obituary, in: *Neue Freie Presse*, 28 April 1930, p. 5.

1269 Josef MELLER, "Hofrat Ernst Fuchs zum 70. Geburtstage", in: *Wien. med. Wochenschr.* 71 (1921), cols. 1041–43.

1270 Ernst Bachstez (1888–1954). Studied at Vienna Univ. (Dr. med. univ. 1912). Joined the 1st Univ. Eye Clinic after a four-month training spell as a surgeon. Worked as a surgeon under Dimmer, 1913–1920 Assist. under Stefan Bernheimer (1861–1918) and his successor, Meller. 1922 Habilitation in Ophthalmology at Vienna Univ.; 1926–1938 Head physician at the Eye Dept. of the Mariahilf Hospital. After Austria's Anschluss with Germany loss of his venia legendi and his hospital post; expelled from the Gesellschaft d. Ärzte and the Ophthalmol. Gesellschaft in Vienna. In August 1945 Restitution of the venia legendi at Vienna Univ.; consultant at two municipal hospitals in Vienna. Cf. *Gedenkbuch für die Opfer des Nationalsozialismus an der Universität Wien 1938* http://gedenkbuch.univie.ac.at/index, last accessed: 20 July 2020); Ernst BACHSTEZ, "Fettsaurer Kalk als Grundlage einer Art von Scintillatio corporis vitrei. Vorläufige Mitteilung", in: *Wien. med. Wochenschr.* 71 (1921), cols. 1044–45.

1271 Rudolf Bergmeister. Son of the ophthalmol. Otto Bergmeister (1845–1918, cf. FN 923). Student under Meller, member of the staff of Meller's clin. lab.; Habil., Head physician in Vienna. (Additional data unverifiable); Rudolf BERGMEISTER, "*Über einen seltenen Fall von epibulbärer Tuberkulose*", in: *Wien. med. Wochenschr.* 71 (1921), cols. 1045–49.

1272 Friedrich DIMMER, "*Über diffuse Rotfärbung des Glaskörpers bei Glaskörperblutungen*", in: *Wien. med. Wochenschr.* 71 (1921), cols. 1049–51.

1273 Adalbert FUCHS, "*Über subkonjunktivale Blutungen*", in: *Wien. med. Wochenschr.* 71 (1921), cols. 1051–53.

1274 Emil von Grósz (1865–1941). Studied at Budapest Univ. (Dr. med. 1887). His grandfather and his father had been well-known ophthalmologists before him. 1888 Study trip to Austria, where he spent several months in Fuchs's Clinic, Germany, and France. Joined the Univ. Eye Clinic No. 1 in Budapest under Vilmos (Wilhelm) Schulek (1843–1905). 1895 Habilitation in Ophthalm. at Budapest Univ. (1900 Assoc. Prof.). 1903 Government commissioner for the management of trachoma. 1905 Full Prof. and Schulek's successor as Dir. of the Univ. Eye Clinic, Budapest, whose new building (1908) is credited to him as are major contributions to the elimination of trachoma. Cf. FISCHER (as in FN 28); HIRSCHBERG, *Geschichte der Augenheilkunde* (as in FN 18), vol. 15/2 [= Reprint, vol. VI], § 1259, pp. 453–454; IBBO (as in FN 18); PAGEL (as in FN 13); Obituary: "Emil de Grosz", in: *Brit. J. Ophthalmol.* 26, 1942, pp. 286–287; Emil v. GRÓSZ, "Unterricht der Augenheilkunde", in: *Wien. med. Wochenschr.* 71 (1921), cols. 1053–55.

1275 Gustav Guist (1892–1967). Originally from Hungary. Studied at Vienna Univ. (Dr. med. 1917). Assist. and habilitation at the 2nd Univ. Eye Clinic of Vienna's Allg. Krankenhaus under Friedrich Dimmer; Gustav GUIST, "Über das Verhalten heller und dunkler Regenbogenhäute auf Homatropin und Atropin", in: *Wien. med. Wochenschr.* 71 (1921), cols. 1055–1058.

[1276] Cf. FN 924; Viktor HANKE, "Doppelperforation des Bulbus und Wanderung eines retrobulbären kleinen Eisensplitters", in: *Wien. klin. Wochenschr.* 71 (1921), cols. 1058–60.

[1277] Paul Kafka, Junior doctor at the Eye Department of the Wiedener Krankenhaus headed by Moriz Sachs (cf. FN 1233); Paul KAFKA, "Epibulbäres Melanosarkom und Radiotherapie", in: *Wien. med. Wochenschr.* 71 (1921), cols. 1060–63.

[1278] Richard Krämer (1878–1937). Studied at Vienna Univ. (Dr. med. 1903). Ophthalmolog. special. under Ernst Fuchs and Friedrich Dimmer at the 2nd Univ. Eye Clinic (Habilitation 1924). Worked in the Ophthalm. Outpatient Clinic of the Kaiser-Franz-Joseph Spital. Cf. TRAGL, *Wien. Krankenanstalten* (as in FN 948), p. 390; Richard KRÄMER; "Keratomalazie bei Erythroderma desquamativa. Ein Beitrag zur Ätiologie der Leiner'schen Erkrankung", in: *Wien. med. Wochenschr.* 71 (1921), cols. 1063–66.

[1279] Hans Lauber (1876–1952). Of Estonian aristocratic extraction. Studied at the Univ. of Marburg and Vienna (Dr. med. 1901). Ophthalm. special. at Vienna's two Univ. Eye Clinics (Fuchs, Schnabel). 1903 Assist. under Schnabel, 1908–1910 Interim Dir. of the 1st Univ. Eye Clinic. 1909 Habilitation, 1922 Assoc. Prof.; after World War I Dir. of the Ophthalm. Dept. of four hospitals in Vienna. 1931 Full Prof. at Warsaw Univ. (1939 Dean of the Med. Fac.). After the occupying power shut down the Univ. Clinic in 1939 Dir. of the Univ. Eye Clinic Krakow. Dir. of the anti-trachoma force in the entire German administered part of Poland (successful sulfonamide therapy). In early 1945 expropriation of his Krakow estate while he was in Vienna on a visit. Visiting Professor at Vienna Univ. when he had already turned 70. Cf. FISCHER (as in FN 28); NDB (as in FN 15); Obituaries, in: *Wien. klin. Wochenschr.* 64 (1952), pp. 904–905 (Arnold Pillat); *Ophthalmologica* 124 (1952), pp. 126–127 (Josef Böck); *Transact. Am. Acad. Ophthalmol. Otolaryngol.* 56 (Sept.–Oct. 1952), pp. 822–824; Hans LAUBER, "*Über die Behandlung oberflächlicher Hornhauterkrankungen mit Radium*", in: *Wien. med. Wochenschr.* 71 (1921), cols. 1066–68.

[1280] Cf. FN 751; Karl LINDNER, "Über die Blenorrhöe des Neugeborenen", in: *Wien. med. Wochenschr.* 71 (1921), cols. 1068–70.

[1281] Josef MELLER, "Über Drucksteigerung im Auge nach Ausziehung des Greisenstares", in: *Wien. med. Wochenschr.* 71 (1921), cols. 1070–76.

[1282] Marie Procksch (biograph. data not retrievable), at that time on the staff of the Ophthal. Dept. of the Wiedener Krankenhaus under Sachs; Marie PROCKSCH, "*Über doppelseitige Keratitis und Iridozyklitis bei Erythema multiforme exsudativum*", in: *Wien. med. Wochenschr.* 71 (1921), cols. 1076–78.

[1283] Adolf PURTSCHER, "Beitrag zur Behandlung der Irisvorfälle", in: Ibid., cols. 1078–79.

[1284] Moriz SACHS, "Bild und Wirklichkeit", in: *Wien. med. Wochenschr.* 71 (1921), cols. 1079–81.

[1285] Maximilian SALZMANN, "*Über Vererbung von Netzhautablösung*", in: Ibid., cols. 1082–84.

[1286] Hubert SATTLER, "*Über einen Fall von Neuritis nervi optici retrobulbaris als Frühsymptom der Basedowschen Erkrankung*", in: Ibid., cols. 1084–88.

[1287] Richard Seefelder (1875–1949). Originally from Bavaria. Studied at the Univ. of Erlangen and Munich (Dr. med. 1898). 1908 Habilitation in Ophthalm. at Leipzig

Univ. (1914 Assoc. Prof.) 1919–1945 Full Prof. and Dir. of the Univ. Eye Clinic Innsbruck as the successor of Josef Meller. 1923/24 Dean of the Med. Fac., 1929/30 Rector of Innsbruck Univ. Illegal Nazi, joined the SS in 1933. 1947 Application for an exemption from the penal provisions mandated by Austria's *Verbotsgesetz 1947* [Prohibition Act 1947]. Application granted. Cf. EULNER (as in FN 13); FISCHER (as in FN 28); ÖBL (as in FN 11); G. OBERKOFLER, Peter GOLLER (eds.), *Die Medizinische Fakultät Innsbruck. Faschistische Realität (1938) und Kontinuität unter postfaschistischen Bedingungen (1945)*. Innsbruck 1999, pp. 159ff.; Franz DAXECKER, Richard Seefelder. Vorstand der Univ. Klinik für Augenheilkunde in Innsbruck von 1919 bis 1945, in: *Klin. Monatsbl. Augenheilk.* 224 (2007), pp. 952–953; Richard SEEFELDER, "Klinische Beobachtungen über Pneumokokkenkonjunktivitis", in: *Wien. med. Wochenschr.* 71 (1921), cols. 1088–91.

1288 Eduard Konrad Zirm (1863–1944). Studied at Univ. Vienna. Ophthalmol. special. under Carl Stellwag v. Carion (cf. FN 165) at Vienna's Allgem. Krankenh. 1892 On the staff of the District Hospital at Olmütz (today Olomouc/Czech Republic), 1894–1928 Dir. of the Eye Dept. Cf. Erna LESKY, "Eduard Konrad Zirm (1863–1944). Zur 100. Wiederkehr seines Geburtstages (18. März 1963)", in: *Wien. klin. Wochenschr.* 7 (1963), pp. 199–201; Eduard ZIRM, "*Über periodischen Exophthalmus und kongenitalen Enophthalmus*", in: *Wien. med. Wochenschr.* 71 (1921), cols. 1091–93.

1289 Cf. FN 769.

1290 Cf. FN 1216, p. 57.

1291 Original document in the Family archive. See also: *Handbuch der Stadt Vienna.* Vol. 82. Verlag für Jugend und Volk. Vienna 1968, p. 327.

1292 Cf. FN 589.

1293 See Hans SLEZAK, "Zur Gründung der Ophthalmologischen Gesellschaft in Vienna (Wie alt ist diese Gesellschaft tatsächlich?)", in: Anton HOMMER, Stephan KAMINSKI (eds.), *100 Jahre Ophthalmologische Gesellschaft in Wien. Wien. med. Wochenschr.* 154 (2004), Suppl. 116, pp. 2–3.

1294 Josef Meller, a former student belonging to Fuchs's inner circle, who had become Dir. of the Univ. Eye Clinic Innsbruck in 1914 and head of 1st Univ. Eye Clinic in Vienna in 1919, was made Vice Chairman, while Arnold Pillat (cf. FN 808), at that time still a junior doctor at the 2nd Univ. Eye Clinic under Fuchs's successor Friedrich Dimmer, was appointed secretary.

1295 Cf. FN 1233.

1296 Friedrich DIMMER, *Der Augenspiegel und die ophthalmoskopische Diagnostik.* Third completely revised and augmented edition. Deuticke, Leipzig 1921.

1297 This book is dedicated to the man who has always been a shining example for us, who has now turned seventy and stands before us, his vigour undiminished, working away tirelessly as ever, to this beacon of the work ethic, for whom work has always been sacred and who has always loved it for its own sake, to our mentor and dear friend Ernst Fuchs.

1298 Josef MELLER, *Augenärztliche Eingriffe. Ein kurzes Handbuch für angehende Augenärzte.* 2nd ed. Josef Šafář, Vienna/Leipzig 1921.

1299 Cf. FN 1216, p. 58.

1300 Ibid., pp. 58–63.

[1301] Ibid., p. 62.

[1302] Ibid., p. 48.

[1303] Ernst FUCHS, "Beleuchtung und Auge. Mit einer historischen Einleitung", in: *Wien. med. Wochenschr.* 71 (1921), cols. 1409–15, No. 32, 6 Aug. 1921 (Verbatim transcript). Cf. "Die Wiener Augenheilkunde aus einer klinischen Vorlesung", in: *Neues Wiener Journal*, 8 Aug. 1921, pp. 2–3.

[1304] Cf. "Offene Korrespondenz", in: *Klin. Monatsbl. Augenheilk.* 66/1 (1921), pp. 134–135. An identical announcement of this conference was inserted at the end of the Fuchs special issue of the *Wien. med. Wochenschr.* of 11 June 1921: "Notizen", in: *Wien. med. Wochenschr.* 71 (1921), cols. 1095–96. See the following announcement and the registrations for the lectures and demonstrations: "Außerordentliche Tagung der ophthalmologischen Gesellschaft in Wien am 4., 5. und 6. August 1921", in: *Zeitschr. Augenheilk.* 46 (1921), pp. 51–54.

[1305] Gabriela SCHMIDT-WYKLICKY, Helmut GRÖGER, "Die Gründung der weltweit ersten Universitäts-Augenklinik in Wien 1812 und ihre Erhebung zum Ordinariat 1818", in: *Spektrum Augenheilk.* 26 (2012), pp. 273–282. The lecture hall was located in Alserstraße 4/Courtyard IV (then in the Vorstadt Alsergrund, today Vienna's 9th district, Alsergrund).

[1306] Cf. "Offene Korrespondenz", in: *Klin. Monatsbl. Augenheilk.* 67/2 (1921), pp. 103–105.

[1307] At the conference the following presentations were made: 1. Wilhelm UHTHOFF (DE), *Klinischer Teil*; 2. Karl WESSELY (DE), *Theoretischer und anatomischer Teil.* The participants in the ensuing discussion were E. Hertel, E. v. Grósz, E. Seidel, M. Wolfrum, H. Sattler, H. Gjessing, N. Blatt, L. Müller, A. Fuchs, Karl Safar, Arnold Pillat and L. Heine. For the presentations, see: *Klin. Monatsbl. Augenheilk.* 67/2 (1921), pp. 293–301.

[1308] Michael Johann-Baptist Baron de Wenzel (1724–1790). Originally from Germany. Established himself as itinerant cataract surgeon in great demand in Paris, from where he was called to other countries such as Austria and Great Britain. He trained a great number of followers all over Europe to perform cataract operations (couchings). Oculist to Britain's King George III. Cf. HIRSCH (as in FN 13); HIRSCHBERG, *Geschichte der Augenheilkunde* (as in FN 18), see index; A. L. WYMAN, "Baron de Wenzel, Oculist to King George III: His Impact on British Ophthalmologists", in: *Medical History* [*Med. Hist.*] 35 (1991), pp. 78–88.

[1309] Joseph Barth (1746–1818). Originally from Malta. Studied at the Univ. of Rome and Vienna (Dr. med. 1772). Initiated into the technique of couching in Vienna by Johann-Baptist Baron de Wenzel (see above), who had been called to Vienna from Paris by the Empress Maria Theresia (1713–1780). 1773 Lecturer in Ophthalmol. and Delicate Anatomy at Vienna Univ. (1774 Full Prof.) 1776 Physician to the Emperor. Establishment of a priv. eye clinic. He is said to have performed 3,000 cataract operations. His interest in ophthalm. was reputedly motivated primarily by financial considerations. It was only when Emperor Joseph II. (1741–1790) offered him a very substantial fee that he consented to train medical doctors as eye specialists. His most well-known disciples were Johann Adam Schmidt, Georg Joseph Beer (cf. FN 525) and Johann Adam Schmidt (1759–1809). Cf. GERABEK et al. (as in FN 13); NDB (as in FN 15); ÖBL (as in FN 11); WURZBACH (as in FN 15).

1310 William ZENTMAYER et al. (eds.), *An International Congress of Ophthalmology*, Washington D. C., April 25–28, 1922. WM. F. Fell Co. Printers, Philadelphia 1922.

1311 "Ausserordentliche Tagung der Ophthalmologischen Gesellschaft in Wien. 4.–6. August 1921". Bericht nach den Manuskripten und Autoreferaten von Dozent Dr. H. Lauber, Wien, in: *Klin. Monatsbl. Augenheilk.* 67/2 (1921), pp. 293–327 (here: p. 293). Cf. Hans LAUBER (ed.), *Verhandlungen der ausserordentlichen Tagung der Ophthalmologischen Gesellschaft in Wien am 4., 5. und 6. August 1921.* Karger, Berlin 1922.

1312 Steward DUKE-ELDER, *A Century of International Ophthalmology 1857–1957.* Written at the Request of the International Council of Ophthalmology, Kimpton 1958, p. 39.

1313 Cf. *Am. J. Ophthalmol.* 5/1 (1922), p. 63 and *The Ophthalmic Year-Book* 18 (1922), p. 589.

1314 Cf. Theodor AXENFELD, "Ausserordentliche Tagung der Wiener ophthalmologischen Gesellschaft vom 4.–6. August 1921 (Offene Korrespondenz)", in: *Klin. Monatsbl. Augenheilk.* 67/2 (1921), pp. 291–292.

1315 Cf. *Bericht ueber die 42. Versammlung der Deutschen Ophthalmologischen Gesellschaft, Heidelberg 1920.* Bergmann, Munich/Wiesbaden 1921, p. 364.

1316 Ibid. Cf. also: Paul JUNIUS, "Außerordentliche Tagung der Ophthalmologischen Gesellschaft in Wien vom 4.–6. August 1921", in: *Zeitschr. Augenheilk.* 46 (1921), pp. 116–118 (Report).

1317 1. W. GILBERT (DE), "Zur herpetischen Augenerkrankung"; 2. H. LARSEN (DK), "Demonstration mikroskopischer Präparate von einem monochromatischen Auge"; 3. A v. PFLUGK (DE), "Die Behandlung von Entzündungen am Auge mit Staphar (Strubell)"; 4. W. GILBERT (DE), "Zur Magnetoperation"; 5. M. MÁRQUEZ (ES), "Versuche über den Mechanismus der Skiaskopie"; 6. C. PASCHEFF (BG) "Ueber eine Streptotrix-Strahlenpilzgeschwulst der Orbita"; 7. F. CANDIAN (IT), "Ueber seltene Makulaerkrankungen"; 8. A. FUCHS (AT), "Sympathisierende Entzündung und Sarkom in einem Auge"; 9. N. BLATT (RO), "Eine neue Chalazionpinzette"; 10. J. BRANA, "Instrumente zur Behandlung des Trachoms"; 11. A. PURTSCHER, G. GUIST (AT), "Benützung der Mikrobogenlampe zur diaskleralen Durchleuchtung"; 12. Josef URBANEK (AT), "Klinischer Beitrag zur Kenntnis der intraokulären Druckschwankungen"; 13. H. LAUBER (AT), "a) Fall von Narbenfixation der Augen nach luetischer Nekrose der nasalen Orbitawand, b) Ein Fall von umschriebener Xerose der Bindehaut des Oberlides mit Kontaktxerose der Hornhaut, c) Eine pigmentierte Geschwulst der linken Papille, d) Ein Fall von erworbenen Venenschlingen auf beiden Papillen"; 14. E. BACHSTEZ (AT), "Eine Ruptur der äusseren Hornhautschichten". Cf. *Klin. Monatsbl. Augenheilk.* 67/2 (1921), pp. 301–304.

1318 1. W. GILBERT (DE), "Ueber Augenerkrankungen bei Nieren- und Gefässleiden"; 2. M. ZUR NEDDEN (DE), "Ueber Glaskörperabsaugungen"; 3. H. RÖNNE (SE), "Die mechanischen Verhältnisse bei den Schieloperationen, speziell bei der kombinierten Vorlagerung"; 4. B. FLEISCHER (DE), "Ueber die Vererbung der myotonischen Dystrophie"; 5. S. HAGEN (SE), "Zur Wirkungsweise der neueren Glaukomoperationen. Die Bedeutung des regenerierten Kammerwassers für die Narbenbildung des Trepanationsdefektes in der Hornhaut und in der Sklerokornea"; 6. F. SCHANZ (DE), "Das Sehen"; 7. A. BIELSCHOWSKY (DE), "Die Genese der dissoziierten Vertikalbewegungen der Augen"; 8. A. JESS (DE) "Die Diaminosäuren der Linsenproteine"; 9. M. GOLDSCHMIDT (DE), "Die Lipoide der Linse"; 10. J. BARRAQUER (E), *Ueber Phakoëresis*; 11. Th. AXENFELD (DE), a) "Tenotomie beider Recti interni in einer Sitzung beim Strabismus convergens; b) Zur Operation der Strangfixation bei kongenitalen Bewegungsdefekten; c) Bunte optisch-kosmetische Tätowierung der durchsichtigen Kornea"; 12. M. MÁRQUEZ (E), "Die Häufigkeit des Biastigmatismus"; 13. E. WEISS (DE), "Die praktische Bedeutung des Unterschiedes zwischen dem Grad der Ametropie und ihrer Brillenkorrektion"; 14. C. H. SATTLER (DE), "Operationen zur Verbesserung der Kosmetik nach Enukleation und deren Ersatzmethoden"; 15. KÖLLNER, HOFFMANN (DE), "Der Einfluss des Vestibulärapparates auf die Aktionsströme der Augenmuskeln"; 16. E. KRAUPA (CZ), "Die Erkenntnis der kongenitalen Lues in ihrer Bedeutung für die Augenheilkunde"; 17. E. HERTEL (DE), "Ueber Extraktion von Fremdkörpern aus dem Augenhintergrund mittelst Pinzette und Magneten"; 18. E. ENGELKING (DE), "Terrainstudien zur Pathologie und Therapie der phlyktänulären Augenentzündung"; 19. K. HEINE (DE), "Zur Biologie der Ziliarepithelien"; 20. A. RADOS (CH), "Ueber Ernährung des Auges"; 21. J. GONIN (CH), "Die Beziehungen der Radiotherapie zur Netzhautablösung"; 22. J. IGERSHEIMER (DE), "Neue Untersuchungen zur Syphilis des Sehapparates"; 23. R. HESSBERG (DE), "Verwendung rostfreien Kruppstahls V 2 A in der Ophthalmochirurgie"; 24. Th. KOPPANYI (HU), "Funktionelle Transplantation von Wirbeltieraugen"; 25. W. KOLMER (AT), "Anatomische Befunde bei den Koppanyischen Versuchen"; 26. G. GUIST (AT), "Ueber wurmförmige Zuckungen der Iris"; 27. J. BRANA (HU), "Beiträge zur Behandlung des Trachoms"; 28. A. v. SZILY (HU), "Morphogenese des Sehnerveneintritts und des Pektens bei Vögeln"; 29. H. ERGGELET (DE), "Zur Raumauffassung bei Aenderung der Augenstandlinie"; 30. A. SCHÜLLER (AT), "Röntgenbefunde bei Sehstörungen"; 31. O. HIRSCH (AT), "Differentialdiagnose der Hypophysentumoren gegenüber Hirntumoren mit besonderer Berücksichtigung der Augensymptome"; 32. L. MÜLLER, CZEPA (AT), "7 Fälle von Hypophysentumor"; 33. N. BLATT (RO), "Experimentelles über Verdauungstherapie bei Hornhautnarben"; 34. E. RUTTIN, E. NOWAK (AT), "Erfahrungen mit der Westschen Operation"; 35. L. MAGGIORE (IT), "Ueber den Mechanismus der Entwicklung der Ora serrata des menschlichen Auges"; 36. B. LIPSCHÜTZ (AT), "*Über Nachweis und Bedeutung der "Zosterkörperchen" und "Herpeskörperchen"* ("α"- und "β-Körperchen") in der geimpften Kaninchenhornhaut"; 37. R. BERGMEISTER (AT), "Ueber die Beziehungen der Glia zum Bindegewebe in mikrophthalmischen Augen"; 38. E. RUTTIN (AT), *Ohrbefunde bei akuter retrobulbärer Neuritis*; 39. E. KLEINSASSER (AT), "Gesichtsfeldstörungen bei Iridozyklitis"; 40. A. PURTSCHER (AT), "Ueber eine neue Art der Verlagerung des M. rectus externus"; 41. E. NOWAK (AT), "Ueber die Partigenauswertung und Behandlung nach Deycke-Much bei tuberkulösen Erkrankungen des Auges"; 42. E. FUCHS (AT), "Ueber Chorioretinitis"; 43. K. FUKALA (AT), "Behandlung der Chorioiditis"; 44. A. KESTENBAUM (AT), *Ueber Fixationsnystagmus*; 45. J. MELLER (AT), "Ueber die Periphlebitis retinalis sympathicans"; 46. M. SALZMANN (AT), "Ueber die Sichtbarkeit der Ora serrata mit Ablösung dieser Gegend und die traumatische Myopie" [Cf. *Klin. Monatsbl. Augenheilk.* 67/2 (1921), pp. 304–327]; 47.O. PALICH–SZÁNTÓ ((HU), "*Über das Auftreten des einseitigen Argyll-Robertsonschen Phänomens*" [Cf. *Zeitschr. Augenheilk.* 46 (1921), pp. 310].

1319 Then on the staff of the 1st Univ. Eye Clinic under Meller. More detailed data concerning person and career not retrievable.

1320 Olga Palich-Száński (1890–1971). Studied medicine at the Univ. of Budapest and Berlin. Ophthalmol. special. as assistant under Emil v. Grosz at the 1st Univ. Eye Clinic in Budapest. From 1919 at the Univ. Eye Clinics in Prague (Elschnig), Vienna (Meller) and Munich (v. Heß). At the time of the WOG conference in 1921 on the staff of the Univ. Eye Clinic in Belgrade (Nesic). 1948 Return to Budapest, later Dir. of the Eye Policlinic of the Johannes Hospital in Budapest. Cf. Obituary, in: *Klin. Monatsbl. Augenheilk.* 160 (1972), pp. 516 (I. Biró).

1321 Cf. Ernst FUCHS, "*Über Chorioretinitis*", in: *Graefes Archiv* 107 (1922), pp. 15–25.

10. Ernst Fuchs as an Innovative Ophthalmic Surgeon and Inventor of New Instruments

Ernst Fuchs was both an ophthalmic pathologist of world-wide renown and a supremely skilled, universally recognised surgeon. A product of Arlt's school, he had acquired a solid surgical training both from his teacher and as a trainee surgeon under Billroth. Arlt set great store by his assistants being able to operate with both hands concurrently and with the same dexterity, in keeping with what had become a proverbial catchphrase, the "watchmaker talent". In this respect, Fuchs proved his teacher's equal. Another product of the Vienna Ophthalmological School, Alexander Jokl[1322] (1895–1965), who made a career in South Africa, saw this skill as a crucial characteristic of the Fuchs school:

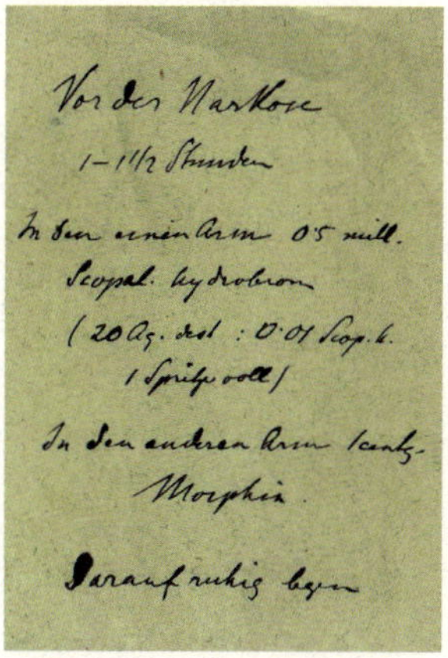
Vor der Narkose
1–1½ Stunden
In den einen Arm 0·5 mill.
Scopol. hydrobrom
(20 Aq. dest : 0·01 Scop. h.
1 Spritze voll)
In den andern Arm 1centg.
Morphin
Darauf ruhig liegen

Fig. 99 Anaesthetic premedication (Personal prescription by Ernst Fuchs)

Ambidexterity, which Fuchs inherited from Arlt, became a hallmark of the Fuchs school.[1323]

Like many other highly gifted surgeons, Fuchs developed new surgical techniques and modifications of existing surgical routines, which have stood the test of time and have been named after him. The same is true of instruments he either modified or developed from scratch, whose practicality has ensured that they are still in use today. Furthermore, Fuchs created a protective dressing to make sure the postoperative phase was not at the mercy of restless patients itching to "lend a hand".

Fuchs formulated guidelines that were put to use at his clinic for dosing medication to prepare patients for anaesthetisation and to make sure they received the necessary care. (Fig. 99) In the postoperative care of cataract patients, too, Fuchs introduced innovations:

He also was an innovator in surgery. Largely through his efforts the age-old custom of a patient after a cataract operation being kept in bed with both eyes covered in a dark room for a week before the dressings were changed, was abandoned. He introduced early ophthalmoscopic examinations after these operations which enabled him to discover that choroidal detachment was far more common than had been imagined.[1324]

In most cases Fuchs made these innovations part of his epoch-making *Lehrbuch* or presented them at specialist meetings, such as the annual conferences of the Ophthalmologische Gesellschaft in Heidelberg. Like any great teacher, he left a great deal for his disciples to try out and publish. They in turn considered it a special honour to be involved in popularising a method of treatment that had been newly developed by their revered mentor and to make sure it was named after him.

Similarly, well-known representatives of the Vienna Ophthalmological School, which owed much of its worldwide reputation to Fuchs, including leading exponents of the universities of Graz, Innsbruck and Prague, made sure that Fuchs's innovations quickly found their way into authoritative handbooks of ophthalmic surgery published during the following decades, raising them to the status of what may properly be called established standard procedures. Important contributions in this direction were made by Wilhelm Czermak,[1325] Anton Elschnig[1326] and Josef Meller.[1327]

Fuchs's disciple Wilhelm Czermak, Chair of Ophthalmology at the German University of Prague, was the author of a monumental, two-volume handbook, *Augenärztliche Operationen*,[1328] which he dedicated to Ernst Fuchs, calling him the "master of ophthalmic surgery". The handbook is the first monograph on ophthalmic surgery as recommended and practised by the Vienna School of Ophthalmology. Its only forerunner, Arlt's ophthalmic *Operationslehre*,[1329] dating as it does to the generation before Fuchs, had been no more than a few chapters in a handbook. After Czermak's premature death in 1906, his successor at the German University of Prague, Anton Elschnig, took charge of the second edition of Czermak's magnum opus.[1330]

1908, the publication year of Elschnig's edition of Czermak's *Augenärztliche Operationen*, also saw the publication of Fuchs disciple Josef Meller's handbook of ophthalmic surgery in English.[1331] It was not published in German until ten years later.[1332] Both in German and in English it retained its status as one of the leading standard textbooks of ophthalmic surgery well into the 1950s.

Surgical Techniques
Blepharorrhaphy/Tarsorrhaphy 1889

In the first edition of the *Lehrbuch* Fuchs described the following modification he had introduced for tarsorrhaphy:

1. Lateral tarsorrhaphy. *In von Walther's*[1333] *method this is performed by paring the upper and lower borders of the lids by ablation of the bed of hair follicles over the space adjoining the external angle of the eye, and then stitching the borders of the lids to each other along the denuded area. As in this way it is only a very narrow raw surface, i.e., the raw edges of the lids over which union is effected, the wound is apt to tear apart under any considerable amount of strain. Hence in these cases I perform the operation in a different way. First, the extent to which it is desired to join the lids together is marked out; then to the same extent the lower lid is split into its two lamina by an intermarginal incision. From the inner extremity of the section a short incision is carried downward through the skin, thus converting the anterior lamina of the bisected portion of the lid into a flap* [...]. *The upper and inner borders of this flap are free, while the lower and outer borders are connected with the skin of the lid. The follicles of the cilia, which lie exposed along the posterior border of the upper end of the flap, are removed by a scissors applied flatwise, this being done so that the cilia may afterward fall out. Then the upper lid is denuded by first making the intermarginal section in the same way as upon the upper lid and ablating the bed of hair follicles thus detached as in Flarer's*[1334] *operation.*[1335] *There is thus produced a raw surface* [...], *to which it is intended that the skin flap of the lower lid shall adhere by its raw surface. In order that adhesion of the raw surfaces themselves, and not just of their edges, shall take place, the suture is applied as follows: Both ends of a thread armed with a needle at each end are carried through the upper lid near its free border, the needles being passed from behind forward. In this way the loop of the thread gets to lie upon the conjunctival side of the lid, while the free ends come out upon the raw anterior surface. These ends are then passed through the base of the skin flap below and are tied upon its anterior aspect over a glass bead. By this suture the base of the flap is kept pressed against the raw surface of the tarsus of the upper lid; then, as an additional precaution, the edges of the skin flap are accurately united to the edge of the wound in the upper lid by means of a few fine sutures. The adhesion of the lids obtained by this method is firm enough to withstand even a powerful strain.*

2. Median tarsorrhaphy, *as devised by Arlt,*[1336] *is performed by excising with the forceps and scissors a narrow strip of skin from both the lower and the upper lid close to their inner angles. The long and slender wounds thus produced should meet in an acute angled at a point on the inside of the inner commissure.* [...]. *They are then united to each other through their entire extent by means of interrupted sutures. If a firmer adhesion is desired, this operation, too, like external tarsorrhaphy, may be made with formation of a small skin flap.*[1337]

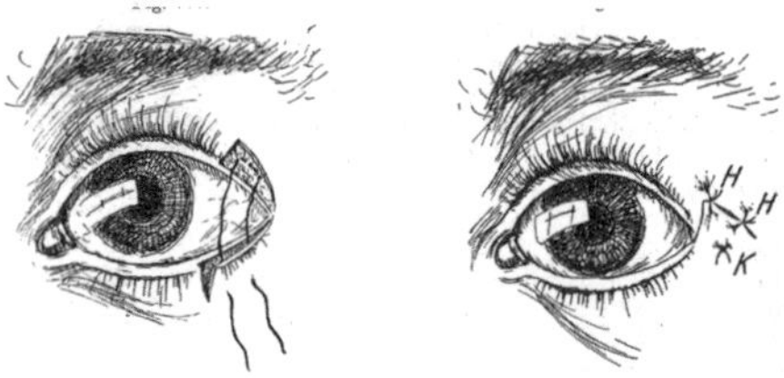

Fig. 100a Blepharorrhaphy according to Fuchs

In his handbook of the most common eye operations, Czermak devotes a detailed section to tarsorrhaphy and the modification of the standard procedure introduced by Fuchs. Guiding the reader step by step through the different phases of the operation with the help of graphic drawings, Czermak makes it clear just where Fuchs departs from Graefe's older method.[1338] (Fig. 100a, b). That Fuchs's modification soon became standard practice in the United States as well is attested by Casey A. Wood[1339] in his *Encyclopedia*, which has already been referred to in the discussion of blepharochalasis. In it, he included an illustrated comparison of the techniques used by von Graefe and Fuchs respectively in his discussion of different blepharoplasty operation techniques.[1340]

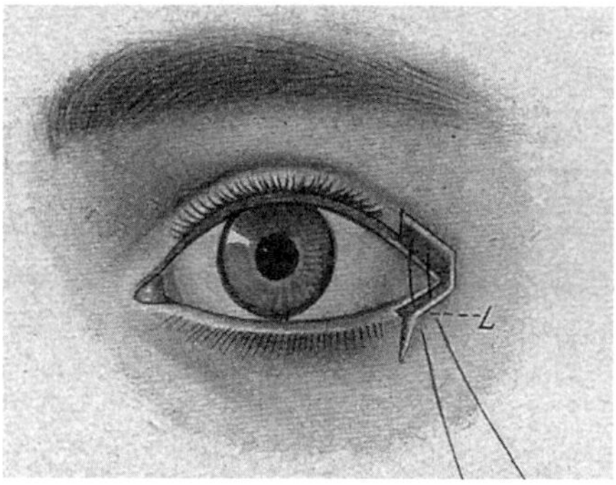

Fig. 100b Lateral tarsorrhaphy according to Fuchs

Transfixion of the Iris 1896

At the 25th Conference of the Deutsche Ophthalmologische Gesellschaft in Heidelberg in 1897, Fuchs presented to the great number of colleagues assembled for the occasion a method of transfixing the iris in cases where the iris has been pushed forward by an elevation of pressure:

I resort to the minor operation I wish to speak about in cases, where, in consequence of the ring-shaped adhesion of the border of the pupil to the lens capsule, aqueous humour has gathered in the posterior chamber and has pushed the iris forward. In these cases, as is well known, iridectomy presents technical difficulties and therefore often produces results that are not entirely satisfactory. Instead of an iridectomy I have sometimes performed the following operation: A Graefe *knife is entered about 1 mm to the inner side of the temporal margin, passed through the anterior chamber, and made to emerge at a spot near the inner margin of the cornea symmetrically situated in respect to the point of entry. The points of entry and exit lie in the horizontal meridian of the cornea, and the knife is held so that its blade is parallel to the base of the cornea. Since the iris is driven forward, the knife as it is being carried through the anterior chamber pierces the most protruding portion of the iris both temporally and nasally and makes holes in it. Those holes remain permanently open and restore the communication between the anterior and posterior chambers; the iris returns to its former position, and intra-ocular pressure becomes normal. As the iris is transfixed in this operation by the knife, I would like to call this operation the* transfixion of the iris. *If the protrusion of the iris is marked enough, one gets to make four holes, all of them located in the horizontal meridian, that is, two each in the nasal and temporal halves of the iris. These holes are minute vertical slits. Often all one gets is three holes if, for example, on one side the two incisions merge at their upper or lower ends, resulting in the formation of a small arched incision in the iris; pulling back the small flap produces a round hole. Or it may happen that on one side the iris slides away from the knife altogether. This is no cause for concern as long as at least some opening has been made in the iris. When I performed this operation for the first time, I asked myself whether these holes would remain permanently open. This was the result I had come to expect as holes in the iris of the sort that often result from its perforation by foreign bodies are not normally filled again. This expectation proved correct and this minor operation has therefore provided me with lasting results in this respect.*

As the idea on which this operation is based is anything but far-fetched, this operation may very well have been described somewhere already, even though I am not aware of it. I therefore believe it is worth being presented to you. I am far from performing this operation in all cases of seclusio pupillae with bulging of the iris; for, as a rule, I prefer iridectomy because I believe that this type of operation, in addition to restoring communication between the two chambers, has a beneficial effect on the nutrition of the eye as a whole. This said, I perform the transfixion, which can also be done under out-patient conditions, in cases where I am loth to create a coloboma, if, for example, the pupil is still unencumbered by a membrane. I performed it on several occasions on patients who had undergone a cataract operation without iridectomy and had later been afflicted with seclusio pupillae without the latter being covered by a membrane. In cases of hump-shaped protrusion of the iris, this operation may consequently be made instead of an iridectomy; and in cases of this sort it may be done as a preliminary operation to an iridectomy, so that the latter can be done later under more favourable conditions.[1341]

Fuchs was right in entertaining the possibility that other ophthalmic surgeons might have expressed a similar or even identical idea before. There is historical evidence for related considerations and therapeutic initiatives dating to the first half of the eighteenth century, starting with British oculist Benedict Duddel(l),[1342] who practised in London and published[1343] the first hints in this direction in 1729.[1344]

D[uddel] describes an operation that resembles FUCHS' *transfixion. He calls the operation* diacope, *while referring to the disease as* diatasis *of the iris. The condition, as we are aware, consists in the protrusion of the iris which is attached to the lens capsule at the border of the pupil.*

'The puncture is performed in a manner that is similar to the cataract operation. The needle is pushed into the tumour, which is comprised of the fleshy fibres of the iris muscles. Spongy and bloated by lost blood, it needs to be moved to behind the iris. This is facilitated by getting the patient to incline his head backward.' [1345]

More than a century later the term transfixion appears to have been common usage in other connections than the iris; it is found, e.g., in the textbook[1346] of the Scottish surgeon Robert Liston (1794–1847).[1347] In 1865, the renowned ophthalmic surgeon William Bowman,[1348] who has already come in for praise in this book, devoted a great deal of his attention to the transfixion of the iris. He was the first to notice the pupillary block and realised that it occurred more frequently after cataract extractions without iridectomy than after that operation accompanied by iridectomy. Bowman described how this condition only ever occurred shortly after the severance of a secondary cataract. Even though he believed that the bulging of the iris was caused by excessive secretion of aqueous humour, he noted that the transfixion of the iris generally put an end to elevated intraocular pressure. [1349]

The method for the transfixion of the iris as devised by Fuchs in 1896, having proved itself, found its way into important ophthalmologic specialist publications and textbooks both in the German-speaking world and worldwide. It may suffice to mention a paper by an aspirant at the Fuchs Clinic, Hugo Aschheim, which was written in 1898, two years after the Heidelberger Conference mentioned above, and published as arguably the first original treatise on his teacher's transfixio iridis in a prestigious ophthalmic journal, the *Archiv für Augenheilkunde*.[1350] The paper reports on several cases in the Fuchs Clinic. As the journal was also published in English, Aschheim's paper was reprinted in translation two years later in *Archives of Ophthalmology*. [1351] The two journals had the same team of editors, Herman(n) Knapp (New York)[1352] and Carl Schweigger (Berlin).[1353] This meant that the knowledge and application of transfixion according to Fuchs spread almost simultaneously in German- and English-speaking specialist circles.

Furthermore, Fuchs's *Lehrbuch* in its wide range of translations contributed decisively to the popularisation of transfixion according to Fuchs. He himself mentioned the transfixion of the iris for the first time in the section on iridotomy of the 8th edition (1900).[1354] It is remarkable, if unsurprising, that Fuchs again forbore from drawing attention to his own achievement in developing or, as one might put it, reinventing this operation method:

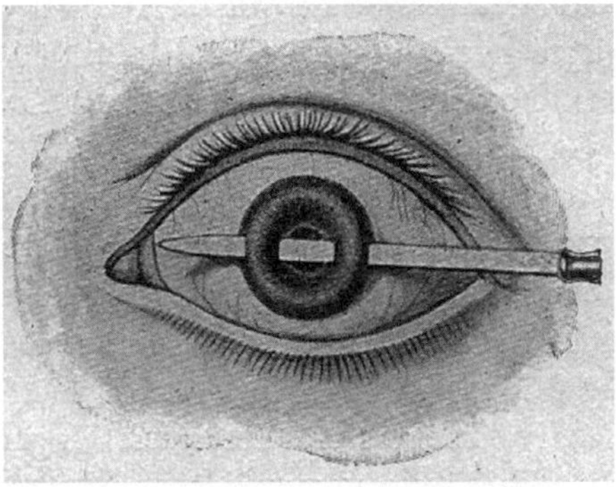

Fig. 101 Transfixion of the iris according to Fuchs

Another case in which it is possible to perform iridotomy when the lens is present, without injuring the latter, is found in a hump-like protrusion of the iris such as results from seclusio pupillae; for here a considerable interspace, namely the enlarged posterior chamber, separates the iris from the lens. Iridotomy in this case may be done by transfixion *of the iris.* [...] *A* Graefe *knife is entered about 1 mm to the inner side of the temporal margin, passed through the anterior chamber, and made to emerge at a spot near the inner margin of the cornea and symmetrically situated with respect to the point of entry. The points of entry and exit lie in the horizontal meridian of the cornea, and the knife is held so that its blade is parallel to the base of the cornea. Since the iris is driven forward, the knife as it is being carried through the anterior chamber pierces the most protruding portion of the iris both temporally and nasally and makes holes in it. Those holes remain permanently open and restore the communication between the anterior and posterior chambers; the iris returns to its former position, and the intra-ocular pressure becomes normal. In cases of hump-shaped protrusion of the iris, this operation may consequently be made instead of an iridectomy; and in cases of this sort it may be done as preliminary operation to an iridectomy, so that the latter can be done later under more favorable conditions.*[1355]

The 2nd edition of Czermak's *Augenärztliche Operationen* of 1908, which was overseen by Anton Elschnig,[1356] features for the first time a chapter devoted to a detailed description of transfixio iridis, divided into subchapters entitled *Execution of transfixio iridis according to E. Fuchs; Dressing; References; and Assessment of the Operation.* Another historic first is the instructive drawing entitled *Transfixio iridis according to E. Fuchs.*[1357] (Fig. 101).

The explanatory text in Meller's ophthalmo-surgical textbook (1908/1918) relies largely on Fuchs's original publication and is supplemented by an instructive drawing, which differs only slightly from the one supplied by Czermak-Elschnig.[1358]

In 1910, Fuchs himself illustrated his transfixion method in the 12th edition of the *Lehrbuch*, with Czermak-Elschnig (1908) serving as a template.[1359] Elschnig's 1922 edition of *Augenärztliche Operationen* featured a significantly expanded explanatory text on the transfixion of the iris, a somewhat simplified drawing and, as a matter of course, the acknowledgement of Fuchs's pioneering role.[1360]

Keratoplastic for ectatic corneal scars

The first successful transplantation of a cornea in humans, in which the transplanted cornea healed permanently and remained transparent, was a feat achieved by Eduard Konrad Zirm (1863–1944)[1361] on December 7, 1905.[1362] It is certainly worth noting that Zirm made a reference to Fuchs early on in his original 1906 publication:

As total keratoplastic for optical purposes has not led to permanent results in any of the cases where it has been attempted, it follows that this operation appears to be performed only rarely. Efforts have been made in a different direction to use it to good effect in line with Fuchs *and* von Hippel[1363], [...] *to counter ulcerous processes of the cornea and their consequences. The idea here was to prevent ectactic scars from forming and to make sure patients retained, if an incapacitated eye, at least one that was as little deformed as possible.*[1364]

In 1894 and 1901 Ernst Fuchs had reported on his attempts at transplanting entire or partial corneas.[1365] Even though the grafted corneas usually clouded over, Fuchs put forward vigorous pleas for the practice to be continued. In support of this, he cited the following observations:

Summing up the results of the operations I have performed myself, I have to admit that the intended goal of restoring sight after total clouding of the cornea has been reached only very unsatisfactorily in some cases and in most cases not at all. This will not prevent me from continuing my attempts in future. In other cases, those of partial staphyloma, I have achieved results that cannot be realised by any other method. We all know how often attenuated ectatic scars defy all attempts at therapy. In all too many cases, excision, cauterisation, iridectomy, etc. fail to put an end to the protrusion of the scar and to elevated pressure, until the eye finally becomes blind. Such cases may be healed permanently, provided the keratoplastic is carried out successfully, and I would like to encourage my colleagues to cultivate keratoplastic surgery especially in these latter cases and to document their experiences with regard to successful outcomes.[1366]

It is highly likely that Fuchs's advocacy of corneal transplantation and the innovative impulse it provided facilitated Eduard Konrad Zirms' epoch-making achievement. In his *Handbook*, which was published three decades after Fuchs had pleaded with his colleagues not to shy away from keratoplastic surgery, Fuchs disciple Josef Meller made this point:

Fuchs was the first to recommend that the fistulous or ectatic cicatrix be excised with a corneal trephine, and that the defect be covered with a piece of cornea removed by a trephine from a freshly enucleated eye.[1367]

Protective Devices

Protective lattice

During his time in Liège Fuchs devised a protective lattice, a contraption to shield newly operated-on eyes:

The idea of the protective lattice came to me during my time in Liège. I had operated on a patient at the clinic for glaucoma. In his sleep the patient hit his eye with his hand, causing the wound to rupture, which in turn filled the chamber with blood, thus delaying healing. When the other eye was due for operation, the patient asked me for a protective device, something in the shape of a muzzle. The device in use at the time was double-sided and relatively heavy. Having presented my lattice on one occasion to the Ophthalmic Section of the Naturforscherkongress in Berlin,[1368] *I subsequently neglected to publish it so that it remained relatively unknown. It was not until many years later that Snellen*[1369] *presented his cup.*[1370]

When he came to write up this episode in his autobiography, Fuchs appears to have forgotten that he in fact presented his protective lattice at a meeting of the Gesellschaft der Ärzte in Vienna on December 16, 1892, when he spoke about new methods applied in cataract operations. He published the

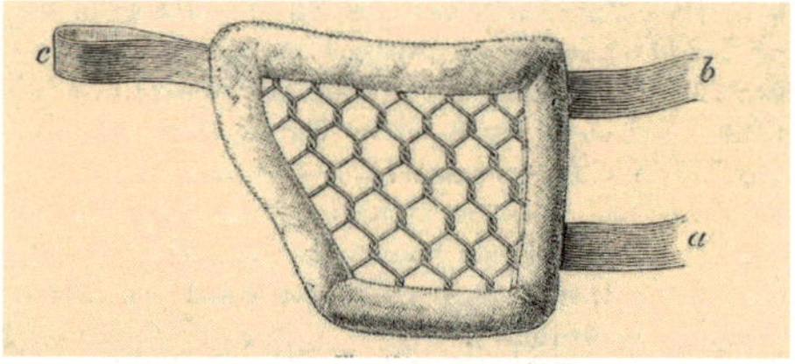

Fig. 102
Protective lattice for the left eye according to Ernst Fuchs (*Lehrbuch* 1894)

paper together with a drawing, as an original contribution in 1893:[1371]

The dressing *is dry and in the form of a gauze flap, which is placed directly upon the closed lid. The eye cavity is then filled with absorbent cotton, which is held in place by a cotton strip whose ends are smeared with collodium to be glued to the patient's forehead and cheek. To prevent the patient from accidentally shifting the dressing or from hitting himself in the eye with his hand, which may easily happen in sleep, a wire lattice is superimposed* […]. *The lattice is slightly arched, its borders fit into the surroundings of the eye and feature a recess for the nose; one must therefore have two lattices in store, one for each eye. The borders of the lattice are sheathed in thick flannel to prevent them from exerting any pressure on the substrate. Straps are tied to the lattice's two temporal corners, one of which* […] *is placed below, the other* […] *above the ear of the appropriate side and slung back to the lattice, across the back of the head and the face half. A loop is attached to the nasal side of the lattice* […] *which the straps are tied to. The lattice can thus be detached and re-attached without the patient having to lift their head from the pillow. I have described this wire lattice in such detail because I have found it to be extremely useful and because I would like to warmly recommend its use to my colleagues. It has the following advantages: 1. It is much lighter and less hot especially in summer than the commonly used monoculus comprised of bandages. 2. It is much superior to the latter when it comes to protecting the eye from involuntarily being touched by the patient's hand. 3. It does not exert even the slightest pressure on the eye. I have no doubt that a monoculus that has been applied too tightly has detrimental consequences owing to the pressure it exerts on the eye. It may by itself cause wound rupture. Many clinics have noticed that wound ruptures occur much more frequently on the watch of young, less experienced assistants. Since I switched to the use of wire lattices, which I first trialled in 1883, wound ruptures at my clinic have become much, much rarer.*[1372]

In the next year Fuchs incorporated the description and a picture of his lattice into his *Lehrbuch*.[1373] (Fig. 102)

To begin with, Fuchs's lattice only became established in the German-speaking world, but its use soon spread. Sensitive to the advantages it offered, Prague University Chair Wilhelm Czermak included a detailed description of its use in *Augenärztliche Operationen*:

In all operations where a major incision opens up the inside of the eye the use of Fuchs's *lattice [...] is to be recommended, as it protects the eye against a blow from the patient's hand. In sleep it may easily happen that the patient, dreaming of his eye, attempts to touch it. Moreover, unreasonable patients may try to dislodge the dressing. This is made much more difficult by this mask.*[1374]

Czermak went on to share his experiences with Fuchs's lattice:

At the time when I was still an assistant at Fuchs's *clinic in Vienna, he realised that the use of roller bandage dressings went hand in hand with a great number of wound ruptures after cataract operations.* Fuchs *therefore adopted the exclusive use of a closed dressing, consisting in a cotton-wool ball placed on the closed eyelids and kept in place by a fitted strip of Arlt's plaster. The lattice Fuchs had invented was then put on top.*
This resulted in a significant reduction in wound ruptures.
I myself made use of this type of dressing for quite a long time at my clinic. However, it was clear that this dressing was neither a pressure dressing nor a closed dressing in the proper sense of the word. As the cotton strip is not elastic, the whole thing mostly worked itself loose within a short time so that patients were able to open their eyes underneath the cotton wool. In the morning, I very often found the cotton-wool ball had shifted to the extreme corner of the eye, even though the cotton strip was still in its proper place. In spite of this, wound ruptures remained exceptional. They were observed almost exclusively after chance events such as sneezing, coughing, vomiting, etc. where they would also have occurred under pressure dressings and in cases where the closed dressing had remained in place.

It is therefore better to make do without the dressing altogether and to relegate that other task which is performed by the closed dressing to prevent light and infectious germs alongside dust and so on from entering through the palpebral fissure from outside to the lattice. This is done by adding thick padding to its rims, by adapting it precisely to each face by bending it so that there is a close fit and by sewing a piece of dense black fabric to its entire outside surface. I have been using this dressing, if that is what it should be called, for more than two years. Never has any shortcoming been in evidence that could be ascribed to the absence of a dressing imposed on the eye lids. Wound healing after cataract operations took place at least as efficiently and with even fewer adverse incidents than under the previous dressing.[1375]

In 1898, Eduard Praun[1376], who had purchased Adolph Weber's (1829–1915)[1377] eye clinic in Darmstadt, reported on the positive experiences he had made with Fuchs's lattice.[1378] In 1892 and 1893 he had been offered

the opportunity to obtain proof of the extraordinary usefulness of FUCHS'S lattice. The straps of the wire mask are placed underneath the patient's head before the operation so that, as he is lying in bed for the operation, not even the slightest movement is required of him; the straps are subsequently tied either in front or at the side temporally. Postoperative treatment is made significantly easier, as there are no endless bandages to be unrolled or to be reapplied between the head of the patient and the cushion. All that needs to be done is to detach the lattice on one side and to tilt it open.

Fuchs has observed moreover that since the deployment of the lattice wound ruptures have become much rarer at his clinic, while irregularly applied dressing involving long bandages and very often insufficiently trained assistants resulted in a much greater number of such ruptures.[1379]

Called to Vienna in 1885, Fuchs replaced at his clinic the dressing that had been used after cataract extractions until then – Arlt's flannel strip dressing imposed on the palpebral fissure closed with strips of adhesive plaster. Praun closed his description of this device with the euphoric words:

This dressing is a blessing for both patient and doctor, sparing the latter a great deal of wasted time, frustration and aggravation and the former a great deal of unnecessary pain.[1380]

A product of the Graz and Vienna Ophthalmological School, the disciple of Isidor Schnabel (1842–1908)[1381] Anton Philipp Elschnig, as Director of the Eye Clinic at the German University of Prague between 1907 and 1933 and Czermak's successor, found words of appreciation in his *Augenpflege* (1915) for a protective lattice for both eyes. While he does not explicitly mention Fuchs's authorship, the illustration he appended makes the matter quite clear:

The use of lattices is recommended when it comes to preventing restless or dazed patients from touching their eye in all cases where it is advisable not to shield the eye with dressing. Lattices and cups must be sterilised before being used.[1382]

Fuchs's lattice remained in use throughout the ensuing decades, as is attested by a report by Hans Lauber[1383] from 1925. As Director of the Eye Department of the City of Vienna's Lainz hospital, Lauber judiciously weighed the pros and cons of this device:

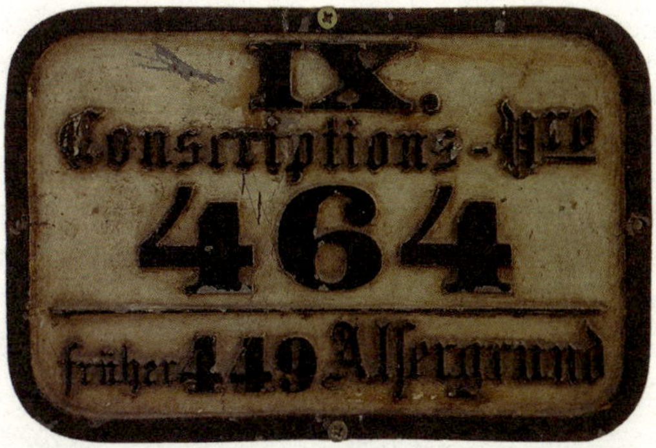

Fig. 103
House number plate of Josef Leitner's firm

Best suited to warding off external force are the Fuchs lattice and the Snellen cup, each with its own specific upsides and downsides. Among the upsides of the Fuchs's lattice I would count its transparency, while its easy slidability is a liability. If one knows how an attentive doctor, who is making his way across a hospital room with a large number of post-operative patients, needs to readjust or re-attach the Fuchs lattice on one or more patients nearly every time, one realises that from this point of view the Fuchs lattice can hardly be called an ideal type of dressing.[1384]

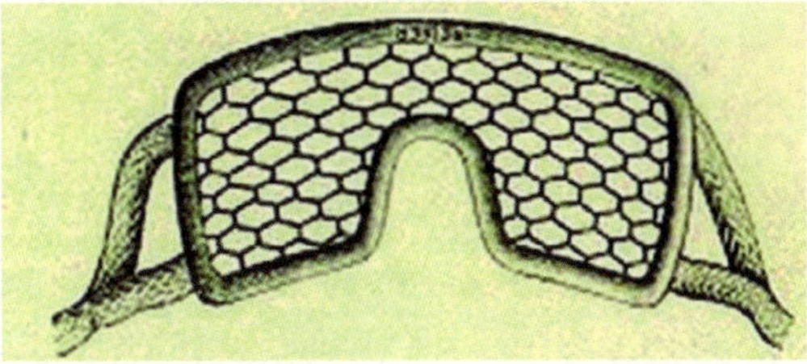

Fig. 104
Protective lattice for both eyes according to Ernst Fuchs (Sales catalogue of the firm of Josef Leitner)

In Vienna Fuchs lattices were produced by Josef Leiter,[1385] a long-established company that manufactured medical instruments and supplied them to the University Clinics, based in Alsergrund (Fig. 103) (today: Mariannengasse 11 in Vienna's 9th district) not far from the Allgemeine Krankenhaus. A 1906 illustrated sales catalogue features it under the designation "Augengitter nach Fuchs" for both eyes or, optionally, for right and left eyes.[1386] (Fig. 104)

The medical instrument maker and manufacturer H. Reiner in Van Swietengasse 10, Alsergrund, next to the Allgemeines Krankenhaus, was another company that manufactured and stocked Fuchs lattices in both variants mentioned above.[1387]

From 1909 onward, the same two variants were available from the renowned Maison Luer, established in 1837 in Paris. The *masque protecteur du Professeur Fuchs en treillis métallique* formed part of that firm's broad range of instruments and devices.[1388]

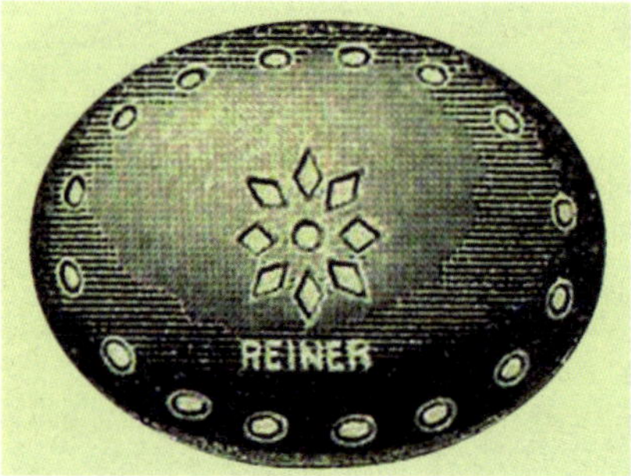

Fig. 105 Protective cup according to Fuchs

At that stage, awareness of the Fuchs lattice had already spread to the United States of America. With *Ophthalmic Surgery* (1908), the first monograph to be published in English on operation techniques practised in the Vienna Ophthalmological School, Meller created a standard reference work.[1389] In it, he refers to what he calls "Fuchs's lattice" as follows:

Bandaging after Operations on the Eye. – We employ Fuchs's lattice in men, and Snellen's cup in women, the cup being attached by strips of adhesive. The latter is not advisable for men, because the plaster will not adhere to the bearded skin. In children and restless patients, bandages are applied, and with the aid of starch a stiff dressing is produced, which will also sufficiently protect the eye against careless contact.[1390]

One year later, Meller gave an *Amerikanerkurs* in English at the Fuchs Clinic,[1391] which was designed to increase awareness of the operative techniques used at the Clinic and of the Fuchs lattice. The lattice is referred to and illustrated as "*wire mask of Fuchs*" in *Ophthalmic Surgery* (1910) by renowned ophthalmic surgeon Charles Heady Beard (1855–1916)[1392] from Chicago.[1393] 1918 saw the publication of Meller's *Ophthalmic Surgery* in German,[1394] which retained multiple references to Fuchs's protective lattice through to its sixth and last edition in 1950.

Protective cup

This device, which Fuchs designed primarily for the protection of injured or inflamed eyes, was on offer in aluminium or celluloid from the firm H. Reiner in Vienna, as can be seen from their 1909 sales catalogue.[1395] (Fig. 105).

Apparatuses and Instruments

Actual Cautery

On the threshold of the introduction of antibacterial chemotherapy in the last quarter of the nineteenth century, when there were as yet only a few locally effective drugs to combat infections of the eye, several ophthalmologists tried to cure abscesses, ulcerations and malign growths of the cornea by the selective application of an electric current. As a refinement of this initially rather crude seeming procedure that made use of red hot wires, Fuchs, at a time when his habilitation was already imminent, developed a significantly more sophisticated and more practicable type of corneal galvanocautery. He presented this innovation on August 13, 1880 at the 48th Conference of the British Medical Association,[1396] presided over by Sir William Bowman. The *British Medical Journal* reported in detail on the presentation:

The Use of Actual Cautery in Ulceration of the Cornea. By Dr. FUCHS (Vienna). – The application of the actual cautery in cases of ulceration of the cornea, so far as Dr. Fuchs knew, just adopted by Martinache[1397] *of San Francisco, and Gayet*[1398] *of Lyons. At the meeting of the German Ophthalmological Society in 1879, Professor Sattler mentioned the success which had attended it;*[1399] *and Dr. Fuchs had since employed it in appropriate cases in Professor Arlt's clinic, with encouraging results. The instrument used by him consisted of a ball of the size of a large pea, with an arm like that used by dentists for the destruction of the dental pulp. It was easily heated red in any good gas flame, and was best applied when the iron was beginning to become black. He had used it in abscesses of the cornea, and in ulcus rodens. The abscesses were partly traumatic and partly spontaneous; some were the result of small-pox. The application was not followed by any serious reaction. He regarded the action of the cautery as that of a powerful caustic, destroying the suppurating parts and the infectious germs contained in them. Its great advantage consisted in its strict limitation of the affected part. Dr. Fuchs believed Paquelin's*[1400] *cautery, or the Galvanocaustic apparatus, liable to become too hot; while the point of the latter was too large for application of the cornea.*[1401]

Half a year later, on February 11, 1881,[1402] Fuchs reported to the Gesellschaft der Ärzte in Vienna on his own mainly positive experiences with the method of cautery of the cornea he had developed himself:

The physicians mentioned earlier, who had been the first to propose this method, had made use of a knitting needle implanted in a piece of cork. Instead of this primitive contraption, which in any case cools much too quickly, I have chosen a small hot iron of the kind used by dentists for the destruction of the dental pulp. An arm a little over 1 cm long, which tapers towards a moderately fine point, is attached obliquely to a ball 7 mm in diameter. This instrument can easily be heated with the help of a Berzelius lamp[1403] *or a gas burner and remains hot for a sufficiently long time, because the ball serves as a heat reservoir. Nor is any great heat required. If one were to touch the cornea with the hot iron while it is*

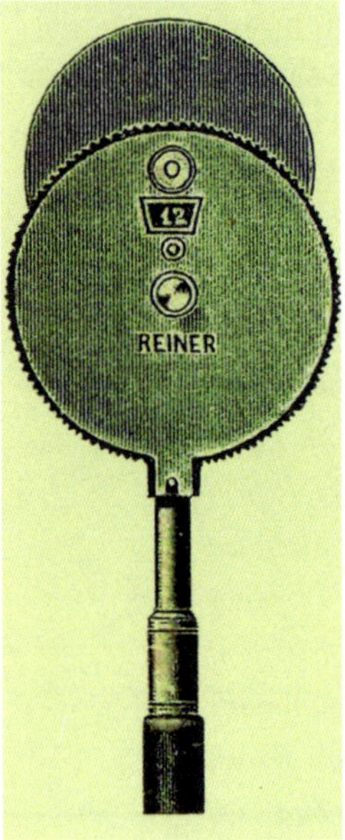

Fig. 106 Ophthalmoscope according to Fuchs

white hot or even only red hot, there would be the danger of perforating the cornea. The best degree of heating seems to me to be weak red hot, when the iron still emits a little light. Then one may touch the cornea at leisure and extensively without having to fear that the etching might penetrate too deeply.

Very recently I have also had the opportunity to use the very finest point of Paquelin's thermocauter. It is capable of good etching but one has to take great care lest the instrument should become too hot. For this reason and because it is much better value, the simple hot iron is arguably preferable for general practitioners.[1404]

Ophthalmoscope

In the wake of Helmholtz's invention of the ophthalmoscope[1405] in 1851, other prominent ophthalmologists took turns over the next years and decades in modifying the basic model in line with their own ideas and needs.[1406] Ernst Fuchs was no exception. His model was offered for sale in the 1909 illustrated sales catalogue of the Viennese medical instrument maker Reiner:

Ophthalmoscope to a design by Professor Fuchs, *consisting of 9 concave and 6 convex correction lenses in a Rekoss*[1407] *disc, 1 large plane mirror and 1 concave mirror, 1 mirror drum in an angular position, 1 large illumination lens in a metal frame* [...]

Each of the two mirrors may be used by itself either in a flat position directly at the ophthalmoscope, or at an angle in the mirror drum.[1408] (Fig. 106)

Operation lamp

Another remarkable contribution Ernst Fuchs made to ophthalmic surgery concerned lighting:

By far the best is the Fuchs *operation lamp, a (frosted) bulb mounted in a sheet housing painted black outside and attached to a long wooden handle that houses the electrical lines. An opening in the sheet housing is fitted with a powerful convex lens that allows moderately divergent light to pass through.*[1409]

Capsule forceps and iris forceps

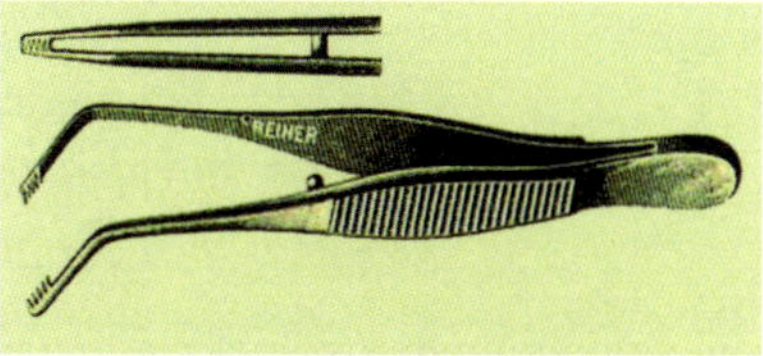

Fig. 107 Capsule forceps according to Fuchs

Another area where Ernst Fuchs made significant contributions was surgical tools. He developed two different forceps types designed to immobilise the eye during operations. While despite the author's best efforts no evidence of the publication of a paper relevant to these particular innovations or of their demonstration within the framework of an ophthalmological conference has been found and while Fuchs himself never referred to them in his epoch-making *Lehrbuch*, proof of their existence does exist, again in the 1909 sales catalogue of H. Reiner, the above-mentioned Viennese firm that specialised in the manufacture of medical-surgical instruments.[1410] (Fig. 107) That the capsule forceps was widely used is attested by its inclusion in the Vienna Ophthalmological School instrument kit, which Meller put together in two versions. Both were included in the Reiner catalogue.[1411]

The Fuchs iris forceps is seven centimeters long, curved, and has two teeth on each of its points. Like the capsule forceps, it is still on sale for use both in human and veterinary surgery.[1412] (Fig. 108)

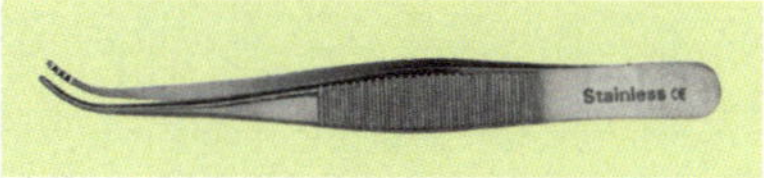

Fig. 108 ReboPharm capsule forceps

In addition, the Reiner catalogue featured a Fuchs eye-washing hose,[1413] which could be flanged to the bibcock of the hard-rubber eye wash, and three different types of the Fuchs-Reuss eye salve stick.[1414]

In obituaries of outstanding ophthalmologists the claim is quite frequently made that the deceased had restored their eyesight to thousands of patients. No one is more entitled to this claim than Ernst Fuchs. That Fuchs successfully extracted thousands of cataracts is a fact, and in the vast majority of cases this operation spared his patients the ordeal of going blind. Equally important is the operation for glaucoma, a disease that in the absence of an operation often leads to blindness. Next in line in the list of life-changing diseases is strabismus, which may result in a disfigurement that tilts the scales for many people, especially for members of the female sex, between happiness and misery. These and all other ophthalmic operations Fuchs had mastered to perfection. […] His excellent training, his experience, his sense of duty, and especially his unflappability made Fuchs an exemplary surgeon. Nothing made him lose his cool. During operations he used to sit on a high three-legged stool next to patient's head. Surrounded by students and physicians who were eager to learn from him, he was often forced to carve out a space for himself with his elbows. His style when performing an operation was targeted and swift, and unforeseen incidents were seen off calmly and securely. Each manipulation, each movement was to the point. There was never too much or too little. One saw an artist at work.[1415]

In today's medical historiography Ernst Fuchs's standing as ophthalmic surgeon is seen as follows:

Even if Fuchs's surgical innovations did not reach the same degree of importance as his clinical research, his studied attention to detail in this field was certainly groundbreaking for its time. As a teacher, he was aware of the fact that surgery can be taught only as a hands-on experience rather than solely through textbooks.[1416]

Notes

1322 Alexander Jokl (1895–1965). Studied at Vienna Univ. (Dr. med. 1919). Ophthalmolog. specialis. at Vienna's Allgem. Krankenhaus, whose two Univ. Eye Clinics were headed by the Fuchs disciples Josef Meller (I) and Friedrich Dimmer (II). Further training at the Univ. of Uppsala and London. 1929 Emigration to South Africa, where he establ. himself as an ophthalmic surg. in Johannesburg in 1930. Among the first members of South Africa's Ophthalmological Society. He left his extensive private library, comprised of ophthalm. and other important, difficult-to-come-by works from a wide range of subjects (ca. 2,000 vols.), which was always accessible to his colleagues, to the Southern Transvaal Group of the Ophthalmic Society of South Africa. In compliance with his wishes, the library was passed on in due course to the Univ. of Witwatersrand in Johannesburg. Cf.: Obituaries, in: *Brit. J. Ophthal.* 49 (1965), p. 385; *S. A. Tydskrif vir Geneeskunde*, 8 Mei 1965, p. 381.

1323 Alexander JOKL, "Ernst Fuchs (1851–1930)", in: NDB (as in FN 15), vol. XV, pp. 142–150.

1324 Ibid.

1325 Cf. FN 43.

1326 Anton Philipp Elschnig (1863–1939). Studied at Graz Univ. (Dr. med. univ. 1886). Assist. at the Univ. Eye Clinic Graz (1892 Habilitation). 1895 Assist. at the 1st Univ. Eye Clinic in Vienna under Isidor Schnabel (cf. FN 602), 1900 Assoc. Prof. 1907–1933 Full Prof. a. d. German Univ. of Prague as the successor of Wilhelm Czermak (cf. FN 43). Accomplished eye surgeon. Developed, among other things, a new surg. procedure for ptosis and keratoplasty. Highly skilled glaucoma and cataract surgeon. Cf. FISCHER (as in FN 28); NDB (as in FN 15, H. Wyklicky); *Münch. Med. Wochenschr.* 80 (1933), p. 1238 (R. Salus); *Med. Klinik* 29 (1933), p. 1127; Obituaries: *Med. Klinik* 35 (1939), p. 1618 (Kubik); *Graefes Archiv* 141 (1940), pp. 338–339.

[1327] Cf. FN 46.

[1328] Wilhelm CZERMAK, *Die augenärztlichen Operationen*. Karl Gerold's Sohn, Vienna 1893–1904.

[1329] Ferdinand ARLT, *Operationslehre*, in: Alfred GRAEFE, Theodor SAEMISCH (eds.), *Handbuch der gesammten Augenheilkunde*. Vol. 3. Pathologie und Therapie. Pt 1. Wilhelm Engelmann, Leipzig 1874, pp. 249–500.

[1330] Anton ELSCHNIG (ed.), Prof. Dr. Wilhelm CZERMAK, *Die augenärztlichen Operationen*. Second enlarged ed. Urban & Schwarzenberg, Berlin/Wien 1908.

[1331] Josef MELLER, *Ophthalmic Surgery. A Handbook of the Surgical Operations on the Eyeball and Its Appendages as Practiced at the Clinic of Prof. Hofrat Fuchs*. P. Blakiston's Son & Co., Philadelphia 1908.

[1332] Josef MELLER, *Augenärztliche Eingriffe. Ein kurzes Handbuch für angehende Augenärzte*. Šafář, Wien 1918.

[1333] Philipp Franz von Walther (1782–1849). Studied medicine at the Univ. of Heidelberg, Vienna and Landshut (Graduation 1803). Ophthalmol. special. espec. under Beer in Vienna. 1804 Prof. of Physiol. and Surg. at Landshut Univ. (1811 Rector). 1818–1830 Prof. of Surg. and Ophthalmol. at Bonn Univ. 1820 Editor of the *Journal f. Chir. u. Augenheilk.* together with Carl (Karl) Ferdinand v. Graefe (1787–1840). 1830 Leading consultant for Surg. and Ophthalmol. at Munich's Städtisches Krankenhaus. Physician to King Ludwig I. of Bavaria. Like his teacher Beer, a vociferous advocate of the autonomy of ophthalmolog. Contributed greatly to the development of science-based surg. and ophthalmolog. in Germany. Trailblazing insights into the nature of cataract. See: GERABEK et al. (as in FN 13); HIRSCH (as in FN 13); HIRSCHBERG, *Geschichte der Augenheilkunde* (as in FN 18), vol. 14/2 (= Reprint vol. III.), §§ 505–508, pp. 205–246; Philipp von WALTHER, *Ectropium anguli externi, eine neue Augenkrankheit, und die Tarsoraphie eine neue Augenoperation*, in: *J. Chir. Augenheilk.* 9 (1826), pp. 86–93. Cf. the reception in the Anglo-American world: (Ed.), *Ectropium anguli oculi externi, cured by the Tarsoraphia, a new operation.* By Prof. WALTHER †, in: *The Lancet* 8/203 (1827), p. 492.

[1334] Franz (Francesco) Flarer (1791–1859). Originally from Dorf Tirol nr. Merano. Initially destined for an ecclesisastic career (Coll. of the Benedictines in Merano, Theol. Fac of Innsbruck Univ.). Studied medicine at the Univ. of Innsbruck, Landshut and Pavia (Dr. med., Dr. chir. 1815). On the advice of the famous anat. and oculist Antonio Scarpa (1752–1832) specialis. in ophthalmol. as a student of Georg Joseph Beer (cf. FN 525) in Vienna (Mag. 1817). 1819 Established the Chair and the Clinic of Ophthalmol. and the Chair of Theoret. and Pract. Ophthalmolog. at the Univ. of Pavia. (1832/33 Rector, 1854 Dean of the Med. Fac.). Of great significance for the surg. development of his specialty was his comprehensive treatment of the diseases affecting the eyelids, where he paid special attention to the operative techniques championed by Friedrich Jaeger v. Jaxtthal (cf. FN 553) and Andrea Vaccà Berlinghieri (1772–1826), for which he proposed a number of modifications (cf. FN 1335). His treatise "*De iritide eiusque speciebus, earumque curatione commentatio*" was awarded a prize in 1836 by the Académie Royale de Médecine in Paris and printed in Pavia in 1841.

[1335] Francesco FLARER, *Riflessioni sulla Trichiasi, sulla Distichiasi e sull'Entropio, avuto particolare riguardo ai metodi di Jaeger e di Vaccà*. Lampato, Milano 1828.

[1336] See also: ARLT, *Operationslehre*, as in FN 1329. Ch. XIX, *"Verkürzung der Lidhaut. (Ausschneiden von Hautfalten)"*, §§ 182–187, pp. 453–458.

[1337] FUCHS, *Lehrbuch*. 1st ed., pp. 780–781. Cf. FUCHS, *Text-Book* (as in FN 810), pp. 941–942.

[1338] CZERMAK, *Die augenärztlichen Operationen* (as in FN 1328), pp. 131–135.

[1339] Cf. FN 908.

[1340] See: WOOD, *American Encyclopedia and Directory of Ophthalmology*, as in FN 909, p. 1049 (Fig. p. 1050).

[1341] *Bericht über die fünfundzwanzigste Versammlung der Ophthalmologischen Gesellschaft Heidelberg 1896*. J. F. Bergmann, Wiesbaden 1897, pp. 179–180.

[1342] Benedict Duddel(l), life data not retrievable. Pioneer in cataract extraction; credited with having been the first to describe keratoconus. See: IBBO (as in FN 18).

[1343] See: GORIN (as in FN 38), p. 52; HIRSCHBERG, *Geschichte der Augenheilkunde* (as in FN 18), vol. 14/I [= Reprint vol. II, 1977), § 391, pp. 125–131.

[1344] Benedict DUDDELL, *A Treatise on the Diseases of the Horny-Coat of the Eye, and the Various Kinds of Cataracts. To which is Prefix'd A Method, entirely New, of Scarifying the Eyes for several Disorders. With Remarks on the Practice of some Oculists both at Home and Abroad*. John Clark, London 1729.

[1345] See: HIRSCHBERG (as in FN 1343), p. 128.

[1346] Robert LISTON, *Elements of Surgery*. Part II. Longman and Company, London; Adam Black, Edinburgh 1831.

[1347] Robert Liston (1794–1847). Originally from Scotland. Studied in Edinburgh; prosector until 1814, then surgeon and prosector at the Royal Infirmary. From 1817 anatom. classes in Edinburgh, where he had established a flourishing practice. 1822 Appointed surgeon at the Royal Infirmary, from 1833 at Univ. College London. See: GERABEK et al. (as in FN 13), HIRSCH (as in FN 13); IBBO (as in FN 18).

[1348] Cf. FN 299.

[1349] William BOWMAN, "On Extraction of Cataract by a Traction Instrument, with Iridectomy; with Remarks on Capsular Obstructions and Their Treatment", in: *Ophthal. Hosp. Rep.* IV (1865), pp. 332–368. See also: Ronnie R. RAY, Richard D. BINKHORST, "The Diagnosis of Pupillary Bloc by Intravenous Injection of Fluorescein", in: *Am. J. Ophthalmol.* 61/3 (1966), pp. 481–483.

[1350] Hugo ASCHHEIM, "Die Transfixion der Iris", in: *Archiv f. Augenheilk.* 37 (1898), pp. 117–124.

[1351] Hugo ASCHHEIM, "Transfixion of the Iris". Translated by Ward A. Holden, in: *Arch. Ophthalmol.* 29 (1900), pp. 507–513.

[1352] Jakob (Jacob) Herman(n) Knapp (1832–1911). Studied at Gießen Univ. (Dr. med. 1854). Ophthalmol. special. in Utrecht (Donders), London (Bowman), Berlin (v. Graefe) u. Heidelberg (v. Helmholtz). 1859 Habilitation in Ophthalm. at Heidelberg Univ., 1859/60–1868 Dir. of the newly founded Univ. Eye Clinic Heidelberg. 1865 Assoc. Prof.). Emigration to the United States. 1869 Foundation of the New York Ophthalmic and Aural Institute (1913–1939 Herman Knapp Memorial Hospital). 1882 Prof. at the New York Univ. Med. College. 1888 Prof. of Ophthalmol. at the

College of Physicians and Surgeons d. Columbia University (1902 Prof. em.). His son Arnold Herman Knapp (1869) also became well-known as an ophthalmologist (cf. FN 1436). See: EULNER (as in FN 13); IBBO (as in FN 18); (Ed.), "Europe in Advance of Us – A Tribute to Hermann Knapp", in: *JAMA* 305/19 (2011), p. 2017 (= Series *JAMA 100 Years Ago*).

1353 Carl (Karl) Ernst Theodor Schweigger (1830–1905). Originally from Halle/Saale. Studied at the Univ. of Erlangen and Halle (Dr. med. 1852). Ophthalmol. special. in Würzburg and Berlin (assistant under v. Graefe, 1860 Habilitation, 1864 Assoc. Prof.). Study trip to Utrecht, London and New York. 1868–1871 Assoc. Prof. of Ophthalm. and Dir. of the newly created Eye Clinic at Göttingen Univ. 1871–1900 Successor of Graefe in Berlin (1873 Full Prof., 1881 newly created clinic and polyclinic). See: EULNER (as in FN 13); HIRSCHBERG, *Geschichte der Augenheilkunde* (as in FN 18), vol. 15/2 [= Reprint vol. VI], § 1105, pp. 44–51; IBBO (as in FN 18); PAGEL (as in FN 13); Jutta HERDE, "Zur Erinnerung an Carl Ernst Theodor Schweigger (1830–1905)", in: *Klin. Monatsbl. Augenheilk.* 222 (2005), pp. 7ff.

1354 FUCHS, *Lehrbuch* (as in FN 787). 8th edition, 1910, pp. 826–827. Cf. FUCHS, *Text-Book* (as in FN 810), pp. 899–900.

1355 Ibid.

1356 Cf. FN 1330.

1357 Ibid., vol. 2, p. 184, Fig. 26.

1358 Cf. FN 1331 and 1332.

1359 FUCHS, *Lehrbuch* (as in FN 787). 12th edition. 1910, p. 955, Fig. 367.

1360 Anton ELSCHNIG (ed.), *Augenärztliche Operationslehre*. In zwei Bänden. In: Theodor AXENFELD, Anton ELSCHNIG, *Handbuch der gesamten Augenheilkunde begründet von A. Graefe und Th. Saemisch fortgeführt von C. Hess.* 2nd and 3rd revised eds. Volume I. Springer, Berlin 1922, pp. 762–764, Fig. 553.

1361 Cf. FN 1288.

1362 Eduard ZIRM, "Eine erfolgreiche totale Keratoplastik", in: *Graefes Archiv* 64/Abtheil. III (1906), pp. 580–583 and ZIRM, "Hornhautpfropfung", in: *Wien. klin. Wochenschr.* 28 (1907), p. 61. (Demonstration in the Gesellsch. d. Ärzte in Wien). See also: Charles SNYDER, "Alois Glogar, Karl Bräuer and Eduard Konrad Zirm", in: *Arch. Ophthalmol.* 74/6 (1965), pp. 871–874; W. J. ARMITAGE, A. B. TULLO, D. F. P. LARKIN, "The first successful full-thickness corneal transplant: a commentary on Eduard Zirm's landmark paper of 1906", in: *Brit. J. Ophthalmol.* 90/10 (2006), pp. 1222–23; Matthias E. ZIRM, Avi A. MANNIS, "Eduard Zirm (1863–1944)", in: Mark J. MANNIS, Avi A. MANNIS (eds.), *Corneal Transplantation: A History in Profiles*. Second Edition. Hirschberg History of Ophthalmology Volume Six. Wayenborgh Publications, Amsterdam 2018, pp. 129–141.

1363 Arthur v. Hippel (1841–1916). Studied at Königsberg Univ. K [today Kaliningrad, Russian exclave betw. Poland and Lithuania] (Dr. med. 1865). Ophthalmol. specialis. under Ferdinand v. Arlt in Vienna and Albrecht v. Graefe in Berlin. Prof. of Ophtlamol. and Director of the Univ. Eye Clinics at Königsberg (1874–1879, 1890–1892), Gießen (1879–1890), Halle (1892–1900) and Göttingen (1900–1914). 1877 Presentation of his corneal trephine utilising the principle of a rotating clockwork to the Ophthalmol. Gesellsch. Heidelberg: Arthur v. HIPPEL, "Eine neue Methode der

Hornhauttransplantation", in: *Graefes Archiv* 34/Abtheil. I. (1888), pp. 108–130. See: EULNER (as in FN 13); FISCHER (as in FN 28); HIRSCH (as in FN 13); IBBO (as in FN 18).

1364 See: ZIRM, "Eine erfolgreiche Keratoplastik" (as in FN 1362), p. 580.

1365 Ernst FUCHS, "Ueber Keratoplastik", in: *Wien. klin. Wochenschr.* 7 (1894), pp. 843–845; FUCHS, "Zur Keratoplastik", in: *Zeitschr. Augenheilk.* 5 (1901), pp. 1–5.

1366 FUCHS, Ibid. (1894), p. 845.

1367 Josef MELLER, *Ophthalmic Surgery. A Handbook of the Surgical Operations on the Eyeball and Its Appendages as Practised at the I. Eye Clinic, University of Vienna.* Edited by William M. Sweet. Third Edition translated from the Second Edition of *Augenärztliche Eingriffe* (Josef Šafar, Vienna). P. Blakeston's Sons & Co., Philadelphia 1923, p. 303.

1368 The reference is to a meeting of the Gesellsch. Dt. Naturforscher u. Ärzte.

1369 Cf. FN 292.

1370 FUCHS, *Augenarzt* (as in FN 2), pp. 91–92.

1371 Ernst FUCHS, "Die neuen Methoden der Staaroperation", in: *Wien. klin. Wochenschr.* 6 (1893), pp. 19–23.

1372 Ibid., pp. 20–21.

1373 The figure in question is appended to the "Operationslehre" in the first chapter under "Allgemeine Bemerkungen" [General remarks]. See: FUCHS, *Lehrbuch* (as in FN 787). 4th ed. 1894, pp. 750–751.

1374 CZERMAK, *Die augenärztlichen Operationen* (as in FN 1328), pp. 95–96 and Fig. 83.

1375 Ibid., pp. 590–591.

1376 Eduard Praun, b. 1868 in Bamberg, 1897 Purchase of Adolf Weber's clinic and ophthalmic practice in Darmstadt (see below).

1377 Adolph (Adolf) Weber (1829–1915). Dr. med. Univ. Gießen 1854. Ophthalmol. special. and later assistant under Albrecht v. Graefe in Berlin. Established a private eye clinic in 1860 in Darmstadt, initially comprised of only one room. 1871 Purchase of a house in Gießen (Frankfurter Straße 42), where he established a significantly more spacious clinic. See: HIRSCH (as in FN 8); HIRSCHBERG, *Geschichte der Augenheilkunde* (as in FN 18), vol. 15/2 [= Reprint vol. VI], §§ 1112–14, pp. 77–89; PAGEL (as in FN 13); Obituaries, in: *Centralbl. Augenheilk.* Sept./Okt. 1915 (Julius Hirschberg); *Klin. Monatsbl. Augenheilk.* 55/2 (1915), pp. 389–398 (Theodor Leber); *Zeitschr. Augenheilk.* 34/Heft 1–2 (1915) (Arthur Ollendorff).

1378 Eduard PRAUN, "Ueber die Verwendbarkeit des von Professor Fuchs zur Nachbehandlung von Star-Operirten angegebenen Drahtgitters", in: *Centralbl. f. prakt. Augenheilk.* 22 (1898), pp. 65–73.

1379 Ibid., p. 66.

1380 Ibid., p. 73.

1381 Cf. FN 602.

1382 Anton Philipp ELSCHNIG, *Augenpflege.* Springer, Berlin/Heidelberg 1915, p. 37 and Fig. 20, p. 36.

1383 Cf. FN 1279.

1384 Hans LAUBER, "Verband und Behandlung nach Staroperation", in: *Wien. med. Wochenschr.* 76 (1925), No. 45.

[1385] Josef Leiter (1830–1892). Apprenticed to a surgical instrument maker in Vienna. Journeyman in Southern Germany, Belgium, England and France, where he received particularly valuable instruction from a med. instrument maker, the German émigré Georges-Guillaume-Amatus Luer (1802–1883), and Joseph-Frédéric-Benoît Charrière (1803–1876) in Paris. Keen interest in electricity and the manufacture of batteries to be incorporated in his models. Return to Vienna, where he took up employment. 1855 Established a small workshop in rented premises opposite the Wr. Allgem. Poliklinik in Alservorstadt, which soon acquired an internat. reputation. 1866 Construction of a factory powered by steam engines. Awarded a medal at the Paris World Exhibition (1873). 1875 Awarded the title *Lieferant der k. k. Universitäts-Kliniken*. Branches set up in Great Britain, Denmark, Sweden, Norway and the United States. Development, together with the Dresden urologist Maximilian Nitze (1848–1906), of the first cystoscope with inbuilt platinum filament to illuminate the bladder. 1879 First Demonstration in the Gesellschaft d. Ärzte in Wien. Seven years later construction of the first cystoscope fitted with an electric light bulb. See: Obituary, in: *Wien. med. Wochenschr.* 42 (1892), cols. 641–642.

[1386] Josef LEITER, *Katalog über ophthalmologische Instrumente und Apparate etc. der Firma Josef Leiter Lieferant für die k. k. Universitätskliniken*. Selbstverlag, Wien 1906, p. 5, Fig. 1114.

[1387] H. REINER, *Verzeichnis über Ophthalmologische Instrumente und Apparate usw.* Selbstverlag, Wien 1909, Nr. 5946 u. 5947, S. 23.

[1388] Maison LUER. Magasin de vente et ateliers: 104, Boulevard Saint-Germain, 104 à Paris. *Catalogue spécial illustré des Instruments d'Ophtalmologie*, Paris 1909, p. 192–193, Figs. 1165 and 1166.

[1389] MELLER, *Ophthalmic Surgery* (as in FN 1331).

[1390] Ibid., p. 244. The first illustration of the Fuchs lattice was included in the second edition of *Ophthalmic Surgery* (1913), p. 152.

[1391] See Ch. 5.

[1392] Charles Heady Beard (1855–1916). Studied at Louisville Univ. (Graduation 1877). Ophthalmolog. special. in New York (Hermann Knapp), London and Vienna. 1886 Established himself as an ophthalmol. in Chicago. Surgeon at the Illinois Charitable Eye and Ear Infirmary and at the Passavant Memorial Hospital. Pres. of the Chicago Ophthalmol. Soc. See: Obituary, in: *The Ophthalmic Record*, Feb. 1916, p. 104.

[1393] Charles H. BEARD, *Ophthalmic Surgery. A Treatise on Surgical Operations Pertaining to the Eye and Its Appendages, with Chapters on Para-Operative Technic and Management of Instruments.* Rebman, London 1910, p. 25.

[1394] Josef MELLER, *Augenärztliche Eingriffe* (as in FN 1332).

[1395] REINER, *Ophthalmologische Instrumente und Apparate* (as in FN 1387), Nos. 5970 and 5971, p. 23.

[1396] *Daily Journal of the British Medical Association Forty-Eighth Annual Meeting, Cambridge 1880.* Friday August 13th, Section H. – Ophthalmology, p. 13. Ernst Fuchs's own programme booklet with handwritten notes and markings. Private collection.

[1397] Narcisse J. Martinache (1834–1892). Studied medicine in Paris (Graduation 1861). Ophthalmol. specialis. uneer de Wecker. 1869 Emigrated to San Francisco. 1873–1881 Prof. of Ophthal. and Otol. at the Med. Dept. of the Univ. of California. 1873 new method of the treatment of corneal ulcers by cauterisation. Cf.

Narcisse J. MARTINACHE, "Ulcers of the cornea, treated by the actual cautery", in: *Pacific Med. Surg. J.*, Nov. 1873, p. 294; MARTINACHE, "De l'emploi du cautère actuel dans les maladies des yeux, et principalement dans les ulcères de la corneé", in: *Annales d'ocul.* 80 (1878), p. 21; IBBO (as in FN 18).

1398 Charles Alphonse Gayet (1832–1904). 1872–1904 Chair of Ophthalm. at Lyon. Univ. Contributed significantly to the general acceptance of Martninache's cauterisation treatment of ulcers of the cornea. See: Charles Alphonse GAYET, "Cauterisation ignée de la cornée", in: *Gazette des Hôpitaux* [= *Gaz. des Hôp.*], No. 11 (1877); IBBO (as in FN 18).

1399 Hubert SATTLER, "Behandlung der Keratitis", in: Bericht d. Ophthalmol. Gesellsch. Heidelberg 1879, S. 140.

1400 Claude-André Paquelin (1836–1905). Initially apothecary for several hospitals in Paris; studied medicine and worked at the Hôpital Saint-Lazare in Paris. Ingenious designer of a wide range of machinery and instruments. His most significant invention was a thermocautery with a platinum point, filled with platin black. Made red hot by being held into a gas flame, the point was made to retain its high temperature by having a petrol-air mixture (or other inflammable gases) being boosted to it by a blower. This opened up a wide range of major innovative possibilities for surgery (e.g. haemostasis). In 1872, in the wake of the Franco-German War, philanthropically inclined Paquelin funded the establishment of the first public polyclinic in Paris, where patients received treatment for free. See: FISCHER (as in FN 28); Obituary: "Claude-André Paquelin", in: *L'Année Scientifique et Industrielle* 49 (1906), pp. 556–557; Cautère-Paquelin (Thermo-Cautère) présenté à l'Académie des Sciences dans la séance du 1er mai 1876.

1401 "Forty-Eighth Annual Meeting of the British Medical Association", in: Brit. Med. J. II (1880), pp. 780ff. (here: p. 781). Cf. also the report in the French specialist press: Annal. d'ocul. 84 (1880), p. 242. See: CZERMAK, Die augenärztlichen Operationen, as in FN 1328, pp. 638 ff.; Fiona ROMAN, "The short history of heat cauterisation of the cornea", in: *Brit. J. Ophthalmol.* 79 (1995), p. 236.

1402 Ernst FUCHS, "Über die Anwendung des Ferrum cadens bei Hornhauterkrankungen", in: *Anzeiger der k.k. Gesellschaft der Ärzte in Wien*, Minutes of the meeting on 11 Feb. 1881, pp. 145–146 (Pres.).

1403 Named after Swed. physician and chemist Jöns Jakob Berzelius (1779–1848). Studied at Uppsala Univ. (Dr. med. 1802). Embarked on wide-ranging electro-chemical studies. 1807 Prof. of Med. and Pharmacy at Stockholm Univ.; 1815–1832 Prof. of Chemistry at the Karolinska Institutet. Pioneer in the field of chem. elementary analysis. Discovered several previously unknown chem. elements. 1811 Initiated the system of abbreviations of chem. elements which is still in use today. Constructed a spirit lamp with a hollow round wick as a heating appliance in the chem. lab. See: Carl Fried. Phil. v. MARTIUS, *Denkrede auf J. J. Berzelius, gehalten in der öffentlichen Sitzung der Königlich Bayerischen Akademie der Wissenschaften am 28. November 1848.* Offprint of *Gelehrte Anzeigen* 1848, Nos. 233–236.

1404 Ernst FUCHS, "Die Anwendung des Glüheisens bei Hornhautleiden", in: *Wien. med. Wochenschr.* 31 (1881), cols. 621–624 (here: col. 621).

1405 See also the entry on *Ophthalmoskopie*, in: Albert EULENBURG (ed.), *Real-Encyclopädie der gesamten Heilkunde. Medizinisch-chirurgisches Handwörterbuch für praktische Ärzte*. Vol. XI. 4th ed. Urban & Schwarzenberg, Berlin/Vienna 1911, pp. 63ff.

1406 Alfred SCHETT, Charles KEELER, *The Ophthalmoscope / Der Augenspiegel*: Ein Beitrag zur Entwicklungsgeschichte bis zum Beginn des 20. Jahrhunderts. Textbook and Atlas. Wayenborgh, Oostende 1996/97.

1407 Instrument mechanic from Königsberg, who in 1852 devised this revolving disc to which the correction glasses are attached.

1408 Cf. REINER, *Ophthalmologische Instrumente und Apparate* (as in FN 1387), No. 5588, p. 6.

1409 Cf. ELSCHNIG (ed.), Prof. Dr. Wilhelm CZERMAK, *Augenärztl. Operationen*, as in FN 1323, pp. 87–88.

1410 Cf. REINER, *Ophthalmologische Instrumente und Apparate* (as in FN 1387), No. 5851, p. 17.

1411 Ibid., No. 5889, p. 19: *Kapselpinzette nach Fuchs im Augeninstrumentenetui zusammengestellt nach den Angaben des Herrn Dozent Dr. Meller, in elegantester Ausführung* and ibid., No. 5890, p. 19: *Augeninstrumentenetui, kleine Zusammenstellung in feinem Holzetui.*

1412 Cf. e. g. the German firms Allgeier Instrumente and Sigmed.

1413 Cf. REINER, *Ophthalmologische Instrumente und Apparate* (as in FN 1387), No. 5989, p. 24.

1414 Ibid., No. 5990, p. 24.

1415 Alexander JOKL, "Ernst Fuchs (1851–1930)" (as in FN 1323), here: p. 146.

1416 MÜLLER, McGHEE, "Professor Ernst Fuchs" (as in FN 218).

11. Highlights of Fuchs's Lecture Tours: United States, Japan and China

In addition to the publication of Fuchs's scientific papers and his epoch-making *Lehrbuch*, which was translated into all major languages,[1417] the worldwide spread of his reputation benefited most from his lecture tours. These and the friendly relations spanning the globe, which he cultivated with former students and with colleagues during his thirty years as Chair and Director of Vienna University's 2nd Eye Clinic, laid the foundation for his reputation as the uncontested leader in the field of scientific ophthalmology. This in turn enhanced the worldwide prestige of the Vienna Ophthalmological School and made it the flagship of this medical specialty for several decades.[1418]

Having decided of his own free will to resign from his university position prematurely in 1915,[1419] Fuchs used the last 15 years of his life to intensify his international teaching. Initially, however, World War I and the increasing dependence of his wife on his care held him back. Julie Fuchs died on 12 June 1919.

After the academic festivities to mark his 70th birthday on June 14, 1921 and the meeting of Vienna's Ophthalmologische Gesellschaft convened in his honour in August 1921[1420] Fuchs embarked on a round-the-world trip lasting several years. The idea behind it was primarily to rebuild his finances from the proceeds of lectures organised by friends and former students. Having invested most of his savings in war bonds, he found himself almost penniless at the end of the war.

As a comprehensive, complete reconstruction of Fuchs's lecture tours would take up more space than is available in this monograph, his sojourns in the United States, Japan, and China are singled out here to serve as examples.

Three Sojourns in the United States of America

In the years before his "habilitation" in 1879, when he was still an assistant under Arlt, Fuchs organised what he and others referred to as *Amerikanerkurse*.[1421] His own extraordinary gift for acquiring foreign languages and, later, that of his assistants – Josef Meller and Maximilian Salzmann need to be mentioned in this context – enabled this group to hold highly specialised ophthalmological courses in English, which attracted an ever growing number of eye specialists and surgeons from all over the world, primarily from the United States, putting Fuchs in contact with a great number of Anglo-American ophthalmologists. This was of course inextricably linked to the great success Fuchs's *Lehrbuch* met with in the Anglo-American world, where it had repeatedly been translated and published in a series of revised editions.[1422]

Lane Lectures (1911)

Fuchs's first invitation to the United States in 1911 was initiated by one of his former private students at Arlt's Clinic, Adolph Barkan.[1423] Having moved to San Francisco in 1872, Barkan became a professor at the Eye, Ear and Throat Department of local Cooper College, which was later to become the Stanford University School of Medicine.[1424] In 1896, the Lane Medical Lectures were established.[1425] Adolph Barkan, whose sons Hans and Otto Barkan[1426] followed in their father's footsteps by becoming Fuchs's students, issued an invitation on behalf of the American Ophthalmological Society in 1911.[1427] It was no doubt an additional incitement for Fuchs that this coincided with the publication of the 4th American edition of the *Lehrbuch* in Alexander Duane's tried and proven translation.[1428]

On my way back from Java I received a telegram in Kandy with the news […] *that Barkan had proposed me as a candidate to give the Lane Lectures in San Francisco. An endowment made by the late Dr Lane provides for ten lectures to be given every other year by a specialist, who is to receive a fee of 2,000 dollars.*[1429] *Up until now this had been the exclusive preserve of Americans and Englishmen. I owed the invitation to Barkan and I accepted it with the greatest pleasure.* […]

The trip to America lasted a full three months, the whole summer, and even though I made a detour to Mexico, I did not spend all the 2,000 dollars.[1430]

Having boarded the steamer *Amerika* of the Hamburg-Amerika-Linie on June 29, 1911, Fuchs reached New York on July 8 via Cuxhaven, Southampton and Cherbourg.[1431] (Fig. 109) Upon arrival, he was sponsored by Alexander Duane. A few days later Fuchs took part as a guest in the 47th Annual Meeting of the American Ophthalmological Society, which was held in New London, a city halfway between New York and Baltimore.[1432] He delivered three lectures there.[1433]

Fuchs then left for San Francisco to give the Lane Lectures, for which he had chosen "The Importance of Ophthalmology in its Relation to Systemic Diseases" as his topic. Between August 21 and 25 he lectured twice a day at

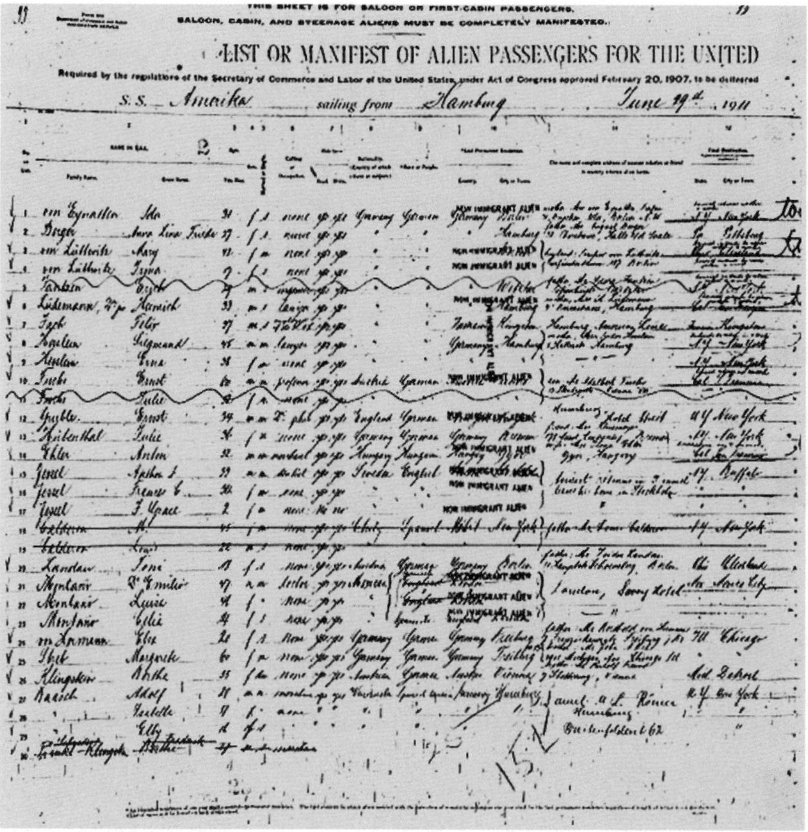
THIS SHEET IS FOR SALOON OR FIRST-CABIN PASSENGERS.
SALOON, CABIN, AND STEERAGE ALIENS MUST BE COMPLETELY MANIFESTED.

LIST OR MANIFEST OF ALIEN PASSENGERS FOR THE UNITED

Required by the regulations of the Secretary of Commerce and Labor of the United States, under Act of Congress approved February 20, 1907, to be delivered

S. S. Amerika sailing from Hamburg June 19th 1911

Fig. 109 Manifest of Ernst Fuchs's voyage to New York in 1911 (entry in lines 10–11)

the Cooper Medical College. His visit had been announced beforehand in several specialist journals and was afterwards reported with a great deal of appreciation.[1434]

Teaching in the States 1921/22

After the Extraordinary Meeting of the Wiener Ophthalmologische Gesellschaft on August 4–6, 1921 to celebrate his 70th birthday,[1435] Fuchs began to prepare for his second spell of teaching in the United States, which was to last a whole year and take in several university metropolises all over the country.

The invitation this time had arisen from an initiative by New York ophthalmologist Arnold Herman Knapp (1869–1956),[1436] the son of the renowned and influential German émigré Hermann Jakob Knapp.[1437]

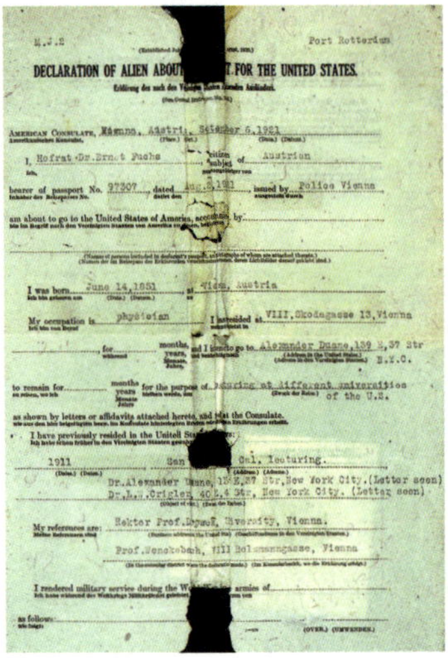

Port Rotterdam

DECLARATION OF ALIEN ABOU… FOR THE UNITED STATES.

AMERICAN CONSULATE, Vienna, Austria, September 6, 1921

I, Hofrat Dr. Ernst Fuchs … citizen subject of Austrian

bearer of passport No. 97307 dated Aug. 2, 1921, issued by Police Vienna

am about to go to the United States of America, accompanied by

I was born June 14, 1851 at Vienna, Austria

My occupation is physician. I have resided at VIII, Skodagasse 13, Vienna

…for … months, years, and I intend to go to Alexander Duane, 139 E, 37 Str N.Y.C.

to remain for … months years for the purpose of lecturing at different universities of the U.S.

as shown by letters or affidavits attached hereto, and that the Consulate.

I have previously resided in the United St…

1911 San … Cal. lecturing.

Dr. Alexander Duane, 139 E, 37 Str, New York City. (Letter seen)

Dr. L. …Crigler, 40 E, 4 Str, New York City. (Letter seen)

My references are: Rektor Prof. Dopsch, University, Vienna.

Prof. Wenckebach, VIII Bolzmanngasse, Vienna

I rendered military service during the W… armies of

as follows:

(OVER.) (UMWENDEN.)

Fig. 110a
Ernst Fuchs's
immigration visa
in 1921 (recto)

I replied that I would be delighted to comply, provided my travel expenses were met. I assumed I would be conducting these courses in the overall context of the postgraduate courses laid on at the Postgraduate [Teaching] *Hospital. I then heard nothing from Knapp for a long time and maybe a year later he wrote to me to say that he and Duane*[1438] *had been at pains to put an independent course together for me in New York and some other cities and so it was arranged that I would arrive in New York for this purpose at the end of September.*

[…]

In the autumn of 1921, I set off on my trip to North America, which was to last much longer than I had anticipated. In addition to the cities where Knapp and Duane had arranged for me to lecture more than a dozen others approached me but I only accepted Houston[1439] *and Minneapolis.*[1440, 1441]

To obtain a visa for the United States Fuchs had to provide "security related information". He did so on September 6, 1921 in Vienna. (Figs. 110a, b) Asked about the purpose of his visit, he indicated that it was *"lecturing at different universities of the U. S."* and pointed to his first sojourn in the States ten years earlier. Again, he named Alexander Duane from New York as his sponsor. Furthermore, Fuchs produced two Austrian testimonies, one issued by the then Rector of Vienna University, the renowned historian Alfons Dopsch,[1442] the other from the distinguished cardiologist and Director of Vienna's 1st Medical University Clinic, Karel Frederik Wenckebach (1864–1940).[1443]

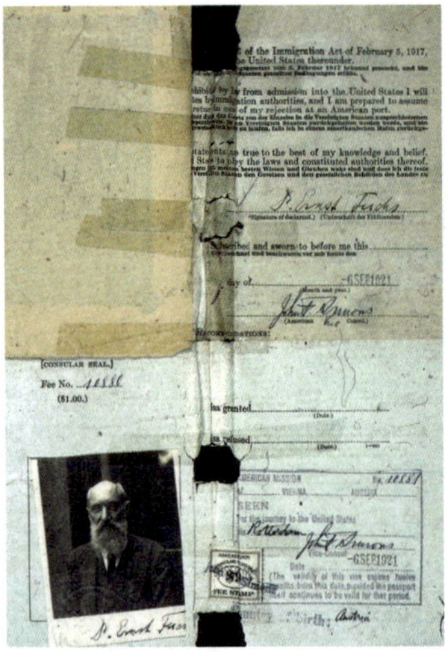

… of the Immigration Act of February 5, 1917, … United States thereunder.

… from admission into the United States I will … immigration authorities, and I am prepared to assume return in case of my rejection at an American port.

… statements are true to the best of my knowledge and belief, … States to obey the laws and constituted authorities thereof.

Dr. Ernst Fuchs
(Signature of declarant.)

Subscribed and sworn to before me this … day of -6SEP1921

(American Vice Consul.)

RECOMMENDATIONS:

[CONSULAR SEAL.]

Fee No. 11886 ($1.00.)

Visa granted … (Date.)

Visa refused … (Date.)

AMERICAN MISSION … VIENNA AUSTRIA

SEEN

For the journey to the United States via Rotterdam

Vice-Consul -6SEP1921

(The validity of this visa expires twelve months from this date, provided the passport shall continue to be valid for that period.)

FEE STAMP

… Birth: Austria

Dr. Ernst Fuchs

Fig. 110b
Ernst Fuchs's
immigration visa
in 1921 (verso)

On September 27 Fuchs went on board the steamer *Rijndam* (Fig. 111) in Rotterdam and arrived in New York on October 7.[1444] On this lecture tour Fuchs was accompanied by his former student Oscar Diem[1445] and Diem's student Henry J. Minsky (1895–1954).[1446]

Immediately after his arrival in New York Fuchs gave a course on the histology and pathology of the eye. Working in close collaboration with Fuchs and with his explicit endorsement, Diem and Minsky prepared a detailed handout,[1447] which described, explained, and partly illustrated the 430 histological preparations Fuchs had brought with him from his collection.[1448] As a guest of the Ophthalmic Section of the New York Academy of Medicine, Fuchs gave a presentation on presbyopia on October 17.[1449]

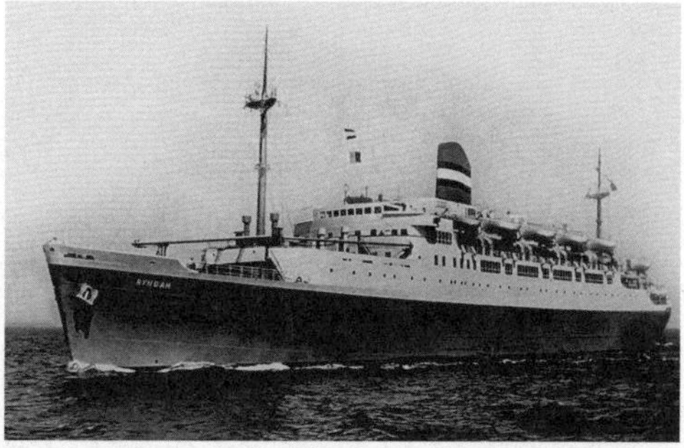

Fig. 111 Steamer Rijndam

Only three days later Fuchs delivered a lecture to the Ophthalmological Section of the College of Physicians of Philadelphia on senile changes of the optic nerve.[1450] Later in the autumn Fuchs gave a course in Boston, which was organised and funded by the New England Ophthalmological Society,[1451] with Fuchs's former student George Strong Derby (1875–1931)[1452] in charge.

During his stay in Boston Fuchs was invited to an extraordinary dinner, which he described in his autobiography as follows:

In November 1921 I had the honour of being invited to a dinner in Boston in celebration of the 50th anniversary of the 'Vienna Dining Club'. In 1871, twelve doctors studying in Vienna had founded this club with the proviso that each month one of them would issue an invitation to dinner in Boston. Members of the club were replaced on their death by other Boston doctors who had studied in Vienna. This resulted in the memory of the time they had spent in Vienna as students being renewed twelve times a year over the course of fifty years. One of the original founders of the club was not only taking part in this dinner, he was doing so with a healthy appetite.[1453]

At the dinner, which took place at the select Algonquin Club, the invitees were offered the chance to purchase a hand-signed portrait photograph of Ernst Fuchs. The revenue from this was $640. Fuchs's lectures and demonstrations yielded $2,575. Most of this was handed over to Fuchs as his fee, and with the rest the New England Ophthalmological Society bought its first slide projector.[1454]

1922 began for Fuchs with a course in Houston/Texas, lasting a fortnight, from January 16 to 30.[1455] (Fig. 112)

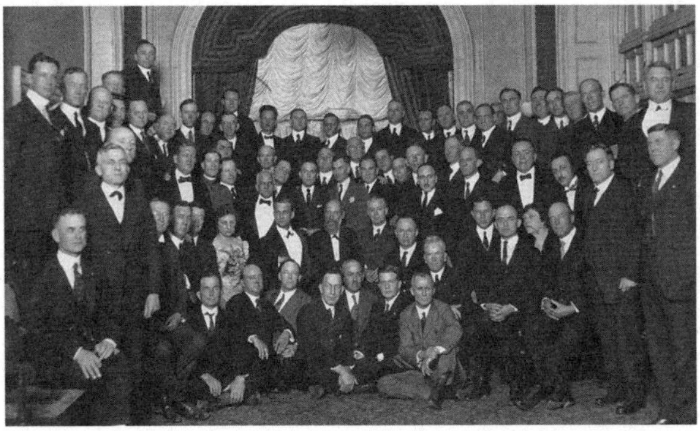

Fig. 112 Course taught by Ernst Fuchs (2nd row, centre) in Houston in 1922, when the Ernst Fuchs Society was founded

The lectures in Houston, where I had perhaps the largest audience – in the region of one hundred –, came about as follows: when I was still in New York, one day Dr Israel[1456] *called on me and asked me if I wanted to lecture in Houston. I told him first that I did not even have a clue where Houston was. Having been put wise on this point, I opined that it was surely unlikely that a sufficient number of ophthalmologists could be got to show an interest in such a course. However, Dr Israel told me that he could guarantee about a hundred participants. I did not believe him but agreed nevertheless,*[1457] *choosing the winter as the time for my course, because it was convenient for me to pass that time of the year in a mild climate. The energetic Israel actually did manage to convene almost one hundred ophthalmologists, for some of whom this involved a 48-hour train journey. In his enthusiasm* [Israel] *and other doctors even founded an Ernst Fuchs Society* [in Houston], *which went belly up after one or two years. Its mission originally was to organise a two-week meeting once a year in a city in one of the southern states with courses in different fields of ophthalmology. They had asked Meller* [to give these courses] *the following year, but Meller had declined. My fee for the course was $50 per participant.*[1458]

Ernst Fuchs's Houston course met with a great deal of appreciation in the specialist press:

The lecture course given by Professor Fuchs at Houston, Texas had an attendance of almost a hundred. The course was well received and the sacrifice made by men, who were in attendance from a distance, was said by all to have been more than worthwhile.[1459]

For the following year the Ernst Fuchs Society announced a meeting in New Orleans, which was scheduled for January 24 to February 9, 1923. In view of the interest this was going to generate the number of participants was limited in advance to 100. Graduate teaching was offered both in ophthalmology and otolaryngology. The list of professors included Arnold Knapp/New York City,[1460] George E. Shambaugh/Chicago (1869–1947),[1461] W. Dean/

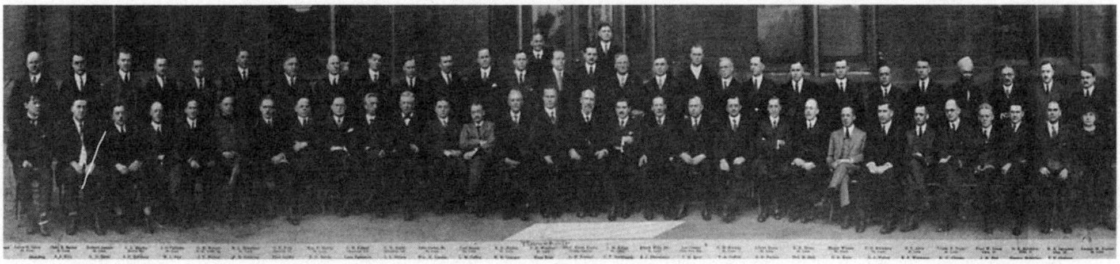

Fig. 113 Course taught by Ernst Fuchs (1nd row, centre) in St. Louis

Iowa City,[1462] Edward Jackson/Denver,[1463] Marcus Feingold/New Orleans (1871–1925),[1464] R. C. Lynch/New Orleans (d. 1930),[1465] in addition to the professors of anatomy, physiology and pathology of Tulane University.[1466]

In February 1922 Fuchs gave a course in St. Louis/Missouri. He was sponsored by the Ophthalmological Section of the Saint Louis Medical Society, which had set up a Fuchs Lecture Committee to take care of organisational matters.[1467] 94 ophthalmologists took part – 61 from Missouri and the rest from other states. A photograph has survived, showing 59 participants, all male with one exception, grouped around Ernst Fuchs. (Fig. 113) Fuchs addressed the St. Louis Medical Society in an additional lecture entitled *The Progress of Ophthalmic Therapeutics from 1870 to the Present Time.*[1468] At the end, Fuchs was made an honorary member of this society.

Since Ernst Fuchs's lecture tour across the United States was a topic that was sure to arouse interest in Austria, the editor-in-chief of the *Wiener medizinische Wochenschrift*, Fuchs's one-time student Adolf Kronfeld,[1469] had asked him while he was still in St. Louis for a report for the journal, focusing on his experiences in the United States. Fuchs replied to this request on February 27, 1922 on paper bearing the letterhead of the University Club Saint Louis:

Sehr geehrter Herr!
As I do not have your Vienna address at hand, I am sending this manuscript to you via my son.[1470] *I am afraid it is badly written because I was confined to my room with a bad bout of influenza when I wrote it down; my state of health was not good and is not good even now. I will send you the travel report you have asked for in the near future. As regards the present manuscript, 20 off-prints will be enough.*
Mit besten Grüssen

Ihr ergebener
Ernst Fuchs

Copy-editing may be left to my son.[1471]

Fuchs's travelogue was published in the *Wiener medizinische Wochenschrift* on May 20, 1922. In it, he gave a brief overview of the hospital system, school education, the study of medicine, and ophthalmological specialisation:

The large hospitals double as teaching hospitals for students of medicine. [Generally speaking], *education is organised as follows: From 6 to 12–14 years Grammar school, which corresponds to our* Volksschule *and* Bürgerschule. *Then four years of High School with Latin, which corresponds to our* Untergymnasium. *This is followed by between two and four years of College, which is usually connected to a university and counts as academic study. College corresponds to our* Obergymnasium, *the only difference being that in addition to subjects of general education it includes those that prepare students for their future profession. In the case of future doctors, this is science, biology, chemistry, physics, etc. The actual study of medicine lasts four years, of which two are devoted to theory and two to clinical practice. In some cases, admittedly the exception rather than the rule, the theoretical subjects take up only three semesters and the clinical subjects get five. School fees both for College and the medical faculty amount to 200 dollars a year. Each state has a state university, but every large city has additional universities, some of which are privately endowed, others by one of the religious denominations. Many universities are located in small towns, which is why medical tuition at university is confined to the two theoretical years. The two clinical years students spend at the medical wards that the universities maintain at the hospitals of the metropolises, in an arrangement where several hospitals provide medical tuition for one university.*

As regards ophthalmology in particular, it does not occupy that outstanding place in medical training it is accorded in our countries. Instead, it is considered to be of the same order as other specialties, such as otology and laryngology. Teaching of ophthalmology varies from institution to institution. Let me give you just two examples. At Columbia University in New York students have in their first clinical year 20, in the second year 12 hours of purely practical and no theoretical tuition. St. Louis University in St. Louis has theoretical tuition three times a week in the first clinical year; in the second [...], *students are divided into groups of eight and receive purely clinical tuition over two semesters at three sessions a week, each lasting one hour. – At the end of the semester and of the academic year there are exams. To be licensed to practise, students need to pass a state exam presided over by a commission. Most young doctors prefer to work at a hospital for between one and several years after the state exam, but this is not obligatory.*

[…]

Specialists have received their training either as assistants in the specialist department of a hospital or from a senior consultant, often a medical doctor who after several years in general practice had felt its demands were getting on top of them. Provided they have the funds required, they then turn to specialisation. Some achieve this by going to clinics in Europe, others to those hospitals in the States that provide specialist training to graduated physicians through postgraduate teaching. This is especially the case in New York, Philadelphia and Boston; other cities are beginning to move in this direction. A case in point is teaching in New York, where the Post Graduate Teaching School and Hospital exclusively serve this purpose with 400 beds and roughly 50,000 outpatients per year. Ophthalmological training takes the form of two courses, lasting 17 weeks, taught by 23 lecturers. There are classes every day and week 17 is devoted to pulling everything together and to discussion. The fee is 500 dollars and each participant is asked to come equipped with certain books and instruments. There are classes in normal and pathological anatomy, histology, physiology and bacteriology of the eye with demonstrations based on the projection of slides, as well as in refraction, muscle anomalies and perimetry, with daily demonstrations involving patients. External eye diseases and ophthalmoscopy are part of the curriculum as well, both in theory and practice and with the involvement of patients. This is complemented with lectures on industrial diseases and the neurology of the eye, and with operations involving practical demonstrations. In Philadelphia the specialisation course lasts between six months and a year. At the end of the course students are required to take an exam but no diplomas are awarded. The design of specialist training courses is subject to ongoing improvement and it may be assumed that in the foreseeable future it will no longer be necessary for medical doctors to travel to Europe for this purpose, with the possible exception of scientific research.[1472]

In early March 1922 Fuchs began a 20-lecture course on "Ocular Pathology" in Philadelphia, organised by the Section on Ophthalmology of the College of Physicians,[1473] where he had already given a lecture on October 20, 1921, immediately after his arrival in the States. It is tempting to assume that the invitation to give this course was a consequence of that first meeting. The local organisation was in the hands of G. Oram Ring (1861–1933).[1474] Together with George Edmund de Schweinitz (1858–1938),[1475] Ring had been one of the driving forces that had brought Fuchs to the United States.

The participants in the course in Philadelphia reacted with enthusiasm:

Professor Fuchs was extensively entertained during his stay in Philadelphia and made a profound impression upon the large group of ophthalmologists of Philadelphia and vicinity, who gave themselves the rare privilege of hearing him.[1476]

On March 29, Fuchs was in Baltimore[1477] to deliver another lecture to the City Medical Society of Baltimore and the State Society of Maryland entitled "Ocular Manifestations of Internal Secretion".[1478]

What is remarkable about the course Fuchs gave in Chicago (April 10–20; May 8–18)[1479] is that the lectures this time were neither organised nor sponsored by a university or a specialist society. The venue was the home of E. V. L. Brown,[1480] who, as has already been mentioned, oversaw eleven years later the last English edition of the *Lehrbuch*.[1481] 110 physicians took part in this course: 86 from Illinois (76 of whom were from Chicago); four from Wisconsin; three from Indiana; two each from Colorado, Kansas, Michigan, Nebraska, North Dakota, Ohio, and Utah; and one each from California, Minnesota, and Oregon.[1482]

On April 21, Fuchs was guest of honour at the Joint Meeting of the Chicago Ophthalmological Society and the Institute of Medicine.[1483] On May 8, the University Club of Chicago gave a festive dinner in honour of Ernst Fuchs and Émile Gallemaerts (1860–1935),[1484] and on May 15 Fuchs was guest of honour at a meeting of the Chicago Ophthalmological Society.[1485]

The insights Fuchs gained in the course of his lecture tour in the United States through his participation in a great number of postgraduate courses resulted in his launching an appeal to his former students and colleagues while he was still in the States to adopt this model for postgraduate courses in ophthalmology in Vienna with a view to offering them to American physicians. An announcement to this effect was made by one of the most influential American ophthalmologists, Edward Jackson,[1486] in his capacity as editor of the *American Journal of Ophthalmology* in the spring of 1922:

The special course here outlined was arranged at the suggestion of Prof. Ernst Fuchs, who during his present visit has come into close touch with the plans for graduate instruction that have recently been developed in the United States. It

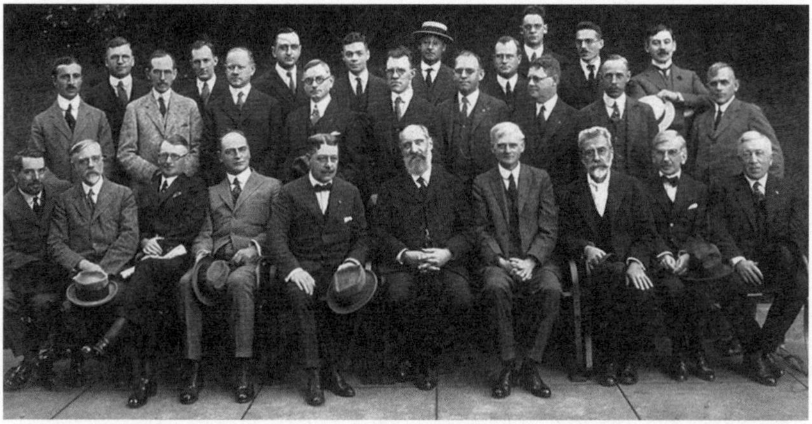

Fig. 114
Course taught by Ernst Fuchs (2nd row, centre) in San Francisco

will be of particular interest at this time because it offers a combination of the enormous clinical advantages of Vienna with intensive systematic instruction by some of the best teachers of ophthalmology in the world.[1487]

From Chicago Fuchs moved on to Denver, where on June 13 he delivered a lecture to the joint meeting of the Colorado Ophthalmological Society and the Denver County Medical Society on "Relations Between Tabes and the Eye".[1488]

Near the end of his lecture tour Fuchs returned to San Francisco. There Fuchs gave his usual three-week course on the pathology of the eye, starting on July 10.[1489] (Fig. 114) His audience included participants from Salt Lake City, Utah.[1490]

Fuchs left San Francisco for the last leg of his tour, embarking on the steamer *President Cleveland* bound for Honolulu on August 12 and arriving five days later.[1491] He spent three weeks in Honolulu and gave two lectures, one on the history of ophthalmology and the other on the diagnostics of arteriosclerosis of the retinal vessels. Both met with an enthusiastic reception.[1492] The Honorary Committee of Queen's Hospital put on a festive lunch for Fuchs, who responded with an undertaking to conduct an "informal clinic" at the surgeries of two local ophthalmologists.

In his autobiography Fuchs sums up his time in the United States as follows:

I had spent almost an entire year in the United States, and been everywhere accorded a most cordial welcome, meeting many kind people. I struck up an especially close friendship with Duane.[1493]

Fuchs departed Honolulu for Yokohama on board the steamer *President Wilson*[1494] on September 8.[1495] This represented a departure from his original plans:

It had not been part of my original plan to return via East Asia after my stay in the United States. This idea only occurred to me after I had set aside a substantial sum of money. I therefore booked a voyage to Siam via Honolulu, China, the Philippines and Borneo.[1496] *I had originally wanted to visit North India, as I had only been to the south before. I had applied* [for a visa] *to the British Colonial Office but my application was rejected. This made me change my plans and instead of India I went to Siam, which was perhaps even more interesting.*[1497]

Even after Fuchs had left the United States in early September 1922, the contacts he had established with American colleagues and friends continued unabated. Arnold Knapp,[1498] for instance, wrote a review of the seventh English edition of the Lehrbuch (1923) in his *Archives of Ophthalmology*:

Fuchs's text-book now appears in its seventh English edition which has been entirely rewritten and rearranged. In some of the changes the translator has had the benefit of consulting with Dr. Fuchs and has drawn on the XIII German edition which was completely revised by Salzmann. […] *Dr. Duane has placed the English-reading ophthalmologist under a great debt, not only by bringing this classical text-book abreast of the times in which he has preserved the spirit, and often the words, of Dr. Fuchs – but also by adding many personal contributions on subjects on which he is an authority.*[1499]

The demand for Fuchs's *Lehrbuch* was such that a new imprint, the 8th edition, was published only one year later.[1500]

Award of the Howe Medal 1924

In 1924, in recognition of his outstanding scientific achievements, the American Ophthalmological Society awarded Fuchs the medal Lucien Howe (1848–1928)[1501] had endowed in 1922.[1502] Fuchs's predecessors in this honour were Carl Koller[1503] in 1922 and Alexander Duane[1504] in 1923.

Ministerial Passport

To facilitate Ernst Fuchs's extensive travels, which were considered to be beneficial to Austria's international reputation at a time when this was badly needed, he was issued a ministerial passport on December 30, 1925 in German and French, valid for six months (Fig. 115a, b), which noted explicitly:

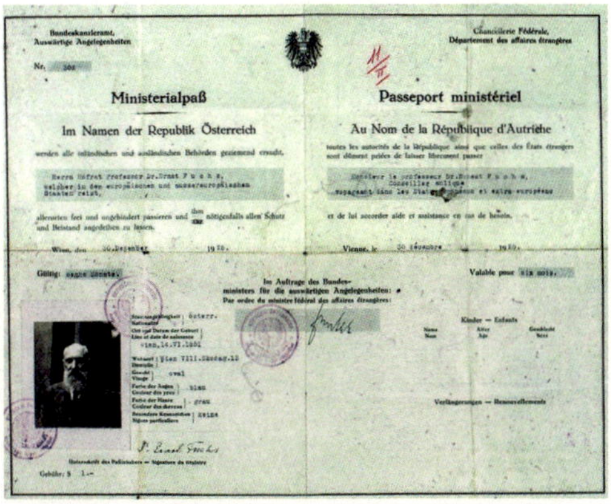

Fig. 115a Ernst Fuchs's ministerial passport, 1925 (recto)

On behalf of the Republic of Austria all domestic and foreign authorities are respectfully requested to grant free and unhindered transit to Herr Hofrat Professor Dr Ernst Fuchs, who frequently travels to European and non-European states, and to give him all kinds of protection and assistance if needed.[1505]

Ernst Fuchs Fund 1926/27

In view of the economic predicament Austria found itself in the postwar years, which made life hard for the new generation of the Vienna Medical School's ophthalmologists, several high-ranking American eye specialists, acting out of a sense of gratitude for the excellent training they had received either at Fuchs's clinic in Vienna or in the postgraduate courses in the United States, decided to do something to at least alleviate this situation. To advertise this across the country and attract the cooperation of the greatest possible number of sympathetic ophthalmologists, they announced the scheme in the *American Journal of Ophthalmology* in 1927:

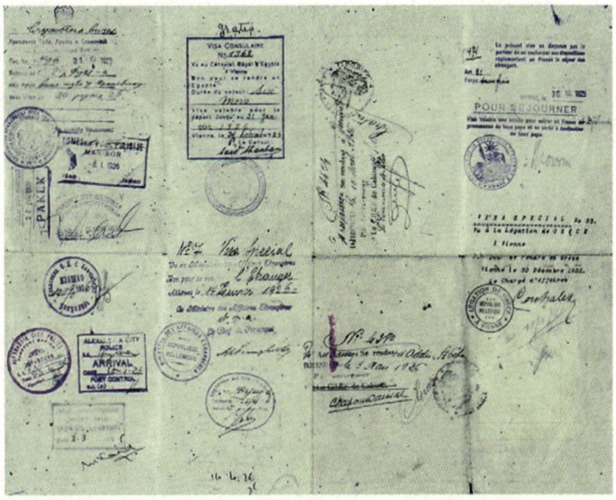

Fig. 115b Ernst Fuchs's ministerial passport, 1925 (verso)

Ophthalmologists for many years have received training and instruction in Vienna. The influence of the Vienna school of ophthalmology is worldwide and its clinical teaching has been of inestimable value, especially in developing ophthalmology in this country.

Unfortunately, owing to the present economic conditions in Austria, the position of the younger ophthalmologists in Vienna, – for the most part, assistants in the two University clinics of ophthalmology in Vienna, – is a very difficult one.

It seemed, therefore, that an opportunity to help the Vienna ophthalmologic school and to preserve its tradition would appeal to those who have had the advantage of studying there.

For this purpose, it is proposed that a fund be collected which will carry the name of ERNST FUCHS and which will have the following purpose:

To give financial aid in experimental investigations.
To help defray the cost of publications, and
To furnish money for attending congresses.

This fund is to be managed by the directors of the two University Eye Clinics in Vienna and by the chairman of the Vienna Ophthalmological Society.

Will you demonstrate your sympathy in this appeal by becoming a subscriber to this Fund?

Communications should be addressed to Dr. E. V. L. Brown, Secy., 122 South Michigan Boulevard, Chicago, Ill.[1506]

This appeal was signed by Adolph Barkan,[1507] Arnold Knapp,[1508] George S. Derby,[1509] E. V. L. Brown,[1510] and Joseph M. Keller.[1511, 1512] The advertisement was placed once again in the journal in early 1928.[1513]

Shortly before his death on November 21, 1930 Ernst Fuchs arranged for the monies in the Fuchs Fund to be transferred to a scholarship foundation for junior ophthalmologists to be overseen by the Academic Senate of the University of Vienna.[1514]

Award of the Leslie Dana Medal and the XIII International Ophthalmological Congress in Amsterdam

Ernst Fuchs took part alongside his son Adalbert in the XIII International Ophthalmological Congress, which was held on September 5 to 13, 1929 in Amsterdam and Scheveningen.[1515] The most important reason for this trip becomes apparent from the following advance notice published on July 29, 1929:

In recognition of 'the most outstanding achievement in the prevention of blindness and the conservation of vision,' Dr. Ernst Fuchs, of Vienna, will be awarded the Leslie Dana Gold Medal. The presentation will be made at the International Ophthalmological Congress in Amsterdam, Holland, September 10, by Dr. William H. Luedde,[1516] *of St. Louis, director of the Prevention of Blindness Department of the Missouri Association for the Blind, through which the medal is offered annually by Mr. Leslie Dana, also of St. Louis.*[1517]

Ernst Fuchs, as was made abundantly clear, was the first non-American to be singled out for this award because of his achievements in the field of the prevention of blindness:

In selecting Dr. Fuchs, there was a departure for the first time from the usual custom of considering only Americans for this honour,' said Mr. Carris, Director of the National Society for the Prevention of Blindness of New York. 'Dr. Fuchs charted the way for all prevention of blindness work accomplished throughout the world in the last 45 years; he did this when he won the prize at the Fifth International Congress for Hygiene at the Hague in 1884 with his essay on 'The Causes and Prevention of Blindness.' Dr. Fuchs was a professor of ophthalmology in the University of Liège at that time; he has been distinguished in his profession for more than half a century.[1518]

On September 10, the roughly 120 participants of the congress listened to speeches detailing the merits Ernst Fuchs had accumulated in his profession over a lifetime. Palpably impressed and in an almost enthusiastic tone so untypical of a man who was notoriously reserved in personal and private matters, Fuchs described the festive occasion and its speakers as follows:

The first [speaker] was Treacher Collins[1519]*, who spoke most impressively on behalf of the Europeans, the second de Schweinitz,*[1520] *who performed the same office equally well for the Americans, then Coppez*[1521] *for Belgium and Rollet*[1522] *for France. I was extolled to the heavens in every way. I could plainly see on that day that I could count on a great deal of sympathy from everyone. After the dinner speeches Dr Luedde from St. Louis presented me with the gold Leslie Dana Medal and said a few words, whereupon I thanked everyone, omitting of course a great deal of what I had been planning to say. The most distinguished ophthalmologists from Germany were present and never in my life have I been honoured in such a way.*[1523]

[…].

At the congress, which was in session for the first five days in Amsterdam, then for three days in Scheveningen, I was the subject of manifold honours, of which I would like to mention only a banquet, organised by the Spanish doctors, a great luncheon, organised by Dr Suker,[1524] *where colleagues from all nations were present and where I was presented with the Leslie Dana Medal by Dr Lüdde and an especially honorific toast given by Dr* Cushing[1525] *at the great banquet at the end of the congress.*[1526]

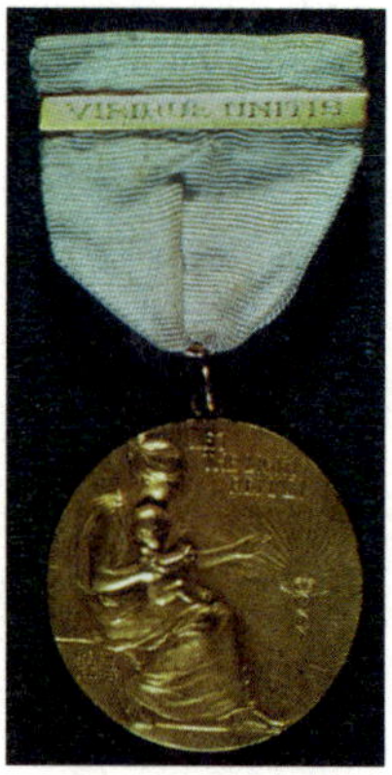

Fig. 116 Leslie Dana Gold Medal

One of Fuchs's American friends, the ophthalmologist Edward Treacher Collins,[1527] has left the following account:

In 1929 [Ernst Fuchs] *motored across Europe, with his old friend Dr. Barkan, some five years his senior, to attend the International Ophthalmological Congress in Amsterdam. Here a great welcome awaited him. To a group of American ophthalmologists attending the congress had occurred the idea of organising a luncheon in honour of this Grand Old Man of Ophthalmology. A large gathering of his friends, pupils and admirers from all countries assembled, with Dr. Suker in the Chair, and when Hofrat Professor Fuchs's health was proposed the toast was received with resounding applause. The opportunity was also taken of presenting to him [with] the Leslie Dana Medal, instituted as an award for work conducive to the prevention of blindness. Fuchs's reply to this enthusiastic reception was characterised by his usual tact and modesty.*[1528]

The medal in question (Fig. 116) had been established in 1925 by the St Louis businessman Leslie Dana (1873–1955). It was designed to honour and encourage social measures to alleviate the lot of the blind and to support initiatives for and research on the prevention of blindness, a cause Dana himself had fostered since 1921 as a member of the Missouri Commission for the Blind.[1529] The award of the medal to Ernst Fuchs was in recognition of his achievements in this cause, notably in the form of his famous monograph, *The Causes and the Prevention of Blindness*, which in 1884 had earned him the prize of the Society for the Prevention of Blindness. The monograph had given the newly founded movement a powerful impulse of international significance.[1530]

The award ceremony was followed by the foundation of the International Association for the Prevention of Blindness, which brought the Amsterdam Congress to a close. Fuchs was immediately elected an honorary member of this association.[1531]

Fuchs, always keen to take in cultural highlights in places he visited on a professional mission, complemented his stay in Amsterdam with a visit to nearby Haarlem.

Keynote Address at the Wilmer Ophthalmological Institute in Baltimore

Ernst Fuchs left Amsterdam for the United States via Montreal on what was his third visit, again lasting several months. After stays in Albany and New York he went on to Baltimore, where he had been asked[1532] to speak at the inauguration of the Wilmer Ophthalmic Institute, named after William Holland Wilmer (1863–1936).[1533] Founded in 1925, it was alternatively known as the Wilmer Ophthalmological Institute or the Wilmer Eye Institute.[1534] The inauguration festivities were scheduled for October 15 and 16, 1929[1535, 1536] and marked the dedication[1537] of a new building, which was to house this prestigious institution. It combined a hospital department with an internationally renowned research venue and had been constrained since its foundation to make do with what little space was available at the world famous Johns Hopkins University School of Medicine.

As he set about preparing his speech in the summer of 1929, Fuchs asked Viennese medical historian Max Neuburger (1868–1955)[1538] to help him find a particular illustration:

Kritzendorf, 19 June 29

Sehr geehrter Herr Kollege!
Would you kindly excuse my inconveniencing you with a request. In the autumn the Wilmer Ophthalmic Institute will be solemnly inaugurated at the Johns Hopkins University in Baltimore and the President of the University has invited me to give one of the two addresses. I am planning a brief overview of the development of ophthalmology since antiquity, with a few slides by way of illustration. One of these pictures would ideally show an itinerant oculist and cataract surgeon in his coach, with a servant or bugler on the box. I have a vague memory of having seen such a picture once, but I don't recall where. If you are aware of such a picture, not necessarily of an oculist but of some other travelling snake oil salesman, I would be extremely grateful if you could let me know where I can find it. If the book in question is in the library of your Institute, would you kindly make it available to me so that I can make a photograph of it.
Mit dem Ausdruck meiner ausgezeichneten Hochachtung

Ihr ergebenster
E. Fuchs[1539]

As the first keynote speaker at the inauguration of the Wilmer Ophthalmic Institute, Fuchs addressed the audience on the topic "The Development of Ophthalmology in Europe"[1540] in the first meeting on October 15, 1929. This address was published in full the next year, which was also the last year of Fuchs's life.[1541]

Annual Conference of the National Society for the Prevention of Blindness 1929

From Baltimore Fuchs travelled once again to St. Louis in response to an invitation to take part in the annual meeting of the National Society for the Prevention of Blindness between November 11 and 13. In the session devoted to a discussion of trachoma[1542] Ernst Fuchs contributed a substantial intervention.[1543] The chairman of the trachoma conference, Harvey J. Howard (1880–1956),[1544] formerly Director of the Eye Department of the Peking Union Medical College and now in charge of the Eye Department of the Washington University School of Medicine, welcomed Fuchs with the following truly memorable words:

I think we are most fortunate in having with us today one who is known the whole world over as the Dean of Ophthalmologists. I fortunately consider him one of the best friends I have ever had. He lived with me in China for a period of six weeks in 1922. I count his association there as one of the high spots of my life. The following year I spent three or four months with him at his home in Vienna. So not only do I have a feeling of great friendship for him, but together with you, I have the conviction that in honoring him we honor the greatest ophthalmologist that ever lived.[1545]

At the Opening Meeting and Reception arranged by the Ophthalmic Section of the St. Louis Medical Society of this annual conference Ernst Fuchs gave an address on the "Subjective Symptomatology of Ocular Disorders".[1546] This was after W. H. Luedde,[1547] Director of the Section for the Prevention of Blindness of the St. Louis Society for the Blind, had found impressive words to describe Ernst Fuchs's historic significance for the prevention of blindness:

It is both an easy and difficult task to introduce Professor Fuchs. It is so easy to do because everybody knows him, and yet it is so difficult because as you know all about him introduction is really impossible. However, relatively few of us who studied his textbook for years know that originally Professor Fuchs made a very important contribution dedicated particularly to the causes and prevention of blindness in a 250-page book that was written nearly fifty years ago. At the Fourth International Congress of Hygiene in 1882 a prize of eighty pounds was offered by some unknown English person for the best essay on the 'Causes and Prevention of Blindness'. The prize was awarded to Professor Fuchs in Paris, France, on the one hundredth anniversary of the Foundation of the First Asylum for the Blind by Huey.[1548] [...]

Let us remember as physicians that while it is true that the practise of ophthalmology in all lands is devoted to the conservation of vision and the prevention of blindness, Professor Fuchs's book clearly demonstrated that the clinic hospital and laboratory alone even at their best are not sufficient for the most successful efforts toward these ends. The intelligent and well-controlled co-operation of physicians, teachers, parents, publicists, architects, hygienists, eugenists, nurses, midwifes, social economists, illuminating engineers, printers, and so forth – in fact, of all the people all the time is needed. [...]

Professor Fuchs's prize essay is out of print. [...] *To those of us who read this remarkable volume today comes the realization that therein is given to the world its 'Decalogue' for the prevention of blindness. It contains the suggestion and often the detailed instructions according to which all that has since been done in this field of human endeavor has been developed. Professor Fuchs is the leader who calls humanity forth from the bondage of darkness, of ignorance and indifference, and points the way toward the promised land where every man shall know how to conserve his own eyesight and all shall work together so that needless blindness may be banished from the face of the earth.*

It is a great honor to introduce Professor Fuchs to you this evening.[1549]

Japan

In the nineteenth century, when Japan first threw open its gates to Western culture and medicine,[1550, 1551] the growing reputation of German-speaking universities and medical training in Germany and Austria put an end to the dominant position Dutch professors had held until then at Japanese universities. Trade and scientific contacts multiplied at pace, and growing numbers of Japanese students spent several semesters at German-speaking universities. This trend was especially pronounced among graduated medical doctors who flocked to Germany, Austria, and Switzerland to deepen their knowledge and subsequently spread it in their native country. Several leading Japanese universities now created positions for German-speaking professors who taught medicine in their own mother tongue:

German is the favourite language of Japanese medical doctors. It was Germans who first brought them the glad tidings of a new medicine that set them free from the ossified forms of East Asian speculation. German [speaking] professors taught at their university in Tokyo. German is the language spoken by their Japanese successors. German is even taught at grammar schools to future students of medicine; and anyone who is given the opportunity of finishing his studies in Germany is considered a darling of fortune by their friends.[1552]

Many Japanese doctors mastered German to a degree that enabled them to publish articles in the most prestigious ophthalmological journals and to give presentations in German on occasions such as the Annual Conference of the Deutsche Ophthalmologische Gesellschaft in Heidelberg. As can be seen from the example of Tatsuya Inouye,[1553] it was the Vienna Ophthalmological School under Arlt that acted as the most powerful magnet in the second half of the nineteenth century. Under Arlt's disciple Ernst Fuchs, Director of the Second University Eye Clinic from 1885 to 1915, relations with Japanese ophthalmologists intensified further. The following guest students of Japanese extraction[1554] who graduated from Vienna University have been identified:

OGATA, Shiujiro (1857–1942)[1555]	Berlin, Vienna 1889–1892 (Dr. med.)
GOU, Kenjuro (1866–1907)[1556]	Vienna, Marburg, Leipzig, Berlin 1892–1897 (Dr. med.)
ASAYAMA, Ikujiro (1861–1915)[1557]	Würzburg, Heidelberg, Berlin, Vienna 1898–1902 (Prof. Univ. of Kyoto)
MURAKAMI, Anzo (1862–1927)[1558]	Breslau, Vienna 1899–1901 (Prof., Univ. of Nagasaki)
INOUYE, Nobuo (1875–1971)[1559]	Leipzig, Würzburg, Heidelberg, Vienna, Bern 1902–1905, 1909–1911 (Prof., Okayama Med. School, Tokyo Med. College)
OGYU, Rokuzo (1859–1914)[1560]	Bern, Vienna 1903–1906 (Prof., Univ. of Chiba)
MIYAHARA, Takekuma (1874–1958)[1561]	Munich, Vienna (Dr. med.) (Miyahara Eye Hosp., Tainan/Taiwan)
AKATSUKA, Toranosuke (1878–1956)[1562]	Vienna, Munich 1910–1912 (Dr. med.) (Ophthalmologist, Osaka)

Table 7: Japanese long-time visitors at the 2nd University Eye Clinic under Ernst Fuchs

After his long stay in the United States Ernst Fuchs arrived in Japan in September 1922. We have diary entries as part of his autobiography, an article on his travels in Japan he published in 1924 with predominantly cultural historical impressions, and a series of photographs, some of which are dated. It is, however, not possible to reconstruct from this evidence the exact route he chose for his travels or the sequence of stopovers he made at Japanese universities and their eye clinics. No information has come down to us as to the topics of lectures or courses he gave during these visits.[1563]

Fuchs's trip to Japan was partly conceived as an attempt to put relations between the German and the Japanese Ophthalmological Societies, which had been severely damaged by the war, on a better footing and to reopen the blocked channels of scientific exchange. The misalignment between Germany and Japan had been caused by Japan entering into the war on the side of the Entente on August 23, 1914. This had resulted in Japan occupying the German colonies in Asia. Even after the armistice between the Entente and the German Empire was concluded on November 11, 1918, Japanese ophthalmologists who had been undergoing training in Germany were still exposed to harassment by the newly installed authorities as they tried to leave what had become the German Republic; some of them were even interned. After the end of the war the scientific societies in all the nations that had been allied against Germany and the Austro-Hungarian Monarchy unanimously decided to ban Germans and Austrians from taking part in international conferences.[1564] The previously highly influential Deutsche Ophthalmologische Gesellschaft felt badly treated by its Japanese sister organisation, to put it mildly, and the originally exceedingly lively mutual contacts – especially the exchange of literature and academic relations – virtually ground to a halt, to Japan's great detriment. Leading professors of Japanese ophthalmology such as Jujiro Komoto (1859–1938),[1565] Chuta Oguchi (1875–1945),[1566] Sousuke Miyashita (1882–1948),[1567] and Yoshizo Koyanagi (1880–1954)[1568] had repeatedly tried in their correspondence with German colleagues they had been friendly with in the past to explain the Japanese point of view as best they could, and to pave the way for a rapprochement. Ernst Fuchs's international reputation made him an ideal mediator.

Prior to his arrival in Tokyo, his stay in Honolulu[1569] had been enhanced by the hospitality of the distinguished pathologist and lepra specialist Eric A. Fennel (1887–1957).[1570] (Fig. 117) When he arrived in Tokyo via Yokohama on September 19, 1922, he was given a cordial welcome by Jujiro Komoto –

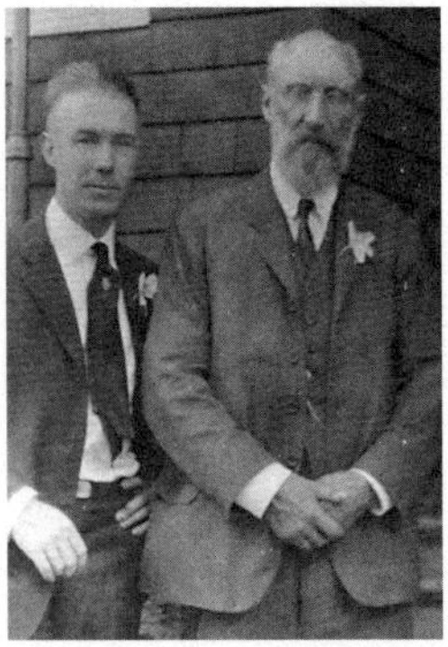
Fig. 117
Ernst Fuchs
with
Eric Fennel

in Fuchs's view Japan's most outstanding ophthalmologist[1571] – at the latter's University Eye Clinic[1572] (Fig. 118) and two days later at Komoto's house, where Fuchs had been invited to tea.[1573] (Fig. 119) On 25 September Fuchs had the privilege of witnessing the solemn return of the Emperor from Nikko to Tokyo.[1574]

The straitened circumstances these doctors were now living in did not prevent them from entertaining me with the lavish kindness and hospitality they had shown Hirschberg so many years ago. The Tokyo Ophthalmological Society had arranged to have colleagues accompany me for the entire month of my travels in the country. I was especially grateful for this, as it enabled me to gain an insight into many things that will remain a closed book for ordinary tourists.[1575]

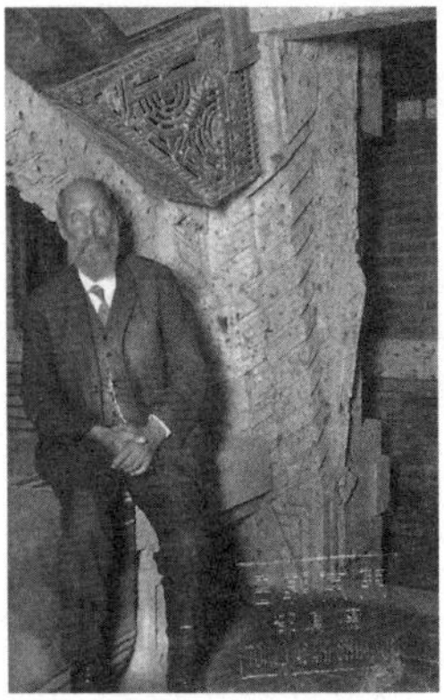
Fig. 118
Ernst Fuchs
in Tokyo, 1922

Fuchs was able to take a close look at Japan's education system, inevitably paying special attention to medical training in general and to that of ophthalmologists in particular:

Education in Japan follows the German model. Children attend primary school between the ages of 8 and 14; for those who want to go on to higher education, this is followed by five years at a secondary school. Among the subjects taught there I would like to single out for emulation not only drawing but painting with water colours. It may well be that the Japanese as an artistic people bring more aptitude to this discipline than our youngsters ever could. But even those who are not gifted artistically are made in this way to sharpen their skills of observation, which will stand budding scientists and medical doctors in good stead later on.

Those who want to go on to university need to attend a crammer for another three to four years; for prospective students of medicine the subjects taught there include science, chemistry, physics, psychology, and biology. One of the most important subjects, however, is German, while the only other languages in the curriculum are Latin and Greek to the extent required for an understanding of medical terminology. The terminology is the same as that in use in Germany, and the students are taught enough German for them to understand and read the language.[1576]

[…]

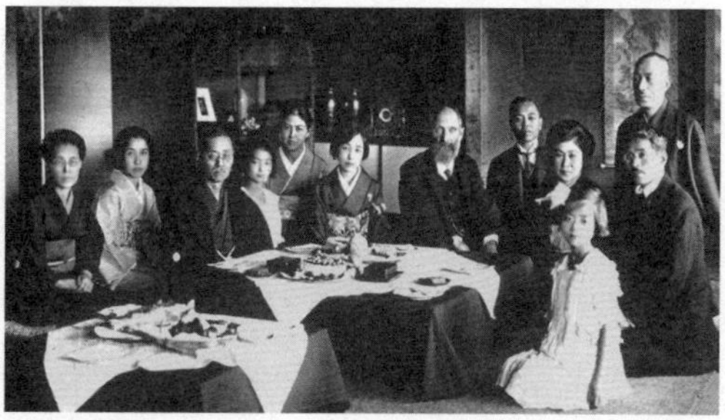

Fig. 119 Ernst Fuchs (1st row, 3rd from right) being hosted by Jujiro Komoto (third from left) on 21 September 1922

The top university in the country is in Tokyo. Until two years ago its Eye Clinic was headed by Professor Komoto, the Japanese doyen of eye specialists who has done so much for ophthalmology in Japan and is revered by his colleagues as the "mother" of ophthalmology in Japan. His successor is Professor Ishihara;[1577] *his clinic has more than 30 beds and a polyclinical patient volume of, on average, 7,000 patients a year. Both the Eye Clinic in Tokyo and those in other cities that I have been able to visit are very well equipped with the latest instruments and apparatuses, and this is also true of the Eye Clinic of Keio, a private university that has 60 beds at its disposal.* [...] *A great deal of assiduous work is being done in the clinics' labs, and I was shown many beautiful microscopic preparations that attest to the technical expertise of the Japanese. In Nagoya, Oguchi's Assistant Professor D[r] Kyozo Majiina*[1578] *showed me pure cultures of chlamydia Prowazekii in a case of trachoma, and I hope that follow-up tests will set the seal on this remarkable find.*[1579]

[...] *The study of medicine lasts four years. A hands-on year after the exams is not mandatory but is an option that most young doctors take up. Instruction in ophthalmology takes the form of two hours of tuition a week in both semesters of Year 3 and of one hour in Year 4; in addition, during those two years the students, divided into groups, practise in the clinic. Instruction is facilitated by a fairly large number of Japanese textbooks of ophthalmology, such as the three volumes written by Professor Suganama*[1580] *and two of his assistants,*[1581] *and an ophthalmoscopic atlas compiled by Professor Ogawa.*[1582]

All the students understand German. The lectures I gave to some medical societies and to students were all in German. The case histories I had the opportunity of seeing in the clinics were sometimes a curious mixture of Japanese and German.[1583]

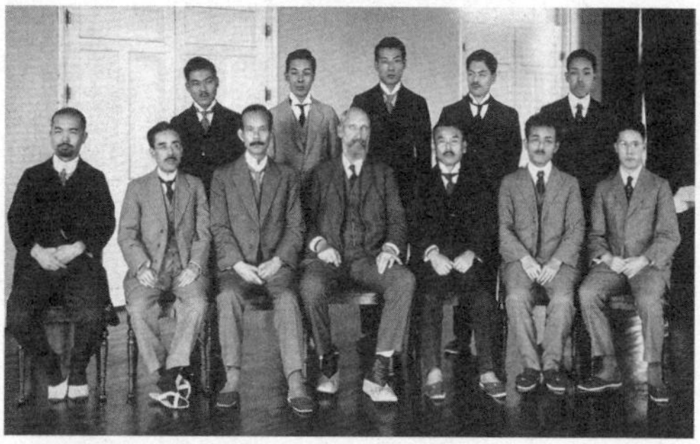

Fig. 120 Ernst Fuchs (1st row, centre) visiting the Nagoya Eye Clinic

From Tokyo Fuchs travelled to Nagoya, where he met Chuta Oguchi.[1584] (Fig. 120) In Kyoto, he visited Kiyoshi Ishikawa[1585] (Fig. 121, 122), before going on to Osaka to call on Sousuke Miyashita[1586] (Fig. 123, 124) at his eye clinic

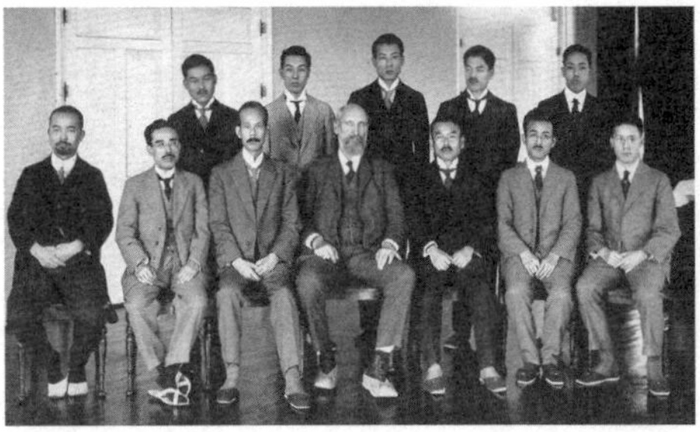

Fig. 120
Ernst Fuchs (1st row, centre) visiting the Nagoya Eye Clinic

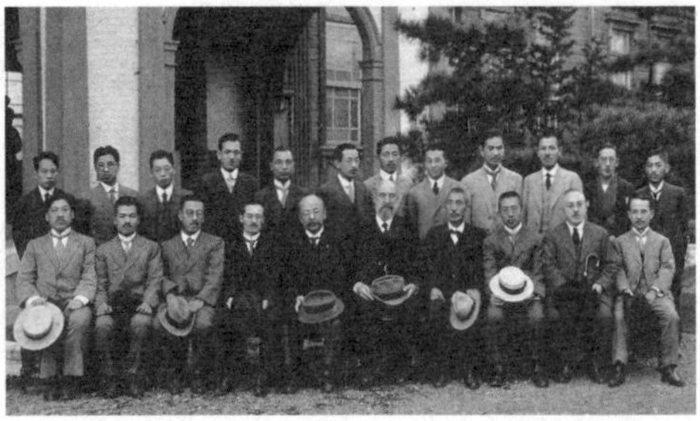

Fig. 121
Ernst Fuchs (1st row, 5th from right) visiting the University of Kyoto

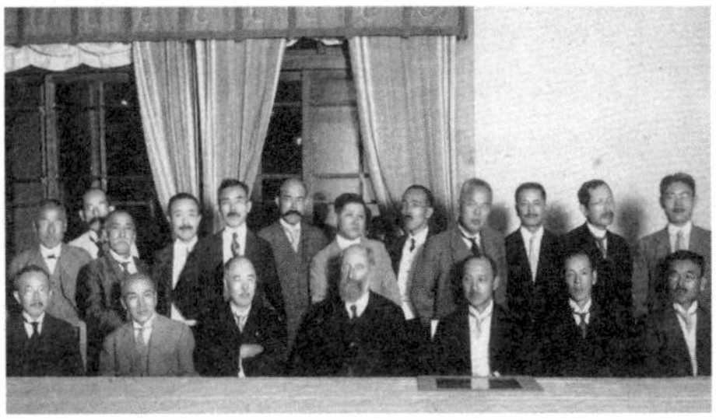

Fig. 122
Ernst Fuchs visiting the Kyoto Eye Clinic

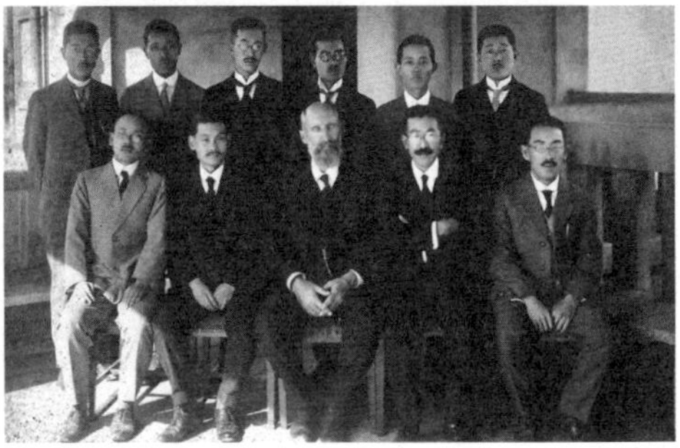

Fig. 123
Ernst Fuchs visiting the Osaka Eye Clinic

and to Hiroshima.[1587] Back in Austria, Fuchs maintained the close scientific and friendly relationships he had formed in Japan. Proof of this, if indeed such proof were needed, are the visit Shigeru Kagoshima (1882–1953),[1588] then in charge of the Eye Clinic of Chiba University, paid Fuchs in Vienna on September 27, 1924 (Fig. 125) and the award to Fuchs of an honorary membership of the Japanese Ophthalmological Society on July 7, 1930, only a few months before Fuchs's death on 21 November 1930.[1589]

China

Having stayed in Japan for three months, Fuchs left the country in late autumn of 1922 for Korea, which was at that time occupied by Japan. Before going on to China he paid a visit to the office Keio University maintained in Seoul.[1590]

While in China at the invitation of the Rockefeller Foundation between November 1922 and early January 1923,[1591] Fuchs relied on the assistance

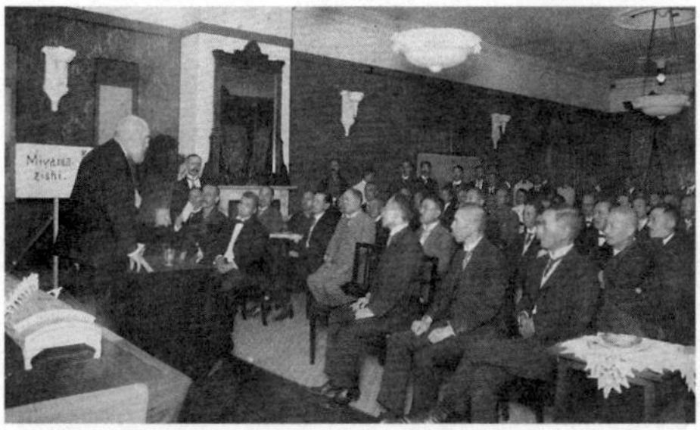

Fig. 124
Ernst Fuchs delivering a lecture at the Eye Clinic of the University of Osaka

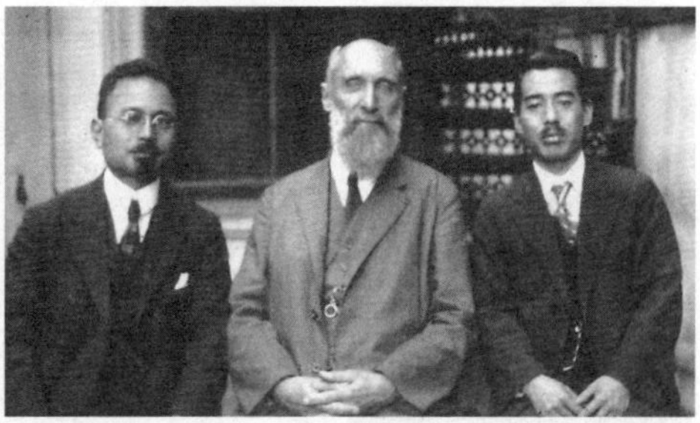

Fig. 125
Professor Kagoshima (on the left of Ernst Fuchs) paying a visit to Vienna, 1924

of medical missionaries such as Arthur Paul Wakefield (1878–1941).[1592] In 1914, the Rockefeller Foundation had established the China Medical Board[1593] with the aim of establishing American medical standards in China, training medical doctors along the lines adhered to by Baltimore's Johns Hopkins University, boosting medical research and improving medical care in China.

Peking Union Medical College

The first step toward realising the ambitious goals of the Rockefeller Foundation was the foundation of the Peking Union Medical College (PUMC) in 1917.[1594] Thereafter a fruitful collaboration was set going between the delegates of the PUMC, the China Medical Board, the China Medical Missionary Association[1595] and representatives of the Chinese government. This resulted in September 1921 in the formal inauguration of the new building of the PUMC, which brought the old Union Medical College, its hospital, the institutes that formed part of it, and the university campus up to date. The inauguration was followed by a conference to highlight the hospital's different departments – general medicine, general surgery, obstetrics, gynaecology, ophthalmology, otolaryngology and neurology – and their operation.[1596]

The Eye Department of the PUMC and the Vienna School of Ophthalmology

The translation in 1911 of Ernst Fuchs's *Lehrbuch* from English to Chinese[1597] by the American James Boyd Neal[1598] made a game-changing contribution to the promotion of European expertise in ophthalmology in China. Between 1917 and 1927 Harvey James Howard[1599] was in charge of the Eye

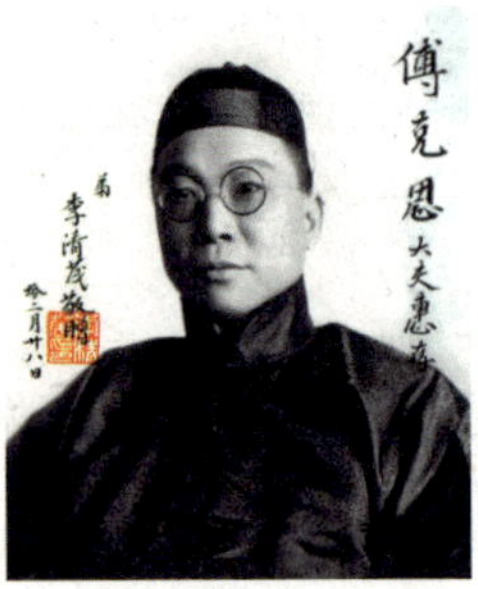

Fig. 126
Tsing-Meu Lin

Department of the PUMC. His first assistant and later Deputy Director was Tsing-Meu Li.[1600] (Fig. 126) Responding to an invitation issued by Howard, Fuchs spent four weeks at the PUMC in the autumn of 1922 as a Visiting Professor.[1601] Howard's reaction was enthusiastic:

The great event of the year was the coming of Professor Ernst Fuchs, of Vienna, who for nearly fifty years has been one of the world's leading ophthalmologists. A postgraduate course covering the period from October 23 to November 22, 1922, was arranged to coincide with Dr. Fuchs's stay in Peking. The feature of the course was the series of lectures and demonstrations on the pathology of the eye given by Dr. Fuchs.[1602]

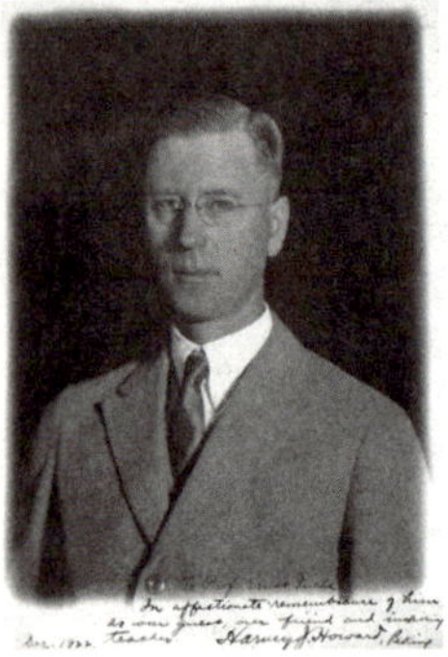

Fig. 127
Harvey J. Howard (1880–1956)

Howard was deeply grateful to Fuchs and in December 1922 sent him a portrait photograph with the following handwritten dedication:

To Professor Ernst Fuchs. In affectionate remembrance of him as our guest, our friend and inspiring teacher.[1603] (Fig. 127)

Ernst Fuchs's visiting professorship at the PUMC ushered in a period lasting more than a decade and a half, during which representatives of the Vienna School of Ophthalmology or former students of that school who had risen to scientific prominence in the United States exerted a formative influence on ophthalmology in Beijing.

Dr Howard's first action was to bring to PUMC for 1 year […] *the world's leading ophthalmologist of that era, Professor Ernst Fuchs of Vienna. At that time, Vienna was the center of the universe for ophthalmology, and for almost 20 years PUMC was a second Vienna.*[1604]

Ernst Fuchs's success as a visiting professor at the PUMC in late autumn of 1922 paved the way in the academic year of 1923/24 for his son Adalbert,[1605] who had "habilitated" at the First University Eye Clinic under Josef Meller in the previous year.

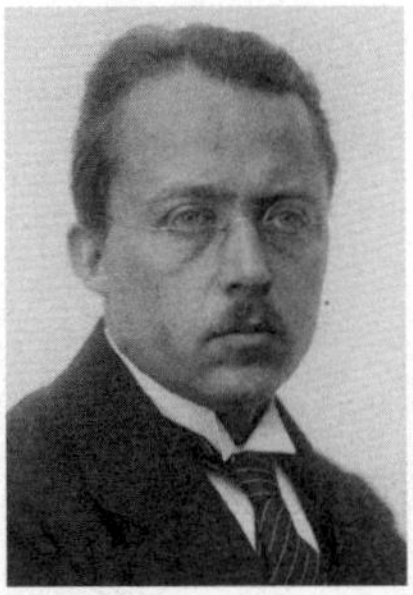

Fig. 128
Arnold Pillat (1891–1975)

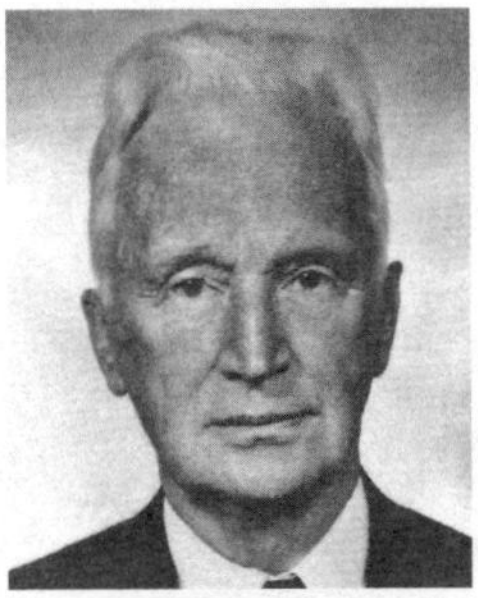

Fig. 129
Ludwig Sallmann (1892–1975)

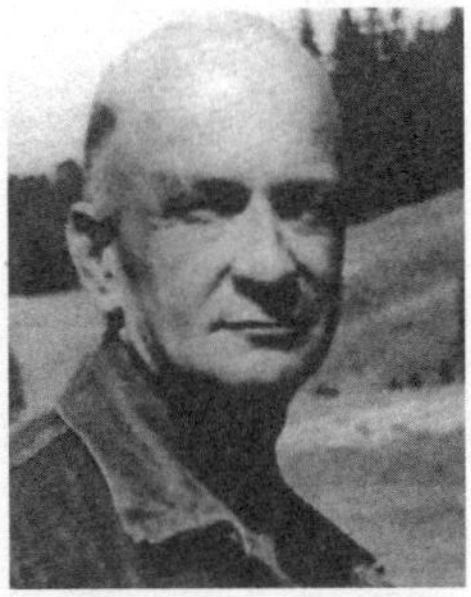

Fig. 130
Peter C. Kronfeld (1899–1980)

For the first time the department has been able to offer a nine month's graduate course in ophthalmology as well as the intensive course at the Chinese New Year. The prominent features of these courses were the series of lectures by Dr. Adelbert [sic] *Fuchs, of Vienna, on ophthalmoscopy, histopathology of the eyes, and ophthalmic surgery, and his clinical demonstrations of cases.*[1606]

Typescript lecture notes[1607] taken during Adalbert Fuchs's lectures and demonstrations of his histological preparations show that his courses were held between September 17, 1923 and June 14, 1924. It appears that the zeal of his students filled him with great satisfaction:

Dr. Adelbert [sic] *Fuchs, an internationally renowned ophthalmologist from Vienna, a visiting professor during 1923–1924, wrote in glowing terms of the students he had guided in studies of the eye, one of China's most pressing health needs.*[1608]

Adalbert Fuchs in turn was succeeded in 1925 by Arnold Pillat,[1609] one of Ernst Fuchs's "grand-disciples".

The first four directors of the Eye Department at the PUMC had all received their training at the two University Eye Clinics of Vienna's Allgemeines Krankenhaus.[1610] When Harvey Howard resigned to become the foundation chair of the Department of Ophthalmology at the Washington University School of Medicine in 1927, Pillat took over for 1928 to 1930 (Fig. 128), serving in 1930 as guest professor at the Manchurian Medical College in Mukden (today Shenyang/China). During his absence another of Ernst Fuchs's "grand-disciples", Ludwig von Sallmann,[1611] (Fig. 129) deputised for him. Even though the Rockefeller Foundation offered Pillat another four-year contract in China

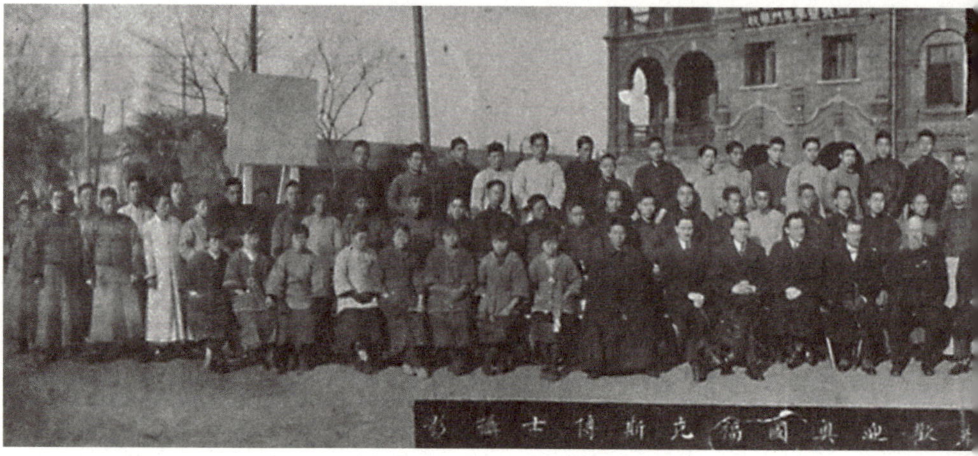

Fig. 131
Ernst Fuchs
(1st row, centre)
paying a visit
to the Dung Day
Medical College
in Shanghai

and, on top of it, an option on the Chair of Ophthalmology at the University of Philadelphia, he returned to Vienna in 1933 to take charge of the Eye Department of Lainz Hospital. He was replaced by Peter C. Kronfeld,[1612] (Fig. 131) who took charge of the Eye Department of the PUMC until 1939. By 1939 Pillat had accepted the Rockefeller Foundation's renewed offer of another stint at the PUMC but was prevented from taking it up by the outbreak of World War II. This spelt the end of the presence of the Vienna School of Ophthalmology at the PUMC.

Ernst Fuchs in Shanghai

In addition to the PUMC, Fuchs paid a visit to Tong Teh (also known as Tong De and Dung Dai) Medical College in Shanghai. (Fig. 131) It has unfortunately proved impossible to ascertain the timing of this visit or any details of any lectures Fuchs may have given there.

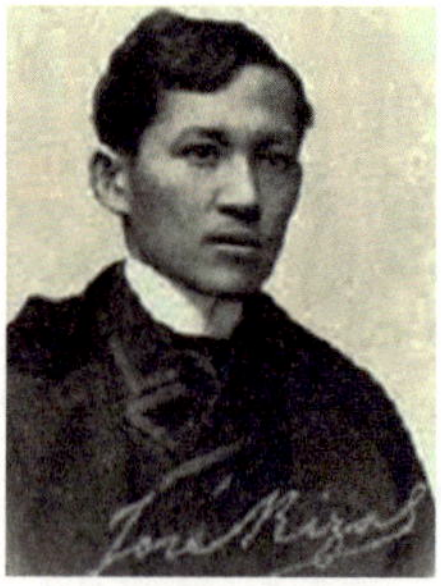

Fig. 132
José Rizal
(1861–1895)

Return to Austria

As he made his way back to Austria, Fuchs spent several weeks in the Philippines.[1613] It is worth pointing out in this context that when he was first appointed chair at Vienna University, Fuchs had a Filipino student who was to acquire tragic fame later on: José Rizal (1861–1896)[1614] (Fig. 132) – a poet, political activist and freedom fighter against the Spanish colonial power and the first ophthalmologist to practise in the Philippines.

In Manila, too, Fuchs made use of the opportunity to hold a course which lasted until January 17, 1923.[1615] A great number of photographs in the Fam-

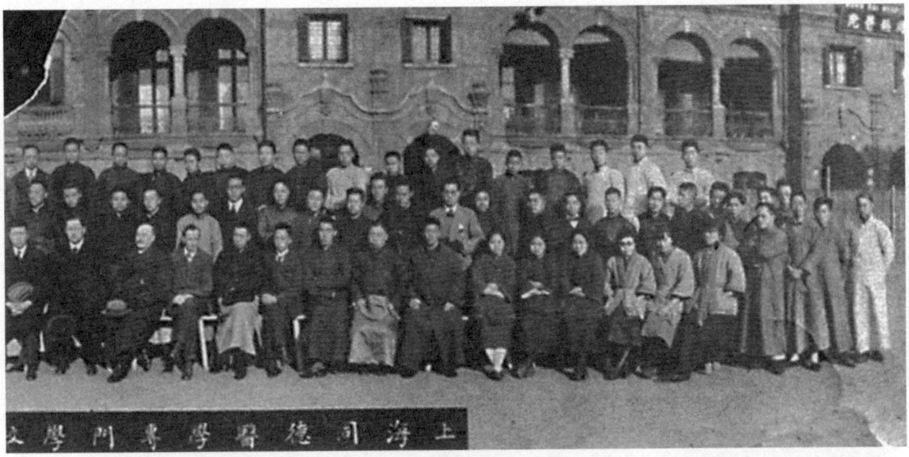

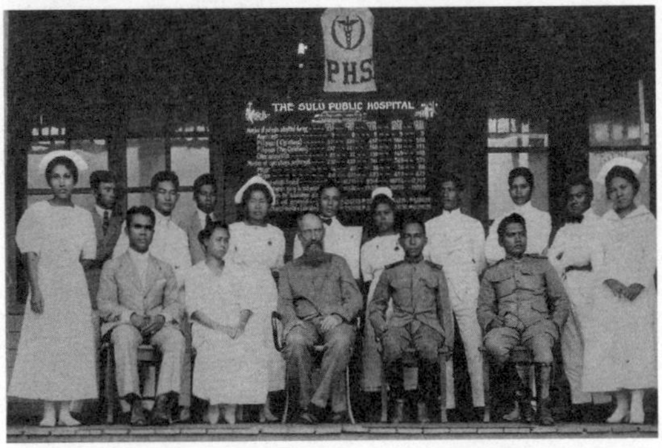

Fig. 133
Ernst Fuchs and Sixto Y. Orosa

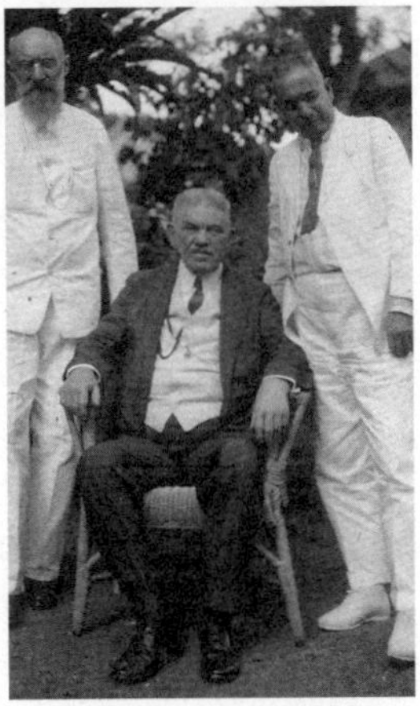

Fig. 134
Ernst Fuchs with F. W. Dudley and Fernando Calderon

ily archive attest the lively contact Fuchs cultivated with local doctors such as Sixto Y. Orosa e Ylagan (1891–1981)[1616] (Fig. 133), F. W. Dudley[1617] and Fernando Calderon[1618] (Fig. 134). As is the rule with all of Fuchs's travelogues, his notes are bound to impress with their exact description of indigenous culture, religious practice, the lifestyle of the inhabitants and natural sights. This lends a great deal of cultural historical significance to his reports as authentic contemporary documents.

On January 19, 1923 the British Vice Consul in Manila issued a transit visa for Fuchs for his return to Austria.[1619] On February 5, he was travelling by train from Singapore to the capital of Siam, Bangkok.[1620] Between February 22 and March 10 he was on his way to Port Said in Egypt, where he boarded

Fig. 135
Ernst Fuchs's passport (1923) with the stamps of the last time he returned to Austria

a steamer on March 30 in Alexandria bound for Brindisi on the Adriatic. On April 6 he reached Feldkirch in Vorarlberg.[1621] (Fig. 135) The precise date of Fuchs's arrival in Vienna cannot be ascertained but what we do know is that Fuchs was issued a new passport on April 11, 1923, valid for two years, stamped inside with "*Länder, für welche dieser Reisepaß gilt/ Pays pour lesquels ce passeport est valable*".[1622]

Notes

[1417] See Ch. 6.

[1418] Gabriela SCHMIDT-WYKLICKY, Helmut GRÖGER, "Die Wiener Ophthalmologische Schule. Geist und Leistung der ersten 150 Jahre", in: Spektrum Augenheilk. 26/6 (2012), pp. 345–356.

[1419] See Ch. 5.

[1420] See Ch. 9.

[1421] See Ch. 2 and FUCHS, *Augenarzt* (as in FN 2), p. 59.

[1422] See Ch. 6.

[1423] Cf. FN 349.

[1424] Hans BARKAN, "Cooper Medical College, founded by Levi Cooper Lane: An Historical Sketch", in: *Stanford Med. Bull.* 12/3 (1954), pp. 145–184.

[1425] The Lane Medical Lectures were established in 1896 by Levi Cooper Lane (1828–1902), the President of Cooper Med. College in San Francisco. Delivered once a year, they featured ten courses on a wide range of med. or surg. topics on five consecutive day. The lectures catered to students, general practitioners and consultants and were entrusted to a renowned specialist either from the United States or from abroad. Cf. "The Lane Medical Lectures for 1911", in: *California State J. of Medicine* 9/7 (1911), p. 306.

[1426] For Hans Barkan (1882–1960), cf. FN 916. Otto Barkan (1887–1958) also trained in Vienna and Munich. 1920 Return to Stanford Univ. Main area of work: Congenital glaucoma. Cf. GORIN (as in FN 38), pp. 346f.; IBBO (as in FN 18).

[1427] Cf. "The Lane Medical Lectures for 1911", in: *California State J. of Medicine* 9/7 (1911), p. 306.

[1428] Ernst FUCHS, *Text-Book* (as in FN 810). See Ch. 6.

[1429] $ 2,000 in 1911 is the equivalent of € 46,340 ($ 55,370) in today's (2021) money (last accessed: 27 Nov. 2020). Interestingly, the fee Fuchs received for the Lane Lectures topped the annual pension Fuchs drew from 1915.

[1430] FUCHS, *Augenarzt* (as in FN 2), p. 106.

[1431] Cf. www.ancestry.com: Hamburg Passenger Lists, 1850–1934; New York, Passenger Lists, 1820–1957 (last accessed: on 6 Sept. 2022). The list of passengers to New York displays the rubber stamp NON IMMIGRANT ALIEN and the memo: *"tourist returns in 3 months"*. The idea was originally for Julie Fuchs to accompany her husband on this trip. This plan had to be abandoned, presumably for health reasons, so that her name was deleted from the passenger list.

[1432] Cf. (Ed.), "Minutes of the Proceedings", in: *Transact. Am. Ophthalmol. Soc.* 12/3 (1911), p. 708.

[1433] Ernst FUCHS, "The Field of Vision in Tabetic Atrophy of the Optic Disc", in: *Transact. Amer. Ophthalmol. Soc.* 12/3 (47th Annual Meeting, New London/Conn. July 11–12, 1911) Part III, pp. 718–736 and *Arch. Ophthalmol.* 40 (1911), pp. 469–475; FUCHS, "Neuroma of the Ciliary Nerves", in: *Transact. Americ. Ophthalmol. Soc.* (47th Annual Meeting, [...], pp. 786–787 (Exhibition of Specimens); FUCHS, "Smallest Sarcoma of the Choroid", in: Ibid., pp. 787–789 (Exhibition of Specimens, Discussion, pp. 789–790).

[1434] Announcement of Courses 1911–1912, *Stanford University 1911*, p. 109, p. 113; *California State Med. J.* 9 (1911), p. 257; *JAMA* 1911; *The Medical World* 29 (1911), p. 354; *The Ophthalmic Record* 20 (1911), p. 336; *Stanford Univ. Bull.* 1912, p. 113; *Canadian J. Med. Surg.* 34 (1913), p. 251; *Annual Announcement, Dep. of Med.*, Stanford Univ. 1913, p. 24; *Annual Register*, Stanford University 1913, p. 179.

[1435] See Ch. 9.

[1436] Arnold Herman Knapp (1869–1956). Studied and trained at Harvard Univ. and the College of Physicians and Surgeons of Columbia Univ./New York. Ophthalmolog. specialis. during study visits to leading European Univ. Eye Clinics, such as Fuchs's clinic in Vienna. He subsequently collaborated with this father Herman(n) Knapp at the New York Ophthalmic and Aural Inst., which, having been founded by Herman(n) Knapp, later had its name changed to Herman Knapp Memorial Eye Hospital. He was active there until 1940 both in teaching and research. 1903–1928 Prof. at Columbia University. Then merger with the Inst. of Ophthalmol. of Presbyterian Hospital, where he served as senior consultant until 1950. Under the aegis of Columbia Univ. foundation of the Knapp Memorial Fund. (Funding of postgraduate teaching, a research lab and a lab for physiol. optics). Cf. Obituaries: *Arch. Ophthalmol.* 55/4 (1956), p. 451–454 (John H. Dunnington); *Brit. J. Ophthalmol.* 40/5 (1956), p. 320.

[1437] Cf. FN 1352.

[1438] Alexander Duane, cf. FN 811.

[1439] For details see below in this chapter.

[1440] See the announcement in: *The Lancet* 42 (1922), p. 322.

[1441] FUCHS, Augenarzt (as in FN 2), p. 108.

[1442] Cf. FN 1221.

[1443] Karel Frederik Wenckebach (1864–1940). Originally from Den Haag/NL. Studied at Groningen Univ. (Dr. med. 1888). Assist. at the Inst. of Zoology, Pathol., Anat. and Physiol. of Utrecht Univ.; 1891 Established himself as a GP in the country. 1896 Return to Utrecht Univ. to study cardiac arrhythmia. 1901–1911 Prof. of Intern. Med. and Dir. of Clinic at Groningen Univ.; 1911–1914 in the same function at Strasbourg Univ. 1914–1929 Full Prof. and Dir. of the 1st Med. Univ. Clinic in

Vienna. One of the first specialists in cardiol. as a subdiscipline of Intern. Med.; outstanding discoveries and descriptions of different forms of cardiac arrythmia on a purely clinical basis (e. g. Wenckebach bundle, Wenckebach period). Deserves credit for relocating the Institute for the History of Medicine to the former military-medical Josephs-Akademie (Josephinum) in Vienna (1920). Cf. CZEIKE (as in FN 13); FISCHER (as in FN 28); GERABEK et al. (as in FN 13); WYKLICKY, *Josephinum*, Ind.; Obituaries: *Münch. med. Wochenschr.* 87 (1940), pp. 1421–1422; *Wien. klin. Wochenschr.* 53 (1940), pp. 1067ff.; Appreciations: Leopold SCHÖNBAUER, "Wenckebachs Verdienste um das Institut für Geschichte der Medizin", in: *Wien. klin. Wochenschr.* 67 (1955), No. 35/36; Gerrit A. LINDEBOOM, "Karel Frederik Wenckebach (1864–1940) und Österreich", in: Erna LESKY (ed.), *Wien und die Weltmedizin* (1974), pp. 214–218; Karl HOLUBAR, "Karel Frederik Wenckebach (1864–1940) und die Domizilierung des Instituts für Geschichte der Medizin im historischen Gebäude der Josephs-Akademie in Vienna: 1990 als doppeltes Gedenkjahr", in: *Wien. klin. Wochenschr.* 102 (1990), pp. 333ff.

[1444] Cf. New York, Passenger Lists, 1820–1957, available on-line at: www.ancestry.com. (last accessed: 6 Sept. 2022).

[1445] Oscar Diem (1875/76–1950). Originally from Switzerland. No data retrievable concerning his studies, graduation or ophthalmol. training. However, there exists an undated original photograph signed by him, which shows him together with Ernst Fuchs and other members of the staff of the 2nd Univ. Eye Clinic, presumably in the garden of the Allgem. Krankenhaus. Cf. Sammlungen d. Med. Univ. Vienna. 1909 Emigration to the United States. 1920 Established himself in New York City. Active at several hospitals, taught at Columbia Univ. and had a private practice. Organised Fuchs's lecture tour together with Henry Minsky (see the next FN), a project in which his German mother tongue stood him in good stead. Cf. 1920, 1930, 1940 United States Federal Census; New York, New York, Extracted Marriage Index, 1866–1937; New York, Death Index, 1880–1956, available at www.ancestry.com (last accessed: 6 Sept. 2022).

[1446] Henry J. Minsky (1895–1959). Originally from New York. Studied at Columbia Univ. College of Physicians and Surgeons (M. D. 1919). Ophthalmol. training and special. as a private student of Fuchs disciple Diem. 1921 Accompanied Fuchs on his lecture tour with Diem. The two carefully documented Fuchs's lectures and later published the typescript as a private imprint (cf. FN 1447). Collaborated several years with Diem, later with Charles H. May (cf. FN 1651), before setting up his own practice in New York. 1921 Assistant ophthalmic surgeon at the New York Eye and Ear Infirmary, 1924 Clinical assistant, later associate ophthalmic surgeon at Mount Sinai Hospital, where he became Dir. of the Eye Department in 1947. Senior consultant at several other hospitals in New York. 1947 Assoc. Clin. Prof. of Ophthalmol. at Columbia Univ. Main area of work: Anat. of the zonula with regard to the pathogenesis of glaucoma and detachment of the retina. Eye manifestations of essential hypertension. Developed a widely used method for the surg. rehabilit. of cuts in and near the eyelid. Cf. Obituaries, in: *New York Med.* 10 (1954), p. 573; *New York State J. Med.* 54/2 (1954), p. 2105; *Arch. Ophthalmol.* 53 (1955), pp. 456–457 (Frederick H. Theodore, Joseph Laval); Appreciation: Arthur H. AUFSES, Barbara NISS, *This House of Noble Deeds: The Mount Sinai Hospital, 1852–2002*. New York University Press 2002, pp. 258–259.

1447 Oscar DIEM, Henry J. MINSKY, *Notes and Remarks on Professor Ernest Fuchs's Lectures on Histology and Pathology of the Eye. Revised by Prof. Fuchs.* New York 1921. Another typescript has come down to us with photographs of 54 histological preparations illustrative of the normal and the pathological anatomy of the eye. The fact that its lettering is identical with the above typescript makes is highly probable that the two share the same source and belong together.

1448 To allow him to have his histol. preparations at hand at all times when he needed them for teaching and/or research purposes Fuchs had a transportable wooden receptacle made (see Fig. 90). On permanent loan in the Sammlungen d. Med. Univ. Vienna.

1449 Cf. "News Items", in: *Am. J. Ophthalmol.* 3/4 (1921), p. 947; Ernst FUCHS, "Presbyopia", in: *Arch. Ophthalmol.* 51 (1922), pp. 21–28; Conrad BERENS, "Report of the Proceedings of the Section on Ophthalmology of the New York Academy of Medicine, Meeting of October 17, 1921", in: *Arch. Ophthalmol.* 51 (1922), pp. 63–67.

1450 Ernst FUCHS, "Senile Changes of the Optic Nerve", in: *Am. J. Ophthalmol.* 3/5 (1922), pp. 215–217. (Original lecture). Rep. by Charles R. Heed, College of Physicians of Philadelphia, Section on Ophthalmology. October 20, 1921.

1451 Cf. "News Items", in: *Am. J. Ophthalmol.* 3/5 (1922), p. 160.

1452 George Strong Derby (1875– 1931). Originally from Boston. Son of Haskett Derby (1835–1914), one of the most highly regarded pioneers of ophthalmol. in the States (M. D. 1858 from Harvard Med. School, ophthalmol. specialis. in Vienna and Berlin). Studied at Harvard Med. School (M. D. 1900). General medical training at the Massachusetts Gen. Hospital. Then ophthalmol. specialis. in a two-year study trip to Europe: London (Moorfields Hospital), Berlin (Th. Axenfeld) and Vienna (Ernst Fuchs), where his emphasis was on the pathohistol. of the eye. Lifelong friendships with Axenfeld and Fuchs. 1903 Return to Boston, establishment of a highly frequented practice. 1904–1907 Assistant Ophthalmic Surgeon, 1907–1913 Ophthalmic Surgeon at Carney Hospital. Continued his career at the Massachusetts General Hospital (1903 Clin. Assist. Surgeon, 1909 Junior Assist. Surgeon, 1914 Assist. Surgeon, 1923 Dir. of the Eye Dept.) and at Harvard Med. School (1913 Assist. Ophthalmol., 1914 Instructor, 1921 Assist. Prof., 1924 Williams Prof. and Dir. of the Eye Dept.) 1912–1924 Secretary of the Section of Ophthalmol. of the Am. Med. Assoc, then its Head. 1924 Pres. of the New England Ophthalmol. Soc.; member of the Ophthalmol. Soc. of the United Kingdom and the Dt. Ophthalmol. Gesellsch. Since 1909 Member of Am. Ophthalmol. Soc. Cf. IBBO (as in FN 18); Obituaries: *Brit. J. Ophthalmol.* (1932), pp. 187–188; *Transact. Am. Ophthalmol. Soc.* 30 (1932), pp. 12.2–17 (F. H. Verhoeff).

1453 Ernst FUCHS, *Wien, das Mekka der amerikanischen Augenärzte*, in: FUCHS, *Augenarzt* (as in FN 2), pp. 335–341 (here: p. 336).

1454 Cf. the website of the New England Ophthalmological Society, accessible online at: http://www.neos-eyes.org/History (last accessed: 6 Sept. 2022).

1455 Cf. a) Advance notice of the beginning of the course on 16 January 1922, in: *JAMA* 78 (1922); b) Original photograph with the inscription: *Ernst Fuchs Society. Houston Texas Jan 16–30–1922* (Family archive).

1456 Sydney Israel. Data regarding lifespan and career not retrievable.

1457 See the local advance notice: (Ed.), "Professor Fuchs to Visit Texas", in: *Texas Med.* 17 (1922), p. 380, and the announcement of the Am. Med. Assoc., from which it becomes clear that the southern states pooled their efforts with those of the Mid-West to prepare for Fuchs's visit. Cf. *JAMA* 78 (1922), p. 118.

1458 FUCHS, *Augenarzt* (as in FN 2), p. 108.

1459 Cf. "Miscellaneous", in: *Am. J. Ophthalmol.* 3/5 (1922), p. 245.

1460 Cf. FN 1436.

1461 George E. Shambaugh (1869–1947). Originally from Iowa. Studied medicine at the Univ. of Pennsylvania (M. D. 1895). Special. in otol. for one year each in Berlin and Vienna. 1902–1935 Otol. u. Laryngol. at Presbyt. Hospital. 1911/12 Dir. of the Section of Otolaryngol. of the Am. Med. Assoc. 1916–1935 Prof. and Dir. of the Dept. of Otol. at Rush Med. College. Between 1918 and the outbreak of World War II organiser of a one-year postgraduate course in otolaryngol. for between 8 and 12 participants. One of the pioneers of otology in the States. Specialis. in the anat. and physiol. of the inner ear. Founder and first editor-in-chief of *Archives of Otolaryngology* (until 1937). Organiser of the Am. Board of Otolaryngol; Pres. of the Am. Otol. Soc. and the Am. Laryngol. Assoc. Cf. Obituaries, in: *Ann. Otol. Rhinol. Laryngol.* 57 (1948), pp. 80–82 (E. W. Hagens); *Arch. Otolarygol.* 47/4 (1948), pp. 526–527.

1462 Lee W. Dean. Prof. of Otol., Laryngol. u. Rhinol. at the Univ. of Iowa. 1918 Chairman of the Section of Otol. Laryngol. u. Rhinol. of the Am. Med. Assoc. Cf. *Transact. of the Section on Laryngol., Otol. and Rhinol. of the Am. Med. Assoc.*, AMA Press, Chicago 1922, List of Officers (n. p.).

1463 Edward Jackson (1856–1942). Studied at the Univ. of Pennsylvania (M. D. 1878). Until 1884 GP, then ophthalmol. special. in Philadelphia. 1888 Prof. of Diseases of the Eye at the Philadelphia Polyclinic Hospital, 1890 Eye surgeon at Willis Hospital and founder of the Ophthalmic Section of the College of Physicians of Philadelphia. 1894 Chairman of the Ophthalm. Section of the American Med. Assoc. (AMA). 1896 First description of cylinder skiascopy to measure astigmatism (Edward JACKSON, *Skiascopy and Its Practical Applications to the Study of Refraction*. Edwards & Docker, Philadelphia 1896). 1903 Pres. of the Am. Acad. of Ophthalmol. and Otolaryngol. 1904 Foundation of the *Ophthalmic Year Book* (Bibliography of ophthalmol. public.). 1905–1921 Prof. at the Univ. of Colorado. Foundation of the Denver Postgraduate Course, which was gradually adopted as a model in many parts of the States. 1912 Chairman of the Am. Ophthalmol. Soc.; 1916 Foundation of the Am. Board of Ophthalm. Certification as the first institution ensuring standardisation and certification of ophthalm. training in the States. From 1918 editor of the 3rd series of *Am. J. Ophthalmol.* Cf. IBBO (as in FN 18); Obituaries, in: *Arch. Ophthalmol.* 29 (1942), pp. 137–140 (Arnold Knapp); *Brit. J. Ophthalmol.* (27) 1943, pp. 190–191; F. T. TOOKE, "Dr. Edward Jackson – A Founder of the Section on Ophthalmology, College of Physicians of Philadelphia. The Personal Appreciation of Burton Chance", in: *Am. J. Ophthalmol.* 26 (1943), pp. 209–214; Appreciations: F. W. NEWELL, *Edward Jackson – a historical perspective of his contributions to refraction and to ophthalmology*, in: Ophthalmol. 95 (1988), pp. 555–558; John Gordon CLARKSON, *Edward Jackson, MD. The Father of Board Certification*, in: Arch. Ophthalmol. 130 (2012), p. 238.

1464 Marcus Feingold (1871–1925). Originally from Romania. Studied at Vienna Univ. (Dr. med. univ. 1896). 1898 Settled in New Orleans; ophthalmol. special.; 1907–1925 Prof. and Dir. of the newly founded Dept. of Ophthalmology at the private

Tulane Univ. in New Orleans. One of the leading ophthalmologists in the States with an impeccable professional reputation. Bequeathed his extensive ophthalmol. library (ca. 2,000 volumes and all relevant specialist journals) to Tulane Univ. Cf. Obituaries, in: *Transact. Ophthalmol. Soc.* 24 (1926), pp. 28–31 (E. Jackson); Am. J. Ophthalmol. 9/6 (1926), pp. 467–469.

1465 R. C. Lynch (d. 1930). Renowned ophthalmol. in New Orleans. Cf. Obituary, in: *Tristate Med. J.* 3–4 (1939), p. 636.

1466 (Ed.), "Ernst Fuchs's Society", in: *Am. J. Ophthalmol.* 3/6 (1923), p. 55.

1467 E. J. GOODWIN, "Prof. Fuchs in St. Louis", in: *Am. J. Ophthalmol.* 3/5 (1922), p. 68.– See the local advance notice issued by the St. Louis Med. Soc., in: *JAMA* 78 (1922), p. 38, and *J. Iowa State Med. Soc.* 12 (1922), p. 77.

1468 Cf. "News Items", in: *Am. J. Ophthalmol.* 3/5 (1922), p. 417.

1469 Cf. FN 818.

1470 Adalbert Fuchs, Cf. FN 807.

1471 The original of this letter is preserved in the Family archive.

1472 Ernst FUCHS, "Amerikanischer Reisebrief", in *Vienna. med. Wochenschr.* 72 (1922), cols. 913–916. (No. 21, Saturday, 20 May 1922, cols. 885–886)

1473 Cf. *JAMA* 77/2 (1921), p. 2129 and *Am. J. Ophthalmol.* 3/5 (1922), pp. 594–595.

1474 G. Oram Ring (1861–1933). Originally from Philadelphia. Studied at the Med. College of Pennsylvania (M. D. 1885). General practitioner. 1885–1889 ophthalmol. special. and assist. at the Eye Dept. of the Univ. of Pennsylvania. 1891–1893 Assistant Surgeon at Willis Hospital. 1895 Fellow of the College of Physicians of Philadelphia (1920/21 Chairman of the Section on OphAtrthalm.). 1901 Member of the Am. Ophthalmol. Soc. Consultant ophthalmol. at several hospitals in his native city. 1922 Diploma of the Am. Board for Ophthalmic Certifications (shortly afterwards himself a member of this body for the approbation of ophthalm. specialists). Repeated study trips to European eye clinics, including Bern (Heinrich Streuli), Paris (Morax, Magitot), Barcelona (Barraquer) and Vienna to work with Ernst Fuchs, whom he regarded especially highly. Cf. Obituaries: *Transact. Am. Ophthalmol. Soc.* 31 (1933), pp. 14.2–17 (Charles E. G. Shannon); *Am. J. Ophthalmol.* 16/4 (1933), p. 356.

1475 Cf. FN 765.

1476 Cf. FN 1459.

1477 Cf. News Items, in: *Am. J. Ophthalmol.* 3/5 (1922), p. 512.

1478 Ernst FUCHS, "Ocular Manifestations of Internal Secretion", in: Arch. Ophthalmol. 5 (1922), pp. 307–320.

1479 See the advance notice in: *Am. J. Ophthalmol.* 3/5 (1922), p. 232. The course took place Monday to Thursday between 5 and 7 p.m.

1480 Cf. FN 815.

1481 See Ch. 6.

1482 Cf. "News Items", in: *Arch. Ophthalmol.* 3/5 (1922), p. 689.

1483 Ibid., p. 417.

1484 Émile Gallemaerts (1860–1935). Studied at Brussels Univ. (1883 Grad. in Philosophy, 1885 Dr. med). Ophthalmol. special. under Jean-Baptiste Coppez (cf. FN 1521). 1905–1925 Coppez' successor. 1896 Foundation of the Belg. Ophthalmol. Society. Main area of work: Pathohistology of the eye. Cf. IBBO (as in FN 18).

1485 Cf. "News Items", in: *Arch. Ophthalmol.* 3/5 (1922), 594 and Robert Von Der HEYDT, "Chicago Ophthalmological Society May 15, 1922", in: *Am. J. Ophthalmol.* 5/9 (1922), pp. 726–731.

1486 Cf. FN 1463.

1487 (Edward JACKSON), "Graduate Study in Ophthalmology at Vienna", in: *Arch. Ophthalmol.* 3/5 (1922), p. 583. The course was scheduled to take place between 2 Oct. and 25 Nov. 1922 at the two Univ. Eye Clinics at Vienna's Allgem. Krankenhaus and was to cater to between 10 and 15 participants. Local organisation was entrusted to Ernst Fuchs's son Adalbert. The fee was $200 per person. The following topics were envisaged: fundus photography (Dimmer), operations (Meller), general diagnostics (Meller), physiol. and optics (Lauber), examinations under red-free light and with the slit lamp (Lauber), refraction (Lindner), bacteriol. (Lindner), retinoscopy (Lindner), pituitary gland (Hirsch), radium therapy (Kummer), muscles (Bachstez), neurol. (Bachstez), external diseases (Bachstez), anat. of the orbita (Adalbert Fuchs), normal histol. (Adalbert Fuchs), pathol. histol. (Adalbert Fuchs), general therapy and local anaesthetics (Adalbert Fuchs) and ophthalmoscopy (Guist).

1488 Cf. *Arch. Ophthalmol.* 3/5 (1922), p. 594.

1489 Ibid., p. 772.

1490 Ibid., p. 931.

1491 Cf. Honolulu, Hawaii, Passenger and Crew Lists, 1900–1959, accessible online at www.ancestry.com (last accessed: 6 Sept. 2022).

1492 Cf. FN 1482 and ibid, p. 987.

1493 FUCHS, *Augenarzt* (as in FN 2), p. 109.

1494 Cf. FN 1283.

1495 See the account of his stay in Japan later in this chapter.

1496 Modern Thailand.

1497 FUCHS, *Augenarzt* (as in FN 2), p. 109.

1498 Cf. FN 1436.

1499 Cf. Book Reviews: (Arnold KNAPP), "Text-Book of Ophthalmology. By Prof. E. Fuchs, Vienna. Translated from the XII German edition, revised and enlarged by Dr. ALEXANDER DUANE, New York. VII edition, 997 pages, 445 illustrations. Philadelphia and London, J. B. Lippincott Co., 1923. Price $9.00", in: *Arch. Ophthalmol.* 52 (1923), p. 308.

1500 Ernest FUCHS, *Text-Book* (as in FN 810).

1501 Lucien (Lucian) Howe (1848–1928). Studied at Harvard Med. School. Ophthalmol. and surg. special. during a study trip to Europe (e.g. under Joseph Lister/Edinburgh and Hermann v. Helmholtz/Berlin and at the Univ. Clinics of the Vienna Allgem. Krankenhaus). 1874 Return to Buffalo. 1876 Foundation of the Buffalo Eye and Ear Infirmary. 1879 Prof. of Ophthalm. at Buffalo Univ.; highly influential activist in the campaign advocating prophylactic instillation of a silver nitrate solution in the eyes of newborn babies to ward off ophthalmia neonatorum (Credé's prophylaxis, as proposed by the Leipzig gynaecologist and obstetrician Carl Sigmund Franz Credé, 1819–1892). 1922 Endowment of what was posthumously called the Howe Medal of the Am. Ophthalmol. Soc., the Society's top award. 1926 Foundation of a lab for research on the biochemistry, genetics and neurobiol. of the eye at the Harvard Med. School (Howe Laboratory of Ophthalmology at Harvard University's Massachusetts

Eye and Ear Infirmary), which soon acquired an outstanding reputation. Prominent advocate of eugenic measures to combat the spread of congenital blindness. 1927 Pres. of the Eugenics Research Assoc. Cf. IBBO (as in FN 18); Obituary, in: *Am. J. Ophthalmol.* 12/2 (1929), pp. 145–147.

1502 Cf. Howe Medal Recipients, accessible online on the website the Am. Ophthlmol. Soc.: https://aosonline.org/annual-meeting/annual-meeting-archives/a-continuation-of-wheelers-first-hundred-years-10/ (last accessed: 6 Sept. 2022).

1503 Cf. FN 591.

1504 Cf. FN 811.

1505 Ministerialpass No. 302, issued by the Federal Chancellery, Foreign Affairs on 30 Dec. 1925. Original in the Family archive.

1506 Cf. Adolph BARKAN, Arnold KNAPP, George S. DERBY, E. V. L. BROWN; Joseph M. KELLER, *Ernst Fuchs Fund*, in: *Am. J. Ophthalmol.* 10 (1927), p. 541.

1507 Cf. FN 349.

1508 Cf. FN 1436.

1509 George Strong Derby (1875–1931). Cf. FN 1452.

1510 Cf. FN 815.

1511 No biographical or career data retrievable.

1512 Cf. FN 1506.

1513 Cf. "News Items", in: *Am. J. Ophthalmol.* 11 (1928), p. 89.

1514 See Ch. 12.

1515 F. FISCHER, "13. Internationaler Ophthalmologischer Kongreß 5.–13. September 1929", in: *Zeitschr. Ophthalm.* 67 (1929), pp. 396–398. (Advance notice with details of registration and conference topics); A. ROSENBERG, "Internationaler Ophthalmologen-Kongreß. Amsterdam, vom 5. bis 13. September 1929", in: *Zeitschr. Ophthalm.* 70 (1930).

1516 William Henry Luedde (1876–1952). Originally from Illinois. Studied at Washington Univ. (M. D. 1900). Ophthalmol. specialis. at Kiel Univ. (two years), 1906 at the Sorbonne in Paris (one year) and several months in London. After his return, he established himself in St. Louis, where he initially worked with other well respected ophthalmol. in their practices before setting up his own practice. Inspired by the contact with Frans Cornelis Donders (Utrecht, cf. FN 38) and Marius Tscherning (Copenhagen, cf. FN 322), he developed a special interest in the mechanism of accommodation. Until 1912 on the staff of the Eye Dept. of Washington Univ. and 1912–1916 of the Eye, Ear, Nose and Throat Infirmary in St. Louis. 1919–1952 Adviser of the United States Public Health Service at the United States Marine Hospital in St. Louis. 1919–1946 Adviser at the United States Veterans Hospital. 1921–1950 Prof. and Dir. of the Eye Dept. of the Univ. of St. Louis. Chairman of the St. Louis Society for the Blind. 1933 Awarded the Leslie Dana Medal for the Prevention of Blindness. He was responsible for bringing the first slit lamps to the United States, followed in 1914 by a Gullstrand ophthalmoscope. Cf. Obituaries, in: *Am. J. Ophthalmol.* 35/6 (1952), pp. 874–875 (Lawrence T. Post); *Transact. Am. Ophthalmol. Soc.* 50 (1952), pp. 31–34 (L. C. Drews).

1517 (Casey Albert WOOD), "Presentation to Dr. Ernst Fuchs. New York City, July 29", in: *Brit. J. Ophthalmol.* 13/9 (1929), p. 474. Similarly worded announcements and reports on the award of the Leslie Dana Medal to Fuchs appeared in local media such as the *J. Missouri State Med. Assoc.* 26 (1929), p. 411; Fred Houdlett ALBEE, Frederik J. ELTON (eds.), *Rehabilitation Review: Devoted to the Restoration and Employment of the Disabled* 3/7 (1929), p. 199; *The Canada Lancet and Practitioner* 1929, p. 28; *Hospital Social Service Assoc. of New York City 1929*, p. 327; *The New Outlook for the Blind.* Vol. 23/24 (1929), p. 46; Fred SMITH HALL, Russell Harold KURTZ, Margaret B. HODGES, *Encyclopedia of Social Work.* Vol. 1 (1930), p. 461; *The New Engl. J. of Med. 205* (1931), p. 1092; *Am. Journal of Public Health and the Nation's Health* 22 (1932), p. 125.

1518 Ibid. (Casey A. Wood).

1519 Cf. FN 320.

1520 Cf. FN 765.

1521 Jean-Baptiste Coppez (1840–1930). Prof. of Ophthalm. at the Vrije Universiteit Brussel. Ophthalmol. special. in Paris under Louis Auguste Desmarres (cf. FN 319), Richard Liebreich (cf. FN 266), Louis de Wecker (cf. FN 252), Xavier Galezowski (cf. FN 257), Arthur Sichel (cf. FN 256), Édouard Meyer (cf. FN 254), and Photinos Panas (cf. FN 258). 1876 Dir. of the Univ. Clinic of Intern. Medicine, with the licence to set up an Eye Clinic at Brussels Univ. 1883 Co-founder of the Société française d'ophtalmologie.1896 Co-founder and first Pres. of the Société d'ophtalmologie de Belgique. Father of the ophthalmol. Henri Coppez (1869–1946), who also trained in Vienna under Fuchs. Cf. Nécrologie, in: *Annales d'Oculistique* 167 (1930), p. 985 (Gallemaerts); Obituary, in: *Am. J. Ophthalmol.* 14 (1931), pp. 167–168 (W. H. Crisp).

1522 Étienne Rollet (1862–1937). Studied at Lyon Univ. (Dr. med. 1888). Ophthalmol. specialis. until 1897. Assoc. Prof. of Ophthalm. at the Med. Fac. of Lyon Univ. and Prof. of Clin. Ophthalm. at the Hospital of the Red Cross. 1905–1932 Dir. of the ophthalmol. Clinic of Lyon Univ.; see: Nécrologie, in: *Presse médicale* 78 (1937), pp. 1381–1382 (E. Velter).

1523 Fuchs, *Augenarzt* (as in FN 2), Tagebuchblätter. Entry of 10 Sept. 1929, p. 326.

1524 George Francis Suker (1869–1933). Senior Ophthalmologist at Cook County Hospital in Chicago.

1525 Harvey Cushing (1869–1939). Originally from Cleveland/Ohio. Studied at Yale and Harvard (M. D. 1895). Surg. specialis. at the Massachusetts Gen. Hospital and the Johns Hopkins Hospital in Baltimore. Specialis. in brain surgery under Sir Victor Alexander Haden Horsley (1857–1916) in London, Theodor Kocher (1841–1917) in Bern and the experim. pathophysiol. Charles Scott Sherrington (1857–1952) in Liverpool. 1912–1932 Prof. of Surgery at the Harvard Med. School in Boston, where he did pioneering work as a neurosurgeon. 1932–1937 Prof. emerit. of Neurol. and the Hist. of Med. at Yale. Pioneering work in the area of anaesthesiol. (Introduction of anaesthesia protocols with obligatory check-ups on all vital parameters). Early adopter of X-rays for diagnostic purposes. Cf. John Farquar FULTON, *Harvey Cushing. A Biography.* Springfield 1946; Nancileigh M. DOYLE et al., "The life and work of Harvey Cushing 1869–1939: A pioneer of neurosurgery, in: *J. Intensive Care Soc.* 18/2 (2017), pp. 157–158

1526 Fuchs, *Augenarzt* (as in FN 2), S. 117.

1527 Cf. FN 320.

1528 Edward TREACHER COLLINS, "Hofrat Professor Ernst Fuchs and His Work", in: Brit. J. Ophthalmol. (1931), pp. 65–75.

[1529] Robert C. DREWS, "The Leslie Dana Gold Medal", in: Am. *J. Ophthalmol.* 105/6 (1988), pp. 683–685.

[1530] See Ch. 3.

[1531] Cf. James E. LEBENSOHN, "Professor Ernst Fuchs (June 14, 1851–November 21, 1930)", in: *Am. J. Ophthalmol.* 34 (1951), pp. 772–774.

[1532] Fuchs wrote in his memoirs: *"While I was still in Italy, [...], I received a letter from Baltimore. The President of the John[s] Hopkins University, Mr. Goodson, invited me to speak at the inauguration of the Wilmer Ophthalmic Institute, offering a travel stipend of $1,500."* Fuchs, *Augenarzt* (as in FN 2), p. 114.

[1533] William Holland Wilmer (1863–1936). Studied at the Univ. of Virginia (M. D. 1885). General training and ophthalmol. specialis. at the New York Poly Clinic, during a study trip to Europe and at the Mount Sinai Hospital in New York. 1889 Establishment of an ophthalmol. private practice in Washington. Taught at Georgetown Univ., leading position at the Episcopal Eye, Ear and Throat Hospital. Developed the first ophthalmol. standards f. pilots during World War I. 1923 Pres. of the Am. Ophthalmol. Soc. 1924, through the intercession of William Henry Welch (1850–1934) [since 1884 Chair of Pathol., 1901 Founding Pres. of the Rockefeller Inst. for Medical Research, 1926 Prof. and Dir. of the Institute of Medical History in Baltimore, which had been founded in that year as the first of its kind in the United States], established the first eye clinic at a US university at the Johns Hopkins Univ. School of Med. in Baltimore. 1925 Inauguration of the Wilmer Ophthalmic Inst., Prof. and head ophthalmol. until 1934 at Johns Hopkins Hospital, which he turned into an institute of worldwide renown. Main area of work: tuberculosis of the eye, glaucoma, relations between systemic illnesses and the eye. Cf. IBBO (as in FN 18); Obituary: *Am. J. Ophthalmol.* 19/8 (1936), pp. 522–523 (E. Jackson).

[1534] Cf. (Ed.) "The Wilmer Ophthalmological Institute", in: *Brit. J. Ophthalmol.* 13 (1929), pp. 621–622; A. E. MAUMENEE, "The History of the Wilmer Ophthalmological Institute", in: *Am. J. Ophthalmol.* 60/5 (1965), pp. 770–783.

[1535] See George S. Derby's advance notice in *Arch. Ophthalmol.* 2/3 (1929), pp. 348–349.

[1536] Fuchs, *Augenarzt* (as in FN 2), p. 327.

[1537] "Dedication of the Wilmer Institute", in: *Bull. Johns Hopkins Hosp.* 47 (1930), pp. 44ff.

[1538] Max Neuburger (1868–1955). Studied at Vienna Univ. (Dr. med. univ. 1893). General medical training at Vienna's Allgem. Krankenhaus, neurol. special. under Moriz Benedikt (1835–1920) at the Allgem. Poliklinik. Disciple of the Professor of Medical History Theodor Puschmann (1844–1899), Habilitation 1898. After Puschmann's death, exponent of the History of Medicine at Vienna Univ. alongside Robert Ritter v. Töply (1856–1947). 1904 Assoc. Prof., 1912 tit. Assoc. Prof.; 1917 Dr. phil. (having completed a course in history at Vienna Univ.) and Full Prof. of the History of Medicine. 1914 Started lobbying for the establishment of a university institute for his specialty at Vienna Univ. He kept his voluminous private collection of histor. books, pictures and documents initially at the Deanery of the Med. Fac., then in a room behind the lecture hall of the 1st Med. Univ. Clinic. Thanks to an initiative of the Dir. of the Clinic, Karel Frederik Wenckebach (1864–1940, cf. FN 1443) establishment of an institute in 1920 in the former med.-surg. Military Acad. (Josephinum). Forced to resign for racist reasons from his position in April 1938 by the Nazi regime. 1939 Emigration to London, where he worked at the Wellcome Historical Museum. 1948 Emigration to join his son Frederick in Buffalo, where he found work at the medical-historical Institute of the Johns Hopkins University in Baltimore. 1952 Return to Vienna. One of the most distinguished historians of medicine in the German-speaking world. Cf. CZEIKE (as in FN 13); GERABEK et al. (as in FN 13); NDB (as in FN 15); Emanuel BERGHOFF, *Max Neuburger. Werden und Wirken eines österreichischen Gelehrten*. Maudrich, Vienna 1948; Gabriela SCHMIDT, "Der Medizinhistoriker Max Neuburger und die Wiener medizinische Fakultät", in: *Wien. klin. Wochenschr.* 105 (1993); pp. 737–739; Michael HUBENSTORF, "Eine 'Wiener Schule' der Medizingeschichte? – Max Neuburger und die vergessene deutschsprachige Medizingeschichte", in: *Medizingeschichte und Gesellschaftskritik*. Festschrift für Gerhard Baader. Matthiesen, Husum 1997, pp. 246–289.

1539 Postcard in a private collection. Only four days later Fuchs wrote the following thank-you letter:
Kritzendorf 23.VI. 29.
Sehr verehrter Herr Kollege!
Thank you most cordially for your kind information. As soon as I get to Vienna, I will take the liberty of calling on you to view the two pictures. Would you kindly tell me at what time you are normally at the Institute and could you let me have your telephone number so that I can call to find out whether you are there.
Yours sincerely, etc.
(Postcard in private collection).

1540 The Wilmer Ophthalmological Institute, as in FN 1534.

1541 Ernst FUCHS, "Development of Ophthalmology in Europe" (Address delivered at the dedication of the Wilmer Ophthalmological Institute, Johns Hopkins Hospital, Baltimore, Oct. 15, 1929), in: *Arch. Ophthalmol.* 3/2 (1930), pp. 133–147.

1542 "Trachoma", in: *Proceedings of the 1929 Annual Conference St. Louis, Missouri November 11–13, 1929. National Society for the Prevention of Blindness.* Publication 65, pp. 123–147.

1543 Ibid., *Discussion*, pp. 136–137.

1544 Harvey James Howard (1880–1956). A descendant of the Duke of Norfolk, born in the federal state of New York. Studied at the Univ. of Pennsylvania (M. D. 1908). 1910 Married and relocated to China on a five-year contract as Dir. of the Eye Clinic of the Univ. Med. School of the Christian College in Canton (today Guangzhou). Returned to the United States. Special. in ophthalmopathol. at Harvard Univ. with a Rockefeller Foundation scholarship (area of special interest: congen. eye anomalies). 1917 Received into the Am. Ophthalmol. Soc. 1917–1927 Dir. of the Eye Dept. at the Peking Union Medical College (PUMC). Initiated a teaching programme that featured invitations to distinguished ophthalmologists as visiting professors. 1921 Visit to Jujiro Komoto (cf. FN 1565) in Tokyo. To thank Howard for inviting Fuchs to the PUMC in 1922 the latter hosted him for several months at the 2nd Univ. Eye Clinic (Director: Fuchs's successor Friedrich Dimmer, cf. FN 44) as his personal guest in 1923/24. In 1925 H. spent ten weeks as the captive of Chinese bandits. Given permission to treat the last Emperor of China (1906–1967) in his palace in the Forbidden City. 1927 First Chair of his specialty at the Washington Univ. School of Medicine/St. Louis, Missouri. 1931–1948 Med. Dir. of the Missouri Commission for the Blind. Cf. Obituary, in: *Am. Med. Assoc. J.* 163 (1957), p. 138; Reginald F. JOHNSTON, *Twilight in the Forbidden City*. Cambridge University Press, 1934, pp. 272–273; David SHAVIT, *The United States in Asia. A Historical Dictionary*. Greenwood Press, New York/Westport, Connecticut/London 1990, p. 247; Harvey J. HOWARD, "A Visit to Dr. J. Komoto of Tokyo", in: *Am. J. Ophthalmol.* 10 (1921), pp. 752–757; HOWARD, "Department of Ophthalmology," in: *Addresses & Papers, Dedication Ceremonies and Medical Conference Peking Union Medical College September 15–22, 1921*. Peking Union Medical College 1922, pp. 385–401; HOWARD, *Ten Weeks with Chinese Bandits*. Dodd, Mead & Co., New York 1926. See the section on Ernst Fuchs's time in China below in this chapter.

1545 Cf. FN 1542, p. 136.

1546 Ibid., p. 169, and Ernst FUCHS, "Subjective Symptomatology of Ocular Disorders. An Address", in: *Amer. J. Ophthalmol.* 13 (1930), pp. 113–117.

1547 Cf. FN 1516.

1548 The reference is to Valentin Haüy (1745–1822), linguist, teacher and translator in Paris. A key experience (blind patients at the Hospice des Quinze-Vingts being mocked and baited during a street festival) had made him decide to teach blind children to read. He was friends with the famous Viennese blind pianist, composer, singer and music teacher Maria Theresia Paradis (1759–1824), who had construed a device on the model of a type case that enabled her to write and print music and give joint music classes to seeing and blind children. Haüy copied this device, using embossed letters. 1784 Presentation of his first student to the Académie des Sciences in Paris. 1785 Foundation of the Institution Nationale des Jeunes Aveugles, Europe's first school for the blind, which fell into disuse during the French Revolution. Established schools for the blind in Berlin and St. Petersburg. 1817 Return to Paris, where he found his school being operated by strangers. The most prominent alumnus of the school founded by Haüy was Louis Braille (1809–1852), who was ten when he joined. In 1825 Braille presented his tactile writing system based on cells and raised dots. Cf. W. H. ILLINGWORTH, *History of the Education of the Blind.* Sampson Low, Marston & Co., London 1910, pp. 4–7.

1549 Cf. FN 1542, pp. 167–169.

1550 W. F. BYNUM, Anne HARDY, Stephen JACYNA, Christopher LAWRENCE, E. M. TANSEY, *The Western Medical Tradition 1800–2000*. Cambridge University Press, Cambridge et al. 2006.

1551 Y. FUJIKAWA, *Geschichte der Medizin in Japan. Kurzgefasste Geschichte der Entwicklung der Japanischen Medizin mit besonderer Berücksichtigung der Einführung der europäischen Heilkunde in Japan.* Ed. by the Imperial-Japanese Ministry of Education. Tokyo 1911.

1552 HIRSCHBERG, *Geschichte d. Augenheilkunde* (as in FN 18), vol. XIV/6 [= Reprint, vol. V], § 994, pp. 377–378.

1553 Cf. FN 842.

1554 Cf. MISHIMA, *History of Ophthalmol. in Japan* (as in FN 838), pp. 294–296.

1555 Shiujiro OGATA (1857–1942). Originally from Osaka. Studied at Tokyo Univ. (Dr. med. 1882). Returned to his native city, where he became Deputy Dir. at Ogata Hospital, founded and headed by his brother. 1889 Foundation of the Ogata Med. Society and its journal. 1889–1892 Ophthalmol. study visits to the eye clinics of the

Univ. of Berlin (Karl Schweigger, cf. FN 1161) and Vienna II (Fuchs). 1893 Co-founder of a specialist ophthalmol. journal (Ganka zasshi) and of the Osaka Jikei Med. School. Cf. IBBO (as in FN 18); MISHI*MA, History of Ophthalmol. in Japan (as in FN 838), p. 277, 294.*

1556 Kenjuro GOU (1866–1907). 1892–1897 Ophthalmol. study visit to the eye clinics of the Univ. of Vienna II (Fuchs), Marburg (Wilhelm Uhthoff), Leipzig (Hubert Sattler), and Berlin (Karl Schweigger). Dir. of his own eye hospital in Kyoto. Cf. MISHIMA (as in FN 838), History of Ophth*almol. in Japan, pp. 294–295.*

1557 Ikujiro ASAYAMA (1861–1915). Studied at Tokyo Univ. (Dr. med. 1884). Appointed teacher at the Med. School in Kyoto, Dir. of the Eye Dept. In the wake of the foundation of the med. school at Kyoto Univ. he was sent to Europe in 1898 by the Imperial Ministry of Education, because he was slated to head the Eye Clinic as its first professor. 1898–1902 ophthalmol, study visits to the eye clinics of the Univ. of Berlin (Karl Schweigger, Richard Greeff), Würzburg (Julius v. Michel), Heidelberg (Theodor Leber) and Vienna I (Isidor Schnabel) and II (Fuchs), where he concentrated on sympath. ophthalmia. Cf. Harvey J. HOWARD, Professor Ikujiro Asayama, in: Am. J. Ophthalmol. Series 3, Vol. 5 *(1922), pp. 926–928;* IBBO *(as in FN 18); MISHIMA, History of Ophthalmol. in Japan (as in FN 838), p. 294–295; Ikujiro ASAYAMA, "Vollständige mikroskopische Untersuchung eines Falles von sympathischer Ophthalmie", in: Graefes Archiv 54/3 (1902), pp. 444ff.*

1558 Anzo Murakami (1862–1927). Studied at Tokyo Univ. (Graduation 1886). 1887–1922 Prof. at the Nagasaki Med. School (today Univ.). 1899–1901 Ophthalmol. study visits to the eye clinics of the Univ. of Breslau/Wroclaw (Wilhelm Uhthoff) and Vienna II (Fuchs). 1901 Dr. med. Univ. of Tokyo with a doct. thesis in German: "Ein Beitrag zu den Netzhautgefäss-Veränderungen bei Leukämie", in: Klin. Monatsbl. *Ophthalm.* 39 (1901), pp. 136ff. 1917–1922 Dean of the Med. Fac. of Nagasaki Univ. Cf. IBBO (as in FN 18); MISHIMA, *History of Ophthalmol. in Japan* (as in FN 838), p. 270, pp. 294–295.

1559 Nobuo INOUYE (1875–1971). Son-in-law of Tatsuya Inouye (cf. FN 842). Studied at Tokyo Univ. (Dr. med. 1901). Ophthalmol. special. under Yujiro Komoto. 1902–1905/1909–1911 Study visits to the Eye Clinics of the Univ. of Freiburg (Theodor Axenfeld), Leipzig (Hubert Sattler), Würzburg (Carl v. Hess), Heidelberg (Theodor Leber), Vienna II (Ernst Fuchs), and Bern (August Siegrist). 1912 Dr. med. sci. Univ. Tokyo. Until 1935 Dir. of the Eye Clinic of the Jutendo Hospital (now Univ.), at the same time Prof. at the Med. School in Tokyo (now Med. Univ. of Tokyo). Cf. IBBO (as in FN 18); MISHIMA, *History of Ophthalmol. in Japan* (as in FN 838), pp. 296–297.

1560 Rokuzo OGYU (1859–1914). Studied at Tokyo Univ. (Grad. 1884). 1885 Prof. at the Chiba Med. School (now Univ.). 1902 Dir. of the Hospital and Dean of the Med. Fac.; 1903–1906 Study visit to the eye clinics of the Univ. of Berlin (Richard Greeff) and Vienna II (Ernst Fuchs). 1907 Dr. med. Tokyo Univ. Cf. IBBO (as in FN 18); MISHIMA (as in FN 838), p. 269, pp. 296–*297.*

1561 Takekuma MIYAHARA (1874–1958). 1904–1907 Ophthalmolog. study visit to the eye clinics of the Univ. of Munich (Oskar Eversbusch, 1853–1911), Vienna I (Isidor Schnabel), and Vienna II (Ernst Fuchs). During the Japan. occupation of Taiwan (1895–1945) foundation of an eye clinic in Tainan. Cf. MISHIMA (as in FN 838), pp. 296–297.

[1562] Toranosuke AKATSUKA (1878–1956). WS 1910/11–WS 1911/12 Ophthalmol. study visits to the eye clinics of the Univ. of Munich (Oskar Eversbusch) and Vienna II (Ernst Fuchs). Ophthalmologist in Osaka.
Cf. MISHIMA (as in FN 838), pp. 296–297; Rudolf HARTMANN, *Japans Studierende in Deutschland 1868–1914.* Electron. data bank CrossAsia Blog, https://blog.crossasia.org (last accessed: 6 Sept. 2022).

[1563] Cf. Family archive; Ernst FUCHS, "Erinnerungen an Japan", in: *Zeitschr. Ophthalm.* 52 (1924), pp. 305–310; *Augenarzt* (as in FN 2), Reise-Tagebuchblätter, pp. 247–252.

[1564] See Ch. 9 for the banning of German as a conference language at the Internat. Ophthalmol. Congress in Washington in 1922.

[1565] Jujiro Komoto (1859–1938). Studied at Tokyo Univ. (Grad. 1883). 1885 Sent to Europe by the government to specialise in ophthalmol. 1886–1889 Study visits to the eye clinics of the Univ. of Freiburg (Wilhelm Manz, 1833–1911), Würzburg (Carl v. Hess), Berlin (K. Schweigger, Julius Hirschberg), Vienna II (Ernst Fuchs), and London. Struck up an especially close friendship with Hirschberg. This resulted in Hirschberg being extensively sponsored by Komoto and T. Inouye in 1892 and in Hirschberg later selling his voluminous private library to Komoto (today the Komoto Library, part of the Univ. Library Tokyo, cf. FN 304). 1889 First Prof. of Ophthalmol. at the Imperial. Univ. of Tokyo (then Japan's only univ.). 1891. Dr. med. sci. 1891–1924 Organ. of one-year postgraduate-courses. In addition to being Dir. of the Univ. Clinic, proprietor and head of a private hospital in Tokyo. 1896 Co-founder of the Japan. Ophthalmol. Society establ. on the model of the Dt. Ophthalmol. Gesellsch. (Heidelberg), with Komoto serving as its first pres. until 1925. Cf. FISCHER (as in FN 28); IBBO (as in FN 18); MISHIMA (as in FN 838), Ind.; Naganori KIRISAWA, "The Komoto Library (Formerly the Hirschberg Library)", in*: Japan. J. Ophthalmol.* 21 (1977), pp. 528–532.

[1566] Chuta Oguchi (1875–1945). Studied at a priv. univ. in Tokyo (Dr. med. 1891), ophthalmol. specialis. under Tetsuzo Suda (1848–1894); postgrad. course under Komoto (see the above FN). Army surgeon in Japan and Taiwan. After the Russo-Japanese War (1904/05) sponsored by Manao Hori (1860–1929), who in his turn had trained at the eye clinics of the Univ. of Berlin (Schweigger), Gießen (M. Burchardt), in Austria and in France between 1893 and 1897. 1893–1897 Publ. of a six-volume work on eye diseases and injuries occurring in the Russo-Japanese war. The statistics were published in German: Chuta OGUCHI, "Augenverletzungen im japanischen Heere während des letzten Krieges", in: *Beiträge z. Augenheilkd.* 83 (1913), pp. 75–303. 1907 First description of congenit. hemeralopia with recess. inheritance (Oguchi disease, eponym coined by Komoto). 1912–1914 Study visit to the univ. eye clinics at Heidelberg (A.Wagenmann) and Munich (C. v. Hess). 1916 Dr. med. sci. Tokyo Univ. 1922–1939 Dir. of the Eye Clinic of Nagoya Univ. Cf. IBBO (as in FN 18); MISHIMA (as in FN 838), pp. 285–286, pp. 298–299.

[1567] Sousuke Miyashita (1882–1948). Studied at Tokyo Univ.; ophthalmol. specialis. under Komoto. 1908–1911 Study visit to the eye clinics of the Univ. of Freiburg (Theodor Axenfeld) and Bern (August Siegrist, 1885–1947), Dr. med. sci. Tokyo Univ. 1913–1926 Dir. of the Univ. Eye Clinic Osaka, followed by a leading position at Tokyo University. Many publications in German. Cf. IBBO (as in FN 18).

[1568] Yoshizo Koyanagi (1880–1954). Studied at Kyoto Univ. (Dr. med. 1908). Ophthalmolog. special. under Ikujiro Asayama (cf. FN 1557). 1912 Ophthalmologist at the Red Cross Hospital in Osaka. 1913 Assoc. Prof. 1917/18 Study visit to Europe. Until 1942 First Professor and Dir. of the Eye Clinic at Tohoku Univ. in Sendai. Together with Kiyoshi Ishikawa (1878–1918) 1912/13 study visits to the eye clinic of Prague Univ. (Anton Elschnig) and to Sadao Suganuma (1879–1946, cf. FN 1580). Author of an outstanding textbook of ophthalm. Cf. MISHIMA (as in FN 838), pp. 298–299.

[1569] Cf. Fuchs, *Augenarzt* (as in FN 2), Reise-Tagebuchblätter, pp. 240–244, entries of 18, 19 and 22 August 1922.

[1570] Eric A. Fennel (1887–1957). Originally from Cincinnati/Ohio. Studied at the College of Med. of the Univ. of Cincinnati (M. D. 1912). Joined the Army Med. Corps during World War I and special. as pathobacteriologist (typhus, pneumococcal infect., lepra). 1919 Set up a practice in Hawaii. From 1920 lifelong collaboration with George Francis (Georg Franz) Straub (1879–1966), a German ophthalmologist, who had emigrated to the United States in 1903 and headed his own clinic in Hawaii. From 1932 responsible for all lepra hospitals in Hawaii. Pioneering pathol. work in Hawaii and seminal influence on the developm. of scient. medicine in the islands. Cf. I. L.TILDEN, "IN MEMORIAM Eric A. Fennel 1887–1967", in: *Am. J. Clin. Pathol.* 30/3 (1966), p. 257.

[1571] Cf. FUCHS, *Erinnerungen an Japan*, as in FN 1563, p. 306.

[1572] Cf. MISHIMA (as in FN 838), Figs. 13–19, p. 316, and the photograph showing Ernst Fuchs in an ornate oriel window, with Fuchs's inscription *"Tokio September 1922"* (see Family archive).

[1573] At the bottom Fuchs wrote: "*Tee im Hause Prof. Komoto's in Tokio.*" Komoto wrote a dedication in the top right-hand corner of the back: "*Meinem verehrten Kollegen Fuchs zur freundlichen Erinnerung und in herzlicher Dankbarkeit Dr. Komoto. Tokio, 21. Sept. 1922.*" [To my esteemed colleague as a souvenir and a token of my heart-felt gratitude, etc.], Fuchs photograph, Sammlungen d. Med. Univ. Wien.

[1574] Fuchs, *Augenarzt* (as in FN 2). Reise-Tagebuchblätter, entry of 25 September 1922, pp. 251–252.

[1575] Cf. FN 1571.

[1576] Ibid., p. 306–307.

[1577] Shinobu Ishihara (1879–1963). Studied at Tokyo Univ. (Grad. 1905). Ophthalmolog. special. under Komoto (cf. FN 1565), then Prof. of Ophthalm. at the Military School of Medicine. 1910–1914 Study visit to the eye clinics of Jena Univ. (Wolfgang Stock, 1874–1956), Freiburg (Theodor Axenfeld) and Munich (Carl v. Hess). 1916 Dr. med. sci. Tokyo Univ. 1922–1941 Successor of Komoto as Dir. of the Tokyo Univ. Eye Clinic. 1928 Dean of the Med. Fac. and Pres. of the Japan. Ophthalmol. Society until 1942. Inventor of a great number of examination instruments and sight tests, espec. the eponymous pseudochromat. test plates he painted himself, designed to aid the diagnosis of colour blindness (1917). The international edition of the Ishihara tables utilises Indo-Arabic numerals. Author of a well-received textbook (1926), which went through more than 20 editions. Cf. IBBO (as in FN 18); MISHIMA (as in FN 838), see Ind.

[1578] The reference is to Kyozo Majima (life data not retrievable).

[1579] See Chuta OGUCHI, Kyozo MAJIMA, "Cytologische Untersuchungen über das Augensekret", in: *Graefes Archiv* 108/1–2 (1922), pp. 86–100 and OGUCHI-MAJIMA, "Neue Ergebnisse der Trachomzellenforschung mit Bezug auf vitale Färbung und Oxydasereaktion", in: Ibid 108/3–4, pp. 359–362; Kyozo MAJIMA, "Studie über PROWAZEKsche Körperchen, besonders die Reinkultur von denselben", in: *Nippon Gankagakkai Zasshi* 29 (1925), p. 5 (in Japanese).

[1580] The reference is to Sadao SUGANUMA (1879–1946). Studied at Kyoto Univ. (Grad. 1906). Ophthalmol. special. under Ikujiro Asayama (cf. FN 1551). 1910 Prof. of Ophthalm. at the Niigata Med. School (now Univ.). 1912–1914 Study visit to Munich. Univ. (Carl v. Hess). 1916 Dr. med. sci. Kyoto Univ. 1919–1941. Prof. and Dir. of the Eye Clinic of newly founded Keio Univ.; highly regarded ophthalmopathol. Cf. IBBO (as in FN 18).

[1581] Including Yoshizo Koyanagi (cf. FN 1568).

[1582] Kenzaburo Ogawa (1871–1933). Studied at Tokyo Univ. (Grad. 1898). Ophthalmol. special. under Komoto (cf. FN 1565). 1904–1906 Study trip to Berlin (Richard Greeff). 1907 Dr. med. sci. Tokyo Univ. Until 1912 Prof. at the Okayama Med. School (now Univ.). Founder and Dir. of an eye hospital in Tokyo. Author of a well-received book on the history of ophthalm. in Japan. Cf. IBBO (as in FN 18); MISHIMA (as in FN 838), pp. 295–296.

[1583] FUCHS, *Erinnerungen an Japan*, as in FN 1556, pp. 308–309.

[1584] Cf. FN 1566.

[1585] MISHIMA (as in FN 838), Ind.

[1586] Cf. FN 1567.

[1587] MISHIMA (as in FN 838), p. 317.

[1588] Shigeru Kagoshima (1882–1953). 1923–1925 Prof. f. Ophthalm. at Chiba Univ., 1925–1941 Dir. of the Eye Clinic at Kumamoto Med. College (now Univ.). Cf. MISHIMA (as in FN 838), p. 307 and 379.

[1589] Letter announcing the award of the honorary membership, signed by the Dir. of the Eye Clinic of Tokyo Univ. and Pres. of the Japan. Ophthalmol. Society, Shinobu Ishihara (cf. FN 1577). Cf. original in the Family archive.

[1590] Cf. Fuchs, *Augenarzt* (as in FN 2), Reise-Tagebuchblätter, p. 252; MISHIMA (as in FN 838), p. 316.

[1591] Ibid., Reise-Tagebuchblätter, pp. 252–268.

[1592] Arthur Paul Wakefield (1878–1941). Originally from Ohio. 1904 M. D., Rush Med. College. 1905–1912 active as a med. doctor on behalf of the Foreign Missionary Soc. of the Christian Church (Disciples of Christ) first in Nanking, then in Luchowfu until 1919. 1917 Rockefeller Foundation Fellow at the Graduate School of Tropical Med. of Harvard. 1919–1927 active on behalf of the Episcopal Am. Church Mission at Boone College of the Central Christian Univ. in Wuchang. Singled out for a Red Cross award for his outstanding work during floods and in the reconstruction of levees at the Yangtsekiang. After his return to the USA he worked in the areas of Public Health and tuberculosis therapy in Massachusetts and Maine. Cf. *Who's Who in Massachusetts*, Larkin, Roosevelt & Larkin 1940, p. 783; *The Living Church* Febr. 25, 1942, p. 24; Frances FRAZEE HAMILTON, "Dr. Arthur Paul Wakefield. Medical Missionary to China, 1904–1927", in: *Ancestral Lines of the Doniphan, Frazee, and Hamilton Families*. Wm. Mitchell Printing Co., 1928, pp. 463–470; *Wakefield Family Papers*: Yale Divinity Library, New Haven.

[1593] Cf. Mary E. FERGUSON, *China Medical Board and Peking Union Medical College. A Chronicle of Fruitful Collaboration 1914–1951.* China Medical Board of New York, Inc., New York 1970; Peter BUCK, *American Science and Modern China.* Cambridge University Press, Cambridge/London et al. 1980; L. A. SCHNEIDER, "The Rockefeller Foundation, the China Foundation, and the development of modern science in China", in: *Soc. Sci. Med.* 16 (1982), p. 1217–1221; Frank NINKOVICH, *The Rockefeller Foundation, China, and Cultural Change*, in: J. Am. Hist. 70 (1984), pp. 799–820; *China Medical Board 100 Years of Philanthropy for Health*, accessible online at: www.chinamedicalboard.org (last accessed: 6 Sept. 2022)

[1594] John Z. BOWERS, *Western Medicine in a Chinese Palace. Peking Union Medical College, 1917–1951.* Josiah Macy, Jr. Foundation 1972; Ricardo K. S. MAK, *Transmitting the Ideal of Enlightenment. Chinese Universities since the Late Nineteenth Century.* University Press of America Inc., Lanham/Maryland, Plymouth 2009, pp. 73–74.

[1595] Cf. FN 875 (Outline of this organisation in Ch. 6 in the context of the translation of the *Lehrbuch* in 1911).

[1596] *Addresses & Papers, Dedication Ceremonies and Medical Conference Peking Union Medical College September 15–22, 1921.* Peking Union Medical College 1922.

[1597] Ernst FUCHS, *Text-Book of Ophthalmology by Ernst Fuchs Vienna. Eleventh Edition Translated from the Third American Edition by James Boyd Neal*, M. A., M. D., Union Medical College, Tsinan. China Medical Missionary Association, Shanghai 1911. See Ch. 6.

[1598] Cf. FN 876.

[1599] Cf. FN 1544.

[1600] Tsing-Meu Li (LI Ching-mo) (b. 1884). Born in Honolulu. Oahu College, Honolulu 1898–1902. Studied at the School of Medicine of St. John's Univ. in Shanghai and at the Univ. of Pennsylvania (1909 M. D.). 1909–1913 Prof. at the Univ. Med. School of Canton. 1915 Diploma of Ophthalm. from the Philadelphia Polyclinic and the College for Graduates of Medicine. 1917 Assistant and later Assoc. Prof. at the PUMC under Harvey Howard (standing in occasionally as acting head of the department) until 1927. Then Visit. Prof. in the United States. Cf. *China Monthly Review* 16 (1921), p. 354; *Annual Report of the Rockefeller Foundation.* China Medical Board 1921, p. 17; T. M. LI, "Report of the Department of Ophthalmology", in: *Sixteenth Annual Report of the Medical Superintendent of the Peking Union Medical College Hospital. For the Year Ending June 30, 1924.* Peking 1924, pp. 64–67; John Benjamin POWELL (ed.), *Who's who in China* [...] *containing the pictures and biographies of China's best known political, financial, business and professional men* [...] The China Weekly Review 1926, p. 454; *Who's who in China 1918–1950.* Vol. 3 (1982), p. 230.

[1601] Cf. FERGUSON (as in FN 1593), p. 47.

[1602] Harvey J. HOWARD, "Report of the Department of Ophthalmology", *in: Fifteenth Annual Report of the Medical Superintendent of the Peking Union Medical College Hospital. For the Year Ending June 30, 1923. Peking 1923,* pp. 50–54 (here: p. 54). Cf. Harvey J. HOWARD, "Professor Fuchs's Visit to Peking", in: *Am. J. Ophthalmol.* 6 (1923), pp. 615–617.

[1603] Original in the Family archive.

[1604] Daniel G. VAUGHAN, "Peking Union Medical College: A Golden Age in Ophthalmology", in: *Transact. Pacific Coast Oto-Ophthalmol. Soc.* 62 (1981), pp. 1–15 (here: p. 7).

[1605] Cf. FN 808.

[1606] Cf. HOWARD, Report of the Department of Ophthalmol., as in FN 1596, pp. 64–67 (here: p. 65).

[1607] *Prof. Fuchs's Lectures Sept. 17, 1923 – June 14, 1924.* Bound typescript, 99 pages. Left-hand side kept free for additional notes. Handwritten note on the inside of the cover and the flyleaf: *K. B. Johnston. Dr. Ad[a]lbert Fuchs First Eye Clinic Allgemeines Krankenhaus Vienna. Histo Pathology Notes. From a course given by Dr. Ad[a]lbert Fuchs at Peking Union Medical College. Nov. 1st 1923 – Mar. 1st 1924.* Private collection. – The owner, Kenneth B. Johnston [b. 1896], a Canadian, studied at McGill Univ. in Montreal. (1918 M. D). 1922–1924 Resident in Ophthalmol. at the PUMC, 1925/26 at Moorfields Hospital (London) and in Vienna under Adalbert Fuchs. Founder member of the Canad. Ophthalmol. Soc. (Pres. 1953). 1950–1956 Prof. and Dir. of the Eye Clinic of McGill Univ. Cf. Sean B. MURPHY, *Portraits of Ophthalmology at McGill University 1876–1990*, pp. 66–67. Available online at: https://www.mcgill.ca/ophthalmology/about-us/history (last accessed: 6 Sept. 2022).

[1608] Mary BROWN BULLOCK, *An American Transplant. The Rockefeller Foundation & Peking Union Medical College*. University of California Press, Berkeley/Los Angeles/London 1980, p. 84.

[1609] Cf. FN 808.

[1610] Cf. BOWERS, *Western Medicine in a Chinese Palace*, as in FN 1594, p. 184; VAUGHAN, as in FN 1604; C. C. CHAN, D. ARDELJAN, "Ten Chairpersons of the Ophthalmology Department at Peking Union Medical College", in: *Asia Pac. J. Ophthalmol.* (Phila) 2 (2013), pp. 3–8.

[1611] Cf. FN 1209.

[1612] Cf. FN 817.

[1613] Fuchs reported on the manifold impressions he had formed of Filipino culture and nature in a popular presentation at the adult education centre Wiener Urania on 5 Nov. 1925. Cf. Ernst FUCHS, "Wanderungen auf den Philippinen". Announcement, in: *Verlautbarungen d. Volksbildungshauses Wiener Urania*, No. 36 of 31 Oct. 1925, p. 4.

[1614] José Rizal (1861–1896). Brilliant student. Early art studies (drawing, painting, sculpture). Brilliant linguist. 1879–1892 Studied medicine, agriculture, philosophy and literature at the Santo Tomas Univ. in Manila. Continued his medical studies at Madrid Univ. until 1884, motivated by his wish to cure his mother, who had been deprived of her eyesight by cataract in both eyes. Further studies in philosophy and literature. Nov. 1885–Febr. 1886 ophthalmol. specialis. as assist. under Louis de Wecker (cf. FN 252) in Paris, then for six months under Arlt disciple Otto Becker (cf. FN 178) at the Univ. Eye Clinic Heidelberg, 1887 under pathologist Rudolf Virchow (1821–1902) in Berlin, who introduced him to the Gesellschaft für Anthropologie, Ethnologie und Urgeschichte, and at the 2nd Univ. Eye Clinic under Ernst Fuchs. During his stay in Germany, he struck up a friendship with *the* expert on the Philippines in the German-speaking world, the Austrian grammar school teacher and ethnographer Ferdinand Blumentritt (1853–1913) based in Leitmeritz/Litoměřice in Bohemia. Blumentritt was learning Tagalog, the Philippine language Rizal had translated Schiller's *Wilhelm Tell* into. He supported Rizal's struggle against Spanish colonial rule. After courses in psychol. and history at Leipzig Univ. Rizal returned to the Philippines via Marseille (Aug.1887 – Febr. 1888 in his hometown Calamba). Nov. 1891– June 1892 practised in Hongkong. 1892–1896 exiled to Dagitan on Mindanao because of his activities against the Spanish colonial power. When he was given permission to emigrate to Cuba to practise there, he returned briefly to the main island. Charged with complicity in the newly ignited rebellion of the Philippine revolutionary movement, he was sentenced to death by a Spanish military tribunal and executed. Hero of the Filipino independence movement. Cf. Harry SICHROVSKY, *Der Revolutionär von Leitmeritz: Ferdinand Blumentritt und der philippinische Freiheitskampf.* Österr. Bundesverlag 1983; Salvador R. SALCEDA, *A Century of Ophthalmology in the Philippines.* Centennial lecture series Univ. of the Philippines Manila 1998, accessible online at: http://www.pao.org.ph/PAO.pdf (last accessed: 23 Aug. 2018); Tracy RAVIN, "José Rizal. Philippine National Hero and Ophthalmologist", in: *Arch. Ophthalmol.* 119/2 (2001), pp. 180–184; Josefina D. HOFILEÑA, *José Rizal and Ferdinand Blumentritt: A Chronology of a Friendship.* Ateneo de Manila 2014; Guido KLUXEN, "José Rizal (1861–1896), Augenarzt und Nationalheld der Philippinen", in: *Mitteilungen der Julius-Hirschberg-Gesellschaft zur Geschichte der Augenheilkunde* 16 (2014), pp. 273–289 (Omits any mention of Rizal's time in Vienna).

1615 Fuchs, *Augenarzt* (as in FN 2), diary entry of 17 Jan. 1923, p. 271.

1616 Sixto Y. Orosa e Ylagan (1891–1981). Studied at Manila University. 1916 Relocated from Manila to Jolo (Sulu), where he was one of the first Christian doctors to work among Muslims. Dir. of Sulu Public Hospital. Renowned physician and writer, author of a several books on his native country. Cf. Carlos QUIRINO, *Who's Who in Philippine History.* Tahanan Books, Manila 1995.

1617 F. W. Dudley. Surg. training in San Francisco. Head surgeon at St. Paul's Hospital in Manila. Assoc. Prof., Philippine Med. School. Cf. *San Francisco Chronicle*; June 21, 1908, p. 7.

1618 Fernando Calderon. First Philippine. Dir. of the Philippine Gen. Hospital in Manila founded in 1908. Leading role on the board of the Manila Med. Soc. Cf. Zoilo M. GALANG, Camilo OSIAS, *Encyclopedia of the Philippines: Builders of the New Philippines.* Philippine Education Company 1936, p. 134; Cristina Evangelista TORRES, *The Americanization of Manila, 1898–1921.* The University of the Philippines Press, 2010, p. 119.

1619 Cf. Entry in Ernst Fuchs's passport, p. 17: Visa No. 22051 … 1923. *Good for transit through British territory en route from the Philippine Islands to Siam and* [illegible] *to Austria.* Document in the Family archive.

1620 Fuchs, *Augenarzt* (as in FN 2), Diary entries from 10 to 16 Feb. 1923, pp. 272–287. See the pertinent entry in his passport (as in FN 1622), p. 18.

1621 Ernst Fuchs's passport (as in FN 1622), p. 18.

1622 [Countries for which this passport is valid: […] All European countries, with the exception of from and to Russia, and all countries overseas. Cf. Reisepass d. Rep. Österr. No. 18071 of 11 April 1923. Document in the Family archive.

12. Sunset, Legacy, and Afterlife

International renown and the recognition of his colleagues was something that came early to Ernst Fuchs in his academic career. What made Ernst Fuchs a household name in ophthalmology was the fact that he was an outstanding clinician, histopathologist, and discoverer of a great number of ophthalmological pathologies, a highly respected academic teacher of worldwide renown and the author of an epoch-making textbook. His extraordinary magnetism inevitably rubbed off on the Vienna School of Ophthalmology as a whole. Particularly in the Anglo-American world Ernst Fuchs the man was identified wholesale with "his" clinic. It was common parlance to refer to Fuchs as the Director of *the* University Eye Clinic in Vienna, regardless of the fact that two University Eye Clinics existed side by side at Vienna's Allgemeines Krankenhaus.

In the autobiography he wrote for his son Adalbert in 1926 he summed up his own life with characteristic modesty:

I had loving parents, a carefree, if work-filled childhood – but then I never was one to shirk work. I wooed a dear wife, and she gave me healthy, good-natured children who grew up to be splendid people. Our daughters are happily married. You, dear Bertl, are not married, which is a pity, but you have been fortunate in that you have come back from the war alive and are now holding a respected position. I have also had my share of external recognition.

It goes without saying that I have not been spared my share of pain. My first loss was the untimely death of my brother,[1623] *to whom I felt very close and who was always my faithful, trusted adviser; then the protracted illness and the relatively early death of my wife.*

I have performed my task in this life. Whether death comes sooner or later is none of my concern. I only hope that the end will not be too bitter.[1624]

Having returned from his third prolonged stay in the United States in the early March of 1930 (see Ch.11), Fuchs spent the next six months partly in Vienna and partly at his Edelhof estate in Kritzendorf. In October 1930 he travelled to South Tyrol and Florence and returned, still outwardly in good health, to his house in Skodagasse 13 in Vienna's 8th district on November 19; the house used to belong to his revered clinical teacher Joseph Škoda.[1625, 1626] Only two days later, on November 21, 1930, 79-year-old Ernst Fuchs succumbed to myocardial infarction, the consequence of coronary heart disease, a condition he had been suffering from for many years.[1627] (Fig. 136)

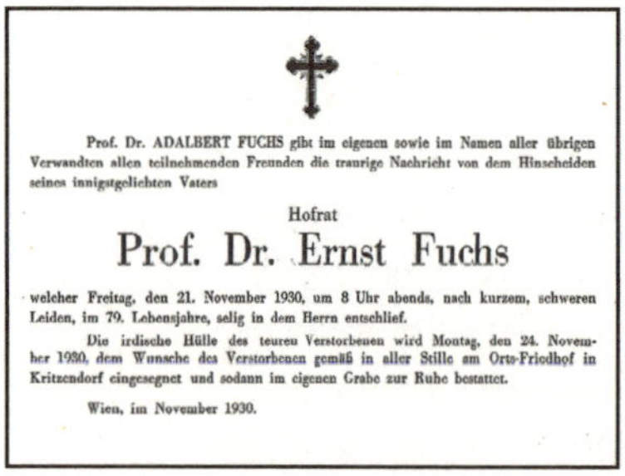

Prof. Dr. ADALBERT FUCHS gibt im eigenen sowie im Namen aller übrigen Verwandten allen teilnehmenden Freunden die traurige Nachricht von dem Hinscheiden seines innigstgeliebten Vaters

Hofrat

Prof. Dr. Ernst Fuchs

welcher Freitag, den 21. November 1930, um 8 Uhr abends, nach kurzem, schweren Leiden, im 79. Lebensjahre, selig in dem Herrn entschlief.

Die irdische Hülle des teuren Verstorbenen wird Montag, den 24. November 1930, dem Wunsche des Verstorbenen gemäß in aller Stille am Orts-Friedhof in Kritzendorf eingesegnet und sodann im eigenen Grabe zur Ruhe bestattet.

Wien, im November 1930.

Fig. 136 Obituary notice of Ernst Fuchs

After a long, beautiful and successful life, my father found what he had been hoping for, a quick and not too bitter end.

Countless friends, colleagues, students, nurses and patients paid their last respects to my father as he was taken to Kritzendorf and interred in the village cemetery[1628] *beneath the stone*[1629] *he had commissioned for his beloved wife, in a tomb he had hoped would also be his own final resting place. From there, the last repose also of his parents and grandparents, one's gaze is free to roam across the Danube and its extensive wetlands, across the gentle hills my father was so attached to and where he loved to wander throughout the many years of his life. Here this man who had time and again been lured to distant lands was put to rest in the place he loved best.*[1630] (Fig. 137)

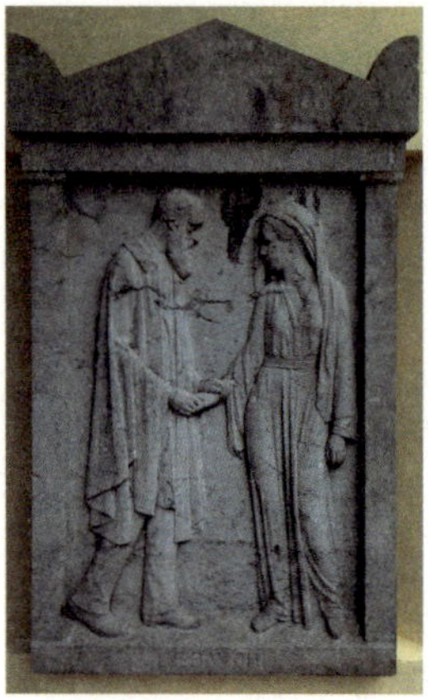

Fig. 137 Headstone at Ernst and Julie Fuchs's tomb

In a way that reflected Ernst Fuchs's international renown and his reputation as a teacher, researcher and member or honorary member of 36 scientific societies,[1631] his disciples and his friends all over the globe expressed their appreciation of his achievements in detailed and often very personal obituaries published by the world's ophthalmological journals.[1632] In Vienna his death was announced in the dailies.[1633] Both the Gesellschaft der Ärzte[1634] and the Wiener Ophthalmologische Gesellschaft[1635] convened mourning sessions.

Hofrat Professor Dr. Ernst Fuchs Scholarship Foundation for Junior Ophthalmologists of the Vienna School (1932)

Six weeks before his death, on October 6, 1930, Ernst Fuchs wrote the following letter, addressed to the Academic Senate of the University of Vienna:

My disciples in the United States of America endowed a foundation in my honour in 1926, the E. Fuchs Fund – Fuchs Foundation.[1636] *As is apparent from the enclosed deed of foundation, which I drafted myself, the interest of the capital is destined to help young Viennese ophthalmologists to complete their scientific training. Based on a capital totalling roughly 34,000 shillings (most of it in a dollar account for donations from the United States), the foundation has been administered by me up until now. To safeguard the foundation's proper use in future I herewith ask the Senate to take charge of it, as the subsidies will as a rule be awarded to members of the University and to assistants and junior doctors associated with the two University Eye Clinics.*

Dr. Ernst FUCHS,
emeritierter Professor der Augenheilkunde[1637]

In its session on July 14, 1931, the Academic Senate of Vienna University adopted the name "Hofrat Professor Dr. Ernst FUCHS-Stipendienstiftung für junge Ophthalmologen der Wiener Schule".[1638] Its purpose was defined as

subsidies as travel bursaries or to facilitate the execution or publication of scientific work done by up-and-coming ophthalmologists of the Vienna School, (preferably assistants and junior doctors of the two University Eye Clinics,) [...] *who do not have the private means needed for such purposes.*[1639]

The bursaries, whose value depended on the interest yielded by the foundation's endowment, were awarded once a year by a committee comprised of the Dean of the Medical Faculty as chairman, the two directors of Vienna's University Eye Clinics and the President of the Wiener Ophthalmologische Gesellschaft.[1640] They were released every year on the anniversary of Ernst Fuchs's death, November 21.[1641] On January 9, 1932, the Rector of Vienna University, pathological anatomist Rudolf Maresch (1868–1936)[1642] and the Dean of the Medical Faculty, hygienist Roland Grassberger (1867–1956),[1643] endorsed the deed of foundation.[1644]

After the Nazi takeover in Austria in 1938 three clauses were added to the deed on March 11, 1941. The most significant one of these decreed that *"the award of individual bursaries requires the consent of the Gauamtsleiter and the Chairman of the Vienna Chamber of Physicians".*[1645]

In 1960 the deed was relieved of this obsolete clause and a new regulation concerning the dissolution of the foundation and the obsolescence of its purpose was introduced. This updated version was put in force on April 17, 1961 by the then Rector of Vienna University, palaeontologist Othmar Kühn (1892–1969).[1646, 1647]

Scientific papers funded by the Foundation were required to declare this fact in their imprint. In around 1988 the Ernst Fuchs Foundation was dissolved

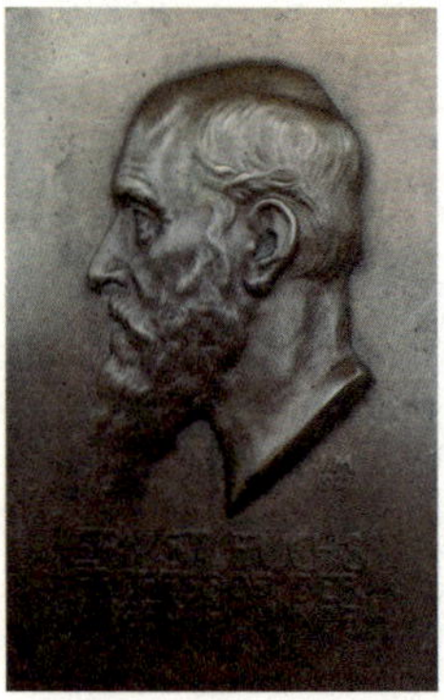

Fig. 138 Bronze plaque with Ernst Fuchs's portrait

because by that time the endowment had become exhausted.[1648] For more than a half century after Fuchs's death it had provided support to a great number of up-and-coming Viennese ophthalmologists connected to the University. A detailed appraisal of the beneficiaries is a project that would be well worth undertaking.

Memorial Plaque

Presumably as Josef Müllner[1649] was already at work on the large-scale marble relief of Fuchs to mark the occasion of his 70th birthday in 1921, he made a small bronze plaque with the same portrait.[1650] Copies of it probably began to circulate before Fuchs's death in November 1930. In 1932 and 1933 his disciple and long-time friend Charles H. May (1861–1943)[1651] told the editor of Archives of Ophthalmology in New York that he had been given such a plaque by Adalbert Fuchs at the behest of Fuchs senior. In collaboration with Adalbert Fuchs May conceived and carried out the plan to have a series of these plaques produced and to make them available to colleagues for a modest fee.[1652] How many of these plaques, each engraved "J. M. 1921", were made is now impossible to tell.[1653] (Fig. 138)

Commemoration of Ernst Fuchs's 100th Birthday in 1951

As had been the case with Ernst Fuchs's 70th birthday on 14 June 1921, the 100th anniversary of the birth of arguably the greatest exponent of the Vienna School of Ophthalmology was celebrated in style.

Transfer of the Müllner Relief to the Arkadenhof

In a public demonstration of the continued appreciation of Fuchs's achievement, the University of Vienna had the marble relief Josef Müllner had created in 1921 for the ophthalmologist's 70th birthday transferred to the Arkadenhof from the Lecture Hall of the First University Eye Clinic.[1654] The result of an initiative put forward jointly by the two Directors of the University Eye Clinics at the Allgemeines Krankenhaus, Arnold Pillat and Karl David Lindner, the transfer was endorsed by the University's Academic Senate on October 21, 1950.[1655] The solemn unveiling ceremony took place on June 21, 1951 in the Great Festival Hall and the Arkadenhof.[1656] In his keynote speech, Karl David Lindner[1657] recalled how the standard Fuchs held his students and his staff to was underpinned by his own example:

Any student who had regularly attended Fuchs's famous lecture course had no need to worry about the professor's notoriously strict style of examination.

[...] *Fuchs was the very model of a strict director. He demanded from his doctors the very best they could give in terms of work and performance of their duty. I myself doubted for quite a while whether I had what it takes to go through with this training. But he himself set the standard by unfailingly attending to what needed to be done and by working himself extremely hard. So we dug in and emulated his example.*[1658]

Anniversary Postcard

A postcard was issued, featuring Müllner's portrait relief, designed to make a non-specialist public aware of the great ophthalmologist.[1659]

Celebratory Meeting on June 22, 1951

On June 22, the day after the unveiling of the relief in the Arkadenhof, Vienna's Ophthalmologische Gesellschaft and the Gesellschaft der Ärzte convened a meeting in honour of Ernst Fuchs at the Billrothhaus at Frankgasse 8 in the 9th district.[1660] The President of the Gesellschaft der Ärzte, Wolfgang Denk (1882–1970),[1661] opened the meeting:

Only to a few mortals is it granted that their achievements and their personalities live on beyond their own death. The Vienna Medical School is fortunate in that it has among its founders a great number of men whose life's work lights the way for the medical generation of today. Ernst Fuchs *belongs to this chosen band. The Gesellschaft der Aerzte, the representatives of medical Vienna, will always loyally and gratefully cherish his memory.*[1662]

In his own keynote speech, the Director of Vienna's First University Eye Clinic, Fuchs's "granddisciple" Arnold Pillat outlined the merits of Vienna's School of Ophthalmology in general and, in a way befitting the occasion, those of Ernst Fuchs as a clinical teacher and researcher in particular.[1663]

Special Issue of the **Wiener klinische Wochenschrift**

The *Wiener klinische Wochenschrift*, the journal co-founded by Fuchs in 1888,[1664] dedicated to him two appraisals, one by his youngest disciple, Karl David Lindner, the other by the dermatologist Leopold Arzt,[1665] the journal's editor,[1666] and a double issue[1667] of scientific papers.[1668]

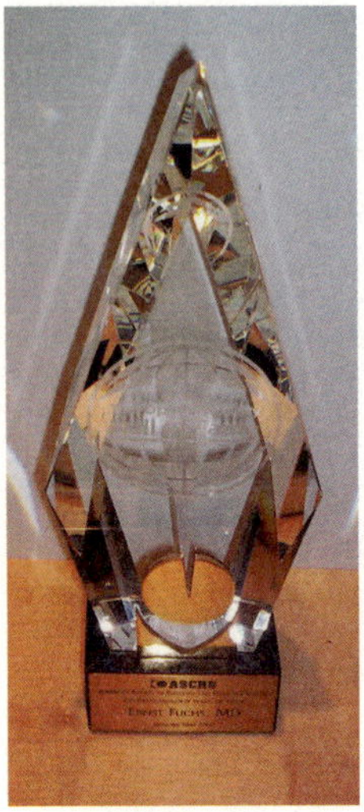

Fig. 139 Ophthalmology Hall of Fame Award for Ernst Fuchs, 2000

Nor was Vienna the only place where note was taken of the 100th anniversary of Fuchs's birthday. Tributes poured in from abroad, especially from the United States and Latin America.[1669]

150th Anniversary of the Foundation of Vienna's University Eye Clinic (1962)

To celebrate the 150th anniversary of the foundation of the world's first university eye clinic, medical historian Erna Lesky (1911–1986)[1670] staged a special exhibition[1671] in June 1962 at the Vienna University Institute for the History of Medicine in the Josephinum, of which she was in charge. In the hope of obtaining highlights for this project, she contacted Fuchs's descendants and was given a representative selection of objects the family had been left by the ophthalmologist. The Institute even obtained on permanent loan Fuchs's unique collection of histological preparations.[1672] It is now part of the Collections of Vienna Medical University.

100th Anniversary of the Foundation of Vienna's Second University Eye Clinic (1983)

The Second University Eye Clinic, whose director Fuchs had been for three decades, celebrated the centenary of its foundation in 1983. Again, the Institute for the History of Medicine under Lesky's successor Helmut Wyklicky (1921–2007)[1673] staged a representative retrospective. While the primary aim was to commemorate the founder, Eduard Jaeger von Jaxtthal, the achievements of Ernst Fuchs and of the subsequent Directors of Clinic were also duly documented.

Induction of Ernst Fuchs into the ARCRS Ophthalmology Hall of Fame (2000)

The American Society of Cataract and Refractive Surgery (ASCRS)[1674] set up a virtual Ophthalmology Hall of Fame in 1999. Since then the Society has singled out for a special award several ophthalmologists, living and dead, who had made a significant contribution to the development of ophthalmology. In the second year of its existence, the Society inducted Ernst Fuchs into this Ophthalmological Hall of Fame, perhaps with an eye on the 150th anniversary of his birthday in 2001.[1675] (Fig. 139)

Fuchs Stiftung zur Förderung der Augenheilkunde – Fuchs Foundation for the Promotion of Ophthalmology (2001)

In 2001, at the initiative of Günther Grabner, then Director of the Landesaugenklinik Salzburg (now Augenklinik der Paracelsus Medizinischen Privatuniversität Salzburg), the private Fuchs Foundation was called into being in collaboration with the Verein zur Förderung der Landesaugenklinik Salzburg. The purpose of this foundation is the advancement of ophthalmology.[1676] This charitable institution,[1677] which has since established an excellent track record, names the following objectives in its 2001 mission statement:

Supporting all kinds of measures that contribute to academic teaching and research in the fields of ophthalmology and optometry;

Organisation, realisation and supplementary funding of medical research and instruction in the fields of ophthalmology and optometry while taking into account border areas ophthalmology shares with other medical specialties;

Supporting research at the Landesaugenklinik and the Verein zur Förderung der Landesaugenklinik; Targeted support for efforts undertaken by various institutions of the Province of Salzburg and Salzburg University to establish a Medical Faculty at Salzburg University;

Targeted support for contacts between the Landesaugenklinik Salzburg and national and international scientific institutions, clinics, and university departments,

General support for in-house training in the fields of ophthalmology and optometry for medical doctors specialising as ophthalmologists and optometrists: for general practitioners; for specialists of other medical specialties; members of other health-related professions, and for staff members of institutions of the health system, administration and scientific research institutions;

Cultivation of the memory of Prof. Dr. Ernst Fuchs and the Second Eye Clinic of the Medical University of Vienna, which he was in charge of;

Medical-historical research on the province of Salzburg with special attention to the St. Johanns-Spital, to the entire province of Salzburg and to ophthalmology.[1678]

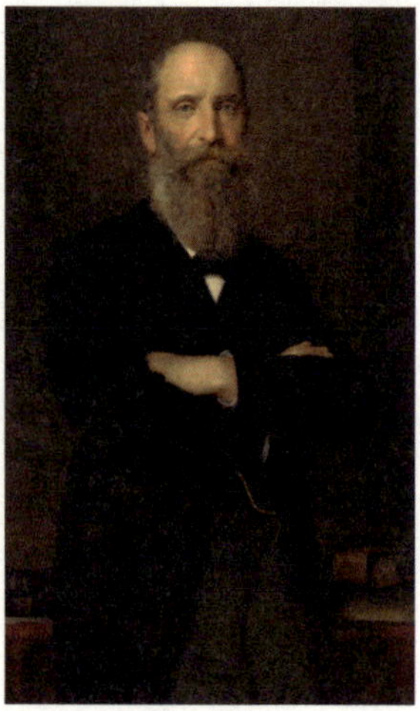

Fig. 140
Portrait of
Ernst Fuchs.
Painting by
R. Bitterlich, 1911

200th Anniversary of the Foundation of Vienna's University Eye Clinic (2012)

Founded in 1812, Vienna's University Eye Clinic changed in 1883 into the "twin clinic" of the First and Second Eye Clinic. It underwent a further change in 2004 when it became the Augenklinik der Medizinischen Universität Wien. In 2012 it solemnised its 200th anniversary. The specialist journal *Spektrum Augenheilkunde*[1679] rose to the occasion by publishing a special issue, which sought to do justice to the scientific and organisational achievements of the clinics' directors from the point of view of the history of medicine. In view of his worldwide reputation it goes without saying that Ernst Fuchs was accorded pride of place.[1680] (Fig. 140).

Notes

[1623] Wilhelm Fuchs, see Ch. 2.

[1624] FUCHS, *Augenarzt* (as in FN 2), p. 113.

[1625] Cf. FN 16.

[1626] Škoda had had this house with garden built in the immediate vicinity of the Allgem. Krankenhaus (9th district, Alserstrasse/Spitalgasse). When he died childless in 1881, ownership passed to his niece, one Baroness Perger. Fuchs purchased the house from her in 1897. Prior to this, when Fuchs returned from Liège to Vienna in the autumn of 1885, he had first set up residence in Alserstraße 28, before moving to nearby Oppolzergasse 9 in 1887. See: FUCHS, *Augenarzt* (as in FN 2), pp. 81–82.

[1627] The cause of death is given as *"arteriosclerosis, angina pectoris"* in the death certificate. See: Toten-Schein. Pfarre Alservorstadt. Sterbe-Buch Tom. 1930, fol. 87. Zahl 518, Pol. Bezirk: Wien, VIII. 10. December 1930. Original in the Family archive.

[1628] Cemetery of the parish of St. Vitus, Kritzendorf/Klosterneuburg. According to the In memoriam card, the funeral took place on 24 November 1930. (Original in the Family archive). For conservation reasons the headstone was transferred to an indoor location some time ago.

[1629] Proficient in ancient Greek since his days at Vienna's Schottengymnasium (see Ch. 1), Fuchs kept alive his interest in all things Greek – literature, history, culture, and art. When his beloved wife [Julie] died, he commissioned the sculptor Richard Bitterlich to make a headstone on the model of a Greek stele. Cf. Fig. 137. See: Maximilian SALZMANN, "Ernst Fuchs †". (Commemorative address, delivered to the mourning session of the Ophthalmol. Gesellsch. in Vienna on 15 Dec. 1930), in: *Zeitschr. Augenheilk.* 73 (1931), pp. 317–325.

[1630] Epilogue by Adalbert Fuchs, in: FUCHS, *Augenarzt* (as in FN 2), p. 118.

[1631] According to an undated list Fuchs compiled himself. Family archive.

[1632] See Ernst Fuchs's chronol. bibliography below.

[1633] (Ed.) "Der berühmte Augenarzt Hofrat Fuchs gestorben", in: *Neue Freie Presse* No. 23776 (evening ed.) of 22 Nov. 1930, p. 3; (Ed.) "Die letzten Säulen", in: *Neues Wiener Tagblatt* No. 23261 of 23 Nov. 1930.

[1634] (Ed.) "Trauersitzung zum Andenken an weil. Prof. Dr. Ernst Fuchs v. 28. November 1930 in der Gesellschaft der Ärzte in Wien: Offizielles Protokoll der Gesellschaft der Aerzte in Wien", in: *Wien. klin. Wochenschr.* (1930), pp. 1517–1520.

[1635] SALZMANN, *Ernst Fuchs †* (as in FN 1629).

[1636] See: Ch. 11: Ernst Fuchs Fund 1926/27.

[1637] Wiener Stadt- u. Landesarchiv (= WSTLA, previously Archiv d. Stadt Wien). Land Wien, Sammlung der Stiftbriefe No. 153, dated 9 January 1932, p. Z. 155 from 1930/31, p. 1. Cf. the Deed of Foundation in the holdings of the University Archive Vienna. Akademischer Senat Sonderreihe, Senat S 144.27. – ATS 34,000 in 1930 would have been the rough equivalent of €120,000 ($145,000) in today's money.

[1638] Ibid., p. 2, § 1.

[1639] Ibid., p. 3, § 3.

[1640] Ibid., § 4.

[1641] Ibid., § 6.

[1642] Rudolf Maresch (1868–1936). Originally from Klattau/Bohemia (today: Klatovy/Czech Republic). Studied at the Germ. Univ. Prag (Dr. med. 1895). Assist. at Prague's Pathol.-Anatom. Inst. under Hans Frh. v. Chiari (cf. FN 101). Continued his training at Vienna's Allgem. Krankenhaus under Karl Gussenbauer (Dir. of the 2nd Chir. Univ. Clinic, cf. FN 27) and Friedrich Schauta (1849–1919, Dir. of 1st Gynaec. Univ. Clinic, cf. FN 102). 1901 at the Serotherapeut. Inst. 1902 Assist. at the Inst. of Bacteriol. and Pathol. Histol. under Richard Paltauf (1858–1924, cf. FN 1228). 1906–1912 Prosector at the Rudolfspital. 1908 Habilitation in Path. Anat. at Vienna Univ. 1912–1925 Dir. of the morgue at Krankenhaus Lainz. 1915 tit. Assoc. Prof., 1923 Full Prof. and Dir. of the Inst. of Pathol. Anat. 1926/27 Dean of the Med. Fac., 1931/32 Rector of Vienna Univ. Deserves credit for the relaunch of his Institute and the Museum. See: CZEIKE (as in FN 13); EULNER (as in FN 13); *Feierl. Inauguration d. Rektors* [...] *1935/36*; FISCHER (as in FN 28); ÖBL (as in FN 11); Obituaries: *Zentralbl. allg. Pathol. u. patholog. Anat.* 65 (1936), pp. 1ff.; *Wien. klin. Wochenschr.* 49 (1936), pp. 497 ff.; *Wien. med. Wochenschr.* 86 (1936), cols. 145ff.; *Almanach Akad. Wissensch. Wien* 1936; *Münch. med. Wochenschr.* 83 (1936), pp. 612–613.

[1643] Roland Grassberger (1876–1956). Studied at Vienna Univ (Dr. med. 1892). From 1897 assist. at the Inst. of Hygiene of Vienna Univ. under Maximilian Ritter v. Gruber (1853–1927, cf. FN 104) and his successor Arthur Schattenfroh (1869–1923). 1902 Habilitation in Hygiene at Vienna Univ. (1906 Assoc. Prof., 1917 tit. Full Prof.). 1924–1936 Dir. of the Inst. of Hygiene of Vienna Univ. See: EULNER (as in FN 13); FISCHER (as in FN 28); NDB (as in FN 15).

[1644] Cf. FN 1637, p. 4.

[1645] Cf. FN 1637, WSTLA. Gau Wien. Sammlung der Stiftbriefe, No. 223; Zahl 489/41, p. 5, § 8.

[1646] Othmar Kühn (1892–1969). Studied sciences at Vienna Univ. (Dr. phil. 1919, botany). Joined the staff of Vienna's Naturhist. Museum. 1951–1964 Full Prof. of Palaeontol. and Palaeobiol. at Vienna Univ. Wien and Dir. of the Palaeontol. Inst.; 1957/58 Dean of the Philosoph. Fac., 1960/61 Rector of Vienna Univ. See: Obituary, in: *Mitteil. d. Geolog. Gesellsch. Wien* 62 (1969), pp. 175–184 (Fritz Steininger, with bibliography).

[1647] WSTLA (Archiv der Stadt Wien). Stiftbriefe 318.

[1648] No documents have come to light yet concerning the Foundation's dissolution.

[1649] Cf. FN 1252.

[1650] See Ch. 9.

[1651] Charles H. May (1861–1943). Originally from Baltimore. 1883 M. D. from Columbia Univ. College of Physicians and Surgeons. 1887 Ophthalmol. and otol. specialis. on a study trip to Halle/Saale and Berlin, where he met Hermann v. Helmholtz (cf. FN 125); to Vienna, where he spent about a year at the 2nd Univ. Eye Clinic under Ernst Fuchs, his assistant Friedrich Dimmer (cf. FN 44), Leopold Königstein (cf. FN 374), Adam Politzer (1835–1920) and Viktor v. Urbantschitsch (1847–1921)]; to Paris (Edmont Landolt, cf. FN 253), Xavier Galezowski (cf. FN 257), Louis de Wecker (cf. FN 252) and Photinos Panas (cf. FN 258)]; and to London (Moorfields Hospital). Lifelong friendship with Ernst Fuchs confirmed by many mutual visits. Consulting ophthalmol. at institutions such as the Mount Sinai Hospital, Bellevue Hospital and the French Hospital in New York City. Shared a practice with Henry Minsky (cf. FN 1446). 1888 Establishment of his own ophthalm. and otol. practice in New York City. Dir. of the Eye Clinic at Columbia University. 1914–1925 Dir. of Eye Service at the Bellevue Hospital, New York. 1900 Inventor of an ophthalmoscope with double disc. 1914 Construction of an electric ophthalmoscope, with was very widely used in his time. See: Charles H. MAY, "A New Electric Ophthalmoscope", in: *Ophthalmol. Record* 23 (1914), pp. 386–389; MAY, *Manual of Diseases of the Eye* (1900), which went through many editions and translations even after May 's death. Cf. IBBO (as in FN 18); Obituaries, in: *Arch. Ophthalmol.* 3 (1944), pp. 103–105 (C. A. Perera); *Brit. J. Ophthalmol.* 28 (1944), pp. 313–314 (K. Herbert); *Transact. Am. Ophthalmol. Soc.* 42 (1944), pp. 18.2–22 (William Brown Doherty).

[1652] Charles H. MAY, "Bronze Plaques of Professor Fuchs available", in: *Arch. Ophthalmol.* 8/5 (1932), p. 760; MAY, "Bronze plate of Professor Ernst Fuchs", in: *Am. J. Ophthalmol.* 16 (1933), p. 71.

[1653] See: "Ophthalmological Numismatics", in: *Arch. Ophthalmol.* 120/2 (2002), p. 246; accessible online at: https://jamanetwork.com (last accessed: 6 Sept. 2022).

[1654] See Ch. 9.

[1655] Cf. UA Wien, Senatsakten, No. 222.13 of 21 Oct. 1950.

[1656] See Ch. 9.

[1657] Karl LINDNER, "Zum 100. Geburtstage von Ernst Fuchs", in: *Wien. klin. Wochenschr.* 63 (1951), pp. 449–450.

[1658] Ibid., p. 450.

[1659] On its back the postcard bears the inscription "Aus der Fuchs-Festschrift / 5. Österreichische Ärztetagung Salzburg (*Wiener klinische Wochenschrift*, 63. Jahrgang/1951, No. 35/36)". Original in private collection.

[1660] "Offizielles Protokoll der Gesellschaft der Aerzte in Wien. Sitzung vom 22. Juni 1951", in: *Wien. klin. Wochenschr.* 63 (1951), p. 500.

[1661] Wolfgang Denk (1882–1970). Originally from Linz. Son of the ophthalmologist Karl Denk. Studied at Vienna Univ. (Dr. med. 1907). Surg. specialis. at the Landeskrankenhaus Linz. 1908 Spent several months working at the Inst. of General and Experim. Pathology under Richard Paltauf. 1908–1924 Assist. at the 1st Surg. Univ. Clinic under Anton v. Eiselsberg (cf. FN 745). 1916 Habilitation in Surgery at Vienna Univ.; tit. Assoc. Prof. 1923. 1924–1928 Dir. of the Surgical Dept. of the Krankenanstalt Rudolfstiftung in Vienna. 1928 Full Prof. and Dir. of the Surg. Univ. Clinic Graz. 1931–1953 in the same function at the 2nd Surg. Univ. Clinic in Vienna. 1946–1968 Pres. of the Gesellschaft d. Ärzte in Wien. 1946–1958 Pres. of the Supreme Medical Council [Oberster Sanitätsrat]. 1948/49 Rector of Vienna Univ.; great interest in research on cancer. Succeeded in the year he became Prof. emerit. in founding the Institut für Krebsforschung, which he headed until 1960. See: CZEIKE (as in FN 13); FISCHER (as in FN 28); Obituaries: *Almanach d. Österr. Akad. d. Wiss. 1971*; *Wien. klin. Wochenschr.* 82 (1970), pp. 245–246 (H. Kunz); 83 (1971), p. 742 (H. Kunz); *Wien. med. Wochenschr.* 120 (1970), pp. 141–142 (G. Salzer); Helmut WYKLICKY, "Historisches zum Krebsproblem. In memoriam Wolfgang Denk", in: *Der praktische Arzt* 37 (1983), pp. 249ff.

[1662] As in FN 1660.

[1663] Arnold PILLAT, "Der Beitrag der Wiener Schule zur Augenheilkunde", in: *Wien. klin. Wochenschr.* 63 (1951), pp. 614–617. Two years later, this keynote was published in English: Arnold PILLAT, "The Contribution of the Vienna School to Ophthalmology", in: *Am. J. Ophthalmol.* 36/1 (1953), pp. 15–25.

[1664] See Ch. 4.

[1665] Leopold Arzt (1883–1955). Studied at Vienna Univ. (Dr. med. 1908). Habilitation in Dermatol. and Syphilidol. 1926 Full Prof. and Dir. of the Univ. Clinic of Skin and Sexually Transmitted Diseases. After Austria's Anschluss dismissed from his post for political reasons and imprisoned. After the end of World War II reinstated as Dir. of Clinic 1945–1954. Reorganised the Gesellschaft d. Ärzte after the end of the Nazi regime, which was in itself a major feat. See: CZEIKE (as in FN 13).

[1666] Leopold ARZT, "Ernst Fuchs, dem Mitbegründer der *Wiener klinischen Wochenschrift* zum 100. Geburtstag", in: *Wien. klin. Wochenschr.* 63 (1951), pp. 449–450.

[1667] *Wien. klin. Wochenschr.* 63 (1951), Nos. 35/36.

[1668] Karl LINDNER, "Einiges über die Keratoplastik", in: Ibid, pp. 627–628; Arnold PILLAT, "Histologische Befunde am Auge bei konnataler Toxoplasmose", in: Ibid., pp. 628–630; Gustav SCHUBERT, "Die Leistungen der Augenmuskeln und ihre Steuerung", in: Ibid., pp. 632–634; Helmut FANTA, "Hochdruck und Auge", in: Ibid., pp. 649–652; Karl HRUBY, *Über die Entwicklung und den gegenwärtigen Stand der Biomikroskopie des Auges*, in: Ibid., pp. 669–672; N. MOSCHIK de REYA, O. EICHHORN, "Zur Registrierung der bioelektrischen Erscheinungen bei Augenbewegungen", in: Ibid., pp. 676–677; Ludwig Bertrand PSENNER, "*Über röntgenologische Veränderungen bei Arachnitis optico-chiasmatis*", in: Ibid., pp. 679–680; H. RIEGER, "Toxoplasmose", in: Ibid., pp. 680–683; H. ROTTER, "Ueber die Verbesserung des Sehvermögens aphaker Augen ohne Starglas durch Mintacol", in: Ibid., pp. 683–684; Ludwig von SALLMANN, Ira S. JONES, Robert L. WIGGINS,

Beatrice D. LOCKE, "Ueber den Einfluß von Cortison auf Wundheilung, Makrophagozytose und Kapillarpermeabilität im Auge", in: Ibid., pp. 684–686; A. ZWIEAUER, "Ueber die Möglichkeit einer Behandlung von entzündlichen Erkrankungen des vorderen Abschnittes mit Tromoxan", in: Ibid., pp. 697–698.; Rudolf BINDER, "Beitrag zur Zellentwicklung im menschlichen Hornhautepithel", in: Ibid., pp. 701–705; U. R. NEMETZ, "Behandlungsversuche mit ACTH bei Augenerkrankungen", in: Ibid., p. 711–713.

1669 See e. g.: James E. LEBENSOHN, "Professor Ernst Fuchs (June 14, 1851–November 21, 1930)", in: *Am. J. Ophthalmol.* 34 (1951), pp. 772–774; B. CARRERAS DURÁN, "Profesor Ernesto Fuchs", in: *Archivios de la Sociedad Oftalmológica Hispano-Americana* (1951); "Prof. Ernest Fuchs", in: *Revista brasileira de oftalmologia 9* (1951), p. 227.

1670 Erna Lesky (1911–1986). Originally from Hartberg/Styria. Studied at the Univ. of Innsbruck and Vienna (Dr. med. univ. 1936). Special. initially in paediatrics. Married Prof. of Classics Albin Lesky (1896–1981). 1949 Began to study history (Dr. phil. 1955). 1957 Habilitation in History of Medicine at the Med. Fac. of Vienna Univ. 1960 Dir. of the Institute for the History of Medicine at the Josephinum; renovation; reorganisation of the Institute's holdings (library, manuscript collection, picture archive). In collaboration with Helmut Wyklicky (cf. FN 1673) relaunch of a museum featuring the history of the Vienna Medical School. This relaunch gave the Institute under Lesky's direction a worldwide reputation. Main works: *Die Wiener Medizinische Schule im 19. Jahrhundert* (1965), *Wien und die Weltmedizin* (1974), *Meilensteine der Wiener Medizin in drei Jahrhunderten* (1980). See: GERABEK et al. (as in FN 13), Obituary: *Wien. klin. Wochenschr.* 99 (1987), pp. 27–30 (Helmut Wyklicky).

1671 Jutta LAUBER, Helmut WYKLICKY, *150 Jahre Wiener Augenheilkunde* (The year 1812 saw the establishment of the world's first University Eye Clinic in Vienna). "Das Institut für Geschichte der Medizin in Wien (Leitung: Doz. E. Lesky) in Verbindung mit der I. Universitäts-Augenklinik Wien (Vorstand: Prof. A. Pillat), II. Universitäts-Augenklinik Wien (Vorstand: J. Böck), Universitäts-Augenklinik der Univ. Graz (Vorstand: K. Hruby) stellt Dokumente, Handschriften, Publikationen, Bilder und Instrumente aus". Exhibition catalogue 1–30 June 1962. Eigenverlag der Wiener medizinischen Akademie für ärztliche Fortbildung, Vienna 1962.

1672 Ibid., p. 15. Extension of the permanent loan agreement dated 25 July 2018. (Person. information passed on to the author by Mag. Dipl.-Ing. Raimund Hofbauer/Kritzendorf).

1673 Helmut Wyklicky (1921–2007). Originally from Troppau (until 1918 located in an Austrian Crownland, the Duchy of Upper and Lower Silesia, today Opava/Czech Republic). Studied at the German University Prague and at Vienna Univ. (Dr. med. univ. 1947). 1948 Emergency doctor with Vienna's Ambulance Service. Junior doctor at the two Univ. Clinics of Intern. Medicine at the Allgem. Krankenhaus. 1959 Internist. From his student days he had worked at the Institute for the History of Medicine under Fritz Lejeune (1892–1966) and Leopold Schönbauer (1888–1963). 1960 Assistant under Erna Lesky (cf. FN 1670). 1975 Habilitation in History of Medicine at the University of Vienna, 1981–1988 Full prof. and Dir. of the Institute. See: Gabriela SCHMIDT-WYKLICKY, "In memoriam Helmut Wyklicky", in: *Wien. med. Wochenschr.* 158 (2008), pp. 745–748.

[1674] See their website: http://ascrs.org.

[1675] Cf. http://ascrs.org/honorees/ernst-fuchs-md (last accessed: 6 Sept. 2022). A list naming all honorees is accessible at: http://ascrs.org/awards/ascrs-ophthalmology-hall-fame (last accessed: 6 Sept. 2022).

[1676] Cf. Fuchs Stiftung zur Förderung der Augenheilkunde (Privatstiftung). St. Johanns-Spital, Müllner Hauptstraße 48, 5020 Salzburg, FN 204652 i. Stiftungsurkunde. Solemn plenary session of the Fuchs Stiftung zur Förderung der Augenheilkunde on 11 October 2001.

[1677] See their website: http://www.fuchsstiftung.at.

[1678] Ibid., p. 2–3.

[1679] Helmut GRÖGER, Gabriela SCHMIDT-WYKLICKY, "200 Jahre Universitäts-Augenklinik Wien", in: *Spektrum Augenheilk.* 26 (2012), pp. 263–356.

[1680] Gabriela SCHMIDT-WYKLICKY, Helmut GRÖGER, "Ernst Fuchs. Vorstand der II. Universitäts-Augenklinik in Wien 1885 bis 1915. Wien als weltweites Zentrum der Ophthalmopathologie", in: Ibid., pp. 312–318.

13. Catalogue of Published Works

A bibliography comprising all the published works by Ernst Fuchs has not been attempted before. Printoffs of original works have not come down to us in the form in which Fuchs had originally caused them to be filed. Only the folder has been preserved in which Ernst Fuchs himself filed works that had been published before he retired.[1681]

More than five decades ago the Vienna medical historian Erna Lesky, sifting through Ernst Fuchs's papers, had asked his son Adalbert for help. In a letter from Merano dated 4 December 1969 Adalbert informed her that to his great regret the bulk of his father's scientific papers had been lost:

The stenogram of my father's autobiography, the 5 bound volumes of my father's Separata,[1682] *the 15 volumes of my father's record of 'special cases', and approx. 20 travel diaries have been stolen from the library of N[ew] Y[ork] U[niversity].*[1683]

To account for Ernst Fuchs's very substantial scientific oeuvre[1684] in a manner that does justice to it required taking account of all available sources in a laborious effort of reconstruction.

1. "Herpes iris conjunctivae". Beobachtet an der Klinik des Professor von Arlt, in: Klin. Monatsbl. Augenheilk. 14 (1876), pp. 333–351.
2. "Ueber Keratitis traumatica". Vorläufige Mitteilung, in: Centralbl. med. Wissensch. 14 (1876), pp. 113–114.
3. "Ueber die traumatische Keratitis", in: Virchows Archiv 66 (1876), pp. 401–445.
4. "Beitrag zur Kenntnis des Froschblutes und der Froschlymphe", in: *Virchows Archiv* 71 (1877), pp. 78–107.
5. "Cysticercus subconjunctivalis". Casuistische Beobachtung aus der Augenklinik des Professor von Arlt in Wien, in: *Klin. Monatsbl. Augenheilk.* 15 (1877), pp. 396–402.
6. "Zur Farbe der Netzhaut", in: *Wien. med. Wochenschr.* 27 (1877), col. 221.
7. "Ruptura retinae", in: *Klin. Monatsbl. Augenheilk.* 15 (1877), pp. 422–431.
8. "Ueber das Chalazion und über einige seltenere Lidgeschwülste", in: *Graefes Archiv* 24. Abtheil. II (1878), pp. 121–168.
9. "Die Lymphgefässe der Lider". Vorläufige Mitteilung, in: *Centralbl. med. Wissensch.* 16 (1878), pp. 497–498.
10. "Zur Anatomie der Blut- und Lymphgefässe der Augenlider", in: *Graefes Archiv* 24/ Abtheil. III (1878), pp. 1–58 and 24/ Abtheil IV (1878), Table IVa.
11. "Chorioiditis bei Glaucom", in: *Bericht über die XI. Versammlung der Ophthalmologischen Gesellschaft*. Heidelberg 1878. Redigirt durch F. C. Donders, W. Hess u. W. Zehender. Universitäts-Buchdruckerei von Adler's Erben. Rostock 1878, pp. 65ff.
12. "Tarsitis syphilitica", in: *Klin. Monatsbl. Augenheilk.* 16 (1878), pp. 21–28.
13. "Verwendung des Pilokarpins in Augenkrankheiten", in: *Wien. med. Wochenschr.* 28 (1878) cols. 997–999 and 1013–1017.

14. "Ueber die Wärmeempfindung der Hornhaut", in: *Medizinische Jahrbücher* herausgegeben von der k. k. Gesellschaft der Ärzte. Wilhelm Braumüller. Wien 1878, pp. 577–579.
15. "Cystöse Erweiterung eines Thränenröhrchens", in: *Klin. Monatsbl. Augenheilk.* 17 (1879), pp. 355–358.
16. "a) Keratitis bullosa. b) Verbreitung des Sarkoms in der Chorioidea (Demonstration)", in: F. C. DONDERS et al. (eds.), Bericht über die XII. Versammlung der Ophthalm. Gesellschaft zu Heidelberg 1879. Univ.-Buchdruckerei von Adler's Erben. Rostock 1880, pp. 212ff.
17. "Neuritis in Folge hereditärer Anlage", in: *Klin. Monatsbl. Augenheilk.* 17 (1879), pp. 332–337.
18. "Homatropinum hydrobromatum", in: *Centralbl. prakt. Augenheilk.* 4 (1880), pp. 182–184.
19. "Dacryocystitis mit Durchbruch in das orbitale Zellgewebe", in: *Centralbl. prakt. Augenheilk.* 4 (1880), pp. 252–253.
20. "Dermoid der Cornea", in: *Klin. Monatsbl. f. Augenheilk.* 18 (1880), pp. 131–134.
21. "Vollständige Sequestration der Cornea nach einfacher Linearextraction", in: *Klin. Monatsbl. f. Augenheilk.* 18 (1880), pp. 134–139.
22. "The use of the actual cautery in ulceration of the cornea", in: *Brit. Med. J.* 1880, II, p. 780 (48th Congress, Brit. Med. Assoc. 1880, Section of Ophthalmology) and *Annal. d'ocul.* 84 (1880), p. 242.
23. "Über die Anwendung des Ferrum cadens bei Hornhauterkrankungen", in: *Anzeiger der k. k. Gesellschaft der Aerzte in Wien*, Minutes of the session on 11 February 1881, pp. 145–146.
24. "Die Anwendung des Glüheisens bei Hornhautleiden", in: *Wien. med. Wochenschschr.* 31 (1881), cols. 621–624.
25. "Zur Behandlung der Conjunctivitis gonorrhoica", in: *Centralbl. prakt. Augenheilk.* 5 (1881), pp. 198–200.
26. "Ueber eine neue entoptische Erscheinung bei Bewegung des Augapfels", in: *Graefes Archiv* 27/ Abtheil. III (1881), pp. 43–46.
27. "Ueber glaukomatöse Hornhauttrübung", in: *Bericht über die Dreizehnte Versammlung der Ophthalmologischen Gesellschaft.* Heidelberg 1881. Ed. by F. C. Donders et al., Universitäts-Buchdruckerei von Adler's Erben. Rostock 1881, pp. 73–79 (Discussion pp. 79–80).
28. "Zur Therapie der Blenorrhoea gonorrhoica", in: *Centralbl. Augenheilk.* 1881.
29. "Ueber die Trübung der Hornhaut bei Glaucom", in: *Graefes Archiv* 27/Abtheil. III (1881), pp. 66–92.
30. "Melanoma iridis", in: *Archiv Augenheilk.* 11 (1882), pp. 435–439.
31. "Aneurysma arterio-venosum retinae", in: *Archiv Augenheilk.* 11 (1882), pp. 440–444.
32. "Beitrag zu den angeborenen Anomalien des Sehnerven", in: *Graefes Archiv* 28/Abth. I (1882), pp. 139–169.
33. *Das Sarcom des Uvealtractus.* Wilhelm Braumüller, Wien 1882. (Habilitation thesis).
34. "Anatomische Miscellen. I. Prolapsus chorioideae. II. Iridodialysis spontanea", in: *Graefes Archiv* 29/Abth. IV (1883), pp. 209–230.
35. "Angeborene Bildungsanomalie in der Chorioidea", in: *Archiv Augenheilk.* 12 (1883), pp. 1–3.
36. "Melanoma of the Iris", in: *Arch. Ophthalmol.* 12 (1883), pp. 26–31.

37. “Arterio-venous Aneurism in the Retina”. (Transl. by William C. Ayres), in: *Arch. Ophthalmol.* 12 (1883), pp. 32–36.
38. “Congenital Anomaly in the Choroid”. (Transl. by S. M. Burnett), in: *Arch. Ophthalmol.* 12 (1883), pp. 37–39.
39. “Beiträge zu den Anomalien der Refraction und Accommodation. (Zur Entstehung der Myopie/ Myopie bei Cataracta senilis incipiens/ Sympathische Accommodationslähmung)”, in: *Klin. Monatsbl. Augenheilk.* 22 (1884), pp. 14–24.
40. “Beiträge zur normalen Anatomie des Augapfels”, in: *Graefes Archiv* 30/Abth. IV (1884), pp. 1–60.
41. “Anatomische Miscellen: III. Glaucoma inflammatorium. IV. Iritis syphilitica”, in: *Graefes Archiv* 30/Abth. III (1884), pp. 123–138 and 139–156.
42. “Klinische Miscellen”, in: *Archiv Augenheilk.* 14 (1884), pp. 385ff.
43. “La prophylaxie de l’ophtalmie du nouveau-né”, in: *Annales d’Oculistique* 101 (1884), p. 187 and *Revue scientifique* 33 (1884), pp. 493–496.
44. “Zur Anatomie der Iris”, in: *Klin. Monatsbl. Augenheilk.* 23 (1885), pp. 467–478.
45. “Angiome de la face et des paupières guérie par l’électrolyse”, in: *Soc. Méd.-Chirurg. de Liège*. Févr. 1885.
46. “Antrittsrede gehalten bei Eröffnung seiner Vorlesungen an der Wiener Universität, Montag den 19. October 1885”, in: *Wien. med. Blätter* 8 (1885), pp. 1301–1304.
47. “Die periphere Atrophie des Sehnerven”, in: *Graefes Archiv* 31/Abth. I (1885), pp. 177–200.
48. “Beiträge zur normalen Anatomie der menschlichen Iris”, in: *Graefes Archiv* 31/Abth. III (1885), pp. 39–86.
49. “Etude microscopique sur le nerf optique”, in: *Arch. d’Ophtalmol.* 1885), p. 173 (Soc. Franç. d’Ophtalmol.) and *Bullet. Soc. Franç. d’Ophtalmol.* 3 (1885), p. 116.
50. “Klinische Miscellen I. Eigenthümliche Form muskulärer Asthenopie”, in: *Arch. Augenheilk.* 14 (1885), pp. 385–391.
51. “Les lésions anatomiques dans l’atrophie du nerf optique”, in: *Bull. Soc. Franç. d’Ophtalmol.* 1885.
52. “Klinische Miscellen. II. Sehstörung durch Anisometropie; III. Angeborene abnorme Kürze der Lider; IV. Freie Cyste in der vorderen Kammer”, in: *Archiv Augenheilk.* 15 (1885), pp. 1–11.
53. “On Congenital Shortness of the Eyelids”, in: *Med. Times and Gaz.* June 13, 1885, p. 776–777.
54. *Die Ursachen und die Verhütung der Blindheit.* Gekrönte Preisschrift. Herausgegeben durch die Society for the Prevention of Blindness in London. J. F. Bergmann, Wiesbaden 1885.
55. *Causes et la prévention de la cécité.* (Mémoire couronné) Traduction par le Docteur Fieuzal. G. Steinheil, Paris 1885.
56. *The Causes and the Prevention of Blindness.* The Essay which gained the Prize of £80 offered by the Society for the Prevention of Blindness in London. Translated by R. E. Dudgeon. With a few notes by M. Roth. Baillière, Tindall & Cox, London 1885.
57. *O prichinakh i preduprezhdenii sliepoty.* Perevod s niemetskavo. E. I. Fyodorov, Kiev 1885.
58. “Discussion über malignes Glaucom”, in: *Bericht über d. XVIII. Versamml. d. ophth. Gesellsch. zu Heidelberg* 1886, p. 11.
59. “Tuberkulose der Conjunctiva”, in: *Wien. med. Presse* (1886), p. 157.
60. “Syphilitische Papel des Ciliarkörpers”, in: *Wien. med. Bl.* (1886), No. 25.

61. "Fall von syphilitischer Geschwulst des Ciliarkörpers", in: *Wien. med. Presse* (1886) No. 26 (Gesellschaft der Ärzte in Wien, Meeting on July 11, 1886).
62. "Zwei Fälle von Melanosarkom der Iris", in: *Münch. med. Wochenschr.* (1887), p. 905.
63. "Ferdinand von Arlt †", in: *Wien. med. Blätter* 10 (1887), pp. 317–321.
64. "Über traumatische Linsentrübung", in: *Wien. klin. Wochenschr.* 1 (1888), pp. 53–57 and 86–88.
65. "Die Entzündungen des Lidrandes", in: *Wien. klin. Wochenschr.* 1 (1888), pp. 773–776 and 807–810.
66. "Zwei Fälle von doppelseitiger Ptosis", in: *Wien. med. Wochenschr.* 39 (1889), No. 52.
67. *Lehrbuch der Augenheilkunde.* Franz Deuticke. Leipzig/Vienna 1889.
68. "Franz Cornelius Donders †", in: *Wien. klin. Wochenschr.* 2 (1889), pp. 271–272.
69. "Keratitis punctata superficialis", in: *Wien. klin. Wochenschr.* 2 (1889), pp. 837–841.
70. "Aus Professor Dr. Ernst Fuchs's Klinik und Ambulatorium für Augenkrankheiten", in: Ernst LANDESMANN, *Die Therapie an den Wiener Kliniken. Ein Verzeichniss der wichtigsten, an denselben gebräuchlichen Heilmethoden und Recepte.* 2nd ed., Franz Deuticke. Leipzig/Vienna 1890, pp. 534–548.
71. "Otto Becker †", in: *Wien. klin. Wochenschr.* 3 (1890), p. 159.
72. "Ueber Blepharophimosis", in: *Wien. klin. Wochenschr.* 3 (1890), pp. 2–3.
73. "Intorno alle cause della cecità ed al modo di prevenirla: Saggio tradotto e pubblicato a cura della società italiana di prevenzione della cecità". Tip. Bonducciana A. Meozzi, Firenze 1890.
74. "Ueber isolirte doppelseitige Ptosis", in: *Graefes Archiv* 36/Abth. I (1890), pp. 234–259.
75. "Tenonitis nach Influenza". (Mitgeteilt in der Sitzung der k. k. Gesellschaft der Aerzte in Wien am 28. Februar 1890), in: *Wien. klin. Wochenschr.* 3 (1890), pp. 206–208.
76. "Zur Anatomie der Pinguecula", in: *Graefes Archiv* 37/Abth. III (1891), pp. 143–191.
77. "Ueber Linsenpräcipitate", in: Richard DEUTSCHMANN, *Beiträge zur Augenheilkunde in Gemeinschaft mit E. Fuchs, O. Haab, A. Vossius.* III. Heft. Hamburg & Leipzig 1890–1891, pp. 201–207.
78. "Gleichzeitige Erkrankung der Thränendrüsen und der Parotiden", in: Richard DEUTSCHMANN (ed.), *Beiträge zur Augenheilkunde.* III. Heft. Leopold Voss, Hamburg/Leipzig 1890–1891, pp. 208–215.
79. "Ueber einen Fall von angeborenen Hornhauttrübungen mit vorderer Synechie bei Mikrophthalmus congenitus", in: Klin. Monatsbl. Augenheilk. 29 (1891), pp. 331–340.
80. *Lehrbuch der Augenheilkunde.* 2nd, enlarged ed., Franz Deuticke, Leipzig/Vienna 1891.
81. *Manuel d'Ophtalmologie.* Traduit sur la deuxième édition allemande par le Docteur C. Lacompte et le Docteur L. Leplat. Georges Carré, Paris 1892.
82. "Der gegenwärtige Stand der Staroperation". (Zuschriften an Landolt), in: Richard DEUTSCHMANN (ed.), *Beiträge zur Augenheilkunde in Gemeinschaft mit E. Fuchs, O. Haab, A. Vossius.* VI. und VII. Heft. Leopold Voss, Hamburg/Leipzig 1892.
83. *Text-Book of Ophthalmology. Authorized translation from the second enlarged and improved German edition by A. Duane.* D. Appleton & Co., New York 1892.
84. "Ueber das Pterygium", in: *Graefes Archiv* 38/Abth. II (1892), pp. 1–90.

85. "Association von Lidbewegung mit seitlichen Bewegungen des Auges, in: R. DEUTSCHMANN (ed.), *Beiträge zur Augenheilkunde in Gemeinschaft mit E. Fuchs, O. Haab, A. Vossius*. XI. Heft. Leopold Voss, Hamburg/Leipzig 1893, pp. 12–30.
86. "Über Aufhellung von Hornhautnarben", in: Richard DEUTSCHMANN (ed.), *Beiträge zur Augenheilkunde in Gemeinschaft mit E. Fuchs, O. Haab, A. Vossius*. IX issue. Leopold Voss, Hamburg/Leipzig 1893, pp. 1–11.
87. *Lehrbuch der Augenheilkunde*. 3rd enlarged ed. Franz Deuticke, Leipzig/Vienna 1893.
88. *Leseproben für die Nähe*. Vienna 1893.
89. "Die neuen Methoden der Staaroperation". Address delivered to the meeting of the k.k. Gesellschaft der Aerzte in Wien on 16 December 1892, in: *Wien. klin. Wochenschr.* (1893), pp. 19–23.
90. "Retinitis circinata", in: *Graefes Archiv* 39 /Abth. III (1893), pp. 229–279.
91. *Tratado de enfermedades de los ojos*. Traducido por D. Victor Cebrián y Diez. Con un prólogo del Dr. Osío. Teodoro, Madrid 1893.
92. "Die ägyptische Augenentzündung", in: *Wien. klin. Wochenschr.* 7 (1894), pp. 211–214.
93. "Egyptian Ophthalmia", in: *The Medical Age. A SemiMonthly Review of Medicine* 12 (1894), pp. 262–267.
94. "Fall von einer angeborenen Trübung der Cornea", in: *Aerztl. Centr. Anz. Wien* 6 (1894), pp. 235.
95. "Ein Fall von angeborener Trübung der Hornhaut", in: *Wien. med. Bl.* 17 (1894), pp. 197–180.
96. "Keratomykosis aspergillina", in: *Wien. klin. Wochenschr.* 7 (1894), pp. 305–307.
97. "Ueber Keratoplastik", in: *Wien. klin. Wochenschr.* 7 (1894), pp. 843–845.
98. *Lehrbuch der Augenheilkunde*. 4. enlarged ed., Franz Deuticke, Leipzig/Vienna 1894.
99. "Episcleritis periodica fugax", in: Sixty-Third Annual Meeting of the British Medical Association: July 30th–August 1st, London 1895. Section of Ophthalmology. *Brit. Med. J.* 2 /1816 (1895), pp. 951–953.
100. "Ueber Episkleritis periodica fugax", in: *Graefes Archiv* 41/Abth. IV (1895), pp. 229–273 and *Wien. klin. Wochenschr.* 8 (1895), pp. 601–603.
101. "Ueber Erythropsie", in: *Bericht über die Vierundzwanzigste Versammlung der Ophthalmologischen Gesellschaft*. Heidelberg 1895. Ed. W. Hess and W. Zehender. (= Ausserordentliches Beilageheft zu den *Klin. Monatsbl. Augenheilk*. Year XXXIII). Ferdinand Enke, Stuttgart 1895, pp. 4–17 and *Aerztl. Centr.-Anz., Wien* 7 (1895), p. 421 and translated in: *Ophthalmol. Rev. London* 14 (1895), p. 241.
102. "Ein Fall von Atrophie der Lidhaut", in: *Wien. med. Wochenschr.* 46 (1895), No. 51.
103. *Lehrbuch der Augenheilkunde*. Japanese Translation by Tatsushichiro Inouye and Y. Morosumi. Asakaya, Tokio 1895
104. *Lehrbuch der Augenheilkunde*. 5th enlarged ed., Franz Deuticke, Leipzig/Vienna 1895.
105. *Leseproben für die Nähe. Jäger's Schriftscalen modifiziert von Professor Dr. E. Fuchs*. 2nd ed. Fritsch, Vienna 1895.
106. "Über Blepharochalasis (Erschlaffung der Lidhaut)". Patient presentation in the meeting of the Gesellschaft der Aerzte in Vienna on 6 December 1895, in: *Wien. klin. Wochenschr.* 9 (1896), pp. 109–110.
107. "Denkrede auf Arlt. Gehalten am 9. Juli 1896 bei der Enthüllung seines Denkmals im Arkadenhof der Universität Wien", in: Anton BETTELHEIM (ed.), *Biographische*

Blätter. Jahrbuch für lebensgeschichtliche Kunst und Forschung. Vol. 2. Hofmann & Co., Berlin 1896, pp. 384–388.

108. "Ueber Erythropsie", in: *Graefes Archiv* 42/Abth. IV (1896), pp. 207–292.
109. "Über Schneeblindheit". Address delivered on 4 March 1896, in: *Schriften des Vereins zur Verbreitung naturwissenschaftlicher Erkenntnisse in Wien*. 36th vol., 1895/96. (= Populäre Vorträge aus allen Fächern der Naturwissenschaft). Ed. Verein zur Verbreitung naturwissenschaftlicher Kenntnisse in Wien. 3. Cyklus. Selbstverlag in Commission bei W. Braumüller & Sohn, pp. 275–299.
110. "Ueber zwei der Retinitis pigmentosa verwandte Krankheiten (Retinitis punctata albescens und Atrophia gyrata chorioideae et retinae", in: *Archiv Augenheilk.* 32 (1896), pp. 111–116.
111. *Lehrbuch der Augenheilkunde*. 6th enlarged ed. F. Deuticke, Leipzig/Vienna 1897.
112. *Manuel d'ophtalmologie*. Seconde édition française, traduite sur la cinquième édition allemande par C. Lacompte et L. Leplat, G. Carré & C. Naud, Paris 1897.
113. *Rukovodstwo k glasnym bolsnjam*. (Textbook of Ophthalmology). Russian translation by A. V. Natanson und L. E. Vorontsova, based on the fifth edition of the *Lehrbuch*, St. Petersburg 1897.
114. "Ueber Pilzrasen auf der Bindehaut", in: *Bericht über die 25. Versammlung der Ophthalmologischen Gesellschaft*. Heidelberg 1896. Bergmann, Wiesbaden 1897, pp. 173–178.
115. "Ueber Transfixion der Iris", in: *Bericht über die fünfundzwanzigste Versammlung der Ophthalmologischen Gesellschaft*. Heidelberg 1896. J. F. Bergmann, Wiesbaden 1897, pp. 179–180.
116. *Trattato di oftalmiatria, ad uso degli studenti e di medici pratici*. Traduzione italiana eseguita sull'ultima edizione tedesca dal dott. Gius. Cirincione, con prefazione del Prof. Carlo de Vincentiis, Casa Edit. Dott. V. Pasquale, Napoli 1897.
117. "Ueber Concremente in der Bindehaut", in: *Graefes Archiv* 46/Abth. I (1898), pp. 103–142.
118. "Two diseases related to retinitis pigmentosa: retinitis punctata albescens and atrophia gyrata choroideae et retinae", in: *Arch. Ophth.* 27 (1898), p. 484–489.
119. *Lehrbuch der Augenheilkunde*. 7th enlarged ed., Franz Deuticke, Leipzig/Vienna 1898.
120. *Text-Book of Ophthalmology*. Authorized Translation from the Second Enlarged and Improved German Edition by A. Duane. D. Appleton and Company, New York 1898.
121. "Zur operativen Behandlung hochgradiger Kurzsichtigkei"t, in: *Wien. klin. Wochenschr.* (1899), p. 125.
122. *Text-Book of Ophthalmology.* Authorized Translation. Revised from the Seventh Enlarged and Improved German Edition by A. Duane. Second American Edition. D. Appleton and Company, New York 1899.
123. "Ablösung der Aderhaut nach Staaroperation", in: *Graefes Archiv* 51 (1900), pp. 199–224.
124. "Ablösung der Aderhaut nach Staaroperation", in: *Bericht über die 28. Versammlung d. Ophthalmol. Gesellsch. Heidelberg* 1900. J. F. Bergmann, Wiesbaden 1901, pp. 84–87.
125. "Über Aufhellung von Hornhautnarben", in: Richard DEUTSCHMANN (ed.), *Beiträge zur praktischen Augenheilkunde*. Issue 44 (1900), pp. 117–118.
126. *Lehrbuch der Augenheilkunde*. 8th enlarged ed. Franz Deuticke, Leipzig/Vienna 1900.

127. "Demonstration von Präparaten eines beginnenden Melanosarkoms der Aderhaut", in: *Bericht über die 28. Versammlung der Ophthalmologischen Gesellschaft Heidelberg 1900*. Bergmann, Wiesbaden 1901, pp. 197–199.
128. "Emphysem am Auge", in: *Wien. klin. Wochenschr.* 14 (1901), No. 4.
129. "Der centrale schwarze Fleck bei Myopie", in: *Zeitschr. Augenheilk.* 5 (1901), pp. 171–178.
130. "Ueber ringförmige und scheibenförmige Keratitis (Keratitis annularis et disciformis)", in: *Klin. Monatsbl. f. Augenheilk.* (1901), pp. 513–523.
131. "Zur Keratoplastik", in: *Zeitschr. Augenheilk.* 5 (1901), pp. 1–5.
132. "Ueber Randsklerose und Randatrophie der Hornhaut", in: *Graefes Archiv* 52 (1901), pp. 317–329.
133. "Ueber die Sichtbarkeit des Schlemm'schen Canals am lebenden Auge", in: *Bericht über die 28. Versammlung der Ophthalmol. Gesellsch. Heidelberg 1900*. Bergmann, Wiesbaden 1901, p. 136.
134. *Text-Book of Ophthalmology*. Authorized translation, revised from the seventh enlarged and improved German edition by A. Duane. D. Appleton and Company, New York 1901.
135. "Das Ulcus atheromatosum corneae (seqestrirende Narbenkeratitis)", in: *Graefes Archiv* 53 (1901), pp. 61–73.
136. "Zur Veränderung der Macula lutea nach Kontusion", in: *Zeitschr. Augenheilk.* 6 (1901), pp. 181ff.
137. "Ablösung der Aderhaut nach Operation", in: *Graefes Archiv* 53 (1902), pp. 375–400.
138. "Ueber Cocain", in: *Wien. klin. Wochenschr.* 15 (1902), pp. 962–964.
139. "On Keratitis". The Bowman Lecture, delivered on June 13, 1902, in: *Transact. Ophthalmol. Soc. of the United Kingdom*, London 22 (1902).
140. "Ueber knötchenförmige Hornhauttrübung", in: *Graefes Archiv* 53 (1902), pp. 423–438.
141. *Lehrbuch der Augenheilkunde*. 9th enlarged ed. Franz Deuticke, Leipzig/Vienna 1903.
142. "Scleritis posterior", in: *Bericht ueber die 30. Versammlung der Ophthalmologischen Gesellschaft in Heidelberg*. 1902, pp. 71–77.
143. "Ueber Ringabscess der Hornhaut", in: *Graefes Archiv* 56 (1903), pp. 1–31.
144. "Anatomische Veränderungen bei Entzündung der Aderhaut", in: *Graefes Archiv* 58 (1904), pp. 391–428.
145. "Ueber sympathisierende Entzündung (nebst Bemerkungen über seröse traumatische Iritis)", in: *Graefes Archiv* 61 (1905), pp. 365–456.
146. "Hypophysentumor", in: *Wien. klin. Wochenschr.* 18 (1905), pp. 236–237.
147. "Kalkeinlagerungen in der Hornhaut", in: *Bericht über die Versammlung der Ophthalmologischen Gesellschaft Heidelberg 1905*. J. F. Bergmann, Wiesbaden 1905, p. 225.
148. *Lehrbuch der Augenheilkunde*. 10th enlarged ed., Franz Deuticke, Leipzig/Vienna 1905.
149. "Kongenitale Ptosis", in: *Wien. klin. Wochenschr.* 18 (1905), p. 923.
150. "Ueber kleine Rupturen an der Corneoskleralgrenze", in: *Wien. klin. Wochenschr.* 18 (1905), pp. 985–989.
151. "Über Komplikationen der Heterochromie", in: *Zeitschr. Augenheilk.* 15 (1906), pp. 191–212.
152. *Manuel d'Ophtalmologie*. Troisième édition française traduite sur la dixième édition allemande par le Dr. L. Leplat et le Dr. C. Lacompte. Steinheil, Paris 1906.

153. "Professor Wilhelm Czermak †", in: *Graefes Archiv* 65 (1906), pp. I–IV.
154. "Zur Aetiologie der Katarakt", in: *Bericht über die 33. Versammlung der Ophthalmologischen Gesellschaft in Heidelberg 1906*. Bergmann, Wiesbaden 1907, pp. 33f. and *Archiv Augenheilk*. 61/1 (1907), pp. 93–94.
155. "Depressione del polo oculare posteriore in seguito ad estrazione della cataratta", in: Clinica Oculistica 8 (1907), pp. 2829–2833.
156. *Lehrbuch der Augenheilkunde*. 11th enlarged ed., Franz Deuticke, Leipzig/Vienna 1907.
157. "Oculomotoriuslähmung ohne Beteiligung der Binnenmuskeln bei peripheren Läsionen", in: Heinrich OBERSTEINER (ed.), *Arbeiten aus dem Neurologischen Institute* (Institut für Anatomie und Physiologie des Centralnervensystems) an der Universität Wien. Vol. 15. Franz Deuticke, Leipzig/Vienna 1907, pp. 1–16.
158. "Auf Xenophons Spuren", in: Heinrich Ritter von WITTEK (ed.), *Festgabe zum 100jährigen Jubiläum des Schottengymnasiums*. Gewidmet von ehemaligen Schottenschülern. Wilhelm Braumüller, Vienna 1907, pp. 95–105.
159. "Zur Frage der Unfallstation für die Wiener chirurgischen Kliniken und der Trachomstation für die Augenklinik", in: *Neue Freie Presse* No. 15813 of 30 August 1908, pp. 3 (together with Anton von Eiselsberg und Julius Hochenegg).
160. "Glaucoma in consequence of cicatrix of cornea with anterior synechia (leukoma adhaerens)", in: *The Ophthalmic Record* 17 (1908), p. 525. (76th Annual Meeting of the Brit. Med. Assoc., July 1908).
161. "Hermann Snellen † 18. Januar 1908", in: *Wien. klin. Wochenschr*. (1908), Nr. 5.
162. "Wucherungen und Geschwülste des Ciliarepithels", in: *Graefes Archiv* 68 (1908) Abth. II, pp. 534–587.
163. "Vordere Synechie und Hypertonie", in: *Graefes Archiv* 69 (1908), pp. 254–271.
164. *Text-Book of Ophthalmology*. Third ed. Translation by A. Duane, Lippincott, Philadelphia & London 1908.
165. "Malformation of the Cornea in Cases of Inherited Syphilis", in: *The Ophthalmic Review* 28 (1909), p. 247ff.
166. "Über Ophthalmia sympathica", in: *Graefes Archiv* 70 (1909) Abth. III, pp. 465–485.
167. "Ueber das Ulcus serpens corneae", in: *Wien. klin. Wochenschr*. 22 (1909), No. 1.
168. "Dystrophia epithelialis corneae", in: *Graefes Archiv* 76 (1910), pp. 478–508.
169. *Lehrbuch der Augenheilkunde*. 12th enlarged ed., Franz Deuticke, Leipzig/Vienna 1910.
170. *Rukovodstwo k glasnym bolsnjam*. (Textbook of Ophthalmology). Russian transl. by E. P. Eberman and S. A. Kaplan of the 11th ed. of Ernst Fuchs. Karzeva, Moskau 1910.
171. (Address delivered by Hofrat Fuchs, at the inauguration of the memorial for Eduard Jaeger at Vienna University on 28 Feb. 1910). (Typescript).
172. "Ueber Sarcom der Aderhaut nebst Bemerkungen über Nekrose der Uvea", in: *Graefes Archiv* 77/III. Abth. (1910), pp. 304–392.
173. "1. Lakunen im Optikus bei Glaukom. 2. Zyste des Ziliarkörpers". (Ophthalmol. Gesellsch. in Wien), in: *Zeitschr. Augenheilk*. 23 (1910), pp. 76ff.
174. "Mikropsie bei Presbyopie", in: *Zeitschr. Augenheilk*. 23 (1910), pp. 277ff.
175. "Varicenbildung auf der Papille", in: *Zeitschr. Augenheilk*. 23 (1910), pp. 504–505.
176. "Zysten der Iris", in: *Klin. Monatsbl. Augenheilk*. 48 (1910), p. 104.
177. "Ueber Dellen in der Hornhaut", in: *Graefes Archiv* 78 (1911), pp. 82–92.

178. “The Field of Vision in Tabetic Atrophy of the Optic Disc”, in: *Transact. Amer. Ophthalmol. Soc.* (47th Annual Meeting, New London/ Conn. July 11–12, 1911) Part III, pp. 718–736 and *Arch. Ophthalmol.* 40 (1911), pp. 469–475.
179. “Neuroma of the Ciliary Nerves”, in: *Transact. Americ. Ophthalmol. Soc.* (47th Annual Meeting, New London/Conn. July 11–12, 1911) 12/Part III, pp. 786–787. (Exhibition of Specimens).
180. “Smallest Sarcoma of the Choroid”. In: *Transact. Americ. Ophthalmol. Soc.* (47th Annual Meeting, New London/Conn. July 11–12, 1911) 12/Part III, p. 787–789 (Exhibition of Specimens, Discussion, pp. 789–790.)
181. “Lochbildung in der Fovea centralis”, in: *Graefes Archiv* 79 (1911), pp. 42–52.
182. “Ueber innere Skleralruptur”, in: *Graefes Archiv* 79 (1911), pp. 53–63.
183. *Text-Book of Ophthalmology.* Authorized Translation from the Twelfth Revised and Greatly Enlarged German Edition with Numerous Additions by Alexander Duane, J. B. Lippincott Company, Philadelphia & London 1911.
184. “Nachtrag zur Arbeit ‘Ueber Sarkom der Aderhaut’ in vol. LXXVII of this archive”, in: *Graefes Archiv* 81 (1912), pp. 556–562.
185. “Tabes und Auge”, in: *Wien. klin. Wochenschr.* 25 (1912), No. 14.
186. “Conglomerattuberkel der Chorioidea”, in: *Beiträge zur Augenheilk.* 79 (1913), pp. 556.
187. “Dystrophie der Hornhaut bei Tabes”, in: *Centralbl. prakt. Augenheilk.* 1913.
188. “Ueber chronische endogene Uveitis”, in: *Graefes Archiv* 84 (1913), pp. 201–292.
189. “Normal pigmentierte und albinotische Iris”, in: *Graefes Archiv* 84 (1913), pp. 521– 529.
190. “Naevus pigmentosus und Naevus vasculosus der Iris”, in: *Graefes Archiv* 86 (1913), pp. 155–169.
191. “De l’opacification du cristallin à la suite de suppuration cornéenne”, in: *Annales d’oculistique* 150 (1913), pp. 81ff.
192. “Lage der Lamina cribrosa und atrophische Exkavation”, in: *Zeitschr. Augenheilk.* 32 (1914), pp. 192ff.
193. “Regarding some unusual varieties of rupture of the cornea”, in: Henry Vanderbilt WÜRDEMANN, Nelson Miles BLACK (eds.), *Ophthalmology: essays, abstracts and reviews.* Vol. 10 (1914), pp. 46–50.
194. “Einfluß der Star-Operation auf die Intelligenz”, in: *Centralbl. prakt. Augenheilk.* 39 (1915), p. 206.
195. “Ueber knötchenförmige Hornhauttrübungen”, in: *Graefes Archiv* 89 (1915), pp. 337–349.
196. “Ueber senile Randatrophie der Hornhaut”, in: *Graefes Archiv* 89 (1915), pp. 386–392.
197. “Ueber Keratitis pustuliformis profunda”, in: *Graefes Archiv* 90 (1915), pp. 13–75 (= Festschrift für Hubert Sattler).
198. “Über Veränderungen des Sehnerven bei ektogener intraokularer Entzündung”, in: *Graefes Archiv* 91 (1915), pp. 1–65.
199. “Ueber die Lamina cribrosa”, in: *Graefes Archiv* 91 (1915), pp. 435–485.
200. “Erkrankung der Hornhaut durch Schädigung von hinten”, in: *Graefes Archiv* 92 (1916), pp. 145–236.
201. “Ueber Schrumpfung der Iris”, in: *Klin. Monatsbl. Augenheilk.* 56/1 (1916), pp. 145–151.

202. "Lymphangiom an Stelle einer zystoiden Narbe", in: *Klin. Monatsbl. Augenheilk.* 56/1 (1916), pp. 152–156.
203. "Limbuskarzinom, unter der Aderhaut wachsend", in: *Klin. Monatsbl. Augenheilk.* 57/2 (1916), pp. 1–8.
204. "Sekundäre Skleritis und Episkleritis", in: *Bericht ueber die 40. Versammlung der Ophthalmologischen Gesellschaft Heidelberg 1916.* J. F. Bergmann, Wiesbaden 1916, pp. 365–387.
205. "Ueber die anatomischen Befunde einiger angeborener Anomalien der Netzhaut und des Sehnerven", in: *Graefes Archiv* 93 (1917, pp. 1–48.
206. "Über Heterochromie nebst Bemerkungen über angeborene Anomalien", in: *Graefes Archiv* 93 (1917), pp. 381–398.
207. "Über Ophthalmoplegia interna", in: *Wien. med. Wochenschr.* 67 (1917), cols. 2016–2017.
208. "Ueber Pigmentierung, Melanom und Sarkom der Aderhaut", in: *Graefes Archiv* 94 (1917), pp. 43–106.
209. "Über eine angeborene Abnormität der Netzhaut nebst Bemerkungen über Scleraleinbuchtung und Aderhautabhebung", in: *Graefes Archiv* 94 (1917), pp. 107–116.
210. "Über pathologische Mitbewegung der Lider", in: Otto MARBURG (ed.), *Feier des 70. Geburtstages von Hofrat Prof. Dr. H. Obersteiner [=Jb. f. Psych. u. Neurol. 38].* Part I. Franz Deuticke, Vienna/Leipzig 1917, pp. 49–78.
211. *Text-Book of Ophthalmology.* Fifth Edition, J. B. Lippincott, Philadelphia and London 1917.
212. "Zur Therapie der nervösen Asthenopie", in: *Klin. Monatsbl. Augenheilk.* 58/1 (1917), pp. 353–360.
213. "Ueber Schleifen der Ziliarnerven", in: *Klin. Monatsbl. Augenheilk.* 60/1 (1918), pp. 3–11.
214. "Ueber Pigmentstreifen im Augenhintergrunde", in: *Klin. Monatsbl. Augenheilk.* 60/1 (1918), pp. 797–801.
215. "Stephan Bernheimer †", in: *Klin. Monatsbl. Augenheilk.* 60 (1918), pp. 814–817.
216. "Ueber Eosinophilie im Auge", in: *Graefes Archiv* 95 (1918), pp. 162–172.
217. "Zur Anatomie des Staphyloma corneae", in: *Graefes Archiv* 95 (1918), pp. 215– 254.
218. "Ueber organische Muskelfasern in der Aderhaut", in: *Graefes Archiv* 95 (1918), pp. 311–313.
219. "Ueber den Sphinkter pupillae", in: *Klin. Monatsbl. Augenheilk.* 61/2 (1918), pp. 1–9.
220. "Ueber gürtelförmige Hornhauttrübung", in: *Klin. Monatsbl. Augenheilk.* 61/2 (1918), pp. 10–14.
221. "Ueber Faltung und Knickung der Hornhaut", in: *Graefes Archiv* 96 (1918), pp. 315–329.
222. "Ueber Beteiligung der Macula lutea an Erkrankungen des Auges", in: *Graefes Archiv* 97 (1918), pp. 57–84.
223. "Ueber luetische Chorioiditis", in: *Graefes Archiv* 97 (1918), pp. 85–104.
224. "Zur pathologischen Anatomie der Glaskörperblutungen", in: *Graefes Archiv* 99 (1919), pp. 202–248.
225. "Nachschrift zur Arbeit: 'Zur pathologischen Anatomie der Glaskörperblutungen'", in: *Graefes Archiv* 99 (1919), p. 397.
226. "Myopische Augen mit dicker Sklera", in: *Klin. Monatsbl. Augenheilk.* 62 (1919), pp. 429–432.

227. "Ueber nasalen Konus", in: *Klin. Monatsbl. Augenheilk.* 62 (1919), pp. 433–438.
228. "Myopie und Glaukom", in: *Klin. Monatsbl. Augenheilk.* 62 (1919), pp. 439–442.
229. "Anatomischer Befund bei angeborener Myopie", in: *Klin. Monatsbl. Augenheilk.* 62 (1919), pp. 559–571.
230. "Direkter oder indirekter Skleralriss?", in: *Klin. Monatsbl. Augenheilk.* 63 (1919), pp. 1–7.
231. *Text-Book of Ophthalmology*. Sixth Edition, J. B. Lippincott, Philadelphia 1919.
232. "Über anatomische Veränderungen bei chronischer endogener Iridochorioiditis", in: Graefes Archiv 98 (1919), pp. 122–140.
233. "Über primäre Tuberkulose der Netzhaut", in: *Graefes Archiv* 101 (1919), pp. 14–23.
234. "Ein Fall von intraokulärer Aktinomykose", in: *Graefes Archiv* 101 (1919), pp. 24–31.
235. "Relaciones entre el ojo y la tabes". Conferencia dada en esta corporación el día 24 de Febrero de 1920, por el Profesor Fuchs (de Viena), in: *Anales de la Real Academia nacional de Medicina [= Anal. R. Acad. Nac. Med.]* 40 (1920), pp. 531–547.
236. "Tiefe Keratitis, hervorgerufen durch eine pathologische Zusammensetzung des Humor aqueus". (Address delivered to the Ophthalmological Society Madrid, 19 Feb. 1920), in: *Arch. de oftalmol. hispano-americ.* 20, No. 230 (1920), pp. 49–53 u. *España oftalmol.* 5 (1920), pp. 121–128 (Spanish) and *Zentralbl. ges. Ophthalmol.* 4 (1920), pp. 522ff.
237. "Netzhautablösung und Drucksteigerung", in: *Graefes Archiv* 102 (1920), pp. 265–298.
238. "Über retinale Pigmentzellen im Irisstroma", in: *Graefes Archiv* 103 (1920), pp. 297–303.
239. "Über senile Veränderungen des Sehnerven", in: *Bericht über die 42. Versammlung der Deutschen Ophthalmologischen Gesellschaft.* Heidelberg 1920, pp. 182–185 and *Graefes Archiv* 103 (1920), pp. 304–330.
240. "Ueber flächenhafte Wucherung des ziliaren Epithels, nebst Bemerkungen über Ektopie der Linse", in: *Klin. Monatsbl. Augenheilk.* 64 (1920), pp. 1–15.
241. "Über seröse Aderhautabhebung", in: *Graefes Archiv* 104 (1921), pp. 247–263.
242. "Beleuchtung und Auge. Mit einer historischen Einleitung", in: *Wien. med. Wochenschr.* 71 (1921), cols. 1409–1415.
243. "Die Wiener Augenheilkunde aus einer klinischen Vorlesung," in: *Neues Wiener Journal* vom 8. 8. 1921, pp. 2–3.
244. "Über Chorioretinitis", in: *Verhandl. der außerordentlichen Tagung der ophthalmologischen Gesellschaft Wien* 4–6 Aug. 1921, pp. 400–402 and *Graefes Archiv* 107 (922), pp. 15–25.
245. "Über kleine entzündliche Herde beider Augen". (Ophthalmologische Gesellschaft Wien, meeting on 13. Dec. 1920), in: *Klin. Monatsbl. Augenheilk.* 66 (1921), pp. 529.
246. Lehrbuch der Augenheilkunde. 13th enlarged ed., revised by Maximilian Salzmann, Franz Deuticke, Leipzig/Vienna 1921.
247. "Über Verziehung der Netzhaut und Papille", in: *Graefes Archiv* 104 (1921), pp. 230–246.
248. "Augensymptome bei Arteriosklerose". (Address delivered to the Dutch Society of Physicians, Rotterdam), in: *Wien. med. Wochenschr.* 72 (1922), cols. 681–684.
249. "Über Chorioretinitis", in: *Graefes Archiv* 107 (1922), pp. 15–25.

250. *Lehrbuch der Augenheilkunde.* 14th enlarged ed., revised by Maximilian Salzmann, Franz Deuticke, Leipzig/Vienna 1922.
251. "Ocular Manifestations of Internal Secretion", in: *Arch. Ophthalmol.* 51 (1922), pp. 307–320.
252. "Postgraduate Medical Instruction in Vienna", in: *JAMA* 78 (1922), pp. 1477–1478.
253. "Presbyopia", in: *Arch. Ophthalmol.* 51 (1922), pp. 21–28.
254. "Amerikanischer Reisebrief", in: *Wien. med. Wochenschr.* 72 (1922), cols. 913–915.
255. "Senile Changes of Optic Nerve", in: *Am. J. Ophthalmol.* 5 (1922), pp. 215–217.
256. "Eine Vorlesung über die Lichtscheu/A Lecture on Photophobia", in: B. LEWIS, *Medizinisches Vademecum für Augenärzte in deutscher und englischer Sprache/Medical Vademecum for Ophthalmologists in German and English.* Im Verlage von B. Lewis/ Published by B. Lewis. Wien/Vienna 1922, pp. 22–36/p. 23–37.
257. "Capsulotomy Operation", in: William Albert FISHER, *Senile Cataract. Methods of Operating. Eye, Ear, Nose and Throat College*, Chicago 1923, pp. 1–12.
258. "Ueber Anomalien der Blutgefässe im Sehnerveneintritt", in: *Klin. Monatsbl. Augenheilk.* 71 (1923), pp. 583–589.
259. "Ocular Manifestations of Internal Secretion", in: *Proc. Inst. Med. Chicago* 4 (1923), pp. 73–84.
260. *Text-Book of Ophthalmology.* Authorized Translation from the Twelfth German Edition. Completely Revised and Reset, with Numerous Additions Specially Supplied by the Author and Otherwise Much Enlarged by Alexander Duane. Seventh Edition Revised and Reset. J. B. Lippincott Company, Philadelphia & London 1923.
261. "Erinnerungen an Japan", in: *Zeitschr. Augenheilk.* 52 (1924), pp. 305–310.
262. "Die ägyptische Augenkrankheit", in: *Wien. klin. Wochenschr.* 37 (1924), pp. 564–566.
263. "Operación por capsulotomía", in: William Albert FISHER: *Catarata senil. Métodos Operatorios.* Traducción por Melchior Parrizas Torres. Imprenta Clarasó, Barcelona 1924, pp. 13–24.
264. *Text-Book of Ophthalmology.* Eighth Edition Revised. Authorized Translation from the Twelfth German Edition. Completely Revised and Reset, with Numerous Additions Specially Supplied by the Author and Otherwise Much Enlarged by Alexander Duane, J. B. Lippincott Company. Philadelphia & London 1924.
265. "Zur Anatomie der Endophthalmitis", in: *Graefes Archiv* 115 (1925), pp. 387–398.
266. "Über Blutaustritte in der Aderhaut", in: *Zeitschr. Augenheilk.* 57 (1925), pp. 1–6.
267. "Erinnerungen", in: *Wien. med. Wochenschr.* 75 (1925), cols. 2475–2477.
268. "Über lymphocytäre Infiltration der Aderhaut", in: *Graefes Archiv* 115 (1925), pp. 584–595.
269. "Über chronische infiltrierende Iritis", in: *Graefes Archiv* 116 (1925), pp. 168–183.
270. "Iritis serosa oder Cyclitis chronica?", in: *Zeitschr. Augenheilk.* 57 (1925), pp. 6–11.
271. "Unbeabsichtigte Nebenverletzungen bei der Staroperation", in: *Zeitschr. Augenheilk.* 65 (1925), pp. 191.
272. *Lehrbuch der Augenheilkunde.* 15. vermehrte und verbesserte Auflage. Bearbeitet von Maximilian Salzmann, Franz Deuticke, Leipzig/Vienna 1926.
273. "Ärztliches aus Abessinien", in: *Wien. klin. Wochenschr.* 39 (1926), pp. 1220–1222.
274. "Gewerbliche Augenverletzungen und deren Verhütung", in: *Wien. med. Wochenschr.* 76 (1926), pp. 307f.
275. "Memories of Vienna Clinics", in: *Amer. J. Ophthalmol.* 9 (1926), pp. 605–607.

276. *Cuestiones oftalmologicas. Cinco lecciones dadas en la Facultad de Medicina de Madrid.* Traducción de T. Arroyo de Márquez, Editorial Paracelso, Madrid 1927.
277. "Die Irrtümer auf dem Gebiete der Augendiagnose mit besonderer Berücksichtigung der klinischen Medizin", in: *Wien. med. Wochenschr.* 77 (1927), pp. 147–149.
278. "Über Ödem und Cysten des ciliaren Epithels", in: *Graefes Archiv* 118 (1927), pp. 681–696.
279. "Über schaumige Einlagerungen in der Aderhaut", in: *Graefes Archiv* 118 (1927), pp. 697–700.
280. "Die Therapie des Trachoms". (Address delivered to trainee physicians), in: *Wien. med. Wochenschr.* 177 (1927), cols. 1615–1618.
281. "Anatomische Befunde nach Tätowierung mit Tusche", in: *Graefes Archiv* 120 (1928), pp. 714–719.
282. "Über den Ciliarmuskel", in: *Graefes Archiv* 120 (1928), pp. 733–741.
283. "Ein Fall zentraler rezidivierender syphilitischer Netzhautentzündung", in: *Zeitschr. Augenheilk.* 40 (1928), pp. 106ff.
284. "Manifestaciones oculares en la sifilis cerebral, en la tabes y paralisis general", in: *Arch. de oft. de Buenos Aires* 2 (1927), No. 8 (Suppl. pp. 1–11) and *Riv. espan. de med. y cir.* 11 (1928), pp. 275–278.
285. "Aus meiner augenärztlichen Praxis", in: *Liječnicki Vjesnik* 50 (1928), pp. 76–82.
286. "Netzhautveränderungen nach Erweichung des Auges", in: *Graefes Archiv* 120 (1928), pp. 694–713.
287. "Über Verschiebung der Netzhaut auf der Aderhaut", in: *Graefes Archiv* 121 (1928), pp. 339–346.
288. "Wien, das Mekka der amerikanischen Aerzte. Die Weltbedeutung der Wiener Schule", in: *Neue Freie Presse* No. 22963 of 19 August 1928 (Special issue).
289. "Der Ciliarkörper bei Luxation der Linse", in: *Graefes Archiv* 122 (1929), pp. 86– 95.
290. "Über die Ciliargefäße", in: *Graefes Archiv* 122 (1929), pp. 219–239.
291. "Über Exsudatbelag bei chronischer Iritis", in: *Graefes Archiv* 123 (1929), pp. 43–51.
292. "Berichtigung meiner Mitteilung: 'Über schaumige Einlagerungen in der Aderhaut'", in: *Graefes Archiv* 123 (1929), pp. 171–172.
293. "Die Augen der Frau Fischer. Aus der Geschichte der Wiener Augenheilkunde", in: *Neues Wiener Tagblatt* No. 322 of 23 Nov. 1930, pp. 6.
294. "Development of Ophthalmology in Europe". (Address delivered at the dedication of the Wilmer Ophthalmological Institute, Johns Hopkins Hospital, Baltimore, Oct. 15, 1929), in: *Arch. Ophthalmol.* 3/2 (1930), pp. 133–147.
295. "Classification of Retinitis", in: *Arch. Ophthalmol.* 3/4 (1930), pp. 393–402.
296. "Consequences of Softening of the Eyeball", in: Arch. Ophthalmol. 3/4 (1930), p. 419–423.
297. "Localization of Pathologic Changes in the Cornea", in: Arch. Ophthalmol. 3/5 (1930), pp. 588–598.
298. "Subjective Symptomatology of Ocular Disorders". An Address, in: *Amer. J. Ophthalmol.* 13 (1930), p. 113–117.
299. *Trattato di oftalmologia.* Traduzione italiana sulla 15ª edizione tedesca aumentata ed elaborata dal Dott. Massimiliano Salzmann, eseguita dal Prof. Mario Pagani. 2ª edizione italiana, Edizione S A V I T, Vercelli 1932.
300. "Capsulotomy Operation", in: William Albert FISHER, *Senile Cataract. Methods of Operating.* 2nd ed. Eye, Ear, Nose and Throat College. Chicago 1933, pp. 1–12.

301. *Diseases of the Eye.* The Fifteenth German Edition of the *Lehrbuch der Augenheilkunde* as Revised by Maximilian Salzmann. Authorized Translation by E.V. L. Brown. Tenth English Edition. J. B. Lippincott, Philadelphia/Montreal/London 1933.
302. *Tratado de oftalmología.* Completado por el Dr. Maximilian Salzmann. Traducción de la 15.ª edición alemana por el Dr. M. Renedo. Con un apéndice a las operaciones oculares por el Dr. Salvador Viusá, Editoral Labor, Barcelona/Madrid/Buenos Aires/ Rio de Janeiro 1935. (Unaltered reprint 1936)
303. "Abessinienreise 1926". Aus dem Tagebuche von Hofrat Professor Dr. Ernst Fuchs †, in: *Sonntagsbeilage der Wiener Zeitung* of 12 Jan. 1936, pp. 1–3 and 19 Jan 1936, pp. 1–3.
304. *Lehrbuch der Augenheilkunde.* Neu bearbeitet von Adalbert Fuchs. 16th enlarged and improved edition. Franz Deuticke, Vienna 1939.
305. *Lehrbuch der Augenheilkunde.* Neu bearbeitet von Adalbert Fuchs. 17th improved edition. Franz Deuticke, Vienna 1944.
306. *Lehrbuch der Augenheilkunde.* Neu bearbeitet von Adalbert Fuchs. 18th improved edition. Franz Deuticke, Vienna 1945.
307. *Wie ein Augenarzt die Welt sah.* Selbstbiographie und Tagebuchblätter. Ed. by Prof. Adalbert Fuchs, Wien, Urban & Schwarzenberg, Vienna 1946.
308. *Oftalmología.* Actualizada por el Dr. Adalbert Fuchs. Tercera Edicion Española. Traducción de la 18.ª edición alemana revisada y ampliada por el Dr. Santiago Vilahur Pedrals, Tomo I + II, Editorial Labor, Barcelona 1958.

Notes

1681 See Fig. 95.

1682 In Albert Fuchs's 1946 introduction to the autobiographical sketch Ernst Fuchs wrote from memory on board the steamer *Anfa* during his voyage from Marseille to Casablanca on 15–19 November 1926, Albert mentions that his father had compiled a catalogue of 245 original works in 5 volumes. Cf. FUCHS, *Augenarzt* (as in FN 2), p. 10, FN 8.

1683 See: Typewritten letter of 4 Dec. 1969, signed A. Fuchs. Handschriftenarchiv/ Sammlungen d. Med. Univ. Wien. On 10 January 2005 the archivist in charge of the Library of New York Univ., Coleen Bradley-Sanders, confirmed to the author of this monograph that this crucial source material remains unaccounted for.

1684 The author of this monograph has followed a policy over many years of purchasing as many of Ernst Fuchs's publications as she could lay hands on and to examine and to have photocopied those that never hit the market. As a result, the catalogue of Fuchs's works presented below runs to a significantly higher number than the 245 mentioned above. Presumably the list Albert mentions comprised only original works and did not make allowance for the many editions of the *Lehrbuch* in German and in other languages. These are included here as separate items in addition to publications and editions of the *Lehrbuch* that appeared posthumously and publications outside specialist journals. Below are listed 308 publications. However, neither completeness nor faultlessness may be taken for granted.

Instead of an epilogue: Ernst Fuchs and His Time

An intensive study of the literature by and about Ernst Fuchs has crystallised into what amounts to a programme: Fuchs, a physician whose work spans two distinct epochs of ophthalmology.

He was already a practising ophthalmologist when there was no such thing yet as antiseptic or aseptic procedures, when his specialty, relying as it mostly did on surgery, did not yet have any practicable anaesthetic at its disposal, and when therapy was in many cases still grounded in humoral-pathological ideas. And yet he was, on the other hand, a disciple of Rokitansky and Škoda, who famously created the 'anatomical clinic' whose influence was to transform medical practice worldwide. It may seem counter-intuitive at first sight to begin with those two images but they may serve to remind us that Fuchs the clinician was at the same time a self-made pathological anatomist. (What kind of pathologist dissects eyes?) The contribution Rokitansky and Škoda made to the Vienna Medical School was equalled by Fuchs alone in the development of contemporary ophthalmology.

At first, methodology apart, Fuchs stood to gain little for his own specialty from these teachers. Arlt, the spiritual father of Fuchs's work, had already endorsed the demands of the anatomical clinic for ophthalmology. But it was left to Fuchs to adapt and fulfil these postulates for his own time and Meller could not emphasize often enough that it was Fuchs who had been the one to initiate the pathological anatomy of the eye. And it was thanks to his unique talents as a teacher – a justified hyperbole in this case – that his *Lehrbuch* lighted the way for eye specialists all over the world during and beyond his lifetime. It was referred to as the "Bible of ophthalmologists" with very good reason. All one needs to do to appreciate the impact this work made is to read the introduction to the first edition.

In the days when Fuchs was still a student under Arlt, humoral-pathological notions were still fighting a rearguard battle with anatomical ideas. A seton like the one pictured in Bartisch's 1583 *Augendienst* was applied by Fuchs himself to a patient when he was an "aspirant" under Arlt. Comparable with bloodletting, which was still frequently resorted to at that time, use of a seton was supposed to drain the body of noxious fluids, the 'materia peccans' thought to be the cause of the disease. In his *Lehrbuch der Krankheiten des Herzens* (1857) even Oppolzer's successor in Vienna, Heinrich Bamberger, recommended the seton as an interval therapy for patients suffering from angina pectoris.

In retrospect Fuchs considered the complete absence of asepsis during his time as an aspirant under Arlt his most disturbing memory. He himself would to go on to provide a remedy. As is still common practice today, Fuchs received his training at a surgical clinic, having become a trainee surgeon at Billroth's clinic in 1874. Even though Billroth, as he said himself, thought very highly of Arlt despite the difference in character between the two men, it appears that Fuchs did not establish any close contact with him. Instead, it was two other men who exerted the most profound influence on him: Joseph Lister, who had come to Vienna from Halle to present his antiseptic operative technique at Billroth's clinic, and Alexander von Winiwarter, the future Chair of Surgery at the University of Liège, then a trainee surgeon under Billroth alongside Fuchs, who was to become a close friend. With his motto "cleanliness to a fault" Billroth himself had anticipated the advent of asepsis as early as 1875, at a time when even antisepsis was not yet fully established. Lister, whose method first came to public attention in 1867, served as Fuchs's assistant in two operations.

"After my two years as a trainee surgeon I would have loved to continue in the craft", Fuchs wrote in his autobiography. We feel involuntarily reminded of the lot of the son of Fuchs's friend and fellow student under Arlt, Karl Denk, who, intending to becoming an ophthalmologist, underwent preparatory surgical training in Linz under Alexander Brenner and remained a surgeon for life. Brenner had registered Wolfgang Denk with Eiselsberg without telling him, redirecting his career in a direction that differed from what Wolfgang's father, the ophthalmologist Karl Denk, had envisaged for him. For Fuchs, however, things worked out differently: the next post of assistant to fall vacant in Arlt's clinic had his name on it, and he remained faithful to ophthalmology. That his surgical training was formative for Fuchs need not come as a surprise for us, seeing that during his traineeship preparations for Billroth's historic pylorus resection were coming to their climax. In 1876 his two friends Gussenbauer and Winiwarter had just completed their mammoth task of digging through 61,248 autopsy protocols for the percentage of metastasis-free pylorus carcinomas Billroth had requested them to provide. The team then carried out the operation seven times on dogs.

After Fuchs's return to Arlt in 1876 he became the driving force behind the introduction of antisepsis at the clinic. Now the seton was consigned to history, now the cataract knife was no longer wetted between the lips of the operator to make it more slippery, now instruments were cleaned before the operation, not just afterwards. This shows Fuchs for the first time bringing about an epochal change of tide: having familiarised himself with antisepsis in surgery, he rang in a new era in ophthalmology.

When he was still an assistant under Arlt Fuchs initiated his second epoch-making leap forward for ophthalmology, laying the foundations for his greatest achievement: the creation of ocular pathohistology. In a travelogue that forms part of his autobiography, he refers to both the origin and the scope of that achievement. *"It had been Arlt's great achievement"*, says Fuchs, *"to put ophthalmology on an anatomical basis as far as he could, limited as he was by having to rely on a magnifying glass"*. "As far as he could, ... having to rely on a magnifying glass": Arlt had therefore shown the way but had been prevented from following it himself by closely drawn limits. It may be permitted here to repeat the words Meller used at the 70th birthday of his teacher: *"Having enriched our science from the very first years of his professional life through the addition of a great number of pathologies masterfully depicted in his characteristic style, with quite a few of them eponymously bearing his name, and having refined in detail our understanding of the normal anatomy of the eye, he became the initiator of the pathological anatomy of the eye."* Meller's words need no amplification. It appears from them that Fuchs was his own prosector. Going beyond the examination of the eye his teacher Arlt had practised, Fuchs was now using the microscope.

The second leap forward he gifted to ophthalmology was arguably facilitated by experiences he had made as a student under Brücke. Alongside Obersteiner and Exner he had done histological work under Brücke's aegis, which flowed into his "habilitation" thesis on the sarcoma of the uveal tract.

A bursary in 1878 allowed Fuchs, while he was still an assistant, to visit Paris and London; in 1877 he had taken part for the first time in the meeting of German ophthalmologists in Heidelberg. There he met Frans Cornelis Donders, the "Olympian", as he was called by his disciples and their peers. The friendship with Donders and Winiwarter was to prove decisive for Fuchs's career within a very short time.

Winiwarter, at one stage trainee surgeon at Billroth's clinic alongside Fuchs, had been appointed Professor of Surgery in Liège in 1878. His job entailed the occasional lecture on ophthalmology, which came with a hospital room with between 8 and 11 beds for eye patients. When one learns from Fuchs that he owed his call to Liège primarily to Winiwarter, one thinks involuntarily of Zurich, and of Horner and Billroth. When no suitable ophthalmologist was to be found in Belgium to follow up on the university's decision to establish a chair for ophthalmology, Donders proposed Fuchs, the disciple of the great Arlt.

Arriving in Liège in 1881, he exchanged, as one might say, the new times he had already helped to pioneer for the past. It came as a shock when he discovered that Theodor Schwann was actually not only still alive but an active member of the faculty. *"I used to believe that he belonged to a by-gone century"*, Fuchs wrote in his autobiography. Schwann had famously discovered pepsin in 1836 and had published his foundational insight that animals and plants were both composed of cells in 1839. Fuchs noted that Schwann, apart from being *"a kind old gentleman and a famous wine connoisseur"*, was *"clerically inclined"*. This raises an interesting point. Schwann published his groundbreaking work about the cell as the basic component only after he had secured the "imprimatur" of the episcopal authority. The physiologist Rothschuh suggested that this was a unique event in the history of science. Yet at the same time this fact makes it clear that Schwann was well aware of the epoch-making significance of his discovery. He did not, after all, apply for an episcopal blessing for the publication of his discovery of pepsin, of his observation that germs played a crucial role in putrefaction and fermentation, or of the role of bile in digestion (he was, incidentally, the first surgeon to apply a biliary fistula).

During Fuchs's time in Liège Arlt had become Professor emeritus in 1883 and been followed by Stellwag. In the same year the Second University Eye Clinic was established for Eduard Jaeger; having been overlooked for many years, this master of ophthalmoscopy died after only one year in office. The Director of the Ophthalmic Policlinic, Arlt disciple August Reuss, now took charge of the Second Eye Clinic on a provisional basis. It was in this place and at that time, in the Second Eye Clinic and during Reuss's deputy leadership, that an event occurred that justifies calling Fuchs an ophthalmologist straddling two epochs: Karl Koller discovered the local anaesthesia of the eye. Now ophthalmology had at its disposal the two crucial preconditions for the development of surgery: freedom from pain and a shield against wound infection.

Compared with the old days, when speedy operating and extraordinary adroitness were of the essence, local anaesthesia allowed surgeons to take more time in their operations. Fuchs and Arlt both had a reputation of being consummately skilled surgeons. Both operated equally skillfully with both hands. What Arlt had said to a non-plussed colleague made absolute sense: *"A good surgeon needs the talents of a watchmaker on top of his scientific grounding."*

The First University Eye Clinic – in historical terms a global first – was now in the hands of Stellwag; Jaeger had died, and Fuchs received the call to Vienna, to which he reacted with mixed feelings. He was successor of Jaeger rather than of his teacher Arlt, even though Jaeger had stood for an approach to ophthalmology that was antithetical to Arlt's. Fuchs's teachers Brücke and Billroth were still members of the Faculty. He was, after all, only 34 at the time.

In 1887 he encouraged Heinrich Bamberger, one of Oppolzer's disciples and his successor at the Second Medical University Clinic, to found a high-quality faculty journal, the Wiener Klinische Wochenschrift, which first saw the light of day in the following year.

In Vienna Ernst Fuchs's teaching unfolded in a way that was then without a parallel. There was, however, one thing that irked him: his students were kept from observing clinical procedures in order to make notes, a situation that was inevitably made even worse by their frequent failure to take note of the salient points. To provide a remedy, Fuchs decided to produce a set of lecture notes. Putting himself in his students' shoes, he felt they were much more likely in future to turn to the familiar lecture notes than to consult an unfamiliar new textbook. He therefore decided to enlarge these lecture notes to a degree that made them suitable as a reference work for the general practitioner. This is how the first edition of the Lehrbuch came into being in 1889, a work which obituarists and keynote speakers alike loved to call the "Bible of ophthalmologists". That it was translated into all the major languages and had seen twelve editions by the time Fuchs resigned from his chair may be taken as read. Salzmann took over from Fuchs as editor and was followed in turn by Adalbert Fuchs, Ernst's son, until 1945.

There is little doubt that Ernst Fuchs was rather headstrong. In his time as an assistant he refused to move into the room that been assigned to him [at the clinic] until a bed was provided that fitted him. When, at the age of 36, he felt dissatisfied with how journalists were doing their job, he vigorously pushed for the foundation of a new specialist journal. And, aged 65, when at the beginning of World War I his staff were being called to the front and students from abroad were forced to stay away, he went to the War Ministry to seek redress. Having failed to obtain it in 1915, he realised a plan he had first announced some time before only to delay its execution temporarily and asked to be retired long before his time. Now he had plenty of time for scientific work. Like Wenckebach, who, having retired before reaching the age limit, devoted himself to the study of the beriberi heart disease, Fuchs continued in his own research.

He was reserved by nature; maybe he resembled Škoda in this respect, who had been his role model when he was a student. Arlt used to drop in at Škoda's house with mutual friends in the evening to relax. Fuchs was later to acquire the house himself. Like Škoda he may have given many people the impression of being aloof and reserved, but his disciples, above all Salzmann, Meller and Lindner, who knew him well, tell a different story. Lindner knew something that only a handful of people were privy to: Fuchs had donated $10,000 to a student hall of residence. Škoda had done something similar. Let me end these minutes of commemoration with this comparison, which to my knowledge has not been made before. Both men practised in their lives unremitting self-discipline; both appeared outwardly – an important qualification – to give science top priority above anything else; both did not simply enrich their specialties but helped to build their very foundations. It is by no means certain that our internal medicine and ophthalmology would ever have excelled as they do had it not been for these two men. They put their entire lives at the service of their specialty, enriching and empowering it with their invaluable insights.

Helmut Wyklicky†

(Slightly edited excerpts from a previously unpublished address given in Salzburg in ca. 1981)

Appendix

I. Bibliography

100 Jahre Wiener Medizinische Akademie. Universimed, Vienna 1996.

Addresses & Papers. *Dedication Ceremonies and Medical Conference Peking Union Medical College September 15–22, 1921.* Peking 1922.

Hans ADLER, "Eduard Jaeger, † 5. Juli 1884", in: *Mittheil. Wien. med. Doct. Coll.* 10 (1884), pp. 212.

Hans ADLER, "Ueber Keratitis subepithelialis centralis, in: *Wien. klin. Wochenschr.* 2 (1889), pp. 713–714 and *Centralbl. prakt. Augenheilk.* Year (1889), p. 289 and 321.

Akademischer Senat der Wiener Universität (ed.), *Geschichte der Wiener Universität von 1848 bis 1898.* Als Huldigungsfestschrift zum fünfzigjährigen Regierungsjubiläum Seiner k. und k. apostolischen Majestät des Kaisers Franz Josef I., Alfred Hölder, Vienna 1898.

Fred Houdlett ALBEE, Frederik J. ELTON (eds.), *Rehabilitation Review: Devoted to the Restoration and Employment of the Disabled* 3/7 (1929).

Daniel M. ALBERT, Harold G. SCHEIE, *A History of Ophthalmology at the University of Pennsylvania.* Charles C. Thomas, Springfield 1965.

Daniel M. ALBERT, *Jaeger's Atlas of Diseases of the Ocular Fundus with new descriptions, revisions and additions.* W. B. Saunders Company, Philadelphia/London/Toronto 1972.

Daniel M. ALBERT, Paul HENKIND, *Men of Vision. Lives of Notable Figures in Ophthalmology.* Gryphon editions, New York 1993.

Daniel ALBERT, Edward W. D. NORTON, Reva HURTES, *Source Book of Ophthalmology.* Blackwell Science 1995.

Daniel M. ALBERT, Diane D. EDWARDS (eds.), The History of Ophthalmology. Blackwell Science, Cambridge 1996.

Daniel M. ALBERT, *Dates in Ophthalmology. A Chronological Record of Progress in Ophthalmology over the Last Millennium.* Landmarks in Medicine Series. The Parthenon Publishing Group, New York/London 2002.

Allgemeiner Bericht über die land- und forstwirthschaftliche Ausstellung zu Vienna im Jahre 1866, in: *Bericht über die von der k. k.Landwirtschafts-Gesellschaft veranstaltete land- und forstwirthschaftliche Ausstellung zu Wien im Jahre 1866.* Herausgegeben durch das Ausstellungs-Comité. Selbstverlag, Vienna 1867.

Allgemeines Beamten-Adressbuch für die k. k.Haupt- und Residenzstadt Wien. Systematische Zusammenstellung sämmtlicher k. k.Hof- und Staats-Aemter, der städtischen Behörden, öffentlichen Anstalten, Vereine etc. und bei denselben angestellten Beamten, Functionäre und Diener, mit Angabe des Namens, der Diensteigenschaft und der Wohnung nebst alphabetischen Registern. 1. Jahrgang. Friedrich Manz, Vienna 1853.

Adolf ALT, *Compendium der normalen und pathologischen Histologie des Auges.* J. F. Bergmann, Wiesbaden 1880.

E. AMMANN, "Ein Fall von Retinitis circinata mit anatomischer Untersuchung", in: *Archiv Augenheilk.* 35 (1897), pp. 123–136.

Gabriel ANTON, "Theodor Meynert, seine Person und sein Werk", in: J. *Psych. Neurol.* 40 (1930), pp. 256ff.

Ferdinand ARLT, *Die Pflege der Augen im gesunden und kranken Zustande, nebst einem Anhange über Augengläser, allgemein fasslich dargestellt.* Prague 1846.

Ferdinand ARLT, *Myopischer Bau des Bulbus.* Vortrag von Professor Arlt im Prag. Med. Doctorencollegium. In: *Dr. Altschuls Monatsschr.* June issue Prague 1854.

Ferdinand ARLT, *Die Krankheiten des Auges, für praktische Ärzte geschildert.* 1st vol. *Die Krankheiten der Binde- und Hornhaut.* F. A. Credner & Kleinbub, Prague 1851; 2nd vol. *Die Krankheiten der Sclera, Iris, Chorioidea und Linse.* F. A. Credner & Kleinbub, Prague 1853; 3rd vol. *Die Krankheiten des Glaskörpers, der Netzhaut, der Augenmuskeln, der Augenlider, der Thränenorgane und der Orbita.* F. A. Credner & Kleinbub 1856.

Ferdinand ARLT, *Die Krankheiten des Auges, für praktische Ärzte geschildert.* Vol 1. *Die Krankheiten der Binde- und Hornhaut.* 2nd unchanged reprint. F. A. Credner & Kleinbub, Prague 1854.

Ferdinand ARLT, "Ueber Retinitis nyctalopica", in: Max TETZER, Lucian RYDEL, Otto BECKER (eds), *Bericht über die Augenklinik der Wiener Universität 1863–1865.* Unter Mitwirkung des Prof. Dr. Ferdinand Arlt. Wilhelm Braumüller, Vienna 1867, pp. 123–132.

Ferdinand ARLT, "Operationslehre", in: Alfred GRAEFE, Theodor SAEMISCH (eds.), *Handbuch der gesammten Augenheilkunde.* Vol 3. *Pathologie und Therapie.* Part 1. Wilhelm Engelmann, Leipzig 1874, pp. 249–500.

Ferdinand Ritter von ARLT, *Ueber die Verletzungen des Auges mit besonderer Rücksicht auf deren gerichtsärztliche Würdigung.* Wilhelm Braumüller, Vienna 1875.

Ferdinand Ritter von ARLT, *Ueber die Ursachen und die Entstehung der Kurzsichtigkeit.* Wilhelm Braumüller, Vienna 1876.

Ferdinand Ritter von ARLT, *Klinische Darstellung der Krankheiten des Auges zunächst der Binde-, Horn- und Lederhaut dann der Iris und des Ciliarkörpers.* Wilhelm Braumüller, Vienna 1881.

Ferdinand ARLT, *Zur Lehre vom Glaukom.* Wilhelm Braumüller, Vienna 1884.

Ferdinand ARLT, *Clinical Studies on Diseases of the Eye Including Those of Conjunctiva, Cornea, Sclerotic, Iris and Ciliary Body.* Translated by Lyman Ware, Blakiston, Philadelphia 1885.

Ferdinand ARLT, *Meine Erlebnisse.* J. F. Bergmann, Wiesbaden 1887.

W. J. ARMITAGE, A. B. TULLO and D. F. P. LARKIN, "The first successful full-thickness corneal transplant: a commentary on Eduard Zirm's landmark paper of 1906", in: *Brit. J. Ophthalmol.* 90/10 (2006), pp. 1222–1223.

George E. ARRINGTON, *A History of Ophthalmology.* MD Publications, Inc., New York 1959.

Leopold ARZT, "Ernst Fuchs, dem Mitbegründer der Wiener klinischen Wochenschrift zum 100. Geburtstag", in: *Wien. klin. Wochenschr.* 63 (1951), p. 613.

Leopold ARZT, "Ferdinand von Hebra und die Dermatologie unserer Zeit", in: *Wien. med. Wochenschr.* 76 (1926), cols. 1316ff.

Hugo ASCHHEIM, "Die Transfixion der Iris", in: *Archiv f. Augenheilk.* 37 (1898), pp. 117–124.

Hugo ASCHHEIM, "Transfixion of the Iris". Translated by Ward A. Holden, in: *Arch. Ophthalmol.* 29 (1900), pp. 507–513.

K. W. ASCHER, "Blepharochalasis mit Struma und Doppellippe", in: *Klin. Monatsbl. Augenheilk.* 65 (1920), pp. 86–97.

Fritz ASK, J. van der HOEVE, "Beiträge zur Kenntnis der Entwicklung der Tränenröhrchen unter normalen und abnormen Verhältnissen, letzteres an Fällen von offener schräger Gesichtsspalte", in: *Graefes Archiv* 105 (1921), pp. 1157–1196.

Arthur H. AUFSES, Barbara NISS, *This House of Noble Deeds: The Mount Sinai Hospital,* 1952–2002. New York University Press 2002.

Au Pays de Liége. Ed. Mathieu Thone, n.p., n.d.

Ausserordentliche Tagung der Ophthalmologischen Gesellschaft in Wien. 4.–6. August 1921. Bericht nach den Manuskripten und Autoreferaten von Dozent Dr. H. Lauber, Vienna, in: *Klin. Monatsbl. Augenheilk.* 67/2 (1921), pp. 293–327.

Außerordentliche Tagung der ophthalmologischen Gesellschaft in Wien am 4., 5. und 6. August 1921, in: *Zeitschr. Augenheilk.* 46 (1921), pp. 51–54.

Austrian Ophthalmologists: *Karl Koller, Eduard Zirm, Joseph Barth, Georg Joseph Beer, Karl Stellwag von Carion, Carl Ferdinand von Arlt.* Books LLC, Memphis 2010.

Theodor AXENFELD, "Kosmetische Immobilisierung des Auges und Tenotomie des Levator palpebrae superioris, nebst Bemerkungen über Operationen an den Obliqui", in: *Graefes Archiv* 105 (1921), pp. 1197–1206.

Theodor AXENFELD, "Ausserordentliche Tagung der Wiener ophthalmologischen Gesellschaft vom 4.–6. August 1921 (Offene Korrespondenz), in: *Klin. Monatsbl. Augenheilk.* 67/2 (1921), pp. 291–292.

E. BAADER, "Dermatostomatitis", in: *Arch. Dermatol. u. Syphilis* 149 (1925), pp. 261–268.

Ernst BACHSTEZ, "Fettsaurer Kalk als Grundlage einer Art von Scintillatio corporis vitrei". Vorläufige Mitteilung, in: *Wien. med. Wochenschr.* 71 (1921), cols. 1044–1045.

Ernst BACHSTEZ, "Über Verfettung in der Hornhaut", in: *Graefes Archiv* 105 (1921), pp. 997–1036.

Jules BADAL, Félix LAGRANGE, "Carcinome primitif des procès et du corps ciliaire", in: *Arch. d'opht.* 12 (1892), p. 143.

Alfred BADER, *Entwicklung der Augenheilkunde im 18. und 19. Jahrhundert mit besonderer Berücksichtigung der Schweiz.* (Nachlass von Prof. Horner, Zürich). Benno Schwabe, Basel 1933.

Karl BÆDEKER, *Belgien und Holland nebst dem Großherzogtum Luxemburg.* Handbuch für Reisende. 22nd ed., Leipzig 1900.

Harold BALME, *China and Modern Medicine. A Study in Medical Missionary Development. United Council for Missionary Education*, London 1921.

Richard BAMBERGER, Franz MAIER-BRUCK (eds.), *Österreich Lexikon in zwei Bänden.* Vol. 1 A–K. Vol. 2 L–Z. Österr. Bundesverlag für Unterricht, Wissenschaft u. Kunst/Verlag Jugend u. Volk, Vienna/Munich 1966/67.

Hans BARKAN, "Cooper Medical College, founded by Levi Cooper Lane: an Historical Sketch", in: *Stanford Medical Bulletin* 12/3 (1954), pp. 145–184.

Martin BARTELS, *Beiträge zur pathologischen Anatomie der Keratitis disciformis.* Inaugural diss., Univ. of Rostock 1907.

Thomas BATEMAN, *A Practical Synopsis of Cutaneous Diseases According to the Arrangement of Dr. Willan, Exhibiting a Concise View of the Diagnostic Symptoms and the Method of Treatment.* Longman, London 1813.

Thomas BATEMAN, *Delineations of Cutaneous Diseases: Exhibiting the Characteristic Appearances of the Principal Genera and Species, Comprised in the Classification of Willan, and Completing the Series of Engravings Began by that Author.* Longman, London 1817.

O. H. BAUMERT, "Zur Kenntnis der Keratitis punctata profunda Mauthner", in: *Klin. Monatsbl. Augenheilk.* 79 (1927), pp. 782ff.

Kurt BAYERTZ, Walter JAESCHKE, Myriam GERHARD, *Weltanschauung, Philosophie und Naturwissenschaft im 19. Jahrhundert.* Vol 1: *Der Materialismusstreit.* Meiner, Hamburg 2007.

Charles H. BEARD, *Ophthalmic Surgery. A Treatise on Surgical Operations Pertaining to the Eye and its Appendages. With Chapters on Para-Operative Technic and Management of Instruments.* Rebman, London 1910 (Copyright 1910 by P. Blakiston's Son & Co.) (= Kessinger Publishing's® Legacy Reprints. La Vergne, TN 21 January 2010).

Charles H. BEARD, "Ophthalmic Semiology and Diagnosis", in: Walter L. Pyle (ed.), *An International System of Ophthalmic Practice.* P. Blakiston's Son & Co., Philadelphia 1914.

Kurt BECK (ed.), *Stefan Zweig auf Reisen.* 2nd ed., S. Fischer Taschenbuch Verlag, Frankfurt am Main 2004.

Otto BECKER (ed.), *Atlas der pathologischen Topographie des Auges.* I. Lieferung. Gezeichnet von Carl Heitzmann.Wilhelm Braumüller, Vienna 1874. II. Lieferung. Gezeichnet von Carl und Julius Heitzmann, Robert Sattler und Friedrich Veith. Lithographirt von Julius Heitzmann. Wilhelm Braumüller, Vienna 1875. III. Lieferung. Gezeichnet von Julius Heitzmann, Hubert Sattler und Friedrich Veith. Lithographirt von Julius Heitzmann.Wilhelm Braumüller, Vienna 1878.

Otto BECKER, *Photographische Abbildungen von Durchschnitten gesunder und kranker Augen.* Gezeichnet von Friedrich Veith, photographirt von J. Schulze in Heidelberg. Wilhelm Braumüller, Wien. I. Serie 1875, II. und III. Serie 1876.

Otto BECKER, *Die Universitäts-Augenklinik Heidelberg. Zwanzig Jahre klinischer Tätigkeit.* J. F. Bergmann, Wiesbaden 1888.

Georg Joseph BEER, *Pflege gesunder und geschwächter Augen, nebst einer Vorschrift, wie man sich bei plötzlichen Zufällen an den Augen, welche nicht eine eigentliche medicinisch-chirurgische Kenntniß fordern, selbst helfen kann. Weidmannsche Buchhandlung, und zu haben bey dem Verfasser.* Vienna and Leipzig 1800.

Georg Joseph BEER, *Lehre von den Augenkrankheiten, als Leitfaden zu seinen öffentlichen Vorlesungen entworfen. Erster Band, welcher die Lehre von der Augen-Entzündung enthält. Camesina Vienna 1813; Zweyter Band, welcher die Lehre von den Nachkrankheiten der Augenentzündung; von dem grauen und schwarzen Staare; und den übrigen in diese Kategorien nicht aufnehmbaren Augenkrankheiten enthält.* Heubner u. Volke, Vienna 1817.

Anton BEHSEL, *Verzeichniß aller in der kaiserl. königl. Haupt- und Residenzstadt Vienna mit ihren Vorstädten befindlichen Häuser, mit genauer Angabe der älteren, mittleren und neuesten Nummerirungen, der dermahligen Eigenthümer und Schilder, der Straßen und Plätze, der Grund-Obrigkeiten, dann der Polizey- und Pfarr-Bezirke.* Carl Gerold, Vienna 1829.

Beiträge zur Ophthalmologie als Festgabe Friedrich Horner zur Feier des fünfundzwanzigsten Jubiläums seiner academischen Lehrthätigkeit gewidmet von Marc Dufour in Lausanne, Otto Haab und Max Knies in Zürich, Julius Michel in Würzburg, Wilhelm Schoen in Leipzig, und O. F. Wadsworth in Boston, U. S. A. J. F. Bergmann, Wiesbaden 1881.

Conrad BERENS, "Report of the Proceedings of the Section on Ophthalmology of the New York Academy of Medicine", Meeting of October 17, 1921, in: *Arch. Ophthalmol.* 51 (1922), pp. 63–67.

Conrad BERENS (ed.), *The Eye and Its Diseases by 82 Authorities.* Saunders, Philadelphia/London 1936.

Emanuel BERGHOFF, *Max Neuburger. Werden und Wirken eines österreichischen Gelehrten.* Maudrich, Vienna 1948.

Otto BERGMEISTER, "Ueber Herpes iris der Conjunctiva", in: *Anzeiger d. k. k.Gesellsch. d. Ärzte* Jg. (1885), pp. 223ff.

Rudolf BERGMEISTER, "Über gliöse Wucherungen im Auge bei Mikrophthalmus congenitus und deren Beziehungen zur Angiomatosis retinae", in: *Graefes Archiv* 105 (1921), pp. 1–38.

Rudolf BERGMEISTER, "Über einen seltenen Fall von epibulbärer Tuberkulose", in: *Wien. med. Wochenschr.* 71 (1921), cols. 1045–1049.

Bericht über die von der k. k.Landwirthschafts-Gesellschaft veranstaltete land- und forstwirthschaftliche Ausstellung zu Wien im Jahre 1866. Herausgegeben durch das Ausstellungs-Comité. Selbstverlag, Vienna 1867.

Bericht ueber die 42. Versammlung der Deutschen Ophthalmologischen Gesellschaft, Heidelberg 1920. J. F. Bergmann, Munich/Wiesbaden 1921.

Peter BERNER, Walter SPIEL, Hans STROTZKA, Helmut WYKLICKY, *Zur Geschichte der Psychiatrie in Wien/Psychiatry in Vienna.* Eine Bilddokumentation/An Illustrated Documentation. Brandstätter, Vienna 1983.

René BERNOULLI, "Über das sogenannte Diktyom – Neuroepithelioma teratoides ciliare", in: *Ophthalmologica* 141 (1961), pp. 386–397.

Alfred BIELSCHOWSKY, "Beitrag zur operativen Behandlung der Vertikalablenkungen der Augen", in: *Graefes Archiv* 105 (1921), pp. 656–687.

J. R. BIERLY, J. P. DUNN, C. R. DAWSON, H. B. OSTLER, I. G. WONG, "Fuchs's superficial marginal keratitis", in: *Am. J. Ophthalmol.* 113/5 (1992), pp. 541–545.

Rudolf BINDER, "Beitrag zur Zellentwicklung im menschlichen Hornhautepithel", in: *Wien. klin. Wochenschr.* 63 (1951), pp. 701–705.

Arthur BIRCH-HIRSCHFELD, "Ein Fall von expulsiver Blutung nach Elliotscher Trepanation mit anatomischem Befund", in: *Graefes Archiv* 105 (1921), pp. 650–655.

Alois BIRNBACHER, *Die pathologische Histologie des menschlichen Auges in Mikrophotogrammen dargestellt.* Erste Lieferung. Bindehaut. Veit & Comp., Leipzig 1899.

Luisa BIZZOTTO, Giorgio RIALDI, "L'attività didattica e scientifica del Fisiologo Maximilian Vintschgau (1832–1902) all'Università di Padova", in: *ActaMed. Hist. Patav.* 22 (1975), pp. 9–20.

Eugene BLAKE, "The Etiology of Retinitis Circinata", in: *Transact. Am. Ophthalmol. Soc.* 14/2 (1916), pp. 753–762.

Hubert BODAMMER, *Die Anfänge der Lokalanästhesie in der Augenheilkunde.* Diss. Med. Hochschule Hannover 1988.

Josef BÖCK, "Ernst Fuchs's Lehre von der posttraumatischen Entzündung des Augeninneren", in: *Wien. med. Wochenschr.* 116 (1965), Special issue (Print-off).

Franz Heinrich BÖCKH (ed.), Wiens lebende Schriftsteller, Künstler, und Dilettanten im Kunstfache. Dann Kunst- und Naturschätze und andere Sehenswürdigkeiten dieser Haupt- und Residenz-Stadt. Ein Handbuch für Einheimische und Fremde. Auf Kosten des Verfassers. Gedruckt bey B. Ph. Bauer, Vienna 1821.

Adelheid BOECKER-REINARTZ, *Die Augen-Kliniken der Universitäten des deutschen Sprachgebietes (1769–1914).* Med. Diss., Universität Köln 1990.

Almut BÖER, "Sir Jonathan Hutchinson (1828–1913)", in: Christoph LÖSER, Gerd PLEWIG (eds.), *Pantheon der Dermatologie.* Springer, Heidelberg 2008, pp. 471–488.

Joseph-Augustin BORLÉE, *Précis clinique et pratique de pathologie chirurgicale spéciale y compris les maladies des yeux.* H. Manceaux, Bruxelles 1872.

Hubert BOURGEOIS, "Alcaloïdes et œil: une longue histoire", in: Julius Hirschberg Gesellschaft (Deutschsprachige Vereinigung für Geschichte der Augenheilkunde) Société francophone d'histoire de l'ophtalmologie, *33 Beiträge zur Geschichte der Augenheilkunde – Contributions à l'histoire de l'ophtalmologie.* Facultas, Vienna 1991, pp. 173–176.

John Z. BOWERS, *Western Medicine in a Chinese Palace. Peking Union Medical College, 1917–1951.* Josiah Macy, Jr. Foundation, Philadelphia 1972.

William BOWMAN, "On Extraction of Cataract by a Traction Instrument, with Iridectomy; with Remarks on Capsular Obstructions and Their Treatment", in: *Ophthal. Hosp. Rep.* IV (1865), pp. 332–368.

Gerhard BOTZ, Ivar Michael POLLAK, Nina SCHOLZ (eds.), *Eine zerstörte Kultur. Jüdisches Leben und Antisemitismus in Wien seit dem 19. Jahrhundert.* Czernin Verlag, Vienna 2002.

Harilaos S. BRILAKIS, Michael L. NORDLUND, Edward J. HOLLAND, *Recurrence of Fuchs Marginal Keratitis Within a Graft*, in: Cornea 23/6 (2004), pp. 639–640.

Mary BROWN BULLOCK, *An American Transplant. The Rockefeller Foundation & Peking Union Medical College*. University of California Press, Berkeley–Los Angeles–London 1980.

Otto BRUCHHÄUSER, *Betrachtungen über Dystrophia epithelialis Corneä*. Med. Diss. Univ. Gießen 1937.

Ernst BRÜCKE, "Anatomische Untersuchungen über die sogenannten leuchtenden Augen bei den Wirbelthieren", in: *Arch. Anat. Physiol. wissenschaftl. Med.* Yr. 1845, pp. 387–406.

Ernst BRÜCKE, "Über den Musculus Cramptonianus und den Spannmuskel der Chorioidea", in: *Arch. Anat. Physiol. wissenschaftl. Med.* Yr. 1846, pp. 370–382.

Ernst BRÜCKE, *Über Gravitation und Erhaltung der Kraft*. K. K. Hof- und Staatsdruckerei, Vienna 1857.

Ernst BRÜCKE, *Vorlesungen über Physiologie. Unter dessen Aufsicht nach stenographischen Aufzeichnungen herausgegeben*. Wilhelm Braumüller, Vienna. Vol.1 1874. Vol. 2 1873.

Ernst Wilhelm von BRÜCKE, **"**Ueber einige Consequenzen der Young-Helmholtz'schen Theorie". 1. Abhandlung, in: *Sitzungsber. d. k. k.Akad. d. Wissensch. Math.-Naturwiss. Cl. Abt. 3,* vol. 80. Gerold, Vienna 1880, pp. 18–72.

Ruth BRUNN-FAHRNI, "Joseph Listers antiseptische Wundbehandlung. Die Listersche Wundbehandlung in der zeitgenössischen Chirurgie", in: *Ciba-Zeitschrift* Nr. 117. Basel, Oktober 1949, pp. 4311–4316.

Ruth BRUNNFAHRNI, Die Listersche Wundbehandlung in der zeitgenössischen Chirurgie, in: *Ciba-Zeitschrift* Nr. 117. Basel, Oktober 1949, pp. 4317–4319.

Robert BUCHBERGER, "Der Billrothsche Hörsaal im Wiener Allgemeinen Krankenhaus. Gemälde von Adalbert F. Seligmann", in: *Wien. klin. Wochenschr*. 78 (1966), pp. 853–856.

Peter BUCK, *American Science and Modern China*. Cambridge University Press, Cambridge et al. 1980.

Clarence Monroe BURTON, *The City of Detroit*. Vol. 5. S. J. Clarke Publ. Comp. 1922.

W. F. BYNUM, Anne HARDY, Stephen JACYNA, Christopher LAWRENCE, E. M. TANSEY, *The Western Medical Tradition 1800–2000*. Cambridge University Press, Cambridge et al. 2006.

David CAHAN (ed.), *Hermann von Helmholtz and the Foundations of Nineteenth-Century Science*. University of California Press, Berkeley/Los Angeles 1993.

Lewis CAMPELL, William GARNETT, *The Life of James Clerk Maxwell. With a Selection of His Correspondence and Occasional Writings and a Sketch of His Contribution to Science*. London, Macmillan 1882.

Cautère-Paquelin (Thermo-Cautère) présenté à l'Académie des Sciences dans la séance du 1er mai 1876.

Víctor CEBRIÁN y DÍEZ, *Patogenia de la glucosuria en sus relaciones con la terapéutica*. Madrid Imp. de Segundo Martínez 1881.

C. C. CHAN, D. ARDELJAN, "Ten Chairpersons of the Ophthalmology Department at Peking Union Medical College", in: *Asia Pac. J. Ophthalmol.* (Phila.) 2 (2013), p. 3–8.

Hans CHIARI, "Eine Erinnerung an Prof. Sigismund Gschwandner", in: Heinrich Ritter von WITTEK (ed.), *Festgabe zum 100jährigen Jubiläum des Schottengymnasiums gewidmet von ehemaligen Schottenschülern*. Wilhelm Braumüller, Vienna 1907.

G. H. CHOA, *"Heal the Sick" Was Their Motto. The Protestant Medical Missionaries in China*. The Chinese University Press, Hong Kong 1990.

Cinquième Congrès International d'Hygiène et de Démographie à La Haye (du 21 au 27 août 1884). Comptes Rendus et Mémoires publiés par le Secrétaire Général avec le concours de MM. les Secrétaires des Sections. Tome I. Imprimerie Sud-Hollandaise, La Haye 1884.

John Gordon CLARKSON, "Edward Jackson, MD. The Father of Board Certification", in: *Arch. Ophthalmol.* 130 (2012), p. 238.

Uwe CLASEN, "Carl Theodor, Herzog in Bayern und Augenarzt (1839–1909)", in: Julius Hirschberg Gesellschaft (Deutschsprachige Vereinigung für Geschichte der Augenheilkunde) Société francophone d'histoire de l'ophtalmologie, *33 Beiträge zur Geschichte der Augenheilkunde – Contributions à l'histoire de l'ophtalmologie*. Facultas, Vienna 1991, pp. 211–220.

Hermann COHN, "Die Ursachen und die Verhütung der Blindheit. Gekrönte Preisschrift. Von Dr. Ernst Fuchs, ordentl. Prof. der Augenheilkunde an der Universität Lüttich. – Herausgegeben von der Society for the prevention of blindness. – Motto: Viribus unitis". Wiesbaden. Verlag von J. F. Bergmann 1885. Preis 2 M. 40 Pf., in: *Dt. Med. Wochenschr.* 11 (1885), pp. 240–241 and 258–259.

J. R. O. COLLIN, C. BEARD, W. H. STERN, D. SCHOENGARTH, "Blepharochalasis", in: *Brit. J. Ophthalmol.* 63 (1979), pp. 542–546.

Wilhelm COMBERG, "Fünfzig Jahre Lokalanästhesie des Auge"s, in: *Münch. Med. Wochenschr.* 81 (1934), pp. 1649.

Comptes-rendues du XII Congrès International de Médecine, Moscou, 7 (19)–14 (26) août 1897. Typ.-lith. Soc. I. N. Kouchnérev & cie, Moscou 1898–1900.

Frederick C. CORDES, "Hans Barkan (1882–1960)", in: *Am. J. Ophthalmol.* 50 (1960), pp. 185–186.

Frederick C. CORDES, "Hans Barkan, M. D"., in: *Trans. Am. Ophthalmol. Soc.* 58 (1960), pp. 7–8. **E. CRAMER, H. KÖLLNER, W. REIS, F. SCHIECK, R.THIEL**, *Kurzes Handbuch der Ophthalmologie*. Vol. 4. Julius Springer, Berlin 1931.

Max de CRINIS, "Meynert in seinem Einfluß auf die moderne psychiatrische Forschung", in: *Wien. klin. Wochenschr.* 55 (1942), pp. 781–782.

Colman W. CUTLER, "Ueber angeborene Nachtblindheit und Pigmentdegeneration", in: *Arch. Augenheilk.* 30 (1895), pp. 92–116.

Colman W. CUTLER, "Drei ungewöhnliche Fälle von Retino-Chorioideal-Degeneration", in: *Arch. Augenheilk.* 30 (1895), pp. 117–122.

S. CZAPSKI, "Mittheilungen aus der Werkstatt von Carl Zeiss in Jena", in: *Zeitschr. wissenschaftl. Mikroskopie u. mikroskop. Technik* 4 (1887), pp. 289–292.

Felix CZEIKE, Historisches Lexikon Wien in 5 Bänden. Kremayr & Scheriau, Vienna 1992–1997, Vol 6 (Supplement) 2004.

Felix F. CZEIPEK, *Wien-Wieden. Historische Bezirksbilder*. Sutton Verlag, Erfurt 2004.

Wilhelm CZERMAK, *Die augenärztlichen Operationen*. Karl Gerold's Sohn, Vienna 1893–1904.

I. CZUKRÁSZ, "Über das Diktyom des Strahlenkörpers", in: *Graefes Archiv* 142 (1941), pp. 619–626.

Albin DALÉN, "Zur Kenntnis der sogenannten Chorioiditis sympathica", in: *Mitteil.Carol. medico- chir. Inst. zu Stockholm* 6 (1904), pp. 6–21.

Franz DAXECKER, "125 Jahre Universitäts-Augenklinik Innsbruck 1869–1994. Ihre Vorstände". (= *Veröffentlichungen der Universität Innsbruck* 201). Universitätsverlag Wagner, Innsbruck 1994.

Franz DAXECKER, "Richard Seefelder. Vorstand der Univ.–Klinik für Augenheilkunde in Innsbruck von 1919 bis 1945", in: *Klin. Monatsbl. Augenheilk.* 224 (2007), pp. 952–953.

Franz DAXECKER, "Das Schicksal des Prof. Ludwig Mauthner (1840–1894). The Fateful Life of Prof. Ludwig Mauthner (1840–1894)", in: *Klin. Monatsbl. Augenheilk.* 225 (2008), pp. 173–174.

Franz DAXECKER, "Geschichte der Innsbrucker Medizinischen Schule. Von Claudia de' Medici bis zur ersten Rektorin 2013", in: *Die Innsbrucker Medizinische Schule*, 2nd ed., Medical University Press, Innsbruck 2013.

Daily Journal of the British Medical Association Forty-Eighth Annual Meeting, Cambridge 1880.

"Dedication of the Wilmer Institute", in: *Bulletin of the Johns Hopkins Hospital* 47 (1930), pp. 44ff.

Erich DEIMER, *Chronik der Allgemeinen Poliklinik in Vienna im Spiegel der Medizin- und Sozialgeschichte*. Göschl, Vienna 1989.

Richard DEUTSCHMANN (ed.), *Beiträge zur Augenheilkunde in Gemeinschaft mit E. Fuchs, O. Haab, A. Vossius*. III issue. Hamburg & Leipzig 1890–1891, pp. 201–207.

Richard DEUTSCHMANN (ed.), *Beiträge zur Augenheilkunde in Gemeinschaft mit E. Fuchs, O. Haab, A. Vossius*. VI and VII issues. Leopold Voss, Hamburg/Leipzig 1892.

Richard DEUTSCHMANN (ed.), *Beiträge zur Augenheilkunde*. IX issue, Leopold Voss, Hamburg–Leipzig 1893.

Richard DEUTSCHMANN (ed.), *Beiträge zur praktischen Augenheilkunde*. Issue 44 (1900).

Richard DEUTSCHMANN, "Seltene Bindehauterkrankungen", in: *Graefes Archiv* 105 (1921), pp. 279–285.

Georg DHOM, *Geschichte der Histopathologie*. Springer, Berlin–Heidelberg 2001.

Charles DICKENS, *Dickens's Dictionary of London 1879*. An Unconventional Handbook. Charles Dickens, London/Macmillan & Co., New York 1879.

Joachim DIEDERICHS, "Von wem stammt die Melodie der österreichischen Bundeshymne?", in: *Österr. Musikzeitschr.* 73, (2018), Issue 1.

Die Deutsche Karl-Ferdinands-Universität in Prague unter der Regierung Seiner Majestät des Kaisers Franz Josef I. Verlag der J. G. Calveschen K. u. K. Hof- u. Universitätsbuchhandlung (Josef Koch), Prague 1869.

Die feierliche Inauguration des Rectors der Wiener Universität für das Studienjahr 1897/98. Selbstverlag d. k. k.Univ. Vienna 1897.

"Die Medizinische Fakultät der Leopold-Franzens-Universität Innsbruck [= Veröffentlichungen der Universität Innsbruck 190]. Universität Innsbruck 1992.

Sven DIERIG, *Wissenschaft in der Maschinenstadt. Emil Du Bois – Reymond und seine Laboratorien in Berlin*. Wallstein, Göttingen 2006.

Friedrich DIMMER, "Ferdinand Ritter von Arlt. Zu seinem hundertsten Geburtstag", in: *Wien. klin. Wochenschr.* 25 (1912), pp. 607–608.

Friedrich DIMMER, "Über diffuse Rotfärbung des Glaskörpers bei Glaskörperblutungen", in: *Wien. med. Wochenschr.* 71 (1921), cols. 1049–1051.

Friedrich DIMMER, *Der Augenspiegel und die ophthalmoskopische Diagnostik*. Third completely revised and enlarged edition. Deuticke, Leipzig 1921.

Friedrich DIMMER, "Über die Lichtempfindung bei geschlossenen Lidern", in: Graefes Archiv 105 (1921), pp. 794–798.

Friedrich DIMMER, Arnold PILLAT, *Atlas photographischer Bilder des menschlichen Augenhintergrundes*. 325 Abbildungen in Lichtdruck nach Photographien vom lebenden Auge. Franz Deuticke, Leipzig/Vienna 1927.

Directory of the American Board for Ophthalmic Examinations. Vol. 2, 1931.

W. DOERR, G. SEIFERT, E. UEHLINGER, *Spezielle pathologische Anatomie*. Vol. 15. Springer-Verlag, Berlin/Heidelberg/New York 1982.

F. C. DONDERS, *On the Anomalies of Accommodation and Refraction of the Eye. With a Preliminary Essay on Physiological Dioptrics.* Translated from the Author's Manuscript by William Daniel Moore. The New Sydenham Society, London 1864.

F. C. DONDERS, *Die Anomalien der Refraction und Accommodation des Auges*. Deutsche Originalausgabe unter Mitwirkung des Verfassers herausgegeben von Dr. Otto Becker. Braumüller, Vienna 1866.

Frans Cornelis DONDERS, "Ueber Farbensysteme", in: *Graefes Archiv* 27/Abth. 1 (1881), pp. 155–223.

Frans Cornelis DONDERS, "Noch einmal die Farbensysteme", in: *Graefes Archiv* 30/Abth. 1 (1884), pp. 15–90.

Nancileigh M. DOYLE, James F. DOYLE, Edward J. WALTER, "The life and work of Harvey Cushing 1869–1939: A pioneer of neurosurgery", in: *J. Intensive Care Soc.* 18/2 (2017), p. 157–158.

Robert C. DREWS, "The Leslie Dana Gold Medal", in: *Am. J. Ophthalmol.* 105/6 (1988), pp. 683–685.

Estelle DU BOIS-REYMOND (ed.), *Jugendbriefe von Emil Du Bois-Reymond an Eduard Hallmann*. Berlin 1918.

Benedict DUDDELL, *A Treatise on the Diseases of the Horny-Coat of the Eye, and the Various Kinds of Cataracts. To which is Prefix'd A Method, entirely New, of Scarifying the Eyes for several Disorders. With Remarks on the Practice of some Oculists both at Home and Abroad.* John Clark, London 1729.

Sir Steward DUKE-ELDER, *A Century of International Ophthalmology 1857–1957*. Written at the Request of the International Council of Ophthalmology, Kimpton 1958.

Arno DUSINI (ed.), Franz GRILLPARZER, *Selbstbiographie*. Residenz Verlag, Salzburg/Vienna 1994.

Daniel van DUYSE, *Coup d'œil sur l'Histoire de l'Ophtalmologie en Belgique au XIXe siècle*. Ad. Host, Gand 1912.

Viktor v. EBNER, "Zum 100. Geburtstage von Theodor Schwann. Gedenkrede, gehalten am 30. September 1910 in der Schlußsitzung des VII. internationalen Physiologenkongresses", in: *Wien. klin. Wochenschr.* 23 (1910), pp. 1404–1406.

(Ed.), "Ectropium anguli oculi externi, cured by the Tarsoraphia, a new operation". By Prof. WALTHER. †, in: *The Lancet* 8/203 (1827), p. 492.

(Ed.), "Barbieri Endowment at Vienna", in: *JAMA*, Feb. 17, 1906, p. 522.

(Ed.), "In Memory of Billroth", in: *BMJ*, Feb. 24, 1906, p. 454.

(Ed.), "The Lane Medical Lectures for 1911", in: *California State J. of Medicine* 9/7 (1911), p. 306.

(Ed.), "Minutes of the Proceedings. Forty-Seventh Annual Meeting. American Ophthalmological Society 1911", in: *Transact. Am. Ophthalmol. Soc.* 12/3 (1911), pp. 708–717.

(Ed.), "The China Medical Missionary Association", in: *The Lancet* 183 (1914), p. 1412.

(Ed.), "Professor Fuchs to Visit Texas", in: *Texas Medicine* 17 (1922), p. 380.

(Ed.), "Ernst Fuchs's Society", in: Am. *J. Ophthalmol.* 6/1 (1923), p. 55.

(Ed.), "The Wilmer Ophthalmological Institute," in: *Brit. J. Ophthalmol.* 13 (1929), pp. 621–622.

(Ed.), "Ophthalmological Society of the United Kingdom. Brief History of the Society", in: *Ann. R. Coll. Surg. Engl.* 56 (1975), pp. 52–53.

(Ed.), "Europe in Advance of Us – A Tribute to Hermann Knapp", in: *J. Am. Med. Assoc.* 305/19 (2011), p. 2017 (= Series *JAMA 100 Years Ago*).

Ambrose Earl EDGERTON, "Circinate Retinitis", in: *Am. J. Ophthalmol.* 19 (1936), pp. 463–469. *Eighth Annual Report of the National Committee for the Prevention of Blindness.* December 31, 1922, New York 1922.

Anton EISELSBERG, *Lebensweg eines Chirurgen*. Tyrolia, Innsbruck 1937. Revised ed., *Lebensweg eines Chirurgen. Eine Autobiographie aus der großen Zeit der Wiener Medizin 1860–1937*. Brandstätter, Vienna 1991, Reprint of the 1st ed. Severus, Hamburg 2010.

Ludwig EISENBERG, *Das geistige Wien*. Künstler- und Schriftsteller Lexikon. Vol. 2: *Medicinisch-naturwissenschaftlicher Theil. Mittheilungen über Wiener Fachschriftsteller und Gelehrte auf dem Gebiete der Medicin (nebst Thierheilkunde und Pharmacie) und Naturwissenschaften*. C. Daberow, Vienna 1893.

(Anton ELFINGER), *Horizontaler Durchschnitt des menschlichen Auges nach Präparaten des Professors Dr. Arlt gezeichnet von Dr. Elfinger*. 1862. Wilhelm Braumüller, Vienna 1875.

Anton ELSCHNIG (ed.), Prof. Dr. Wilhelm CZERMAK, *Die augenärztlichen Operationen*. 2nd enlarged ed. Urban & Schwarzenberg, Berlin/Vienna 1908.

Anton ELSCHNIG, *Augenpflege*. August Hirschwald, Berlin 1915.

Anton ELSCHNIG, "Die Grundlage der Spätinfektion nach Trepanation und der Wagenmannschen Infektion", in: *Graefes Archiv* 105 (1921), pp. 599–604.

Anton ELSCHNIG (ed.), *Augenärztliche Operationslehre*. In two vols. In: Theodor AXENFELD, Anton ELSCHNIG, *Handbuch der gesamten Augenheilkunde begründet von A. Graefe und Th. Saemisch fortgeführt von C. Hess*. 2nd and 3rd revised editions. I. Julius Springer, Berlin 1922.

Carl EMANUEL, "Ein Fall von Gliom der Pars ciliaris retinae nebst Bemerkungen zur Lehre von den Netzhaut-Tumoren", in: *Graefes Archiv* 161/II (1900), pp. 338–364.

Isolde EMICH, "In memoriam Dr. med. Anton Elfinger (geb. 15. Januar 1821, gest. 18. Januar 1864). Zu Leben und Werk des Wiener Mediziners und Karikaturisten 'Cajetan'", in: *Materia therapeutica* 17 (1971), pp. 117–144.

W. ENGELMAYR, G. K. KRIEGLSTEIN, *Pilokarpin. Ein Jahrhundert in der Glaukomtherapie*. Kaden, Heidelberg 1980.

W. EPPACHER, "Die Tschurtschenthaler, ein uraltes Tiroler Geschlecht", in: *Amtsblatt d. Landeshauptstadt Innsbruck* 23/Nr. 9, September 1960.

Albert ESSER, *Geschichte der Deutschen Ophthalmologischen Gesellschaft*. Zur ersten Säkularfeier im Auftrage der Gesellschaft geschrieben. J. F. Bergmann, Munich 1957.

Hans-Heinz EULNER, *Die Entwicklung der medizinischen Spezialfächer an den Universitäten des deutschen Sprachgebietes. (= Studien zur Medizingeschichte des neunzehnten Jahrhunderts Bd. IV/ ed. Walter ARTELT, Walter RÜEGG)*. Ferdinand Enke, Stuttgart 1970.

John N. EVANS (Book Review), Diseases of the Eye. Hofrat Ernst Fuchs. Fifteenth German edition, rev. by Maximilian Salzmann and transl. by E. V. L. Brown, M. D. 10th English edition, Philadelphia: J. P. Lippincott, 1933. 641 pp., in: *The Sight-Saving Review*, Vol. 3, Nr. 4 (1933), pp. 307–308.

Oskar EVERSBUSCH, "Zum 70. Geburtstag von Dr.med. Carl, Herzog in Bayern", in: *Münch. med. Wochenschr*. 56 (1909), pp. 1648–1649.

Karl EWALD, "Eduard Albert (20. 1. 1841 bis 25. 9. 1900) und die Chirurgie seiner Zeit", in: 91 (1941), cols. 79ff. and cols. 121ff.

Sigmund EXNER, "Ernst v. Brücke und die moderne Physiologie", in: *Wien. klin. Wochenschr*. 3 (1890), pp. 807–812.

Sigmund EXNER, "Das neue physiologische Institut in Wien". Keynote delivered on 2. May 1904, in: *Wien. klin. Wochenschr*. 17 (1904), pp. 712–716.

Exposition Universelle Liége 1905.

F. A. J., "Professor Dr. Josef Meller (Vienna)", in: *Brit. J. of Ophthalmol*. 33 (1949), pp. 653–654.

Helmut FANTA, "Hochdruck und Auge", in: *Wien. klin. Wochenschr.* 63 (1951), pp. 649–652.

Wolfgang FASCHINGER, "Zum 150. Geburtstag von Maximilian Salzmann (1862–1954)", in: *Spektrum Augenheilkd.* 27 (2013), pp. 153–156.

Stella FATOVIĆ-FERENČIĆ, "Anton Elfinger (1821–1862)", in: Christoph LÖSER, Gerd PLEWIG (eds.), *Pantheon der Dermatologie.* Springer, Heidelberg 2008, pp. 256–259.

Stella FATOVIĆ-FERENČIĆ, "Carl Heitzmann (1836–1896)", in: Christoph LÖSER, Gerd PLEWIG (eds.), *Pantheon der Dermatologie.* Springer, Heidelberg 2008, pp. 433–437.

Mary E. FERGUSON, *China Medical Board and Peking Union Medical College. A Chronicle of Fruitful Collaboration 1914–1951.* China Medical Board of New York, Inc., New York 1970.

"Feier des 70. Geburtstages Ernst Fuchs's am 14. Juni 1921 in Wien", in: *Zeitschr. Augenheilk.* 47 (1922), pp. 47–63.

Festschrift Julius Hirschberg von Schülern und Freunden aus Anlass seiner fünfundzwanzigjährigen Wirksamkeit als Professor an der Universität Berlin in Verehrung überreicht. Veit & Comp., Leipzig 1905.

Festschrift zur Feier des siebzigsten Geburtstages Herrn Hofrat Prof. Dr. Ernst Fuchs in Wien gewidmet von Freunden und dankbaren Schülern [= Graefes Archiv 105 (1921)].

Festschrift für Leopold v. Schrötter, in: *Wien. med. Wochenschr.* 87 (1937), cols. 141–152, 157–160 and 163–164.

Noël FIESSINGER, R. RENDU, "Sur un syndrome caractérisé par l'inflammation simultanée de toutes les muqueuses externes coexistant avec une éruption vésiculeuse des quatre membres, non douloureuse et non récidivante", in: *Paris médicale* 25 (1917), pp. 54–58.

Fifteenth Annual Report of the Medical Superintendent of the Peking Union Medical College Hospital. For the Year Ending June 30, 1923. Peking 1923.

F. FISCHER, "13. Internationaler Ophthalmologischer Kongreß 5.–13. September 1929", in: *Zeitschr. Augenheilk.* 67 (1929), pp. 396–398.

Isidor FISCHER (ed.), "Theodor Billroth und seine Zeitgenossen. In Briefen an Billroth". Aus dem Archiv der Gesellschaft der Ärzte in Wien. Urban & Schwarzenberg, Berlin/Vienna 1929.

Isidor FISCHER, *Geschichte der Geburtshilfe in Wien.* Franz Deuticke, Leipzig and Vienna 1909.

Isidor FISCHER, "Zur Vorgeschichte der Wiener Augenkliniken", in: *Zeitschr. Augenheilk.* 85 (1935), pp. 226–236.

Isidor FISCHER (ed.), *Biographisches Lexikon der hervorragenden Ärzte der letzten fünfzig Jahre. Zweite und dritte unveränderte Auflage. Zugleich Fortsetzung des Biographischen Lexikons der hervorragenden Ärzte aller Zeiten und Völker.* Urban & Schwarzenberg, Munich/Berlin 1962.

W. A. FISHER, "Senile Cataract. Methods of Operating". With the collaboration of Prof. E. FUCHS, Vienna, Austria; Prof. L. BARRAQUER, Spain, Lt. Col. Henry SMITH, London, England; Dr. H. T. HOLLAND, Shikarpur, Sindh, India; Dr. John Westley WRIGHT, Columbus, O. Chicago Eye, Ear, Nose and Throat College, Chicago 1923.

Francesco FLARER, *Riflessioni sulla Trichiasi, sulla Distichiasi e sull'Entropio, avuto particolare riguardo ai metodi di Jaeger e di Vaccà.* Lampato, Milano 1828.

Franciscus FLARER, *De iritide eiusque speciebus, earumque curatione commentatio a celeberrima societate medico-practica Parisiensi in primo certamine di XXVII Septembr. Anni MDCCCXXXVI numismate aureo publice donate.* Ticini Regii, Typographia Bizzoni 1841.

H. J. FLIERINGA,"Der Ringabszess in der Hornhaut", in: *Klin. Monatsbl. Augenheilk.* 69/2 (1922), pp. 241–248.

Marcel FLORKIN, *Naissance et déviation de la théorie cellulaire dans l'œuvre de Théodore Schwann*. Hermann, Paris 1960.

Marcel FLORKIN, "Les origines de l'Hôpital de Bavière", in: Marcel FLORKIN, Léon-E. HALKIN (eds.), *Chronique de l'Université de Liège*. Université, Liège 1967, pp. 9–22.

Marcel FLORKIN, "La personnalité de Théodore Schwann", in: ibid, pp. 147–167.

Marcel FLORKIN, "Le passage de Théodore Schwann de la Faculté de médecine de Louvain à celle de Liège", in : ibid., pp. 169–179.

Marcel FLORKIN, "Apports viennois à la Faculté de médecine de Liège", in: ibid., pp. 217–230.

Marcel FLORKIN, "L'enseignement clinique au Vieux-Bavière et au Nouveau-Bavière", in: ibid, pp. 407–431.

Marcel FLORKIN, Léon-E. HALKIN (eds.), *Chronique de l'Université de Liège*. Université, Liège 1967.

Marcel FLORKIN, "Le 150e anniversaire de l'Université de Liège et l'histoire de sa Faculté de médecine", in: *Médecine et Hygiène* 25 (1967), p. 537–538.

Marcel FLORKIN, "Les Années de Professorat de Karl Gussenbauer, d'Alexander von Winiwarter et d'Ernst Fuchs à la faculté de médecine de Liège", in: Erna LESKY (ed.), *Wien und die Weltmedizin*. Hermann Böhlaus Nachfolger. ,Vienna/Cologne/Graz 1974, pp. 196–203.

"Forty-Eighth Annual Meeting of the British Medical Association", in: *Brit. Med. J.* II (1880), pp. 780ff.

Benedikt FÖGER, Klaus TASCHWER, *Die andere Seite des Spiegels. Konrad Lorenz und der Nationalsozialismus*. Czernin-Verlag 2001.

Carl F. R. FÖRSTER, *Ophthalmologische Beiträge*. Enslin, Berlin 1862.

(Alexander FRAENKEL), "Domenico Barbieri", in: *Wien. klin. Wochenschr.* 19 (1906), p. 53.

E. FRANKE, "Zur Kenntnis des Lymphangioms der Bindehaut", in: *Graefes Archiv* 105 (1921), pp. 1058–1068.

Léon FREDERICQ, J.-P. NUEL, *Élements de physiologie humaine à l›usage des étudiants en médecine*. Gand et Paris 1883.

Sigmund FREUD, "Beitrag zur Kenntnis der Cocawirkung", in: *Wien. med. Wochenschr.* 35 (1885), cols. 129–133.

Gustav FREUDENTHAL, "Ueber das Sarcom des Uvealtractus", in: *Graefes Archiv* 37/Abth. I (1891), pp. 137–184.

Irmgard FREY, Lenore LÜBKE-SCHMID, Walter WENZEL, *Krankenpflegehilfe. Alle Fächer für Ausbildung und Praxis*. 11th rev. ed., Georg Thieme Verlag, Stuttgart 2002.

Heinz FREYLER, "Die I. Universitäts-Augenklinik in Wien von Arlt bis heute – zur 175-Jahr-Feier", in: *Spektrum Augenheilk.* 2/2A (1988), pp. 9–17.

George FRICK, *A Treatise on the Diseases of the Eye; Including the Doctrines and Practise of the Most Eminent Modern Surgeons and particularly those of Professor Beer*. Fielding Lucas Jr., Baltimore 1823.

Edward FRIDENBERG, "A Case of Retinitis Circinata", in: *Transact. Am. Ophthalmol. Soc.* 8 (1897), pp. 181–185.

Jonas pp. FRIEDENWALD, "The contributions of Professor Ernst Fuchs to ophthalmic pathology", in: *Am. J. Ophthalmol.* 14 (1931), pp. 138–140.

Theodor von FRIMMEL, "Erinnerungen an Josef Hyrtl", in: Alois TROST (ed), *Alt-Wiener Kalender für das Jahr 1919*. Kunstverlag Anton Schroll & Co., Vienna 1919, pp. 53–57.

Adalbert FUCHS, *Amtlicher Bericht über die im Mai 1857 abgehaltene fünfzigjährige Jubelfeier der k. k.Landwirthschafts-Gesellschaft in Wien an ihre allgemeine Versammlung am 26. Jänner*

1858 erstattet im Auftrage des General-Comité von dessen Schriftführer, dem beständigen Secretär der Gesellschaft, Prof. Dr. Ad. Fuchs. K. K. Hof- und Staatsdruckerei, Vienna 1858.

Adalbert FUCHS, "Über subkonjunktivale Injektionen", in: *Wien. med. Wochenschr.* 71 (1921), cols. 1051–1053.

Adalbert FUCHS, "Zur Pathogenese und Anatomie der Netzhautcysten", in: *Graefes Archiv* 105 (1921), pp. 333–375.

Adalbert FUCHS, *Atlas der Histopathologie des Auges*. Franz Deuticke, Leipzig and Vienna 1923.

Adalbert FUCHS, "Über einige seltene luetische Erkrankungen des Auges", in: *Zeitschr. Augenheilk.* 8 (1926), pp. 315–342.

Adalbert FUCHS, "Pathological Dimples ('Dellen') of the Cornea", in: *Americ. J. Ophthalmol.* 12 (1929), p. 877–883.

Adalbert FUCHS, *Die Erkrankungen des Augenhintergrundes*. Franz Deuticke, Vienna 1943.

Adalbert FUCHS (ed.), *Ernst Fuchs. Wie ein Augenarzt die Welt sah.* Selbstbiographie und Tagebuchblätter. Urban & Schwarzenberg, Vienna 1946.

Adalbert FUCHS, *Diseases of the Fundus Oculi.* Translated by Erich Pressburger. Edited by Abraham Schlossman. First English Edition. The Blakiston Company, London 1949 (Reprint H. K. Lewis & Co., London 1951).

Adalbert FUCHS, Erich PRESSBURGER, "Myopia inversa", in: *Arch. Ophthalmol.* 37 (1947), pp. 722–739.

Adalbert FUCHS, *Geography of Eye Diseases*. Notring d. wissenschaftl. Verbände Österreichs. Vienna 1962.

Albert FUCHS, *Geistige Strömungen in Österreich 1867–1918*. Mit einem Essay von Friedrich Heer. Löcker, Vienna 1996.

Carolus FUCHS, *Dissertatio inauguralis medico-practica de Endocarditide quam consensu et auctoritate illustrissimi ac magnifici domini Praesidis et Directoris, perillustris ac spectabilis domini Decani, nec non clarissimorum et celeberrimorum D. D. Professorum, pro doctoris medicinae laurea summisque in medicina honoribus ac privilegiis rite et legitime obtinendis in antiquissima ac celeberrima Universitate Vindobonensi publicae eruditorum disquisitioni submittit.* Schmid 1837.

Ernst FUCHS, "Herpes iris conjunctivae. Beobachtet an der Klinik des Professor von Arlt", in: *Klin. Monatsbl. Augenheilk.* 14 (1876), pp. 333–351.

Ernst FUCHS, "Ueber Keratitis traumatica". Vorläufige Mitteilung, in: *Centalbl. med. Wissensch.* 14 (1876), pp. 113–114.

Ernst FUCHS, "Ueber die traumatische Keratitis", in: *Virchows Archiv* 66 (1876), pp. 401–445.

Ernst FUCHS, "Beitrag zur Kenntnis des Froschblutes und der Froschlymphe", in: *Virchows Archiv* 71 (1877), pp. 78–107.

Ernst FUCHS, "Chorioiditis bei Glaukom", in: Frans Cornelis DONDERS, Wilhelm HESS, Wilhelm

ZEHENDER (eds.), *Bericht über die elfte Versammlung der Opthalmologischen Gesellschaft Heidelberg 1878*. Universitäts-Buchdruckerei von Adler's Erben. Rostock 1878, pp. 65.

Ernst FUCHS, "Ueber die Verwendung des Pilocarpins in Augenkrankheiten", in: *Wien. med. Wochenschr.* 28 (1878), cols. 997–999 and 1013–1017.

Ernst FUCHS, "Vollständige Sequestration der Cornea nach einfacher Linearextraktion", in: *Klin. Monatsbl. f. Augenheilk.* 18 (1880), pp. 134–139.

Ernst FUCHS, "Über die Anwendung des Ferrum cadens bei Hornhauterkrankungen", in: *Anzeiger d. k. k.Gesellschaft d. Aerzte in Wien*, Protokoll der Sitzung vom 11. Februar 1881, pp. 145f. (Pres.).

Ernst FUCHS, "Die Anwendung des Glüheisens bei Hornhautleiden", in: *Wien. med. Wochenschr.* 31 (1881), cols. 621–624.

Ernst FUCHS, "Ueber glaukomatöse Hornhauttrübung", in: *Bericht über die Dreizehnte Versammlung der Ophthalmologischen Gesellschaft.* Heidelberg 1881. Redigirt durch F. C. Donders, W. Hess u. W. Zehender. Universitäts-Buchdruckerei von Adler's Erben. Rostock 1881, pp. 73–79 (Discussion pp. 79–80).

Ernst FUCHS, "Ueber die Trübung der Hornhaut bei Glaucom", in: *Graefes Archiv* 27/III (1881), pp. 66–92.

Ernst FUCHS, "Beitrag zu den angeborenen Anomalien des Sehnerven", in: *Graefes Archiv* 28/ Abth. I (1882), pp. 139–169.

Ernst FUCHS, *Das Sarcom des Uvealtractus.* Wilhelm Braumüller, Vienna 1882.

Ernst FUCHS, "Anatomische Miscellen: III. Glaucoma inflammatorium", in: *Graefes Archiv* 30/ Abth. III (1884), pp. 123–138.

Ernst FUCHS, "Beiträge zur normalen Anatomie des Augapfels", in: *Graefes Archiv* 30/Abth. IV (1884), pp. 1–60.

Ernst FUCHS, "Beiträge zu den Anomalien der Refraction und Accommodation. (Zur Entstehung der Myopie/ Myopie bei Cataracta senilis incipiens/Sympathische Accommodationslähmung)", in: *Klin. Monatsbl. f. Augenheilk.* 22 (1884), pp. 14–24.

Ernst FUCHS, "Antrittsrede gehalten bei Eröffnung seiner Vorlesungen an der Wiener Universität Montag den 19. October 1885", in: *Wien. med. Bl.* 8 (1885), cols. 1301–1304.

Ernst FUCHS, "Die periphere Atrophie des Sehnerven", in: *Graefes Archiv* 31/Abth. I (1885), pp. 177–200.

Ernst FUCHS, "Zur Physiologie und Pathologie des Lidschlusses", in: Graefes Archiv 31/Abth. II (1885), pp. 97–120.

Ernst FUCHS, "Zur Anatomie der Iris", in: *Klin. Monatsbl. Augenheilk.* 23 (1885), pp. 467–478.

Ernst FUCHS, "Beiträge zur normalen Anatomie der menschlichen Iris", in: *Graefes Archiv* 31/ Abth. III (1885), pp. 39–86.

Ernst FUCHS, *Die Ursachen und die Verhütung der Blindheit.* Gekrönte Preisschrift. Herausgegeben durch die Society for the Prevention of Blindness in London. Bergmann, Wiesbaden 1885.

Ernst FUCHS, *The Causes and the Prevention of Blindness by Dr. Ernst Fuchs, Professor of Ophthalmology in the University of Liege. VIRIBUS UNITIS. The Essay which gained the Prize of £80 offered by the Society for the Prevention of Blindness in London.* Translated by R. E. Dudgeon [...]. With a Few Notes by Dr. M. Roth. Ballière, Tindall & Cox, London 1885.

Ernst FUCHS, *Causes et prévention de la cécité. (Mémoire couronné).* Traduction par le Docteur Fieuzal. G. Steinheil, Paris 1885.

Ernst FUCHS, O prichinakh i preduprezhdenii sliepoti. Perevod s *niemetskavo.* E. I. Fyodoroff, Kiev 1885.

Ernst FUCHS, "Ferdinand Ritter von Arlt †", in: *Wien. med. Bl.* 10 (1887), pp. 317–321.

Ernst FUCHS, "Über traumatische Linsentrübung", in: *Wien. klin. Wochenschr.* 1 (1888), pp. 53–57 and 86–88.

Ernst FUCHS, "Die Entzündungen des Lidrandes", in: *Wien. klin. Wochenschr.* 1 (1888), pp. 773–776 and 807–810.

Ernst FUCHS, "Franz Cornelius Donders †", in: *Wien. klin. Wochenschr.* 2 (1889), pp. 271–272.

Ernst FUCHS, *Lehrbuch der Augenheilkunde.* 1st.–18th eds., Franz Deuticke 1889–1945.
Ernst FUCHS, "Keratitis punctata superficialis", in: *Wien. klin. Wochenschr.* 2 (1889), pp. 837–841.
Ernst FUCHS, "Otto Becker †", in: *Wien. klin. Wochenschr.* 3 (1890), pp. 159.
Ernst FUCHS, *Intorno alle cause della cecità ed al modo di prevenirla. VIRIBUS UNITIpp. Saggio che ottenne il Premio di L. 2000 dalla Società inglese di Prevenzione della Cecità.* Tradotto e pubblicato a cura della medesima società italiana. Tipografia Bonducciana – A. eozzi, Firenze 1890.
Ernst FUCHS, "Ueber isolierte doppelseitige Ptosis", in: *Graefes Archiv* 36/Abtheil. I (1890), pp. 234–259.
Ernst FUCHS, *Text-Book of Ophthalmology by Dr. Ernest Fuchs.* Authorized Translation from the Second Enlarged and Improved German Edition by A. Duane, M. D. D. Appleton and Company, New York 1892. (Reprints: 1893, 1898).
Ernst FUCHS, *Manuel d'Ophtalmologie.* Traduit sur la deuxième édition allemande par le Docteur C. Lacompte et le Docteur L. Leplat. Georges Carré, Paris 1892.
Ernst FUCHS, *Tratado de enfermedades de los ojos por el Dr. E. Fuchs catedrático ordinario de oftalmología en la Universidad de Viena traducido por Don Víctor Cebrián y Díez medico de número del Hospital de Madrid.* Con un prologo del Doctor Osío y 74 figuras intercaladas en el texto. Tomo I + II. Biblioteca escogida del Siglo Médico, Madrid 1893.
Ernst FUCHS, "Ueber das Pterygium", in: *Graefes Archiv* 38 (1892), Abtheil. II, pp. 1–90.
Ernst FUCHS, "Über Aufhellung von Hornhautnarben", in: Richard DEUTSCHMANN (ed.), Beiträge zur Augenheilkunde. IX. Heft, Leopold Voss, Hamburg–Leipzig 1893, pp. 1–11.
Ernst FUCHS, "Die neuen Methoden der Staaroperation", in: *Wien. klin. Wochenschr.* 6 (1893), pp. 19–23.
Ernst FUCHS, "Retinitis circinata", in: *Graefes Archiv* 39 /Abth. III (1893), pp. 229–279.
Ernst FUCHS, "Die ägyptische Augenentzündung", in: *Wien. klin. Wochenschr.* 7 (1894), pp. 211–214.
Ernst FUCHS, "Egyptian Ophthalmia", in: The Medical Age. A Semi-Monthly Review of Medicine 12 (1894), pp. 262–267.
Ernst FUCHS, "Episcleritis periodica fugax", in: *Brit. Med. J.*, Oct. 19, 1895, pp. 951–953.
Ernst FUCHS, "Ueber Episcleritis periodica fugax", in: *Wien. klin. Wochenschr.* 8 (1895), pp. 601–603.
Ernst FUCHS, "Ueber Episcleritis periodica fugax", in: *Graefes Archiv* 41/Abtheil. I (1895) pp. 229–273.
Ernst FUCHS, *Lehrbuch der Augenheilkunde*: Japanese Translation by Tatsushichiro Inouye and Y. Morosumi. (Parts 1 and 2). Asakaya, Tokio 1895.
Ernst FUCHS, *Leseproben für die Nähe. Jäger's Schriftscalen modifiziert von Professor Dr. E. Fuchs.* Fritsch, Vienna 1895.
Ernst FUCHS, "Ueber Blepharochalasis (Erschlaffung der Lidhaut)", in: *Wien. klin. Wochenschr.* 9 (1896), pp. 109–110.
Ernst FUCHS, "Denkrede auf Arlt. Gehalten am 9. Juli 1896 bei der Enthüllung seines Denkmals im Arkadenhof der Universität Wien", in: Anton BETTELHEIM (ed.), *Biographische Blätter. Jahrbuch für lebensgeschichtliche Kunst und Forschung.* Vol. 2. Ernst Hofmann & Co. Berlin 1896, pp. 384–388.
Ernst FUCHS, "Ueber zwei der Retinitis pigmentosa verwandte Krankheiten (Retinitis punctata albescens und Atrophia gyrata chorioideae et retinae)", in: Archiv Augenheilk. 32 (1896), pp. 111–116.

Ernst FUCHS, *Rukovodstwo k glasnym bolsnjam. (Lehrbuch der Augenheilkunde).* Russian translation by A. V. Natanson and L. E. Vorontsova, according to Fuchs's 5th ed. St. Petersburg 1897.

Ernst FUCHS, *Manuel d'ophtalmologie. Seconde édition française, traduite sur la cinquième édition allemande par G. Lacomte et L. Leplat.* G. Carré & C. Naud, Paris 1897.

Ernst FUCHS, *Trattato di oftalmiatria, ad uso degli studenti e di medici pratici.* Traduzione italiana eseguita sull'ultima edizione tedesca dal dott. Gius. Cirincione, con prefazione del Prof. Carlo de Vincentiis, Casa Edit. Dott. V. Pasquale, Napoli 1897.

Ernst FUCHS, "Two diseases related to retinitis pigmentosa: retinitis punctata albescens and atrophia gyrata choroideae et retinae", in: *Arch. Ophth.* 27 (1898), pp. 484–489.

Ernst FUCHS, Text-Book of Ophthalmology by Dr. Ernest Fuchs. Authorized Translation, Revised from the Seventh Enlarged and Improved German Edition by A. Duane, M. D. Second American Edition. D. Appleton and Company, New York 1899.

Ernst FUCHS, "Ablösung der Aderhaut nach Staaroperation", in: *Graefes Archiv* 51 (1900), pp. 199–224.

Ernst FUCHS, "Ablösung der Aderhaut nach Staaroperation", in: *Bericht über die 28. Versammlung d. Ophthalmol. Gesellsch. Heidelberg 1900.* Bergmann, Wiesbaden 1901, pp. 84–87.

Ernst FUCHS, "Ueber ringförmige und scheibenförmige Keratitis (Keratitis annularis et disciformis)", in: *Klin. Monatsbl. Augenheilk.* 39 (1901), pp. 513–523.

Ernst FUCHS, "Ueber Randsklerose und Randatrophie der Hornhaut", in: *Graefes Archiv* 52 (1901), pp. 317–329.

Ernst FUCHS, "Das Ulcus atheromatosum corneae (sequestrirende Narbenkeratitis)", in: *Graefes Archiv* 53 (1901), pp. 61–73.

Ernst FUCHS, "Der centrale schwarze Fleck bei Myopie", in: *Zeitschr. Augenheilk.* 5 (1901), pp. 171–178.

Ernst FUCHS, "Ablösung der Aderhaut nach Operation", in: *Graefes Archiv* 53 (1902), pp. 375–400.

Ernst FUCHS, "Ueber Cocain", in: *Wien. klin. Wochenschr.* 15 (1902), pp. 962–964.

Ernst FUCHS, "On Keratitis. Being the Bowman Lecture". Delivered on June 13, 1902, in: *Transact. Opthalmol. Soc. United Kingdom* 22 (1902), pp. 15–34.

Ernst FUCHS, "Ueber knötchenförmige Hornhauttrübung", in: *Graefes Archiv* 53 (1902), pp. 423–438.

Ernst FUCHS, "Über Ringabscess der Hornhaut", in: *Graefes Archiv* 61 (1903), pp. 1–31.

Ernst FUCHS, "Scleritis posterior", in: *Bericht über die 30. Versammlung der Ophthalmologischen Gesellschaft Heidelberg 1902.* Bergmann, Wiesbaden 1903, pp. 71–77.

Ernst FUCHS, "Anatomische Veränderungen bei Entzündung der Aderhaut", in: *Graefes Archiv* 58 (1904), pp. 391–428.

Ernst FUCHS, **"**Über sympathisierende Entzündungen (nebst Bemerkungen über seröse traumatische Iritis), in: *Graefes Archiv* 61 (1905), pp. 365–456.

Ernst FUCHS, *Manuel d'Ophtalmologie. Troisième édition française traduite sur la dixième édition allemande par le Dr. L. Leplat et le Dr. C. Lacompte.* Steinheil, Paris 1906.

Ernst FUCHS, "Über Komplikationen der Heterochromie", in: *Zeitschr. Augenheilk.* 15 (1906), pp. 191–212.

Ernst FUCHS, *Lehrbuch der Augenheilkunde.* 11th ed. Wilhelm Maudrich, Leipzig/Vienna 1907.

Ernst FUCHS, "Auf Xenophons Spuren", in: Heinrich R. v. WITTEK (ed.), F*estgabe zum 100jährigen Jubiläum des Schottengymnasiums gewidmet von ehemaligen Schottenschülern.* Wilhelm Braumüller, Vienna 1907, pp. 96–106.
Ernst FUCHS, "Hermann Snellen † (1834–1908)", Obituary, in: *Wien. klin. Wochenschr.* 21 (1908), pp. 157.
Ernst FUCHS, "Wucherungen und Geschwülste des Ciliarepithels", in: *Graefes Archiv* 68/Abth. II (1908), pp. 534–587.
Ernst FUCHS, "Über Ophthalmia sympathica", in: *Graefes Archiv* 70/Abth. III (1909), pp. 465–485.
Ernst FUCHS, "Dystrophia epithelialis corneae", in: *Graefes Archiv* 76 (1910), pp. 478–508.
Ernst FUCHS, *Lehrbuch der Augenheilkunde.* 12. Auflage. Maudrich, Leipzig/Vienna 1910.
Ernst FUCHS, *Rukovodstwo k glasnym bolsnjam.* (Lehrbuch der Augenheilkunde). Russian translation by E. P. Eberman and S. A. Kaplan from Fuchs's 11th ed. A. A. Karzeva, Moscow 1910.
Ernst FUCHS, "Über Sarcom der Aderhaut nebst Bemerkungen über Nekrose der Uvea", in: *Graefes Archiv* 77/III. Abth., (1910), pp. 304–392.
Ernst FUCHS, "Über Dellen in der Hornhaut", in: *Graefes Archiv* 78 (1911), pp. 82–92.
Ernst FUCHS, "Smallest Sarcoma of the Choroid", in: *Transact. Americ. Ophthalmol.* Soc. 12/ Part III, pp. 787–789 [47th Annual Meeting, New London/Conn. July 11–12, 1911. Exhibition of Specimens, Discussion, pp. 789–190.].
Ernst FUCHS, *Text-Book of Ophthalmology by Ernst Fuchs Vienna.* Eleventh Edition Translated from the Third American Edition by James Boyd Neal, M. A., M. D., Union Medical College, Tsinan. China Medical Missionary Association, Shanghai 1911.
Ernst FUCHS, "Nachtrag zur Arbeit 'Ueber Sarkom der Aderhaut' im LXXVII. Band dieses Archivs", in: *Graefes Archiv* 81 (1912), pp. 556–562.
Ernst FUCHS, "Über chronische endogene Uveitis", in: *Graefes Archiv* 84 (1913), pp. 201–292.
Ernst FUCHS, "Normal pigmentierte und albinotische Iris", in: *Graefes Archiv* 84 (1913), pp. 521–529.
Ernst FUCHS, "Über senile Randatrophie der Hornhaut", in: Graefes Archiv 89 (1915), pp. 386–392.
Ernst FUCHS, Über Keratitis pustuliformis profunda, in: *Graefes Archiv* 90 (1915), pp. 13–75.
Ernst FUCHS, "Erkrankung der Hornhaut durch Schädigung von hinten", in: Graefes Archiv 92 (1916), pp. 145–236.
Ernst FUCHS, "Über den anatomischen Befund einiger angeborener Anomalien der Netzhaut und des Sehnerven", in: *Graefes Archiv* 93 (1917), pp. 1–48.
Ernst FUCHS, "Über Heterochromie nebst Bemerkungen über angeborene Anomalien", in: *Graefes Archiv* 93 (1917), pp. 381–398.
(Ernst FUCHS), "Relaciones entre el ojo y la tabes". Conferencia dada en esta corporación el día 24 de Febrero de 1920, por el Profesor Fuchs (de Viena), in: *Anales de la Real Academia Nacional de Medicina [= Anal.R. Acad. Nac. Med.]* 40 (1920), pp. 531–547.
Ernst FUCHS, "Über senile Veränderungen am Sehnerven", in: *Graefes Archiv* 103 (1920), pp. 304–330.
Ernst FUCHS, "Beleuchtung und Auge. Mit einer historischen Einleitung", in: *Wien. med. Wochenschr. 71* (1921), cols. 1409–1415.
Ernst FUCHS, "Über Chorioretinitis", in: *Graefes Archiv* 107 (1922), pp. 15–25.
Ernst FUCHS, "Senile Changes of the Optic Nerve", in: *Am. J. Ophthalmol.* 5 (1922), pp. 215–217.(Original lecture, College of Physicians of Philadelphia, Section on Ophthalmology. October 20, 1921).

Ernest FUCHS, *Text-Book of Ophthalmology*. Authorized Translation from the Twelfth German Edition, Completely Revised and Reset, with Numerous Additions Specially Supplied by the Author and Otherwise Much Enlarged by Alexander Duane. Seventh Edition Revised and Reset. J. B. Lippincott Company, Philadelphia & London 1923.

Ernst FUCHS, "Die ägyptische Augenkrankheit", in: *Wien. klin. Wochenschr.* 37 (1924), pp. 564–566.

Ernest FUCHS, *Text-Book of Ophthalmology*. Translated from the XII German edition by Dr. Alexander Duane. Eighth Revised Edition. J. B. Lippincott Co., Philadelphia and London 1924.

Ernst FUCHS, "Erinnerungen an Japan", in: *Zeitschr. Augenheilk.* 52 (1924), pp. 305–311.

Ernst FUCHS, "Zur Anatomie der Endophthalmitis", in: *Graefes Archiv* 115 (1925), pp. 387–398.

Ernst FUCHS, "Erinnerungen", in: *Wien. med. Wochenschr.* 75 (1925), pp. 2475–2477.

Ernst FUCHS, "Memories of Vienna Clinics", in: *Am. J. Ophhalmol.* 9 (1926), pp. 605–607.

Ernst FUCHS, *Lehrbuch der Augenheilkunde*. 15 ed. Ed. by Maximilian Salzmann. Vienna 1926.

Ernst FUCHS, *Cuestiones Oftalmologicas (Cinco lecciones dadas en la facultad de medicina de Madrid)*. Traduccíon de la Dra. T. Arroyo de Márquez. Editorial Paracelso, Madrid 1927.

Ernst FUCHS, "Die Therapie des Trachoms", in: *Wien. med. Wochenschr.* 177 (1927), cols. 1615–1618.

Ernst FUCHS, "Wien, das Mekka der amerikanischen Aerzte. Die Weltbedeutung der Wiener Schule", in: *Neue Freie Presse* No. 22963 of 19 August 1928.

Ernst FUCHS, "Development of Ophthalmology in Europe". (Address delivered at dedication of the Wilmer Ophthalmological Institute, Johns Hopkins Hospital, Baltimore, Oct. 15, 1929), in: *Arch. Opthalmol.* 3/2 (1930), pp. 133–147.

Ernst FUCHS, "Subjective Symptomatology of Ocular Disorders". An Address, in: *Amer. J. Ophthalmol.* 13 (1930), p. 113–117.

Ernst FUCHS, "Die Augen der Frau Fischer. Aus der Geschichte der Wiener Augenheilkunde", in: *Neues Wiener Tagblatt* No. 322 of 23 November 1930.

Ernst FUCHS, *Trattato di oftalmologia del Prof. Dott. Ernst Fuchs*. Traduzione italiana sulla 15ª edizione tedesca aumentata ed elaborata dal Dott. Massimiliano Salzmann, Professore di Oculistica nell' Università di Graz eseguita dal Prof. Mario Pagani libero docente. Edizione S.A.V.I.T, Vercelli 1932.

Ernst FUCHS, *Diseases of the Eye*. The Fifteenth German Edition of the Lehrbuch der Augenheilkunde as Revised by Maximilian Salzmann. Authorized Translation by E. V. L. Brown. Tenth English Edition. J. B. Lippincott, Philadelphia–Montreal–London 1933.

Ernst FUCHS, *Tratado de Oftalmología por el Prof. Dr. Ernst Fuchs† completado por el Maximilian Salzmann Profesor de Oftalmología en la Universidad de Graz*. Traducción de la 15.ª Edición Alemana por el Dr. M. Renedo Jefe del Servicio de Oftalmologiá del Hospital Militar de Madrid–Carabanchel con un Apéndice a las Operaciones oculares por el Dr. Salvador Viusá. Editorial Labor, S. A. Barcelona/Madrid/Buenos Aires/Rio de Janeiro 1935.

Ernst FUCHS† *Oftalmología actualizada por el Dr. Adalbert Fuchs Profesor de Oftalmología en la Universidad de Viena*. Tercera Edición Española. Traducción de la 18.ª edición alemana revisada y ampliada por el Dr. Santiago Vilahur Pedrals Jefe de Clinica Oftamolólogica de Hospital Provincial M. de la Real Academia de Medicina. Editorial Labor, S. A. Barcelona/Madrid/Buenos Aires/Rio de Janeiro/México/Montevideo 1958.

Wilhelm FUCHS, *Das Ehehinderniss des bestehenden Ehebandes nach österreichischem Rechte und seine Umgehung*. Alfred Hölder, Vienna 1879.

Wilhelm FUCHS, *Die Rechtsvermuthung der ehelichen Vaterschaft nach römischem und neuerem Rechte mit besonderer Berücksichtigung des österreichischen Rechtes.* Alfred Hölder, Vienna 1880.

Wilhelm FUCHS, *Die Karten und Marken des täglichen Verkehres.* Manz, Vienna 1881.

Wilhelm FUCHS (ed.), *Rechtsfälle zum Allgemeinen Bürgerlichen Gesetzbuche. Für den akademischen Gebrauch bearbeitet.* Alfred Hölder, Vienna 1881.

Wilhelm FUCHS, *Die sogenannten Siebenbürgischen Ehen und andere Arten der Wiederverehelichung geschiedener österreichischer Katholiken.* Manz, Vienna 1889.

Wilhelm FUCHS, *Beiträge zur Lehre von der Religionsfreiheit in der Praxis.* Manz, Vienna 1894.

Fünfundzwanzigste Versammlung der ophthalmologischen Gesellschaft Heidelberg 1896. J. F. Bergmann, Wiesbaden 1897.

Y. FUJIKAWA, *Geschichte der Medizin in Japan. Kurzgefasste Geschichte der Entwicklung der Japanischen Medizin mit besonderer Berücksichtigung der Einführung der europäischen Heilkunde in Japan.* Herausgegeben vom Kaiserlich-Japanischen Unterrichtsministerium. Tokyo 1911.

John Farquar FULTON, *Haryey Cushing.* A. Biography. Springfield 1946.

Gustav GAERTNER, "Die Entdeckung der Lokalanästhesie", in: *Der neue Tag* Yr. 1, No. 137, Vienna, Saturday, 9 August 1919, pp. 6.

Zoilo M. GALANG, Camilo OSIAS, *Encyclopedia of the Philippines: Builders of the New Philippines.* Philippine Education Company 1936.

Rudolf-Josef GASSER (ed.), *Der Anatom Joseph Hyrtl 1810–1894.* Wilhelm Maudrich, Vienna/Munich/Bern 1991.

Friedrich GATTI, *Geschichte der K. K. Ingenieur- und K. K. Genie-Akademie 1717–1869.* Wilhelm Braumüller, Vienna 1901.

Charles Alphonse GAYET, "Cauterisation ignée de la cornée", in: *Gaz. des Hôp.*, No. 11 (1877).

Genealogisches Handbuch des Adels. Vol. 58. C. A. Starke, Limburg 1974.

"Genf. Preisaufgabe über die Verhütung der Blindheit", in: *Klin. Monatsbl. f. Augenheilk.* 21 (1883), pp. 25–27.

Werner E. GERABEK, Bernhard D. HAAGE, Gundolf KEIL, Wolfgang WEGNER (eds.), *Enzyklopädie Medizingeschichte.* Walter de Gruyter, Berlin 2005.

Francisco GIBRAL, *Ciencia española en el exilio (1939–1949). El exilio de los científicos españoles.* Editorial Anthropos, Barcelona 1994.

W. GILBERT, "Zur Histologie des Aderhautsarkoms", in: *Graefes Archiv* 105 (1921), pp. 159–176.

Siegmund GINSBERG, *Grundriss der pathologischen Histologie des Auges.* S. Karger, Berlin 1903.

Harald G. A. GJESSING, "Über Tonometrie", in: *Graefes Archiv* 105 (1921), pp. 221–242.

Rickman GODLEE, "Sir Jonathan Hutchinson, F. R. S. (1828–1913)", in: *Brit. J. Ophthalmol.* June 1925/9, pp. 257–281 [= British Masters of Ophthalmology Series 15].

M. GOLDSCHMIDT, "Beitrag zur Pharmakologie des Optochins", in: *Graefes Archiv* 105 (1921), pp. 456–464.

Wilhelm GOLDZIEHER, "Ueber die Hutchinson'sche Veränderung des Augenhintergrundes", in: *Wien. med. Wochenschr.* 37 (1887), cols. 861–865.

Wilhelm GOLDZIEHER, "Einfachstes Verfahren gegen Ptosis und Entropium spasticum senile", in: *Centralbl. prakt. Augenheilk.* 14 (1890), pp. 34–36.

Wilhelm GOLDZIEHER, "Die Hutchinson'sche Veränderung des Augenhintergrundes. (Retinitis circinata Fuchs)", in: *Arch. Augenheilk.* 34 (1897), pp. 112–134.

Peter GOLLER, Die Matrikel der Universität Innsbruck. Vol. 1 1869–1900. Universitätsverlag Wagner, Innsbruck 1995.

Peter GOLLER, "Osttiroler Studenten an der Philosophischen Fakultät der Universität Innsbruck in der zweiten Hälfte des 19. Jahrhunderts (1848–1904)", in: *Osttiroler Heimatblätter [= Heimatkundliche Beilage des "Osttiroler Boten"]* 70 (2002), No. 11 [n.p.].

M. GOERIG, "Aus dem Nachlass von Carl Koller. Aufzeichnungen zu seinen Experimenten mit Kokain", in: *Der Anaesthesist* 64/6 (2015), pp. 469–477.

E. J. GOODWIN, "Prof. Fuchs in St. Louis", in: *Am. J. Ophthalmol.* 3/5 (1922), p. 68.

George GORIN, *History of Ophthalmology. Publish or Perish*, Wilmington 1982.

Alfred GRAEFE, Theodor SAEMISCH (eds.), *Handbuch der gesammten Augenheilkunde*. Vol. 3. Pathologie und Therapie. Part 1. Wilhelm Engelmann, Leipzig 1874.

Malcolm V. GRAHAM, Graham J. WAKEFIELD, "Bitemporal visual field defects associated with anomalies of the optic discs", in: *Brit. J. Ophthalmol.* 57 (1973), pp. 307–314.

Richard GREEF, *Anleitung zur mikroskopischen Untersuchung des Auges*. August Hirschwald, Berlin 1898.

Richard GREEFF, "Flocculi am Pigmentsaum der Iris", in: *Graefes Archiv* 105 (1921), pp. 134–136.

John GREEN, "Nodular Opacity of the Cornea with Special Reference to Its Etiology", in: *J. Am. Med. Assoc.* 53 (1909), pp. 151ff.

Franz GREHN, Gerd GEERLING, Frank KROGMANN, Michael STOLBERG (eds.), *Geschichte der Augenheilkunde in Würzburg*. Akamedon-Verlag, Würzburg 2007.

Dietmar GRIESER, *Weltreise durch Wien. Lebensstationen berühmter Persönlichkeiten*. Deutscher Taschenbuch Verlag, Munich 2006.

Arthur GROENOW, "Knötchenförmige Hornhauttrübungen (Noduli corneae)", in: *Graefes Archiv* 21 (1890), pp. 281–289

Arthur GROENOW, "Knötchenförmige Hornhauttrübungen", in: *Graefes Archiv* 46 (1898), pp. 85–102.

Bernhard GROIS, *Das Allgemeine Krankenhaus in Vienna und seine Geschichte*. Wilhelm Maudrich, Vienna 1965.

Richard GRONER, *Wien wie es war. Ein Auskunftsbuch für Freunde des alten Wien*. 3rd ed. (Otto Erich Deutsch). Hain, Vienna 1934.

Helmut GRÖGER, "Carl Toldt. Hervorragender Anatom und Anthropologe der Wiener medizinischen Schule", in: *APIS (= Arzt und Patient in Südtirol)* 3 (1990), pp. 44ff.

Helmut GRÖGER, Eberhard GABRIEL, Siegfried KASPER (eds.), *Zur Geschichte der Psychiatrie in Wien*. Brandstätter, Vienna 1997.

Helmut GRÖGER, Gabriela SCHMIDT-WYKLICKY, "Carl Koller und die Entdeckung der Lokalanästhesie 1884", in: *Spektrum Augenheilk.* 26 (2012), pp. 309–311.

Helmut GRÖGER, Gabriela SCHMIDT-WYKLICKY, "Isidor Schnabel. Vorstand der I. Universitäts-Augenklinik in Wien von 1895 bis 1908", in: *Spektrum Augenheilk.* 26 (2012), pp. 321–324.

Helmut GRÖGER, Gabriela SCHMIDT-WYKLICKY, "Friedrich Dimmer. Vorstand beider Universitäts-Augenkliniken in Wien: I. Augenklinik 1910 bis 1915. II. Augenklinik 1916 bis 1926", in: *Spektrum Augenheilkd.* 26 (2012), pp. 325–329.

Helmut GRÖGER, Gabriela SCHMIDT-WYKLICKY, "Josef Meller. Vorstand der I. Universitäts-Augenklinik in Wien 1919 bis 1944", in: *Spektrum Augenheilkd.* 26 (2012), pp. 332–335.

Helmut GRÖGER, Gabriela SCHMIDT-WYKLICKY, "Karl David Lindner. Vorstand der II. Universitäts-Augenklinik von 1927 bis 1953", in: *Spektrum Augenheilk.* 26 (2012), pp. 336–340.

Helmut GRÖGER, Gabriela SCHMIDT-WYKLICKY, "Arnold Pillat. Vorstand der I. Universitäts-Augenklinik in 'Wien 1944 bis 1963", in: *Spektrum Augenheilkd.* 26 (2012), pp. 341–344.

V. GRÖNHOLM, "Über prä-äquatoriale Sklerektomie bei Netzhautablösung", in: *Graefes Archiv* 105 (1921), pp. 899–915.

Emil v. GRÓSZ, "Über einige Operationsmethoden an der königlich-ungarischen Universitäts-Augenklinik Nr. 1 in Budapest", in: *Graefes Archiv* 105 (1921), pp. 1075–1083.

Emil v. GRÓSZ, "Unterricht in der Augenheilkunde", in: *Wien. med. Wochenschr.* 71 (1921), cols. 1053–1055.

Gustav GUIST, "Über das Verhalten heller und dunkler Regenbogenhäute auf Homatropin und Atropin", in: *Wien. med. Wochenschr.* 71 (1921), cols. 1055–1058.

Eduard Vincenz GULDENER Edl. v. LOBES, *Sammlungen der Sanitäts-Verordnungen für das Erzherzogthum Oesterreich unter der Enns, als Fortsetzung der v. Ferro'schen Sammlung. Fünfter Theil, enthaltend die Verordnungen vom Jahre 1818 bis Ende des Jahres 1824.* Gerold, Vienna 1825.

Allvar GULLSTRAND, "Demonstration der Nernst-Spaltlampe", in: *Bericht über die Siebenunddreissigste Versammlung der Ophthalmologischen Gesellschaft Heidelberg*, Bergmann, Wiesbaden 1911, pp. 374–376.

Walter GUTTMANN, *Medizinische Terminologie. Ableitung und Erklärung der gebräuchlichsten Fachausdrücke aller Zweige der Medizin und ihrer Hilfswissenschaften.* Sechste und siebente umgearbeitete und erweiterte Auflage. Urban & Schwarzenberg, Berlin 1913.

Ingrid HACKSTOCK, *Die wissenschaftlichen Illustrationen der Wiener Medizinischen Schule vom Ende des 18. bis Mitte des 19. Jahrhunderts.* Phil. Diss. Univ. Vienna 1988.

Ingrid HACKSTOCK, "Carl Heitzmann (1836–1896): physician and illustrator", in: *Intern. J. Dermatol.* 37 (1998), pp. 235–240.

Eïsaburo HADANO, *Über die Behandlung von Hornhauterkrankungen mit dem scharfen Löffel.* Med. Diss. Univ. Rostock 1903.

Eïsaburo HADANO, "Beitrag zur Kenntnis der Keratitis disciformis", in: Zeitschr. Augenheilk. 10 (1903), pp. 500–504.

A. HADWIGER, *Geschichte der Wiener Augenklinik.* J. B. Wallishauser, Vienna 1836.

F. Herbert HAESSLER, "Heterochromia Irides", in: *Arch. Ophthalmol.* 2/3 (1929), pp. 333–347.

Sigurd HAGEN, "Zur Ätiologie der transitorischen Hypermetropie bei Diabetes mellitus", in: *Graefes Archiv* 105 (1921), pp. 243–240.

Michael HAGNER, Bettina WAHRIG-SCHMIDT (eds.), *Johannes Müller und die Philosophie.* Akademie-Verlag, Berlin 1992.

Dieter HALBWIDL, "Life and Times of Count Thun", in: *Mensch–Wissenschaft–Magie/ Mitteilungen der Österreichischen Gesellschaft für Wissenschaftsgeschichte* 30 (2013), pp. 111–131.

Léon HALKIN, Paul HARSIN (eds.), *LIBER MEMORIALIS. L'Université de Liége de 1867 à 1935. Notices biographiques.* Tome III. *Faculté de Médecine.* Rectorat de l'Université, Liége 1936.

Léon-E. HALKIN, "Trasenster contre Kurth", in: Marcel FLORKIN, Léon.E. HALKIN (eds.), *Chronique de l'Université de Liège.* Université, Liège 1967, pp. 319–333.

Carl HAMBURGER, "Glaukomprobleme", in: *Klin. Monatsbl. Augenheilk.* 78 (1927), pp. 189–205.

Franz HAMBURGER, "Theodor Escherich", in: *Wien. med. Wochenschr.* 82 (1932), cols. 1216ff.

Handbuch der Stadt Wien. Bd. 82.Verlag für Jugend und Volk. Vienna 1968.

Viktor HANKE, "Zur Aetiologie des Ringabszesses der Kornea", in: *Klin. Monatsbl. Augenheilk.* 42 (1904), pp. 172–173. (Ophthalmol. Gesellsch. in Wien. Bericht v. Doz. Dr. Wintersteiner. 2. Sitzung v. 11. November 1903).

Viktor HANKE, "Ein bisher unbekannter Bacillus, der Erreger des typischen Ringabszesses der Cornea", in: *Zeitschr. Augenheilk.* 10 (1904), pp. 373ff.

Viktor HANKE, Rudolf TERTSCH, "Einige seltene Infektionen des Auges", in: *Klin. Monatsbl. Augenheilk.* 45 (1907), pp. 545–560.

Viktor HANKE, "Doppelperforation des Bulbus und Wanderung eines retrobulbären kleinen Eisensplitters", in: *Wien. med. Wochenschr.* 71 (1921), cols. 1058–1060.

Viktor HANKE, "Septische Metastasen in der Chorioidea", in: *Graefes Archiv* 105 (1921), pp. 851–864.

Hugo HANTSCH, *Die Geschichte Österreichs*. 2 vols. Styria, Graz/Vienna/Cologne. 2nd ed. 1955.

Henry HARRIS, *The Birth of the Cell*. Yale University Press, New Haven/London 1999.

Christian HARTMANN (ed.), "Albrecht von Graefe. Berlin 1828 bis 1870". Gedächtnisband anläßlich des 125-jährigen Todestages. ad manum medici, Germering 1996.

Thilo von HAUGWITZ, "Augenheilkunde im 20. Jahrhundert. Ergebnisse und Ereignisse im deutschsprachigen Raum", in: G. O. H. NAUMANN, H.-J. MERTÉ, B. GLOOR, R. ROCHELS, *Bücherei des Augenarztes Bd. 127 (= Beihefte der Klinischen Monatsblätter für Augenheilkunde)*. Ferdinand Enke, Stuttgart 1991.

Reinhard HAUPENTHAL, *Die Wien-Aufenthalte von Lazar Markovic Zamenhof (1859–1917) und seine ophthalmologischen Studien bei Ernst Fuchs (1851–1930): ein Beitrag zum 150. Geburtstag Zamenhofs*. Ed. Iltis, Saarbrücken 2009.

Josef HÄUSLER, *Die Entwicklung der K. K. Landwirtschafts-Gesellschaft in Vienna während ihres hundertjährigen Bestandes*. Österreichische Land- und Forstwirtschaftsgesellschaft, Vienna 1907.

Ferdinand HEBRA, "Das umschriebene Eczem. Eczema marginatum", in: Rudolf VIRCHOW, *Handbuch der speciellen Pathologie und Therapie*. Abth. I. Ferdinand Enke, Erlangen 1860, pp. 361–363.

Ferdinand HEBRA, *Atlas der Hautkrankheiten*. Nach der Natur gemalt von Anton Elfinger. Lithographiert von Carl Heitzmann. Lieferung 1–10. Lfg. 1 in Kommission bei Braumüller 1856; Lfg. 2–10 in Kommission bei Gerold 1858–1876.

Charles R. HEED (Ref.), College of Physicians of Philadelphia, Section on Ophthalmology. October 20, 1921, in: *Am. J. Ophthalmol.* 5 (1922), p. 211–217.

Dieter HEID, *Personalbibliographien der Professoren und Dozenten der Augenheilkunde an der Medizinischen Fakultät der Universität Wien, im Zeitraum 1812 bis 1884*. Med. Diss. Erlangen/Nürnberg 1972.

Gottfried HEINDL, *Wien. Brevier einer Stadt*. Paul Neff Verlag, Vienna/Berlin 1972.

Otto HEINRICY, *Klinische Beiträge zur Degeneratio circinata retinae [Retinitis circinata (Fuchs)] mit besonderer Berücksichtigung der atypischen Formen dieses Krankheitsbildes*. Med. Diss. Univ. Tübingen, Wilhelm Engelmann 1913.

Carl HEITZMANN, "20 Jahre wissenschaftliche Thätigkeit in Amerika", in: *Wien. klin. Wochenschr.* 8 (1895), pp. 561ff.

Joseph Alexander Frh. von HELFERT, *Österreichisches Jahrbuch*. Vol. 7. Verlag des Österreichischen Volksschriften-Vereins in Kommission bei Kubasta & Voigt, Vienna 1883.

Hermann HELMHOLTZ, "Ueber die Erhaltung der Kraft". Eine physikalische Abhandlung, vorgetragen in der Sitzung der Physikalischen Gesellschaft zu Berlin am 23. Juli 1847. G. Reimer, Berlin 1847.

Hermann HELMHOLTZ, *Beschreibung eines Augen-Spiegels zur Untersuchung der Netzhaut am lebenden Auge*. A. Förstner, Berlin 1851.

Hermann von HELMHOLTZ, "Ueber die Theorie der zusammengesetzten Farben", in: *Arch. Anat. Physiol. wiss. Med.* Yr. 1852, pp. 461–482 and *Ann. Phys. Chem.* 87 (1852), pp. 45–66.

Johann Nepomuk Frh. v. HEMPEL-KÜRSINGER, *Handbuch der Gesetzeskunde im Sanitäts- und Medicinal-Gebiethe in alphabetisch-chronologisch und materienweiser Zusammenstellung für Sanitäts- und Polizeybeamte im Allgemeinen und insbesondere für Aerzte, Wundärzte, Geburtshelfer, Hebammen und Apotheker*. Vol. 1 A–I, Vienna 1830.

Jutta HERDE, "Zur Erinnerung an Carl Ernst Theodor Schweigger (1830–1905)", in: *Klin. Monatsbl. Augenheilk.* 222 (2005), pp. 7ff.

Ernst HERTEL, "Über die Bestimmung der Wasserstoffionenkonzentration im Kammerwasser", in: *Graefes Archiv* 105 (1921), pp. 421–427.

Paul HERTZ, Moritz SCHLICK (eds.), *Hermann von Helmholtz. Schriften zur Erkenntnistheorie*. Springer, Berlin 1921.

Wilhelm HERZIG, *Das medicinische Wien. Wegweiser für Aerzte und Naturforscher, vorzugsweise für Fremde. Nach Originalquellen*. Braumüller & Seidel, Vienna 1844.

Wilhelm HERZIG, *Das medicinische Wien. Wegweiser für Aerzte und Naturforscher, vorzugsweise für Fremde. Nach Originalquellen bearbeitet*. 3rd ed., Wilhelm Braumüller, Vienna 1863.

Carl v. HESS, "Die relative Rotsichtigkeit und Grünsichtigkeit", in: *Graefes Archiv* 105, pp. 137–153.

Robert von der HEYDT, Chicago Ophthalmological Society May 15, 1922, in: *Am. J. Ophthalmol.* 5/9 (1922), pp. 726–731.

Blida HEYNOLD von GRAEFE, *Albrecht von Graefe: Mensch und Umwelt*. Stapp, Berlin 1969. (Reprint 1991).

J. HILLEMANN, G. NAUMANN, "Beitrag zum benignen Epitheliom (Fuchs) des Ziliarkörpers", in: *Ophthalmologica* 164 (1972), pp. 321–335.

Arthur v. HIPPEL, "Eine neue Methode der Hornhauttransplantation", in: *Graefes Archiv* 34/ Abtheil. I. (1888), pp. 108–130.

Eugen v. HIPPEL, "Beiträge zur pathologischen Anatomie seltener Augenerkrankungen", in: *Graefes Archiv* 105 (1921), pp. 1037–1049.

August HIRSCH, *Geschichte der Augenheilkunde. [= GRAEFE und SAEMISCH, Handbuch der Augenheilkunde, vol. VII]*. Wilhelm Engelmann, Leipzig 1877.

August HIRSCH (ed.), *Biographisches Lexikon der hervorragenden Aerzte aller Zeiten und Völker*. Vol. 3. Urban & Schwarzenberg, Vienna/Leipzig 1886 (Reprint Martino Publishing, Mansfield 2002).

Julius HIRSCHBERG (ed.), *Professor A. v. Graefe's klinische Vorträge über Augenheilkunde*. A. Hirschwald, Berlin 1872.

Julius HIRSCHBERG, "Zur Prognose der Aderhautsarcome", in: *Virchows Archiv* 90/Abth. I (1882), pp. 1–23.

Julius HIRSCHBERG, *Um die Erde. Eine Reisebeschreibung*. Georg Thieme, Leipzig 1894.

Julius HIRSCHBERG, *Geschichte der Augenheilkunde*. Reprint, Georg Olms, Hildesheim/New York 1977 = Theodor SAEMISCH (ed.), GRAEFE-SAEMISCH, *Handbuch der gesammten Augenheilkunde*. 2nd revised edition.
Vol. I = 12th volume 1899, 13th volume. Wilhelm Engelmann, Leipzig 1908.
Vol. II= 14th volume/I. Wilhelm Engelmann, Leipzig 1911.
Vol. III= 14th volume/II and III. Wilhelm Engelmann, Leipzig 1911 und 1912.
Vol. IV= 14th volume/IV and V. Wilhelm Engelmann, Leipzig and Berlin 1914 and 1915–1918.
Vol. V= 14th volume /VI and VII. Wilhelm Engelmann, Leipzig 1915–1918.
Vol. VI= 15th volume /I. Julius Springer, Berlin 1918.
Vol. VII= 15th volume /II. Julius Springer, Berlin 1918.

Julius HIRSCHBERG, "Alkmaion's Verdienst um die Augenheilkunde", in: *Graefes Archiv* 105 (1921), pp. 129–133.

Julius v. HOCHENEGG, *Dem Andenken Eduard Alberts*. Vienna 1909.

Jakob HOCK, "Fall von Cysticercus cellulosae unter der Bindehaut des Augapfels", in: *Mittheil. d. aerztl. Vereins in Wien* 3 (1874), pp. 89–95.

J. van der HOEVE, "Augengeschwülste bei der tuberösen Hirnsklerose (Bourneville)", in: *Graefes Archiv* 105 (1921), pp. 880–898.

Hof- und Staats-Schematismus des österreichischen Kaiserthums. II. Theil. K. K. Hof- u. Staats-Aerarial-Druckerey, Vienna 1822.

Hof- undStaatsschematismus des österreichischen Kaiserthumes. II. Theil. K. K. Hof- u. Staats-Aerarial-Druckerey, Vienna 1843.

Andreas HÖFERLIN, "Der Chirurg Anton Wölfler (1850–1917). Sein Leben und sein Werk mit besonderer Berücksichtigung seiner Arbeiten zur Schilddrüsenchirurgie". Med. Diss. Univ. Mainz 1989.

Joseph HOFFMANN, *Das Wiener k. k.allgemeine Krankenhaus*. K. K. Hof- und Staatsdruckerei, Vienna 1873.

Josefina D. HOFILEÑA, *José Rizal and Ferdinand Blumentritt: A Chronology of a Friendship*. Ateneo de Manila 2014.

Walter HÖFLECHNER (ed.), *Publikationen aus dem Archiv der Universität Graz 18*. Graz 1986.

Eugen HOFMOKL, *Wiener Heilanstalten*. [= *Beilage zur Wochenschrift Das Österreichische Sanitätswesen*]. Vienna 1910.

Joh. W. HOLCZABEK, Adalbert WINTER, *Sagen und geschichtliche Erzählungen der Stadt Wien. Nebst einer kurzen Geschichte der k. k.Reichshaupt- und Residenzstadt Vienna und der Vororte. Nach besten Quellen bearbeitet. Unveränderter Nachdruck der Ausgabe 1900*. Geyer Edition Wien 1978.

F. HOLLWICH, "Zur Differentialdiagnose der Heterochromiezyklitis", in: *Klin. Monatsbl. Augenheilk*. 142 (1963), pp. 129–139.

Karl HOLUBAR, "Ferdinand von Hebra und das Allgemeine Krankenhaus in Wien", in: *Wien. med. Wochenschr*. 132 (1982), cols. 423ff.

Karl HOLUBAR, "Hyperkeratosis follicullaris et parafollicularis in cutem penetrans. Josef Kyrle and 'his' disease", in: *Americ. J. Dermatopathol*. 7 (1985), pp. 261–264.

Karl HOLUBAR, Klaus WOLFF, "The Genesis of American Investigative Dermatology from Its Roots in Europe", in: *J. Invest. Dermatol*. 92 (1989), Suppl. No. 4, pp. 14ff.

Karl HOLUBAR, "Karel Frederik Wenckebach (1864–1940) und die Domizilierung des Instituts für Geschichte der Medizin im historischen Gebäude der Josephs-Akademie in Wien: 1990 als doppeltes Gedenkjahr", in: *Wien. klin. Wochenschr*. 102 (1990), pp. 333ff.

Karl HOLUBAR, "Anton von Rosas (1791–1855): On the occasion of the bicentennial of his birth". Part 1; in: *Wien. klin. Wochenschr.*103 (1991), pp. 470–472.

Karl HOLUBAR, Cathrin SCHMIDT, "Art in dermatology versus dermatology in art. Anton Elfinger (1821–1864) and Carl Heitzmann (1836–1896). Hebra's forgotten painter-physicians", in: *Int. J. Dermatol.* 33/5 (1994), pp. 385–387.

Karl HOLUBAR, "Salomon Stricker (1834–98) pioneer experimental pathologist", in: *American Journal of Dermatopathology* [= *Americ. J. Dermatopathol.*] 9 (1997), pp. 147ff.

Karl HOLUBAR, Stella FATOVIĆ-FERENČIĆ, Gerd PLEWIG, Looking at Eyes and Faces. Ophthalmologic watercolours drawn largely by physician-artists Vienna [sic!] late 18th and 19th centuries. Austrian Academy of Sciences Press, Vienna 2006.

E. HOLZMAIR, "Die Sammlung Brettauer", in: Otto ZEKERT, *Kunst in Medizin und Pharmazie. HMW-Jahrbuch 1956.* Heilmittelwerke Vienna 1956, pp. 76–79.

Anton HOMMER, Stephan KAMINSKI (ed.), "100 Jahre Ophthalmologische Gesellschaft in Wien", in: *Wien. med. Wochenschr.* 154 (2004), Supplement 116.

Heinrich HONEGGER, Herbert HESSLER, "Die Entdeckung der Lokalanästhesie durch Karl Koller (I–III)", in: *Klin. Monatsbl. Augenheilk.* 157 (1970), pp. 428–438, 569–578 and 714–723.

Karl HOOR, "Eine eigenartige Veränderung der Netzhaut um die Macula lutea und die Retinitis circinata Fuchs", in: *Zeitschr. Augenheilk.* 3 (1900), pp. 26–31.

E. HORNIKER, "Augenspiegelstudien bei Kriegsnephritis", in: *Graefes Archiv* 105 (1921), pp. 104–128.

Herbert HÖRZ, *Physiologie und Kultur in der zweiten Hälfte des 19. Jahrhunderts. Briefe an Hermann von Helmholtz.* Basilisken-Presse/Verlag Natur & Text 1994.

Hospital Social Service Association of New York City 1929.

Harvey J. HOWARD, "A Visit to Dr. J. Komoto of Tokyo", in: *Am. J. Ophthalmol.* 10 (1921), pp. 752–757.

Harvey J. HOWARD, "Professor Ikujiro Asayama", in: *Am. J. Ophthalmol.* 5 (1922), pp. 926–928.

(Harvey J. HOWARD), "Department of Ophthalmology", in: Adresses & Papers, Dedication Ceremonies and Medical Conference Peking Union Medical College September 15–22, 1921. Peking Union Medical College 1922, pp. 385–401.

Harvey J. HOWARD, "Professor Fuchs's Visit to Peking", in: *Am. J. Ophthalmol.* 6 (1923), pp. 615–617.

Harvey J. HOWARD, "Report of the Department of Ophthalmology", in: *Fifteenth Annual Report of the Medical Superintendent of the Peking Union Medical College Hospital. For the Year Ending June 30, 1923.* Peking 1923, pp. 50–54.

Harvey J. HOWARD, *Ten Weeks with Chinese Bandits.* Dodd, Mead & Co., New York 1926.

Karl HRUBY, "Über die Entwicklung und den gegenwärtigen Stand der Biomikroskopie des Auges", in: *Wien. klin. Wochenschr.* 63 (1951), pp. 669–672.

Karl HRUBY, "Wurde Dr. Carl Koller 1885 aus Wien vertrieben?", in: *Wien. klin. Wochenschr.* 98 (1985), pp. 155f.

Michael HUBENSTORF, "Eine 'Wiener Schule' der Medizingeschichte? – und Max Neuburger und die vergessene deutschsprachige Medizingeschichte", in: *Medizingeschichte Gesellschaftskritik.* Festschrift für Gerhard Baader. Matthiesen, Husum 1997, pp. 246–289.

Heinz HUBER, *Geschichte der Medizinischen Fakultät Innsbruck und der medizinisch-chirurgischen Studienanstalt (1673–1938).* Unter Mitarbeit von Verena Plankl. Böhlau, Vienna/Cologne/Weimar 2010.

Albert HÜBL, *Geschichte des Unterrichtes im Stifte Schotten in Wien*. Herausgegeben anläszlich der Zentenarfeier des k. k.Schottengymnasiums. Carl Fromme, Vienna 1907.

Walter HUMMELBERGER, Kurt PEBALL, *Die Befestigungen Wiens*. [= Peter PÖTSCHER (ed.), *Wiener Geschichtsbücher* vol. 14]. Paul Zsolnay Verlag, Vienna/Hamburg 1974.

Suzan HUNT, "Leben und Werk von Hermann Kuhnt (1850–1937) und Paul Junius (1871–1948)", in: *Klin. Monatsbl. Augenheilk.* 224/8 (2007), pp. 678–682.

Jonathan HUTCHINSON," On the different forms of inflammation of the eye consequent to inherited syphilis", in: *Ophthalmic Hospital Reports*, London 1 (1858), pp. 191–203 and pp. 226–244; ibid. 2 (1859), pp. 54–105; ibid. 3 (1860), pp. 258–283.

Jonathan HUTCHINSON, *Clinical Memoir on Certain Diseases of the Eye and the Ear Consequent on Inherited Syphilis*. John Churchill, London 1863.

Jonathan HUTCHINSON, "New facts and opinions as to inherited syphilis", in: *London Hospital Reports II* (1865), pp. 145–204.

Franz HUTER (ed.), *Hundert Jahre Medizinische Fakultät Innsbruck 1869 bis 1969*. Part II. *Geschichte der Lehrkanzeln, Institute und Kliniken*. (= *Forschungen zur Innsbrucker Universitätsgeschichte* 7). Österr. Kommissionsbuchhandlung, Innsbruck 1969.

Joseph HYRTL, "Die materialistische Weltanschauung unserer Zeit". Rede bei dem Antritte der Rectorswürde an der Wiener Universität am 1. October 1864. Adolf Holzhausen, Vienna 1865.

Josef IGERSHEIMER, Walter PRINZ, "Gedanken und Untersuchungen zur Pathogenese der phlyktänulären Augenentzündungen und zum Schicksal skrofulöser Augenpatienten", in: *Graefes Archiv* 105 (1921), pp. 640–649.

Josef IGERSHEIMER, "Syphilis und Auge", in: J. JADASSOHN, *Handbuch der Haut- und Geschlechtskrankheiten*. Vol. 17/2, Springer, Berlin/Heidelberg 1918.

Die feierliche Inauguration des Rektors der Universität Vienna für das Studienjahr 1924/25. Univ. Vienna 1924.

IN MEMORIAM Dr. Georges Haltenhoff, Professeur d'Ophtalmologie à l'Université de Genève. 8 juin 1843–25 avril 1915. Lausanne, Imprim. Hoirs Borgeaud 1915. (With contributions by J. Reverdin, Weber, E. Götz, Rehfous, G. Porte, C. Picot, A. Bernoud, Gourfein-Welt and P.-G. Piccard).

Tatsushichiro INOUYE, "Ueber die eigenthümliche Farbe des Augenhintergrundes der mongolischen Race", in: *Centralbl. f. Augenheilk.* 20 (1896), pp. 200–205.

Tatsushichiro INOUYE, "Bericht über einen neuen Netzhautreflex", in: *25. Versammlung d. ophthalmol. Gesellsch. Heidelberg*. J. F. Bergmann, Wiesbaden 1897, pp. 297–299.

Tatsushichiro INOUYE, "Ein Fall von Veränderungen des Augenhintergrundes durch Filixvergiftung", in: ibid., pp. 300–301.

Tatsushichiro INOUYE, "Ueber einen Fall von Augenverletzung durch stumpfe Gewalt und insbesondere ueber Linsenkapsel-Abhebung", in: *Centralbl. Augenheilk.* 21 (1897), pp. 147–149.

Tatsushichiro INOUYE, "Ueber einen Fall von Retinitis albuminurica ohne ausgesprochene Nephritis bei einem Neger." Aus der Augenklinik Leipzig, in: *Klin. Monatsbl. Augenheilk.* 36 (1898), pp. 297–309.

Alexander IWANOFF, "Ueber Conjunctivitis und Keratitis phlyctaenularis", in: *Klin. Monatsbl. Augenheilk.* 7 (1869), pp. 462–470.

Edward JACKSON, "Skiascopy and Its Practical Applications to the Study of Refraction". Edwards & Docker, Philadelphia 1896.

(Edward JACKSON), "Graduate Study in Ophthalmology at Vienna", in: *Arch. Ophthalmol.* 5 (1922), p. 583.

Edward JACKSON, "Adolph Barkan. A Pioneer Ophthalmologist", in: *Am. J. Ophthalmol.* 19/3 (1936), p. 260–262.

Joseph JADASSOHN, *Handbuch der Haut- und Geschlechtskrankheiten.* Vols. 1–23. Springer, Berlin 1927–1934.

Eduard JAEGER, *Ueber die Behandlung des grauen Staares an der ophthalmologischen Klinik der Josephs-Akademie.* Carl Ueberreuter, Vienna 1844.

Eduard JAEGER, *Ueber Staar und Staaroperationen nebst anderen Beobachtungen und Erfahrungen aus seines Vaters Dr. Friedrich Jaeger, k. k.Professors etc. etc. und aus der eigenen ophthalmologischen Praxis.* L. W. Seidel, Vienna 1854 (Habilitation thesis).

Eduard JAEGER, *Beiträge zur Pathologie des Auges. Mit Abbildungen im Farbendruck.* Kaiserlich-Königliche Hof- und Staatsdruckerei, Vienna 1855.

Eduard JAEGER, *Ergebnisse der Untersuchung des menschlichen Auges mit dem Augenspiegel.* Braumüller, Vienna 1855.

(Eduard JAEGER), *Schrift-Scalen des Prof. Jaeger jun.* 2nd enlarged edition. K. K. Hof- und Staatsdruckerei. Vienna 1857.

Eduard von JAEGER, Ophthalmoskopischer Hand-Atlas. K. K. Hof- und Staatsdruckerei. Vienna 1869.

Eduard von JAEGER, *Über die Einstellungen des dioptrischen Apparates im menschlichen Auge.* Seidel, Vienna 1871.

Jahrbuch für Landeskunde von Niederösterreich. Vols. 56–58 (1991).

Jahresbericht der Allgem. Poliklinik für 1924. Eigenverlag Poliklinik 23 (1925).

Jahresverzeichnis der an den deutschen Universitäten erschienenen Schriften XVIII. 15. August 1902 bis 14. August 1903. A. Asher & Co., Berlin 1903.

Adolf JARISCH, "Zur Geschichte des Pharmakologischen Instituts der Universität Innsbruck", in: Forschungen u. Forscher d. Tiroler Ärzteschule (1948–1950). Vol 2. Oberösterr. Landesverlag, Wels 1950.

Alireza JAVADZADEH, Davood GHARABAGHI, "Gyrate atrophy of the choroid and retina with hyper-ornithinemia responsive to vitamin B6: a case report", in: *J. Med. Case Reports* 1 (2007), p. 27.

Émile JAVAL, *Entre Aveugles. Conseils à l'usage des personnes, qui viennent de perdre la vue.* Masson et Cie., Paris 1903.

Émile JAVAL, *Der Blinde und seine Welt. (Entre Aveugles). Ratschläge zum Nutzen für Erblindete.* Übersetzt von Dr. med. J. Türkheim. Leopold Voss, Hamburg/Leipzig 1904.

A. JESS, "Die moderne Eiweißchemie im Dienste der Starforschung (1. Teil)", in: *Graefes Archiv* 105 (1921), pp. 428–455.

Dieter JETTER, *Wien von den Anfängen bis um 1900* [= *Geschichte des Hospitals* vol. 5]. Franz Steiner, Wiesbaden 1982.

Reginald F. JOHNSTON, *Twilight in the Forbidden City.* Cambridge University Press, 1934.

Alexander JOKL, "Ferdinand Arlt and Ernst Fuchs. Two Representatives of the Vienna School of Ophthalmology", in: *Suid-Afrikaanse Tydskrip vir Geneeskunde/South African Med. Journal*, 15 Maart 1958, pp. 301–303 and *Internat. Rec. Med.* 170 (1957), pp. 702–707.

Alexander JOKL, "Ernst Fuchs (1851–1930)", in: *Neue Österreichische Biographie ab 1815.* Große Österreicher. Vol. XV. Amalthea, Vienna/Munich/Zürich 1963, pp. 142–150.

Paulus T. V. M. de JONG, "A Historical Analysis of the Quest for the Origins of Aging Macula Disorder, the Tissues Involved, and Its Terminology", in: *Ophthalmology and Eye Diseases* [= *Ophthalmol. Eye Dis.*] 8/Suppl. 1 (2016), pp. 5–14.

Paulus T. V. M. de JONG, "Elusive drusen and changing terminology of AMD", in: *Eye* 32 (2018), pp. 904–914.

JULIUS HIRSCHBERG-GESELLSCHAFT (Deutschsprachige Vereinigung für Geschichte der Augenheilkunde) Société francophone d'histoire de l'ophtalmologie, *33 Beiträge zur Geschichte der Augenheilkunde – Contributions à l'histoire de l'ophtalmologie*. Facultas, Vienna 1991.

Paul JUNIUS, "Zur Frage der Keratitis disciformis", in: *Klin. Monatsbl. Augenheilk.* 67/2 (1921), pp. 110–112 (Report of the meeting).

Paul JUNIUS, "Über Keratitis disciformis. Ein Beitrag zur Klinik und zur Entstehungsweise der Krankheit", in: *Graefes Archiv* 105 (1921), pp. 177–204. (= *Festschrift zur Feier des siebzigsten Geburtstages Herrn Hofrat Prof. Dr. Ernst Fuchs in Vienna gewidmet von Freunden und dankbaren Schülern*).

Paul JUNIUS (Ref.), "Außerordentliche Tagung der Ophthalmologischen Gesellschaft in Vienna vom 4.–6. August 1921", in: *Zeitschr. Augenheilk.* 46 (1921), pp. 116–118.

Paul JUNIUS, Hermann KUHNT, *Die scheibenförmige Entartung der Netzhautmitte: Degeneratio maculae luteae disciformis.* S. Karger, Berlin 1925.

Johann JURENITSCH, Claudia MÜLLER, Kurt SCHNEIDER, Wolfgang KUBELKA, *200 Jahre Pharmakognosie in Wien. Eine Wissenschaft im Dienst der Arzneimittelsicherheit.* Facultas Universitätsverlag, Vienna 1998.

Paul KAFKA, "Epibulbäres Melanosarkom und Radiotherapie", in: *Wien. med. Wochenschr.* 71 (1921), cols. 1060–1063.

Paul KAFKA, "Über einen eigenartigen Pupillenbefund", in: *Graefes Archiv* 105 (1921), pp. 384–389.

Dewey KATZ, "Maximilian Salzmann, 1862–1954", in: *Am. J. Ophthalmol.* 38 (1954), pp. 738–740.

Herbert E. KAUFMAN, "Ludwig von Sallmann", in: *Invest. Ophthalmol. Vis. Sc.* 9 (1970), pp. 1–2.

Richard KEELER, "Allvar Gullstrand: Dioptics of the Eye and the Slit Lamp", in: Michael F. MARMOR, Daniel ALBERT (eds.), *Foundations of Ophthalmology. Great Insights that Established the Discipline*. Springer Internat. Publ. 2017.

Friedrich KERSCHBAUMER, *Die Blinden des Herzogthums Salzburg nebst Bemerkungen über die Verbreitung und die Ursachen der Blindheit im Allgemeinen. Eine Studie für Aerzte, Hygieniker und Nationalökonomen.* J. F. Bergmann, Wiesbaden 1886.

Alfred KESTENBAUM, "Der Mechanismus des Nystagmus", in: *Graefes Archiv* 105(1921), pp. 799–843.

S. J. KIMURA, M. J. HOGAN, P. THYGESON, "Fuchs's syndrome of heterochromic cyclitis", in: *Arch. Ophthalmol.* 54 (1955), pp. 179–186.

Salomon KIRCHENBERGER, *Lebensbilder hervorragender österreichisch-ungarischer Militär- und Marineärzte* (= *Militärärztliche Publikationen* Nr. 150). Šafář, Vienna/Leipzig 1913.

Naganori KIRISAWA, "The Komoto Library (Formerly the Hirschberg Library)", in: *Japan. J. Ophthalmol.* 21 (1977), pp. 528–532.

Salomon KLEIN (BÄRINGER), "Gedenkrede zu Ehren Prof. Eduard v. Jaegers anläßlich der Enthüllung seines Denkmals in der Universität am 28. Februar 1910", in: *Wien. klin. Wochenschr.* 23 (1910), pp. 410–413.

Bertha A. KLIEN, "Diktyoma retinae", in: *Arch Ophthalmol.* 22/3 (1939), pp. 432–438.

Guido KLUXEN, "José Rizal (1861–1896), Augenarzt und Nationalheld der Philippinen", in: *Mitteilungen der Julius-Hirschberg-Gesellschaft zur Geschichte der Augenheilkunde* 16 (2014), pp. 273–289 (Rizal's sojourn in Vienna is not mentioned).

Arnold KNAPP, "Dystrophia epithelialis corneae (Fuchs), with report of a case", in: *Transact. Am. Ophthalmol. Soc.* 12 (1911), pp. 745–747.

(Arnold KNAPP), *Text-Book of Ophthalmology. By Prof. E. Fuchs, Vienna. Translated from the XII German edition, revised and enlarged by Dr. ALEXANDER DUANE, New York.* VII edition, 997 pages, 445 illustrations. Philadelphia and London, J. B. Lippincott Co., 1923, in: *Arch. Ophthalmol.* 52 (1923), p. 308.

Max KNIES, "Über sympathische Augenerkrankung", in: *Beiträge zur Ophthalmologie als Festgabe Friedrich Horner zur Feier des fünfundzwanzigsten Jubiläums seiner academischen Lehrthätigkeit gewidmet von Marc Dufour in Lausanne, Otto Haab und Max Knies in Zürich, Julius Michel in Würzburg, Wilhelm Schoen in Leipzig, und O. F. Wadsworth in Boston, U. S.* A. J. F. Bergmann, Wiesbaden 1881, pp. 53–97.

Anton KÖHLER (ed.), *Curiositäten- und Memorabilien-Lexicon von Wien. Ein belehrendes und unterhaltendes Nachschlag- und Lesebuch in anekdotischer, artistischer, biographischer, geschichtlicher, legendarischer, pittoresker, romantischer u. topographischer Beziehung.* Vol. 1. Realis, Vienna 1846.

Leo KOENIGSBERGER, *Hermann von Helmholtz.* Reprint of the edition of 1902/03. 3 vols., Thoemmes Press 2001.

Leopold KÖNIGSTEIN, "Das Sarkom des Uvealtraktus. Von Dr. Ernst Fuchs, Professor der Augenheilkunde in Lüttich", in: *Wien. med. Presse* 22 (1881), cols. 1612–1614.

Leonard KOEPPE, "Keratitis epithelialis punctata", in: *Graefes Archiv* 95 (1917), pp. 250ff.

Walter KOERTING, Die Deutsche Universität in Prag. Die letzten 100 Jahre ihrer Medizinischen Fakultät [= *Schriftenr. d. Bayer. Landesakademie vol.* 11]. Richard Pflaum Verlag, Munich 1968.

Moriz KOHN, "Zur Aetiologie des Erythema multiforme und des Herpes iris sowie zur Frage über die Identität der die Mykosen bedingenden Pilze", in: *Arch. Dermatol. u. Syphilidol.* 3 (1871), pp. 381–396.

Carl KOLLER, "Vorläufige Mittheilung über lokale Anästhesirung am Auge", in: *Klin. Monatsbl. Augenheilk.* 22 (1884), Supplement [= *Bericht über d. XVI. Versammlg. d. Ophthalmol. Gesellschaft Heidelberg* 16 (1884)], pp. 60–63, Meeting on 15 Sept. 1884.

Carl KOLLER, "Ueber die Verwendung des Cocaïn zur Anästesirung am Auge", in: *Wien. med. Wochenschr.* 34 (1884), cols. 1275–1278 and cols. 1309–1311 (Sitzung d. k. k.Gesellschaft d. Ärzte v. 15. Oktober 1884 (ssee also: *Anzeiger d. k. k.Gesellsch. d. Aerzte in Wien*, Nr0 2, 23. October 1884).

Karl KOLLER, "Historische Notiz über die ersten Anfänge der lokalen Anästhesie", in: *Wien. med. Wochenschr.* 78 (1928), cols. 601–602. [Reprint ibid. 84 (1934), cols. 1179–1180].

Karl KOLLER, "Nachträgliche Bemerkungen über die ersten Anfänge der Lokalanästhesie", in: ibid. 85 (1935), cols. 7–8.

Hortense KOLLER BECKER, "Carl Koller and Cocaine", in: *Psychoanalytic Quarterly* 32 (1963), pp. 309–373.

Gustav KOLMER, *Parlament und Verfassung in Österreich.* Third volume 1879–1885. Carl Fromme, Vienna/Leipzig 1905.

A. E. KOMERS (ed.), *Jahrbuch für österreichische Landwirthe.* 1st and 2nd year. J. G. Calve'sche k. k.Universitäts-Buchhandlung, Prague 1863.

Oskar KOPETZKY von RECHTPERG, "Ringförmiges Sarkom der Iris und des Ciliarkörpers", in: *Graefes Archiv* 52 (1901), pp. 330–335.

W. KOSTER Gzn., "Schädigung des Auges durch Wasserstoffperoxyd (H2O2)", in: *Graefes Archiv* 105 (1921), pp. 538–541.

W. KOZUSCHEK, D. LORENZ, H. THOMAS (eds.), *Theodor Billroth – Ein Leben für die Chirurgie.* Mit Beiträgen zur Entwicklung der Magenchirurgie. Karger, Basel 1992.

Richard KRÄMER, "Die optischen Grundlagen der 'scheinbaren Spiegelung der Pupille in der Hornhaut' (nebst Bemerkungen über konstruktive Optik); in: *Graefes Archiv* 105 (1921), pp. 1091–1108.

Richard KRÄMER, "Keratomalazie bei Erythrodermia desquamativa. Ein Beitrag zur Ätiologie der Leiner'schen Erkrankung", in: *Wien. med. Wochenschr.* 71 (1921), cols. 1063–1066.

Fritz KRAFT (ed.), *Grosse Naturwissenschaftler. Biographisches Lexikon. Mit einer Bibliographie zur Geschichte der Naturwissenschaften.* 2nd ed. Verlag d. Vereins dt. Ing., Düsseldorf 1986.

Ernst KRAUPA, "Pigmentierungen der Hornhauthinterfläche bei 'Dystrophia epithelialis' (Fuchs)', in: *Zeitschr. Augenheilk.* 44 (1920), pp. 247–250.

Ernst KRAUPA, "Beiträge zur Morphologie des Augenhintergrundes II", in: *Graefes Archiv* 105 (1921), pp. 865–879.

Gertrud KRETSCHMAR, Monsignore Joseph Greuter und die Tiroler Konservativen. Diss. Univ. Vienna 1949.

Frank KROGMANN, "Ferdinand von Arlt (1812–1887) unter dem Aspekt seiner Beziehungen zu deutschen Wissenschaftlern", in: *Würzb. medizinhist. Mitteil.* 13 (1995), pp. 60–66.

Frank KROGMANN, "Streifzug durch die Geschichte der Augenheilkunde in Wien", in: *Mitteilungen der Österreichischen Gesellschaft für Wissenschaftsgeschichte* 18 (1998), pp. 124–152.

Adolf KRONFELD (ed.), *Führer durch das Medizinische Wien. Geschichte und Organisation.* Moritz Perles, Vienna 1911.

Peter C. KRONFELD, "Maximilian Salzmann", in: *Am. J. Opthalmol.* 36 (1953), pp. 128–129.

Lorenz KRÜGER (ed.), *Universalgenie Helmholtz. Rückblick nach 100 Jahren.* Akademie-Verlag, Berlin 1994.

Gerhard KLUMBIES, "Konrad Lorenz 1903–1989. Verhaltensforscher – Professor in Königsberg (1940–45) – Nobelpreis 1973". In: Dietrich RAUSCHNING, Donata v. NERÉE (eds.): *Die Albertus-Universität zu Königsberg und ihre Professoren. Aus Anlaß der Gründung der Albertus-Universität vor 450 Jahren.* Duncker & Humblot, Berlin 1995.

Hans Joachim KÜCHLE, *Augenkliniken deutschsprachiger Hochschulen und ihre Lehrstuhlinhaber im 19. und 20. Jahrhundert.* Biermann, Cologne 2005.

Andreas KÜNZLI, *L. L. Zamenhof (1859–1917). Esperanto, Hillelismus (Homaranismus) und die jüdische Frage in Ost und West.* Otto Harrassowitz Verlag, Wiesbaden 2010.

R. KUHTE, S. GINSBERG, "Malignes Epitheliom d. Ciliarkörpers bei einem fünfjährigen Kinde", in: *Beiträge zur Augenheilkunde. Festschrift Julius Hirschberg von Schülern und Freunden aus Anlass seiner fünfundzwanzigjährigen Wirksamkeit als Professor an der Universität Berlin in Verehrung überreicht.* Veit & Comp., Leipzig 1905, pp. 127–160.

Kunst des Heilens. Aus der Geschichte der Medizin und Pharmazie. Katalog der Niederösterreichischen Landesausstellung in der Kartause Gaming vom 4. Mai bis 27. Oktober 1991. Katalog des Niederösterreichischen Landesmuseums. N. F. 276. – Wien: Amt der Niederösterreichischen Landesregierung, Kulturabteilung 1991.

Toshima KURAWA, "Ueber eine eigenthümliche Art von Keratitis superficialis punctata nach Influenza", in: *Centralbl. prakt. Augenheilk.* Sept. 1902.

Josef KYRLE, "Tabes und negativer Liquor," in: *Graefes Archiv* 105 (1921), pp. 390–400.

W. B. LAFFER, "Blepharochalasis. Report of a case of this trophoneurosis, involving also the upper lip", in: *Cleveland Med. J.* 8 (1909), pp. 131–135.

Leo LASKER, *Ein Beitrag zur Retinitis circinata.* Med. Diss. Univ. Leipzig 1904.

Hans LAUBER, "Außerordentliche Tagung der Ophthalmologischen Gesellschaft in Vienna 4.–6. August 1921", in: *Zeitschr. Augenheilk.* 46 (1921), pp. 223–242 and pp. 293–310.

Hans LAUBER, "Über die Behandlung der oberflächlichen Hornhauterkrankungen mit Radium", in: *Wien. med. Wochenschr.* 71 (1921), cols. 1066–1068.

Hans LAUBER, "Klinische und anatomische Untersuchungen im Sehnervenkopf", in: *Graefes Archiv* 105 (1921), pp. 567–589.

Hans LAUBER, "Verband und Behandlung nach Staroperation", in: *Wien. med. Wochenschr.* 75 (1925), No. 45.

Hans LAUBER (ed.), *Verhandlungen der ausserordentlichen Tagung der Ophthalmologischen Gesellschaft in Vienna am 4., 5. und 6. August 1921.* Karger, Berlin 1922.

Jutta LAUBER, Helmut WYKLICKY, *150 Jahre Wiener Augenheilkunde (1812 wurde in Wien die erste Universitäts-Augenklinik der Welt begründet). Das Institut für Geschichte der Medizin in Wien (Leitung: Doz. E. Lesky) in Verbindung mit I. Univ.-Augenklinik Vienna (Vorstand: Prof. A. Pillat), II. Univ.-Augenklinik Vienna (Vorstand: J. Böck), Univ.-Augenklinik Graz (Vorstand: K. Hruby) stellt Dokumente, Handschriften, Publikationen, Bilder und Instrumente aus.* Exhibition catalogue 1 – 30 June 1962. Eigenverlag der Wiener medizinischen Akademie für ärztliche Fortbildung, Vienna 1962.

James E. LEBENSOHN, "The Eye and Sleep", in: *Arch. Ophthalmol.* 25 (1941), pp. 401–411.

James E. LEBENSOHN, "Professor Ernst Fuchs (June 14, 1851–November 21, 1930)", in: *Americ. J. Ophthalmol.* 34 (1951), pp. 772–774.

James E. LEBENSOHN, "The Application of Cocaine to the Eye as an Anesthetic", in: James E. LEBENSOHN, *An Anthology of Ophthalmic Classics*. Williams & Wilkens Co., Baltimore 1969, pp. 324–329.

Pierre LEBRUN, "Tumeur sarcomateuse de l'iris. Extirpation du globe". Guérison. in: *Annales d'Oculistique* 1869.

Pierre LEBRUN, "New Mode of Operating for Cataract by Median-Sphero-Cylindrical Flap", in: Henry P. MENESES, George CRITCHETT (eds.), Report of the Fourth International Ophthalmological Congress held in London, August, 1872. Vol. 4, Savill, Edwards 1873, p. 205.

Alfred LECHNER, *Geschichte der Technischen Hochschule in Vienna (1815–1940).* Vienna 1942.

Emilie LEHMUS, *Die Erkrankungen der Macula lutea bei progressiver Myopie.* Inaug.-Diss. Univ. Zürich 1875.

Bernfried LEIBER et al. (eds.), *Die klinischen Syndrome. Syndrome, Sequenzen und Symptomenkomplexe.* 8th ed. Urban & Schwarzenberg 1996.

Josef LEITER, *Katalog über ophthalmologische Instrumente und Apparate etc. der Firma Josef Leiter Lieferant für die k. k. Universitätskliniken.* Selbstverlag, Vienna 1906.

Carola LEITNER, Kurt HAMTIL (eds.), *Wiens 4. Bezirk Wieden in alten Fotografien.* Carl Ueberreuter, Vienna 2007.

Lucien LEPLAT, Ernest FUCHS (1882), in: Léon HALKIN, Paul HARSIN (Ed.), LIBER MEMORIALIpp. L'Université de Liége de 1867 à 1935. Notices biographiques. Tome III. Faculté de Médecine. Rectorat de l'Université, Liége 1936, p. 122–124.

Alphonse LE ROY, Liber Memorialis. L'Université de Liége depuis sa fondation. Ouvrage rédigé et publié en vertu d'une décision du Conseil Académique, à l'occasion du premier jubilé semi-séculaire de l'Université (3 Novembre 1867). Carmanne, Liége 1869.

Erna LESKY, Joseph Skoda, in: Wien. klin. Wochenschr. 68 (1956), pp. 726–729.

Erna LESKY, Aus dem Nachlaß Ferdinand von Arlts im Wiener medizinhistorischen Institut, in: Klin. Monatsbl. Augenheilk. 139 (1961), pp. 847–856.

Erna LESKY, "Die Wiener ophthalmologische Schule", in: *Wien. klin. Wochenschr.* 74 (1962), pp. 529–532.

Erna LESKY, "Eduard Konrad Zirm (1863–1944). Zur 100.Wiederkehr seines Geburtstages (18. März 1963)", in: *Wien. klin. Wochenschr.* 75 (1963), pp. 199–201.

Erna LESKY, "Die Errichtung der beiden Wiener Unfallstationen im Jahre 1909", in: *Acta chir. Austriaca* 2 (1970), pp. 3–6.

Erna LESKY, "Purkiněs Weg. Wissenschaft, Bildung und Nation", in: Sitzungsber. d. ÖAW. Phil.–hist. Kl. 265. Bd., 5. Abhandl. [= *Veröffentlichungen d. Kommission für Geschichte d. Erziehung u. d. Unterrichtes* Issue 12]. Hermann Böhlaus Nachf., Vienna/Cologne/Graz 1970.

Erna LESKY (ed.), *Wien und die Weltmedizin. 4. Symposium der Internationalen Akademie für Geschichte der Medizin veranstaltet im Institut für Geschichte der Medizin der Universität Wien 17.–19. September 1973.* Hermann Böhlaus Nachfolger, Vienna/Cologne/Graz 1974.

Erna LESKY, *The Vienna Medical School of the 19th Century. Translated from the German Die Wiener Medizinische Schule im 19. Jahrhundert by L. Williams and I. S. Levij.* The Johns Hopkins University Press, Baltimore/London 1976.

Erna LESKY, *Die Wiener Medizinische Schule im 19. Jahrhundert.* 2nd ed. Böhlau, Graz/Cologne 1978.

Erna LESKY, *Meilensteine der Wiener Medizin. Große Ärzte Österreichs in drei Jahrhunderten.* Wilhelm Maudrich, Vienna/Munich/Bern 1981.

L. LEVY-WOLFF, "Zur Genese der 'gutartigen Epithelwucherung des Ziliarkoerpers' nach Fuchs", in: *Klin. Monatsbl. Augenh.* 89 (1932), pp. 593ff.

F. PARK LEWIS, "Giuseppe Cirincione. Leader of Italian ophthalmology", in: *Am. J. Ophthalmol.* 13 (1930), pp. 707–709.

T. M. LI, "Report of the Department of Ophthalmology", in: *Sixteenth Annual Report of the Medical Superintendent of the Peking Union Medical College Hospital. For the Year Ending June 30, 1924.* Peking 1924, pp. 64–67.

L. v. LIEBERMANN, "Kaustische Resektion der trachomatösen Tarsalbindehaut", in: *Graefes Archiv* 105 (1921), pp. 542–550.

Liège et son Université. Georges Thone 1929.

J. G. LINDBERG, "Zwei Fälle von sogenannten 'Dellen' in der Hornhaut", in: *Acta Ophthalmol.* 9 (1931), pp. 88–93.

Gerrit A. LINDEBOOM, "Karel Frederik Wenckebach (1864–1940) und Österreich", in: Erna LESKY (ed.), *Wien und die Weltmedizin* (1974), pp. 214–218.

E. LINDGREN, "Neuroretinitis eclamptica", in: *Graefes Archiv* 105 (1921), pp. 286–298.

Karl LINDNER, "Die freie Initialform der Prowazek'schen Einschlüsse", in: *Wien. klin. Wochenschr.* 22 (1909), pp. 1697–1698.

Karl LINDNER, "Über den jetzigen Stand der Trachomforschung", in: *Wien. klin. Wochenschr.* 22 (1909), pp. 1742–1746.

Karl LINDNER, "Zur Färbung der Prowazek'schen Einschlüsse", in: *Centralbl. Bakt. Parasitol. Infektionskrankh.* 55 (1910), pp. 429–432.

Karl LINDNER, *Die freie Initialform der Prowazek'schen Einschlüsse*, in: *Graefes Archiv* 76 (1910), pp. 559–567.

Karl LINDNER, "Gonoblenorrhoe, Einschlussblenorrhoe, Trachom," in: *Graefes Archiv* 78 (1911), pp. 348–380.

Karl LINDNER, "Über die Blenorrhöe des Neugeborenen", in: *Wien. med. Wochenschr.* 71 (1921), cols. 1068–1070.

Karl LINDNER, "Über die Topographie der parasitären Bindehautkeime", in: *Graefes Archiv* 105 (1921), pp. 726–777.

Karl LINDNER, "Über die Schwierigkeiten der Trachomforschung", in: *Zeitschr. Augenheilk.* 57 (1925), pp. 508–556.

Karl LINDNER, "Ist das Bacterium granulosis Noguchi der Erreger des Trachoms?", in: *Zeitschr. Augenheilk.* 67 (1929), pp. 374–376.

Karl LINDNER, "Ist das Bacterium granulosis Noguchi der Erreger des Trachoms?", in: *Graefes Archiv* 122 (1929), pp. 391–414.

Karl LINDNER, "Trachoma", in: Conrad BERENS (ed.), *The Eye and Its Diseases by 82 Authorities*. Saunders, Philadelphia/London 1936, pp. 399–417.

Karl David LINDNER, "Zur Geschichte der Kurzsichtigkeit von Kepler bis Arlt", in: *Klin. Monatsbl. Augenheilk.* 107 (1941), pp. 320–328.

Karl LINDNER, "Hermann Helmholtz, zum 50. Todestag", in: *Wien. med. Wochenschr.* 94 (1944), p. 433.

Karl LINDNER, "Zum 100. Geburtstage von Ernst Fuchs", in: *Wien. klin. Wochenschr.* 63 (1951), pp.449–450.

Karl LINDNER, "Einiges über die Keratoplastik", in: *Wien. klin. Wochenschr.* 63 (1951), pp. 627–628.

Karl LINDNER, *Lehrbuch der Augenheilkunde*. Urban & Schwarzenberg, Vienna 1952.

Karl LINDNER, "Ueber das Verschwinden des Trachoms und die Abnahme der infektiösen Bindehautentzündungen in Oesterreich", in: *Wien. klin. Wochenschr.* 65 (1953), pp. 759–760.

Arthur LINKSZ, "The Development of Visual Standards: Snellen, Jaeger, and Giraud-Teulon", in: *Bull. N. Y. Acad. Med.* 51/2 (1975), pp. 277–285.

C. S. F. LINCOLN, "Medical Missionary Association of China", in: *JAMA* 44/12 (1905), p. 970.

Karl LISCH, "Beziehungen von Otmar Purtscher zu Julius Hirschberg und zur Reform der Augenheilkunde", in: *Spektrum Augenheilk.* 1 (1988), pp. 157–159.

Joseph LISTER, "A Method of Antiseptic Treatment of Wounded Soldiers in the Present War", in: BMJ 2 (1870), pp. 243–244.

Robert LISTON, *Elements of Surgery.* Part II. Longman and Company, London; Adam Black, Edinburgh 1831.

J. H. LIU, Wu-Lien TEH, Yui C. VOONPING, "Western Ophthalmology in China", in: *Nat. Med. J. of China* 17 (1931), pp. 120–121.

Gaetano LODATO, "Blefarocalasi. Contribuito clinico ed anatomico-patologico", in: *Archivio d'ottalmologia* (1903), Special edition.

Adolf LORENZ, *Ich durfte helfen. Mein Leben und Wirken*. Albrecht, Vienna 1949.

Christoph LÖSER, Gerd PLEWIG (ed.), *Pantheon der Dermatologie*. Springer, Heidelberg 2008.

Irene LOEWENFELD, H. Stanley THOMPSON, "Fuchs's Heterochromic Cyclitis. I. Clinical Characteristics of the Syndrome", in: Surv. Ophthalmol.17 (1973), p. 394–414.

Irene E. LOEWENFELD, H. Stanley THOMPSON, "Fuchs's Heterochromic Cyclitis: A Critical Review of the Literature. II. Etiology and Mechanisms", in: *Surv. Ophthalmol* 18 (1973), pp. 2–61.

Irene E. LOEWENFELD, Otto LÖWENSTEIN, *The Pupil: Anatomy, Physiology, and Clinical Applications*. Vols. 1+2. Iowa State University Press, 1993.

Carlos LÓPEZ DE LETONA, "El Profesor Ernesto Fuchs y España (1931)", in: *Arch. Soc. Esp. Oftalmol.* 78/9 (2003), pp. 517–518.

Albert LORENZ, *Wenn der Vater mit dem Sohne … Erinnerungen an Adolf Lorenz.* Franz Deuticke, Vienna 1952.

Arnold LÖWENSTEIN, "Über den Einfluß einseitiger Beschränkung des Lichteinfalles auf die Sehschärfe", in: *Graefes Archiv* 105 (1921), pp. 844–850.
Erwin LUCIUS, Arslan TERZIOGLU (ed.), "Österreichisch-türkische medizinische Beziehungen. Berichte d. Symposions v. 28. u. 29. 4. 1986 in Istanbul". Istanbul 1987.
Kathrin McEWEN, *Antisemitismus in Wien um 1900: Eine Diskursanalyse der christlichsozialen und deutschnationalen Presse*. VDM Verlag Dr. Müller 2010.
Hunter McGUIRE, "Gyrate Atrophy of the Choroid and Retina (FUCHS)", in: *Arch. Ophthalmol.* 8/3 (1932), pp. 372–379.
Thomas MAISEL, *Gelehrte in Stein und Bronze. Die Denkmäler im Arkadenhof der Universität Wien*. Böhlau, Vienna/Cologne/Weimar 2007.
Maison LUER. *Catalogue spécial illustré des Instruments d'Ophtalmologie*. Paris 1909.
Kyozo MAJIMA, "Studie über PROWAZEKsche Körperchen, besonders die Reinkultur von denselben", in: *Nippon Gankagakkai Zasshi* 29 (1925), p. 5. (Japan.)
Sadhan MAJUMDER (Ed.), *Stem Cells and Cancer*. Springer, New York 2009.
Ricardo K. S. MAK, *Transmitting the Ideal of Enlightenment. Chinese Universities since the Late Nineteenth Century*. University Press of America Inc., Lanham, Maryland/Plymouth 2009.
Manifestations en l'honneur de M. le professeur Th. Schwann. Liège, 23 juin 1878.
Gunter MANN (ed.), *Naturwissen und Erkenntnis im 19. Jahrhundert: Emil Du Bois-Reymond*. Gerstenberg, Hildesheim 1981.
Mark J. MANNIS, Avi A. MANNIS (eds.), *Corneal Transplantation: A History in Profiles*. 2nd ed. Hirschberg History of Ophthalmology Volume Six. Wayenborgh Publications, Amsterdam 2018.
Kenneth G. MANTON, Igor AKUSHEVICH, Julia KRAVCHENKO, *Cancer Mortality and Morbidity Patterns in the U. S. Population. An Interdisciplinary Approach*. Springer, New York 2009.
Otto MARBURG, "Einiges über Grundlagen, Komplikationen und Erfolge der Sehnervenscheiden-Trepanation nach Müller", in: *Graefes Archiv* 105 (1921), pp. 590–598.
Michael F. MARMOR, Daniel ALBERT (eds.), Foundations of Ophthalmology. Great Insights that Established the Discipline. Springer Internat. Publ. 2017.
W. MARTIN, *Zur Prognostik der Uvealsarcome*. Med. Diss. Univ. Halle 1885.
Narcisse J. MARTINACHE, "Ulcers of the cornea, treated by the actual cautery", in: *Pacific Med. Surg. J.*, Nov. 1873, p. 294.
Narcisse J. MARTINACHE, "De l'emploi du cautère actuel dans les maladies des yeux, et principalement dans les ulcères de la cornée", in: *Annales d'ocul.* 80 (1878), p. 21.
Carl Fried. Phil. v. MARTIUS, "Denkrede auf J. J. Berzelius, gehalten in der öffentlichen Sitzung der Königlich Bayerischen Akademie der Wissenschaften am 28. November 1848". Separatabdruck aus den gelehrten Anzeigen 1848, Nos. 233–236.
H. MASCHKE, *Ein Beitrag zur Lehre der Aderhautsarcome*. Med. Diss. Univ. Königsberg 1884.
Erwin MATSCH, *Geschichte des Auswärtigen Dienstes von Österreich (-Ungarn) 1720–1920*. Böhlau, Vienna/Graz/Cologne 1980.
A. E. MAUMENEE, "The History of the Wilmer Ophthalmological Institute", in: *Am. J. Ophthalmol.* 60/5 (1965), pp. 770–783.
Ludwig MAUTHNER, *Gehirn und Auge*. Bergmann, Wiesbaden 1881 (= MAUTHNER Vorträge aus dem Gesammtgebiete der Augenheilkunde für Studirende und Aerzte. Issues IX–XI, 1881–1882).
Ludwig MAUTHNER, *Die Lehre vom Glaukom*. Bergmann, Wiesbaden 1882.
Charles Henry MAY, *Manual of Diseases of the Eye for Students and General Practitioners*. Williams & Wilkins, Baltimore 1900.

Charles H. MAY, "A New Electric Ophthalmoscope", in: *Ophthalmol. Record* 23 (1914), pp. 386–389.
Charles H. MAY, "Bronze Plaques of Professor Fuchs available", in: *Arch. Ophthalmol.* 8/5 (1932), p. 760.
Charles H. MAY, "Bronze plate of Professor Ernst Fuchs", in: *Am. J. Ophthalmol.* 16 (1933), p. 71.
Hunter McGUIRE, "Gyrate Atrophy of the Choroid and Retina (FUCHS)", in: *Arch. Ophthalmol.* 8/3 (1932), pp. 372–379.
Josef MELLER, "Die histologischen Veränderungen des Auges bei der Keratitis disciformis", in: *Klin. Monatsbl. f. Augenheilkunde* 43 (1905), pp. 335–352.
Josef MELLER, *Ophthalmic Surgery. A Handbook of the Surgical Operations on the Eyeball and Its Appendages as Practiced at the Clinic of Prof. Hofrat Fuchs*. P. Blakiston's Son & Co., Philadelphia 1908.
Josef MELLER, *Augenärztliche Eingriffe. Ein kurzes Handbuch für angehende Augenärzte*. Šafář, Vienna 1918.
Josef MELLER, "Zur Ätiologie der Keratitis pustuliformis profunda", in: *Centralbl. prakt. Augenheilk.* 42 (1918), pp. 1–8.
Josef MELLER, *Augenärztliche Eingriffe. Ein kurzes Handbuch für angehende Augenärzte*. 2nd ed. Josef Šafář, Vienna/Leipzig 1921.
Josef MELLER, "Chronische Iridocyclitis und Neuritis retrobulbaris", in: *Graefes Archiv* 105 (1921), pp. 299–332.
Josef MELLER, "Hofrat Ernst Fuchs zum 70. Geburtstage", in: *Wien. med. Wochenschr.* 71 (1921), cols. 1041–1043.
Josef MELLER, "Über Drucksteigerung im Auge nach Ausziehung des Greisenstares", in: *Wien. med. Wochenschr.* 71 (1921), cols. 1070–1076.
Josef MELLER, *Ophthalmic Surgery. A Handbook of the Surgical Operations on the Eyeball and Its Appendages as Practised at the I. Eye Clinic, University of Vienna*. Edited by William M. Sweet. Third Edition translated from the Second Edition, *Augenärztliche Eingriffe* (Josef Šafar, Vienna). P. Blakeston's Sons & Co., Philadelphia 1923.
Josef MELLER, "Gedenkworte zum 50. Jahrestage des Vortrages von Dr. Karl Koller über das Kokain vor der Gesellschaft der Ärzte in Wien", in: *Wien. klin. Wochenschr.* 47 (1934), pp. 1313–1317.
Josef MELLER, "Über die Entwicklung der Lehre von der sympathischen Ophthalmie in der Wiener ophthalmologischen Schule", in: *Wien. klin. Wochenschr.* 48 (1935), pp. 622–629.
Josef MELLER, Josef BÖCK (ed.), *Augenärztliche Eingriffe. Eine kurzgefasste Operationslehre.* Mit einem Beitrag v. K. Kofler. Springer, Vienna 1950.
Friedrich MERKEL, *Jakob Henle: Ein deutsches Gelehrtenleben, nach Aufzeichnungen und Erinnerungen.* Friedrich Vieweg und Sohn, Braunschweig 1891.
Robert MESSNER, *Wien vor dem Fall der Basteien. Häuserverzeichnis und Plan der Inneren Stadt vom Jahre 1857.* Österr. Bundesverlag, Vienna 1958.
Robert MESSNER, *Der Alsergrund im Vormärz. Historisch-topographische Darstellung der nordwestlichen Vorstädte und Vororte Wiens auf Grund der Katastralvermessung.* Notring d. wissenschaftl. Verbände Österr., Vienna 1970.
Robert MESSNER, *Mariahilf im Vormärz. Historisch-topographische Darstellung der westlichen Vorstädte (südliche Hälfte) auf Grund der Katastralvermessung (= Topographie von Alt-Wien VI. Teil).* Verband der Wissenschaftlichen Gesellschaften Österreichs, Vienna 1982.
Michel MEULDERS, *Helmholtz. From Enlightenment to Neuroscience. Translated and edited by Laurence Garey*. MIT Press 2010.

Meyers Lexikon. 7th ed., Bibliograph. Inst. Leipzig 1924–1930.

Julius von MICHEL, *Die histologische Struktur des Irisstromas.* Universitätsprogramm, Erlangen 1875.

Julius von MICHEL, "Ueber Iris und Iritis", in: *Graefes Archiv* 27, Abth. II (1881), pp. 171–282.

Edoardo MIDENA, "Anton von Rosas (1791–1855): On the occasion of the bicentennial of his birth. Part 2: A survey of his scientific works with special emphasis on specific topics", in: *Wien. klin. Wochenschr.* 103 (1991), pp. 473–476.

B. MILDER, "As I remember: Edward Vail Lapham Brown", in: *Eye Ear Nose Throat Mon.* 54/12 (1975), pp. 465–467.

B. MILDER, "A remembrance of Edward Vail Lapham Brown", in: *Surv. Ophthalmol.* 43/2 (1998), pp. 188–191.

Militär-Schematismus des österreichischen Kaiserthumes. K. K. Hof- und Staats-Druckerey, Vienna 1837.

John Stuart MILL, *A System of Logic, Ratiocinative, and Inductive, Being a Connected View of the Principles of Evidence, and the Methods of Scientific Investigation.* John W. Parker, London 1843.

Minerva. Jahrbuch der gelehrten Welt. Yr. 2 1892–1893. Karl J. Trübner, Strassburg 1893.

Ministerium für Cultus und Unterricht (ed.), *Unterrichtsanstalten, Wissenschaftliche und Kunst- Institute in Wien und Niederösterreich.* K. K. Schulbücherverlag, Vienna 1917.

Saiichi MISHIMA, *The History of Ophthalmology in Japan.* G. Schmidt, Oostende 2004.

Philipp Christiaan MOLHUYSEN, Petrus Johannes BLOK (eds.), *Nieuw Nederlandsch Biografisch Woordenboek.* Sijthoff, Leiden 1911–1936.

N. MOSCHIK de REYA, O. EICHHORN, "Zur Registrierung der bioelektrischen Erscheinungen bei Augenbewegungen", in: *Wien. klin. Wochenschr.* 63 (1951), pp. 676–677.

H. MÜHLENDYCK, M. HUNDEIKER, "Blepharochalasis (Fuchs) und Laffer-Ascher-Syndrom", in: *Hautarzt* 29 (1978), p. 474.

Johannes MÜLLER, *Zur vergleichenden Physiologie des Gesichtssinnes des Menschen und der Thiere nebst einem Versuch über die Bewegungen der Augen und über den menschlichen Blick.* Leipzig 1826.

Wolfgang MÜNCHOW, "Geschichte der Augenheilkunde," in: Karl VELHAGEN (ed.), *Der Augenarzt.* Vol IX. 2nd ed. Georg Thieme, Leipzig 1983.

J. Fraser MUIRHEAD, "Adolph Barkan (1845–1935), European ophthalmologist in San Francisco", in: *JAMA Ophthalmol.* 132/3 (2014), pp. 346–349.

Anzo MURAKAMI, "Ein Beitrag zu den Netzhautgefäss-Veränderungen bei Leukämie", in: Klin. Monatsbl. Augenheilk. 39 (1901), pp. 136ff.

Sean B. MURPHY, *Portraits of Ophthalmology at McGill University 1876–1990.*

OBITUARIES

Eduard Albert, in: *Wien. klin. Wochenschr.* 13 (1900), pp. 995ff. (Karl Gussenbauer).

Karl Wolfgang Ascher, in: *Klin. Monatsbl. Augenheilk.* 101 (1972), pp. 126–128.

Otto Becker, in: *Wien. klin. Wochenschr.* 2 (1890), p. 159 (Ernst Fuchs).

Otto Becker, in: Centralbl. prakt. Augenheilk. 14 (1890), pp. 60–62 (Julius Hirschberg).

Edouard van Beneden, in: *Naturwiss. Rundschau* 25 (1910), pp. 362–363.

Carl Braun R. v. Fernwald, in: *Wien. med. Wochenschr.* 41 (1891), cols. 628–629.

Ha(n)ns Frh. v. Chiari, in: *Wien. klin. Wochenschr.* 29 (1916), pp. 688ff.

Ha(n)ns Frh. v. Chiari, in: *Centralbl. Allg. Pathol. u. pathol. Anat.* 27 (1916), pp. 289ff.
Ha(n)ns Frh. v. Chiari, in: *Münch. med. Wochenschr.* (1916), pp. 1080ff.
Ottokar Frh. v. Chiari, in: *Internat. Zentralbl. Laryngol. Rhinol.* 34 (1918), pp. 151f–152.
Ottokar Frh. v. Chiari, in: *Wien. med. Wochenschr.* 68 (1918), pp. 917–918.
Ottokar Frh. v. Chiari, in: *Monatsschr. Ohrenheilk. u. Laryngo–Rhinol.* 53 (1919), pp. 81ff.
Wilhelm Czermak, in: *Graefes Archiv* 65 (1906), pp. I–IV (Ernst Fuchs).
Johan Albin Dalén, in: *Acta Ophthalmol.* 18 (1940), pp. 221–223 (Fredrik Berg).
Viktor Ebner R. v. Rofenstein, in: *Wien. med. Wochenschr.* 75 (1925), col. 89.
Viktor Ebner R. v. Rofenstein, in: *Wien. klin. Wochenschr.* 38 (1925), pp. 441ff.
Viktor Ebner R. v. Rofenstein, in: *Anat. Anzeiger* 64 (1927), pp. 1ff.
Theodor Escherich, in: *Zeitschr. Kinderheilk.* 1 (1911), pp. 423ff.
Ernst Fuchs, in: *Zeitschr. Augenheilk.* 73 (1931), pp. 317–325. (Memorial speech delivered to the mourning session of the Ophthalmologische Gesellschaft in Vienna on 15. Dec 1930). (Maximilian Salzmann).
Ernst Fuchs, in: *Wien. klin. Wochenschr.* 42 (1931), pp. 1493–1495 (Josef Meller).
Allvar Gullstrand, in: *Dt. Opt. Wochenschr.* 16 (1930), pp. 546–548.
Allvar Gullstrand, in: *Zeitschr. Ophthalmol. Optik* 18 (1930), pp. 129–134 (Moritz von Rohr).
Allvar Gullstrand, in: Zeitschr. Augenheilk. 73 (1931), pp. 326–330 (Heinrich Erggelet).
Ferdinand Herbert Haessler, in: *Transact. Am. Ophthalmol.* Soc. 64 (1966), pp. 5–6.
Ferdinand Herbert Haessler, in: Am. J. Ophthalmol. 61 (1966), pp. 357–358.
Ludwig Halberstätter, in: *Zeitschr. Haut- u. Geschlechtskrankh.* 7 (1949), p. 39.
Eduard R. v. Hofmann, in: *Wien. klin. Wochenschr.* 10 (1897), pp. 797ff.
Eduard R. v. Hofmann, in: *Prag. Med. Wochenschr.* 22 (1897), pp. 453ff.
Eduard R. v. Hofmann, in: *Wien. med. Blätter* 20 (1897), p. 584.
Tatsuya Inouye, in: *Centralbl. Augenheilk.* 19 (1895), pp. 200–205 and pp. 286–287 (Julius Hirschberg).
Leopold Königstein, in: *Die feierliche Inauguration des Rektors der Universität Vienna für das Studienjahr1924/25. Univ. Wien 1924*, pp. 22–23 (Moriz Sachs).
Othmar Kühn, in: *Mitteil. d. Geolog. Gesellsch. Wien* 62 (1969), pp. 175–184 (Fritz Steininger).
Hans Kundrat, in: *Wien. klin. Wochenschr.* 6 (1893), pp. 323ff.
Hans Kundrat, in: *Wien. med. Wochenschr.* 43 (1893), cols. 810–811.
Josef Kyrle, in: *Wien. klin. Wochenschr.* 39 (1926), pp. 377–378.
Josef Kyrle, in *Wien. med. Wochenschr.* 76 (1926), pp. 48ff.
Josef Kyrle, in: *Die feierliche Inauguration des Rektors der Universität Vienna für das Studienjahr 1926/27*, pp. 54–55.
Karl Langer, in: *Wien. med. Wochenschr.* 37 (1887), col. 1657 (Carl Toldt).
Karl Langer, in: *Wien. med. Blätter* 10 (1887), pp 1597 (Ferdinand Hochstetter).
Karl Langer, in: *Almanach Akad. Wissensch.* 38 (1888), pp. 185ff. (Eduard Suess).
Josef Leiter, in: *Wien. med. Wochenschr.* 42 (1892), cols. 641–642.
Karl David Lindner, in: *Wien. klin. Wochenschr.* 73 (1961), pp. 429–430 (J. Böck).
Karl David Lindner, in: *Wien. med. Wochenschr.* 111 (1961), pp. 473–474 (H. Fanta).
Karl David Lindner, in: Graefes Archiv 163 (1961), pp. 489–492 (K. Hruby).
Karl David Lindner, in: *Klin. Monatsbl. Augenheilk.* 139 (1961), pp. 383–384 (A. Pillat).
Irene Loewenfeld, in: *Neuro-Ophthalmol.* 34 (2010), p. 78 (Neil R. Miller).
Adolf Lorenz, in: *Wien. klin. Wochenschr.* 58 (1946), pp. 96–97.
Ernst Ludwig, in: *Wien. med. Wochenschr.* 65 (1915), cols. 1593–1594 and 1825ff.
Ernst Ludwig, in: *Almanach Akad. Wissensch.* 66 (1916), pp. 323ff.
Otto Marburg, in: *Wien. med. Wochenschr.* 98 (1948), pp. 461–462

Otto Marburg, in: *Die feierliche Inauguration des Rektors der Uni.versität Wien für das Studienjahr 1948/49*, pp. 43ff.
Otto Marburg, in: *Wien. Zeitschr. Nervenheilk.* 2 (1949), pp. 1ff.
Rudolf Maresch, in: *Zentralbl. allg. Pathol. u. patholog. Anat.* 65 (1936), pp. 1ff.
Rudolf Maresch, in: *Wien. klin. Wochenschr.* 49 (1936), pp. 497ff.
Rudolf Maresch, in: *Wien. med. Wochenschr.* 86 (1936), cols. 145ff.
Rudolf Maresch, in: *Almanach Akad. Wissensch.* Vienna 1936.
Rudolf Maresch, in: *Münch. med. Wochenschr.* 83 (1936), pp. 612–613.
Theodor Meynert, in: *Wien. med. Wochenschr.* 42 (1892), cols. 938f–939.
Theodor Meynert, in: *Münch. Med. Wochenschr.* 39 (1892), pp. 495–496.
Albert Mosetig R. v. Moorhof, in: *Die feierliche Inauguration des Rektors der Universität Wien für das Studienjahr 1907/1908*. Selbstverlag der Universität, Vienna 1908, pp. 45ff.
Albert Mosetig R. v. Moorhof, in: *Wien. klin. Wochenschr.* 20 (1907), pp. 545–546.
Albert Mosetig R. v. Moorhof, in: *Wien. med. Wochenschr.* 57 (1907), cols. 251–252.
Albert Mosetig R. Moorhof, in: *Wien. med. Presse* 37 (1896), pp. 156–157.
Franz Mraček, in: *Wien. klin. Wochenschr.* 21 (1908), p. 633.
Franz Mraček, in: *Münch. med. Wochenschr.* 55 (1908), p. 832.
Albert Neisser, in: *Dermatol. Wochenschr.* 131 (1955), pp. 214–216.
Mario Pagani, in: *Boll. oculist.* 52 (1973), p. 170.
Olga Palich-Szánto, in: *Klin. Monatsbl. Augenheilk.* 160 (1972), p. 516 (Biró).
Richard Paltauf, in: *Wien. klin. Wochenschr.* 37 (1924), pp. 487ff.
Richard Paltauf, in: *Die feierl. Inauguration des Rektors der Universität Wien für das Studienjahr 1924/25* (with bibliogr.).
Arnold Pillat, in: *Wien. med. Wochenschr.* 126 (1976), pp. 26f.
Arnold Pillat, in: *Klin. Monatsbl. f. Augenheilk.* 168 (1976), pp. 152–153 (F. C. Blodi).
Olga Prager, in: *Neue Freie Presse* of 28. April 1930, p. 5.
Stanislaus v. Prowazek, in: *Verhandl. Zoolog.-Botan. Gesellsch. Wien* 65 (1915), pp. 65ff.
Otmar Purtscher, in: *Wien. med. Wochenschr.* 77 (1927), col. 1760.
Otmar Purtscher, *Zeitschr. Augenheilk.* 64 (1928), pp. 346f. (Josef Meller).
Otmar Purtscher, Klin. Monatsbl. Augenheilk. 80 (1928), pp. 99–100 (Richard Krämer).
August Leopold Ritter von Reuss, in: *Die feierl. Inauguration d. Rektors d. Wiener Universität für d. Studienjahr 1924/25*. Eigenverlag Univ. Vienna 1924, pp. 33–34 (Viktor Hanke).
August von Reuß, in: *Wien. klin. Wochenschr.* 37 (1924), pp. 1171–1172 (Julius Mannaberg).
August L. v. Reuß, in: *Jahresbericht der Allgem. Poliklinik für 1924*. Eigenverlag Poliklinik 23 (1925), pp. 4–6 (Julius Mannaberg).
Theodor Saemisch, in: *Centralbl. f. Augenheilk.* Jan. 1910 (J. Hirschberg).
Theodor Saemisch, in: *Klin. Monatsbl. Augenheilk.* 48 (1910), p. 86 (Zur Nedden).
Theodor Saemisch, in: *Archiv Augenheilk.* 45 (1910), p. 268.
Theodor Saemisch, in: *Zeitschr. Augenheilk.* 23 (1910), p. 90.
Friedrich Schauta, in: *Monatsschr. Geburtsh. Gynäkol.* 49 (1919), pp. 151ff.
Friedrich Schauta, in: *Arch. Gynäkol.* 111 (1919), pp. XXI ff.
Friedrich Schauta, in: *Zentralbl. Gynäkol.* 43 (1919) pp. 129ff (Josef Halban).
Friedrich Schauta, in: *Wien. klin. Wochenschr.* 32. (1919), pp. 98ff. (Ludwig Adler).
Friedrich Schauta, in: *Med. Bl.* 41 (1919), pp. 29–30.
Friedrich Schauta, in: *Die feierliche Inauguration des Rektors der Universität Wien für das Studienjahr 1919/20*. Vienna 1919, pp. 46–47.
Leopold Schrötter R. v. Kristelli, in: *Wien. med. Wochenschr.* 58 (1908), cols. 961–962.
Leopold Schrötter R. v. Kristelli, in: *Wien. klin. Wochenschr.* 21 (1908), 641–642.

Leopold Schrötter R. v. Kristelli, in: *Med. Klinik* 4 (1908), pp. 715–717.
Leopold Schrötter R. v. Kristelli, in: *Internat. Centralbl. f. Laryngol., Rhinol, u. verwandte Wiss.* 24 (1908), pp. 281–87 (with bibliogr.).
Guntram Schrutka-Rechtenstamm, in: *Mitteil. Astronom. Gesellsch.* 79 (1996), p. 9 (Hermann Haupt).
Hermann Snellen, in: *Wien. klin. Wochenschr.* 21 (1908), pp. 157 (Ernst Fuchs).
Salomon Stricker, in: *Münch. med. Wochenschr.* 45 (1898), pp. 568–569.
Salomon Stricker, in: *Wien. med. Wochenschr.* 48 (1898), cols. 712–713 and cols. 911ff.
Carl Toldt, in: *Wien. klin. Wochenschr.* 33 (1920), pp. 1041ff.
Carl Toldt, in: *Wien. med. Wochenschr.* 70 (1920), col. 2045.
Édouard Van Beneden, in: *Naturwiss. Rundschau* 25 (1910), pp. 362–363.
Adolf Vossius, in: *Zeitschr. Augenheilk.* 67 (1925), pp. 153–154.
Julius Wagner R. v. Jauregg, in: *Monatsschr. f. Psychiatr. u. Neurol.* 103 (1940), pp. 186ff.
Karel Frederik Wenckebach, in: *Münchner med. Wochenschr.* 87 (1940), pp. 1421–1422.
Karel Frederik Wenckebach, in: *Wien. klin. Wochenschr.* 53 (1940), pp. 1067ff.
Hugo Wintersteiner, in: *Centralbl. prakt. Augenheilk.* 43 (1919), p. 188.
Helmut Wyklicky, in: *Wien. med. Wochenschr.* 158 (2008), pp. 745–748 (Gabriela Schmidt-Wyklicky).
Emil Zuckerkandl, in: *Wien. med. Wochenschr.* 60 (1910), cols. 1323–1324.
Emil Zuckerkandl, in: *Anat. Anzeiger* 37 (1910), pp. 86ff. (J. Tandler).
Emil Zuckerkandl, in: *Wien. klin. Wochenschr.* 23 (1910), pp. 789ff.
Emil Zuckerkandl, in: *Almanach Akad. Wiss.* 61 (1911), pp. 364ff.
Emil Zuckerkandl, in: *Archiv f. Ohrenheilk.* 84 (1911), pp. 7–8 (A. Politzer).

Arin NAMAL, Arnold REISMAN, "Joseph Igersheimer (1879–1965): a visionary ophthalmologist and his contributions before and after exile", in: *J. Med. Biogr.* 15/4 (2007), pp. 227–234.

NÉCROLOGIES

Jean-Baptiste Copppez, in: *Annales d'Oculistique* 167 (1930), p. 985 (Gallemaerts).
Camille Lacompte, in: *Archive d'ophthalmol.* 47 (1930), p. 576.
Claude-André Paquelin, in: *L'Année Scientifique et Industrielle* 49 (1906), p. 556–557.
Étienne Rollet, in: *Presse médicale* 78 (1937), pp. 1381–1382 (E. Velter).
Pietro Baiardi, in: *Archivio di ottalmologia giornale mensile* 1922, pp. 89–96.
James Boyd NEAL, *Report of the Chinanfu Medical Work. In Charge of the American Presbyterian Mission, Chinanfu, China for Six Years 1891–1896.* American Presbytarian Mission Press 1897.
James Boyd NEAL, "Medical Training in China", in: *CMMJ* 11/2 (1897), pp. 89–91.
H. V. NEMA, *Ophthalmic Syndromes.* Butterworth & Co., London et al. 1973, pp. 94–96.
U. R. NEMETZ, "Behandlungsversuche mit ACTH bei Augenerkrankungen," in: *Wien. klin. Wochenschr.* 63 (1951), pp. 711–713.
Max NEUBURGER, *Hermann Nothnagel. Leben und Wirken eines deutschen Klinikers.* Rikola, Vienna et al. 1922.
Max NEUBURGER, "Rokitansky als Vorkämpfer der mechanistischen Forschungsmethode und der idealistischen Weltanschauung", in: *Wien. klin. Wochenschr.* 47 (1934), pp. 12–13.

Neue Deutsche Biographie [= NDB]. Hgg. v. d. Hist. Komm. bei d. Bayer. Akad. d. Wissensch. Duncker & Humblot, Berlin 1953ff.

Neuester Plan von Vienna und seinen Vorstädten. Artaria & Comp., Vienna 1856.

Josef NEUWIRTH (ed.), *Die K. K. Technische Hochschule in Vienna 1815–1915.* Selbstverlag der K. K. Technischen Hochschule in Wien in Kommission bei Gerold & Co. Vienna 1915.

F. W. NEWELL, "Edward Jackson – a historical perspective of his contributions to refraction and to ophthalmology", in: *Ophthalmol.* 95 (1988), p. 555–558.

Frank NINKOVICH, "The Rockefeller Foundation, China, and Cultural Change", in: *J. Am. Hist.* 70 (1984), pp. 799–820.

Nick J. NIVELL, "Thomas Bateman (1778–1821)", in: Christoph LÖSER, Gerd PLEWIG (eds.), *Pantheon der Dermatologie.* Springer, Heidelberg 2008, pp. 57–66.

Nobel Lectures, Physics 1901–1921. Elsevier Publishing Company, Amsterdam 1967.

Pierre NOLF, "Notice sur Constant Vanlair", in: *Annuaire Académie royale des Sciences, des Lettres et des Beaux-Arts de Belgique* 89 (1923), pp. 125–150.

J. W. NORDENSEN, "Über die Größe der Doppelbrechung der Hornhautsubstanz", in: *Graefes Archiv* 105 (1921), pp. 721–725.

Jeremy M. NORMAN (ed.), *Morton's Medical Bibliography. An Annotated Check-List of Texts Illustrating the History of Medicine* (Garrison and Morton). Fifth Edition. Scolar Press, Aldershot, Reprint 1993.

M. NORN, O. A. JENSEN, "Marius Tscherning (1854–1939): his life and work in optical physiology", in: *Acta Ophthalmol. Scand.* 82 (2004), pp. 501–508.

Hermann NOTHNAGEL, *Topische Diagnostik der Gehirnkrankheiten.* Eine klinische Studie. A. Hirschwald, Berlin 1879.

Notiz, in: *Wien. med. Presse* 26 (1885), pp. 1037.

Notiz, in: *Wien. med. Wochenschr.* 35 (1885), col. 1025.

Notiz, in: *Wien. med. Bl.* 8 (1885), col. 1140, 9 September 1885.

Notiz, in: *Wien. med. Wochenschr.* 44 (1894), col. 1365.

Jean-Pierre NUEL, "De la kératide punctuée superficielle", in: *Arch. d'Ophtalmol.* 14 (1894), p. 145.

James J. O'DONNELL, "Gyrate atrophy of the retina and choroid is an inborn error of metabolism of ornithine aminotransferase", in: *Neurochemistry International* 1 (1980), pp. 459–463.

Gerhard OBERKOFLER, Peter GOLLER, *Die Medizinische Fakultät Innsbruck. Faschistische Realität (1938) und Kontinuität unter postfaschistischen Bedingungen (1945).* Innsbruck 1999.

OBITUARIES

James Edward Adams, in: *Brit. Med. J.* February 1, 1890, pp. 271–272.

Karl Wolfgang Ascher, in: *Transact. Am. Ophthalmol. Soc.* 69 (1971), pp. 5–9.

Karl Wolfgang Ascher, in: *Am. J. Ophthalmol.* 73 (1972), p. 140.

Adolph Barkan M. D., in: *Brit. Med. J.* 20 (1936), pp. 188–189.

Pietro Baiardi, in: *Am. J. Ophthalmol.* 5 (1922), p. 416, p. 842.

Charles Heady Beard, in: *The Ophthalmic Record*, Feb. 1916, p. 104.

William Arthur Brailey, M. A., M. D. Cantab., Consulting Ophthalmic Surgeon, Guy's Hospital, in: *Brit. Med. J.* 1915 Apr 17; 1 (2833), p. 701.

Edward Vail Lapham Brown, in: *Arch. Ophthalmol.* 50/2 (1953), pp. 270–271 (F. Brawley).

Edward Vail Lapham Brown, in: *Proc. Inst. Med. Chic.* 19/13 (1953), p. 291–293 (E. B. Fowler).
Edward Vail Lapham Brown, in: *Trans. Am. Ophthalmol. Soc.* 51 (1953), p. 3–5 (Peter C. Kronfeld).
Edward Vail Lapham Brown, *Edward Vail Lapham Brown; in: Am. J. Ophthalmol. 36 (1953), pp.* 865–867 (Peter C. Kronfeld).
Jean-Baptiste Coppez, in: *Am. J. Ophthalmol.* 14 (1931), pp. 167f–168.
Colman Ward Cutler, in: *Transact. Am. Ophthalmol. Soc.* 33(1935), pp. 24–25. (Conrad Berens).
George Strong Derby, in: *Brit. J. Ophthalmol.* 15 (1932), p. 187–188.
George Strong Derby, in: *Transact. Am. Ophthalmol. Soc.* 30 (1932), pp. 12.2–17 (F. H. Verhoeff).
Alexander Duane, in: *Am. J. Ophthalmol.* 9/12 (1926), p. 917–922 (Conrad Berens).
Alexander Duane, in: *Transact. Am. Ophthal. Soc.* 24 (1926), pp. 18–20 (John E. Weeks).
Alexander Duane, in: *Arch. Ophthalmol.* 56 (1927), p. 66.
Alexander Duane, in: *Brit. J. Ophthalmol.* 11/5 (1927), pp. 255–256.
Robert Ellis Dudgeon, in: *Med. Cent.* 12 (1904), p. 352.
Daniel van Duyse, in*: Brit. J. Ophthalmol.* 1925 Jan; 9/1, p. 42.
Marcus Feingold, in: *Transact. Ophthalmol. Soc.* 24 (1926), p. 28–31 (Edward Jackson).
Marcus Feingold, in: *Am. J. Ophthalmol.* 9/6 (1926), pp. 467–469.
Eric A. Fennel, in: *Am. J. Clin. Pathol.* 30/3 (1966), pp. 257–258 (I. L. Tilden).
Emil de Grosz, in: *Brit. J. Ophthalmol.* 1942 Jun; 26(6), pp. 286–287.
Robert Marcus Gunn, in: *The Lancet*, Dec. 11, 1909, pp. 1786–1787.
Robert Marcus Gunn, in: *Brit. Med. J.* 2 (1909), pp.1719–1721.
Robert Marcus Gunn, in: *Am. J. Ophthalmol.* 27 (1910), p. 49.
Ludwig Halberstätter, in: *Brit. J. Radiol.* 22 (1949), pp. 347.
Ludwig Halberstätter, in: *Brit. Med. J. I* (1949), p. 871.
Ludwig Halberstätter, in: *Lancet I* (1949), p. 845.
Harvey J. Howard, in: *Am. Med. Assoc. J.* 163 (1957), p. 138.
Lucien Howe, in: *Am. J. Ophthalmol.* 12/2 (1929), pp. 145–147.
Josef Igersheimer, in: *Trans. Am. Ophthalmol. Soc.* 64 (1966), p. 7–8. (Albert E. Sloane).
Edward Jackson, in: *Arch. Ophthalmol.* 29 (1942), pp. 137–140 (Arnold Knapp).
Edward Jackson, in: *Brit. J. Ophthalmol.* (27) 1943, pp. 190–191.
Alexander Jokl, in: *Brit. J. Ophthal.* 49 (1965), p. 385.
Alexander Jokl, in: *S. A. Tydskrif vir Geneeskunde*, 8 Mei 1965, p. 381.
Carl Koller, in: Arch. Ophthalmol. 31 (1944), p. 344f. (pp. Bloom)
Samuel Thomas Knaggs, in: *Med. J. of Australia*, 16 Apr. 1921, p. 320–321.
Arnold Herman Knapp, in: *Arch. Ophthalmol.* 55/4 (1956), pp. 451–454 (John H. Dunnington).
Arnold Herman Knapp, in: *Brit. J. Ophthalmol.* 40/5 (1956), p. 320.
Peter C. Kronfeld, in: Transact. *Am. Ophthalmol. Soc.* 78 (1980), pp. 11–12. (William F. Hughes).
Gaetano Lodato, in: *Am. J. Ophthalmol.* 20 (1937), p. 205 (Melchiore Lombardo).
R. C. Lynch, in: *Tri-state Med. J.* 3–4 (1939), p. 636.
Otto Marburg, in: *JAMA* 138 (1948), p. 375.
Otto Marburg, in: J. *Neuropathol. Exp. Neurol.* 8 (1949), pp. 247ff.
Philip Henry Mules, in: *Brit. Med. J.* Sept. 9, (1905), p. 610.
Charles H. May, in: *Arch. Ophthalmol.* 31/1 (1944), pp. 103–105 (Charles A. Perera).
Charles H. May, in: *Brit. J. Ophthalmol.* 28 (1944), pp. 313–314. (K. Herbert).
Dr. Charles H. May, in *Transact. Am. Ophthalmol. Soc.* 42 (1944), pp. 18.2–22 (William Brown Doherty).

Henry Minsky, in: *Arch. Ophthalmol.* 53 (1955), pp. 456–457 (F. H. Theodore, J. Laval).
Henry Minsky, in: *New York Med.* 10 (1954), p. 573.
Henry Minsky, in: *New York State J. Med.* 54/2 (1954), p. 2105.
James Boyd Neal, in: *Nat. Med. J. of China* 11 (1925), p. 147.
James Boyd Neal, in: *The Chinese Recorder* 56 (1925), pp. 255–256.
Stanilslaus v. Provazek, in: *J. Parasitol.* 2 (1915), pp. 51–53.
G. Oram Ring, in: Transact. *Am. Ophthalmol.* Soc. 31 (1933), pp. 14.2–17 (Charles E. G. Shannon).
G. Oram Ring, in: *Am. J. Ophthalmol.* 16/4 (1933), p. 356.
Ludwig von Sallmann, in: *Trans. Am. Ophthalmol. Soc.* 74 (1976), pp. 8–11 (Peter C. Kronfeld).
Ludwig von Sallmann, in: *Arch. Ophthalmol.* 94/4 (1976), p. 685 (G. Richard O'Connor).
Maximilian Salzmann, in: *Arch. Ophthalmol.* 52 (1954), pp. 808–809 (A. B. Reese).
George E. de Schweinitz, in: *Transact. Am. Ophthalmol. Soc.* 37 (1939), pp. 14.2–21 (John D. Carpenter).
George E. Shambaugh, in: *Ann. Otol. Rhinol. Laryngol.* 57 (1948), pp. 80–82 (E. W. Hagens).
George E. Shambaugh, in: *Arch. Otolarygol.* 47/4 (1948), pp. 526–527.
Priestley Smith, in: *Brit. J. Ophthalmol.* Yr. 1933, pp. 442–444 (Wilfrid Allport).
Auguste Swaen, in: *JAMA* 92/25 (1929), pp. 2118–2119.
Prof. E. Van Beneden, in: *Nature* 83 (1910), p. 344.
Casey Albert Wood, in: *Arch. Ophthalmol.* 27/4 (1942), pp. 779–781 (Frank Brawley).
Casey Albert Wood, in: *Brit. J. Ophthalmol.* 26/6 (1942), pp. 287.

Louis OBROWSKY, *Historische Betrachtung der sozialmedizinischen Einrichtungen in Wien vom Beginn des 20. Jahrhunderts bis zum Ende der Ersten Republik.* [= *Beiträge zur neueren Geschichte Österreichs* Vol 21]. Peter Lang, Frankfurt am Main/Vienna et al. 2005.
Öffentliche Vorlesungen an der k. k.Universität zu Wien im Winter-Semester 1868/9. K. K. Hof- und Staatsdruckerei, Vienna 1868.
Öffentliche Vorlesungen an der K. K. Universität zu *Wien im Winter-Semester 1869/70.* K. K. Hof- und Staatsdruckerei, Vienna 1869.
Öffentliche Vorlesungen an der K. K. Leopold-*Franzens-Universität zu Innsbruck im Winter-Semester 1873/74.* Wagner'sche Universitäts-Buchdruckerei, Innsbruck 1873.
Öffentliche Vorlesungen an der K. K. Universität zu *Wien im Sommer-Semester 1881.* Kaiserlich-Königliche Hof- und Staatsdruckerei, Vienna 1881.
Öffentliche Vorlesungen an der K. K. Universität zu *Wien im Winter-Semester 1881/82.* Kaiserlich-Königliche Hof- und Staatsdruckerei, Vienna 1881.
Öffentliche Vorlesungen an der k. k.Universität zu *Wien im Wintersemester 1885/86.* Kaiserlich-Königliche Hof- und Staatsdruckerei, Vienna 1885.
Öffentliche Vorlesungen an der K. K. Universität zu *Wien im Sommersemester 1886.* Kaiserlich-Königliche Hof- und Staatsdruckerei, Vienna 1886.
Öffentliche Vorlesungen an der k. k.Universität zu *Wien im Wintersemester 1886/87.* Kaiserlich-Königliche Hof- und Staatsdruckerei, Vienna 1886.
Öffentliche Vorlesungen an der K. K. Universität zu *Wien im Winter-Semester 1887/78.* Kaiserlich-Königliche Hof- und Staatsdruckerei, Vienna 1887.
Öffentliche Vorlesungen an der K. K. Universität zu *Wien im Sommer-Semester 1891.* Kaiserlich-Königliche Hof- und Staatsdruckerei, Vienna 1891.
Öffentliche Vorlesungen an der K. K. Universität zu *Wien im Sommer-Semester 1893.* Adolf Holzhausen, Vienna 1893.

Öffentliche Vorlesungen an der K. K. Universität zu *Wien im Sommer-Semester 1897.* Adolf Holzhausen, Vienna 1897.

Chuta OGUCHI, "Augenverletzungen im japanischen Heere während des letzten Krieges", in: *Beiträge z. Augenheilkd.* 83 (1913), pp. 75–303.

Chuta OGUCHI, Kyozo MAJIMA, *Cytologische Untersuchungen über das Augensekret*, in: *Graefes Archiv* 108/1–2 (1922), pp. 86–100.

Chuta OGUCHI, Kyozo MAJIMA, "Neue Ergebnisse der Trachomzellenforschung mit Bezug auf vitale Färbung und Oxydasereaktion", in: *Graefes Archiv* 108/3–4 (1922), pp. 359–362.

Walter ÖHLINGER (ed.), *Rundpanorama von Wien. Ansicht der k. k.Haupt- und Residenzstadt Wien vor Beginn der Stadterweiterung und Demolierung der Basteien im Jahre 1858 von C. Zacijek.* Edition Winkler-Hermaden, Schleinbach 2010.

Walter ÖHLINGER (ed.), *Die Pläne der k. k.Haupt- und Residenzstadt Vienna von Carl Graf Vasquez.* Edition Winkler-Hermaden, Schleinbach 2011.

Johann Nepomuk OELLER, *Atlas der Ophthalmoskopie. Atlas of Ophthalmoscopy.* Translated into English by A. H. Knapp. J. R. Bergmann, Wiesbaden 1896–1899.

Johann Nepomuk OELLER, *Atlas seltener ophthalmoskopischer Befunde. Zugleich Ergänzungstafeln zu dem Atlas der Ophthalmoskopie. Atlas of Rare Ophthalmoscopic Conditions and Supplementary Plates to the Atlas of Ophthalmoscopy.* The Text translated into English by Thos. Snowball. J. F. Bergmann, Wiesbaden 1900/12.

Österreichische Krebshilfe (ed.), *100 Jahre Österreichische Krebshilfe 1910–2010.* Verlagshaus der Ärzte, Vienna 2010.

Österreichisches Biographisches Lexikon 1815–1950 [= ÖBL]. Herausgegeben von der Österreichischen Akademie der Wissenschaften (Leo SANTIFALLER/Eva OBERMAYER-MARNACH). Hermann Böhlaus Nachfolger, Graz/Cologne 1957ff.

"Ophthamological Numismatics", in: *Arch Ophthalmol.* 120/2 (2002), p. 246.

Max OPPEL (ed.), *100 Jahre Augenklinik Herzog Carl Theodor. Festschrift zum 100-jährigen Bestehen der Augenklinik Herzog Carl Theodor in Munich 1995.* Stiftung Augenklinik Herzog Carl Theodor, Munich 1995.

Reinhard OTTO, "Über das Vorkommen Fuchs›scher peripherer Atrophie des Sehnerven", in: *Untersuchungen über Sehnervenveränderungen bei Arteriosclerose.* Springer, Berlin 1893, pp. 123–128.

Ouverture solennelle des cours, 17 octobre 1881. Des cours et rapport de M. le recteur Trasenster. Liège 1881.

Maria PACOLT, *Sagen aus Alt-Wien.* Alexa & Co, Vienna 1946.

Julius PAGEL (ed.), *Biographisches Lexikon hervorragender Ärzte des neunzehnten Jahrhunderts. Mit einer historischen Einleitung.* Urban&Schwarzenberg, Berlin/Vienna 1901 (Reprint Karger, Leipzig 1989).

Stephen PAGET, "The Distribution of Secondary Growths in Cancer of the Breast", in: *The Lancet* 67/1 (1889), pp. 571–573.

James N. PARKER, Philip M. PARKER (eds.), *The Official Patient's Sourcebook on FUCHS'S DYSTROPHY. A Reference Manual for Self-Directed Patient Research.* ICON Group International, Inc., San Diego 2002.

Viktor PATZELT, "Carl Wedl, der erste Vorstand einer deutschsprachigen Lehrkanzel für Histologie", in: *Anat. Anz.* 100 (1953/54), pp. 147–156.

Viktor PATZELT, "Zum 100jährigen Bestand der Wiener Lehrkanzel für Histologie", in: *Wien. klin. Wochenschr.* 66 (1954), pp. 775–779.

Au Pays de Liége. Mathieu Thone. Liège, n.d.

Walter PERKO, "Der akademische Bildhauer Josef Müllner (1879–1968)". *Katalogblätter des Rollettmuseums Baden.* Vol. 16. 2nd ed. 2004.

Personalstand und Ordnung der öffentlichen Vorlesungen an der K. K. Leopold-Franzens-Universität zu Innsbruck im Sommer-Semester 1873.

Personalstand und Ordnung der öffentlichen Vorlesungen an der K. K. Leopold-Franzens-Universität zu Innsbruck im Sommer-Semester 1874. Wagner'sche Universitäts-Buchdruckerei, Innsbruck 1874.

Albert PETERS, "Über traumatische Hornhauterkrankungen (Erosionen, Keratitis disciformis und Ulcus serpens) und ihre Beziehungen zum Herpes corneae", in: *Graefes Archiv* 57 (1904), pp. 93–137.

Albert PETERS, "Zur Frage der Keratititis disciformis", in: Klin. Monatsbl. Augenheilk. 43/II (1905), pp. 535ff.

Albert PETERS, "Zur Kenntnis des Kapselstares", in: Graefes Archiv 105 (1921), pp. 154–158.

E. PFLÜGER, "Moskau. Internationaler medicinischer Congress", in: *Klin. Monatsbl. Augenheilk.* 35 (1897), pp. 391–397.

F. PHINIZY CALHOUN, "A Classification of Corneal Affections", in: *Am. J. Ophthalmol.* 3/5 (1922), pp. 8–13.

Albert v. PFLUGK, "Über Brillenmünzen und Medaillen", in: *Graefes Archiv* 105 (1921), pp. 688–707.

H. T. PI, "A Brief Historical Sketch of Native Ophthalmology in China". In: *Nat. Med. J. of China* 15 (1929), pp. 604–613.

Arnold PILLAT, "Zur Topographie der saprophytären Bindehautkeime des menschlichen Auges", in: *Graefes Archiv* 105 (1921), pp. 778–793.

Arnold PILLAT, "Report of the Ophthalmological Service", in: *Twenty-Fourth Annual Report of the Medical Superintendent June 30, 1932.* Peiping Union Medical College Hospital. Formerly the Peking Union Medical College Hospital. P. U. M. C. Press 1932, pp. 45–47.

Arnold PILLAT, "Der Beitrag der Wiener Schule zur Augenheilkunde", in: *Wien. klin. Wochenschr.* 63 (1951), pp. 614–617. (Address delivered to the Commemorative Meeting of the Gesellschaft der Aerzte Wien, on Ernst Fuchs's 100th birthday on 22 June 1951).

Arnold PILLAT, "Histologische Befunde am Auge bei konnataler Toxoplasmose", in: *Wien. klin. Wochenschr.* 63 (1951), pp. 628–630.

Arnold PILLAT, "The Contribution of the Vienna School to Ophthalmology", in: *Am. J. Ophthalmol.* 36 (1953), pp. 15–25.

Arnold PILLAT, "Zur Geschichte der beiden Lehrkanzeln für Augenheilkunde in Wien", in: Beiträge *zur Geschichte der Ophthalmologie/Contributions to the History of Ophthalmology/Contributions à l›Histoire de l›Ophtalmologie = Suppl. ad. Ophthalmologica* 134 (1957), pp. 76–84.

Arnold PILLAT, "Lebenslauf von Professor für Augenheilkunde Dr. Arnold Pillat. Meinen Freunden und Schülern gewidmet". Eigenverlag, Vienna 1971.

Adriano PIRIS, Manfred MIHM," Mechanisms of Metastasis: Seed and Soil. Cancer Metastasis and the Lymphovascular System: Basis of Rational Therapy", in: Stanley P. L. LEONG (eds.), *Cancer Treatment and Research.* Springer, New York 2007.

Plan de la Ville de Liége. Guide-Notice. J. Claesen, Bruxelles, n.d.

Joseph Jakob PLENCK, *Doctrina de morbis oculorum.* Rud. Graeffer. Viennæ 1777.

(Joseph Jacob PLENCK), *Verhandeling over de Ookziekten door den Heer Joseph Jakob Plenck door Martinus Pruys.* Rotterdam, Pols & Knap 1787.

(Joseph Jakob PLENCK), *Ganka Shinso (New Work on Ophthalmology).* Edo/Osaka/Kyoto 1815.

Ferdinand PLENK, "Bericht über die k. k.Augenklinik der Univ. zu Innsbruck für das Studienjahr 1871/72", in: *Berichte d. naturwissenschaftl.-med. Vereins in Innsbruck*, 3 (1873), pp. 223–230.

Margarete POCH-KALOUS, *Cajetan. Das Leben des Wiener Mediziners und Karikaturisten Dr. Anton Elfinger.* Wiener Bibliophilen-Gesellschaft, Vienna 1966.

Leo POLLNOW, "Beiträge zur Retinitis circinata und zur Lochbildung in der Makula", in: *Zeitschr. Augenheilk.* 70 (1930), pp. 257–264.

Konstantin POLLOK, *Kants* Metaphysische Anfangsgründe der Naturwissenschaft. *Ein kritischer Kommentar.* (= *Kant-Forschungen* 13). Meiner, Hamburg 2001.

Ludwig POPPER, "Jakob Pal 1863–1936. Zur hundertsten Wiederkehr seines Geburtstages", in: *Wien. klin. Wochenschr.* 75 (1963), pp. 606–608.

George POSTE, Linda PARUCH, "Stephen Paget, M. D., F. R. C. S. (1855–1926). A retrospective", in: *Cancer and Metastasis Reviews* 8 (1989), pp. 1–97.

Benjamin POWELL (ed.), Who's who in China [...] *containing the pictures and biographies of China's best known political, financial, business and professional men* [...] The China Weekly Review 1926.

Karl PORTELE, "Dr. med. Anton Elfinger, ein vergessener medizinischer Modelleur", in: *Ann. Naturhistor. Mus. Wien* 78 (1974), pp. 95–102.

E. PRAUN, "Ueber die Verwendbarkeit des von Professor Fuchs für die Nachbehandlung von Staroperierten angegebenen Drahtgitters", in: *Centralbl. prakt. Augenheilk.* 52 (1897), pp. 65ff.

Georg PREYSS, "Rede zum Andenken Georg Josef Beer's, gehalten bei Gelegenheit der siebenten Jahresfeier der wissenschaftlichen Thätigkeit des Doctoren-Collegiums der Wiener medicinischen Facultät am 18. April 1857". Ditmarsch, Vienna 1857.

Georg PREYSS, "Das Leben und Wirken des k. k.Raths, Stabsfeldarzts und Professors der Augenheilkunde am Josefinum Dr. Friedrich Jaeger Ritter von Jaxtthal". Memorial Address [...], Gesellschafts-Buchdruckerei Vienna 1877.

Proceedings of the 1929 Annual Conference St. Louis, Missouri November 11–13, 1929. National Society for the Prevention of Blindness. Publication 65 (Self published).

Marie PROCKSCH, "Über doppelseitige Keratitis und Iridozyklitis bei Erythema multiforme exsudativum", in: *Wien. med. Wochenschr.* 71 (1921), cols. 1076–1078.

Programm (Foundation of the Wien. klin. Wochenschr.), in: *Wien. klin.Wochenschr.* Yr. 1, No. 1 of 5 April 1888, first page without pagination.

Ludwig Bertrand PSENNER, "Über röntgenologische Veränderungen bei Arachnitis opticochiasmatis", in: *Wien. klin. Wochenschr.* 63 (1951), pp. 679–680.

Adolf PURTSCHER, "Beitrag zur Behandlung der Irisvorfälle", in: *Wien. med. Wochenschr.* 71 (1921), cols. 1078–1080.

Adolf PURTSCHER, "Scheinbare Spiegelung der Iris und Pupille in der Hornhaut, ein bisher unbekanntes Phänomen", in: *Graefes Archiv* 105 (1921), pp. 1084–1090.

Ernst PURTSCHER, "Zur Aetiologie der 'spontanen' Aderhautabhebung und der 'serösen Tenonitis'", in: *Zeitschr. Augenheilk.* 94 (1938), pp. 141–151.

Otmar PURTSCHER, "Angiopathia retinae traumatica, Lymphorrhagien des Augengrundes", in: *Graefes Archiv* 82 (1912), pp. 347–37.

Otmar PURTSCHER, "Angeborene Mißbildung bei einem Brüderpaar", in: *Graefes Archiv* 105 (1921), pp. 39–47.

Otmar PURTSCHER, *Erinnerungen aus meinem Berufsleben.* Artur Kollitsch, Klagenfurt 1926.

Theodor PUSCHMANN, *Die Medicin in Wien während der letzten 100 Jahre.* Moritz Perles, Vienna 1884.

Rosa PUTJATA-KERSCHBAUMER, *Das Sarkom des Auges*. J. F. Bergmann, Wiesbaden 1890.
Walter L. PYLE (ed.), *An International System of Ophthalmic Practice*. P. Blakiston's Son & Co., Philadelphia 1914.
Carlos QUIRINO, *Who's Who in Philippine History*. Tahanan Books, Manila 1995.
Carl RABL, *Édouard van Beneden und der gegenwärtige Stand der wichtigsten von ihm behandelten Probleme*. F. Cohen, Bonn 1915.
Andreas RADOS, "Über die Veränderungen im Frühstadium der Retinitis exsudativa externa", in: *Graefes Archiv* 105 (1921), pp. 973–996.
A. RASTEIRO, "L'impact de l'ophtalmologie européenne sur le Japon au XVIeme siècle", in: Julius Hirschberg Gesellschaft (Deutschsprachige Vereinigung für Geschichte der Augenheilkunde) Société francophone d'histoire de l'ophtalmologie, *33 Beiträge zur Geschichte der Augenheilkunde – Contributions à l'histoire de l'ophtalmologie*. Facultas, Vienna 1991, pp. 114–117.
Maurice-P. RAVAULT, *Syndromes en Ophtalmologie (Guide-Dictionnaire)*. Doin-Deren, Paris 1970.
G. RAVIN, "In the Kingdom of the Shah: Treacher Collins' Persian adventure", in: *Surv. Ophthalmol.* 43 (1999), pp. 361–367.
Tracy RAVIN, "José Rizal. Philippine National Hero and Ophthalmologist", in: *Arch. Ophthalmol.* 119/2 (2001), pp. 180–184.
Ronnie R. RAY, Richard D. BINKHORST, "The Diagnosis of Pupillary Bloc by Intravenous Injection of Fluorescein", in: *Am. J. Ophthalmol.* 61/3 (1966), pp. 481–483.
L. RAZZAQ et al., "Fuchs's adenoma of the choroid simulating a choroidal hemangioma", in: *Case Rep. in Ophthalmol.* 3/1 (2012), pp. 83–86.
Reallexikon der Medizin und ihrer Grenzgebiete. 6 vols. Urban & Schwarzenberg, Munich/Berlin/Vienna 1966–1977.
(Red.), "Errichtung einer stehenden Klinik für Augenkranke", in: *Med. Jahrb.* II (1814), pp. 8–11.
(Red.), "Errichtung ordentlicher öffentlicher Lehrkanzeln und Kliniken für die Augenheilkunde an den Universitäten zu Wien und Prag", in: Med. Jahrb. V/I (1818), pp. 7–8.
(Red.), "Regulirung des Studiums der Augenheilkunde", in: Eduard Vincenz GULDENER Edl. v. LOBES, *Sammlungen der Sanitäts-Verordnungen für das Erzherzogthum Oesterreich unter der Enns, als Fortsetzung der v. Ferro'schen Sammlung. Fünfter Theil, enthaltend die Verordnungen vom Jahre 1818 bis Ende des Jahres 1824*. Gerold, Vienna 1825, pp. 46–47.
(Red.), "Errichtung einer ordentlichen öffentlichen Lehrkanzel und Klinik für die Augenheilkunde", in: Johann Nepomuk Frh. v. HEMPEL-KÜRSINGER, *Handbuch der Gesetzeskunde im Sanitäts-und Medicinal-Gebiethe in alphabetisch-chronologisch und materienweiser Zusammenstellung für Sanitäts- und Polizeybeamte im Allgemeinen und insbesondere für Aerzte, Wundärzte, Geburtshelfer, Hebammen und Apotheker.* Vol. 1: A–I, Vienna 1830, pp. 114–117.
(Red.), "Zur Besetzungsfrage der Augenklinik", in: *Wien. med. Wochenschr.* 34 (1884), col. 1477.
(Red.), "Zur Besetzung der ophthalmologischen Klinik an der Wiener Universität", in: *Wien. med. Presse* 26 (1885), p. 1011.
(Red.), "Zur Besetzung der ophthalmologischen Klinik in Wien", in: *Wien. med. Presse* 26 (1885), p. 1041.
(Red.), "Zur Besetzung der II. Klinik für Augenheilkunde in Wien". in: *Allg. Wien. med. Zeitg.* 30 (1885), p. 367.

(Red.), "Die Ursachen und die Verhinderung der Blindheit. Gekrönte Preisschrift von Dr. Ernst Fuchs, Professor der Augenheilkunde an der Universität Lüttich. Herausgegeben durch die Society for the prevention of blindness in London". (Wiesbaden 1885, J. Bergmann, 8°. pp. VI and 243. Mit einer Steindrucktafel.), in: *Wien. med. Presse* 26 (1885), cols. 1031–1033.

(Red.), "Feier des 70. Geburtstages Ernst Fuchs's am 14. Juni 1921", in: *Zeitschr. Augenheilk.* 47 (1921), pp. 47–63.

(Red.), "Die Wiener Augenheilkunde aus einer klinischen Vorlesung", in: *Neues Wiener Journal*, 8 Aug. 1921, pp. 2–3.

(Red.), "Der berühmte Augenarzt Hofrat Fuchs gestorben", in: *Neue Freie Presse* No. 23776 (Evening paper), 22 November 1930, p. 3.

(Red.), "Die letzten Säulen", in: *Neues Wiener Tagblatt* No. 23261, 23 November 1930.

(Red.), "Trauersitzung zum Andenken an weil. Prof. Dr. Ernst Fuchs v. 28. November 1930 in der Gesellschaft der Ärzte in Wien: Offizielles Protokoll der Gesellschaft der Aerzte in Wien", in: *Wien. klin. Wochenschr.* (1930), pp. 1517–1520.

Reden, gehalten bei der feierlichen Inauguration des für das Studienjahr 1869/70 gewählten Rectors des k. k.polytechnischen Institutes, Dr. Adalbert Fuchs am 12. October 1869. Vienna 1870.

H. REINER, *Verzeichnis über Ophthalmologische Instrumente und Apparate usw.* Selbstverlag, Vienna 1909.

W. REIS, **"**Über Ophthalmomalacie", in: *Graefes Archiv* 105 (1921), pp. 617–639.

Hans REMKY, "Albrecht von Graefe – Facets of His Work", in: *Graefes Arch. Clin. Exper. Ophthalmol.* 233 (1995), pp. 537–548.

R. RENDU, "Sur un syndrome caractérisé par l'inflammation simultanée de toutes les muqueuses externes (conjunctivale, nasale, linguale, buccopharyngée, orale et balanopréputiale) coexistant avec une éruption varicelliforme puis purpurique des quatre membres", in: *Rev. Gen. Clin. Ther.* 30 (1916), pp. 351–358.

August v. REUSS, "Ophthalmologische Mittheilungen. Aus der zweiten Universitäts-Augenklinik in Wien. I. Abtheilung", in: *Wien. med. Presse* 26 (1885), p. 2.

August R. v. REUSS, **"**Keratitis maculosa", in: *Wien. klin. Wochenschr.* 2 (1889), pp. 665–666.

August REUSS, "Lehrbuch der Augenheilkunde. Von Dr. Ernst Fuchs, o. ö. Professor der Augenheilkunde an der Universität Wien. [...] Leipzig und Wien, Franz Deuticke, 1889", in: Wien. klin. Wochenschr. 3 (1890), pp. 256–257.

August REUSS, "Lehrbuch der Augenheilkunde. Von Dr. Ernst Fuchs, [...] Zweite vermehrte Auflage [...]. Leipzig und Wien, Franz Deuticke, 1891", in: *Wien. klin. Wochenschr.* 4 (1891), pp. 425.

Domenico RIBATTI, G. MANGIALARDI, A. VACCA, "Stephen Paget and the 'seed and soil' theory of metastatic dissemination", in: Clin. Exp. Med. 6 (2006), pp. 145–149.

H. RIEGER, "Toxoplasmose", in: *Wien. klin. Wochenschr.* 63 (1951), pp. 680–683.

Shirley ROBERTS, *Sir James Paget – the Rise of Clinical Surgery.* Royal Society of Medicine Services Ltd., London 1989.

Victor ROBINSON, *The Life of Jacob Henle.* Medical Life Company, New York 1921.

G. F. ROCHAT, "Sympathische Ophthalmie ohne Iridocyclitis auf dem verletzten Auge", in: *Graefes Archiv* 105 (1921), pp. 614–616.

Jens Martin ROHRBACH, "Ophthalmopathology between yesterday and tomorrow", in: *Klin. Monatsbl. Augenheilk.* 221/2 (2004), pp. 87–91.

Fiona ROMAN, "The short history of heat cauterisation of the cornea", in: Brit. J. Ophthalmol. 79 (1995), p. 236.

Henning RÖNNE, "Pseudoglaukomatöse Exkavation der Papille", in: *Graefes Archiv* 105 (1921), pp. 465–468.

Henning RÖNNE, "Über Stauungspapille mit doppelseitiger plötzlicher Erblindung und deren eventuellen Behandlung mit Palliativtrepanation", in: *Graefes Archiv* 105 (1921), pp. 605–613.

Gill ROPER-HALL, "Historical Vignette: Robert Marcus Gunn (1850–1909): Scottish Ophthalmologist, Skilled Observer, and Gifted Teacher", in: *Am. Orthoptic J.* 65/1 (2015), pp. 121–127.

Anton ROSAS, *Handbuch der theoretischen und practischen Augenheilkunde.* 3 vols. J. B. Wallishausser, Vienna 1830.

Anton ROSAS, *Lehre von den Augenkrankheiten. Zum Gebrauche für practische Aerzte und Wundärzte, wie auch zur Benutzung als Leitfaden beim klinischen Unterrichte abgefasst.* Wien, J. B. Wallishausser, Vienna 1834.

L. ROSENZWEIG, "Zwei Fälle von Keratitis punctata nach Influenza", in: *Centralbl. prakt. Augenheilk.* May 1890.

Fritz RÖSSLER, "Der blinde Fleck in schielenden Augen", in: *Graefes Archiv* 105 (1921), pp. 48–103.

Sarah ROTHBÜHR, Thorsten ZUBERBIER, "Edward Nettleship (1845–1913)", in: Christoph LÖSER, Gerd PLEWIG (eds.), *Pantheon der Dermatologie.* Springer, Heidelberg 2008, pp. 738–741.

Karl Eduard ROTHSCHUH, "Hyrtl contra Brücke. Ein Gelehrtenstreit im 19. Jahrhundert und seine Hintergründe", in: Erna LESKY (ed.), Wien und die Weltmedizin. 4. Symposium der Internationalen Akademie für Geschichte der Medizin veranstaltet im Institut für Geschichte der Medizin der Universität Vienna 17.–19. September 1973. Hermann Böhlaus Nachfolger. Vienna/Cologne/Graz 1974, pp. 159–169.

H. ROTTER, "Ueber die Verbesserung des Sehvermögens aphaker Augen ohne Starglas durch Mintacol", in: *Wien. klin. Wochenschr.* 63 (1951), pp. 683–684.

Helmut RUMPLER, "Eine Chance für Mitteleuropa. Bürgerliche Emanzipation und Staatsverfall in der Habsburgermonarchie", in: Herwig WOLFRAM (ed.), *Österreichische Geschichte 1804–1914.* Ueberreuter, Vienna 1997, pp. 419–422.

Helmut RUMPLER, Helmut DENK (eds.), *Carl Freiherr von Rokitansky 1804–1878. Pathologe, Politiker, Philosoph, Gründer der Wiener Medizinischen Schule des 19. Jahrhunderts.* Wien, Böhlau 2005.

Paul E. RUNGE, "Eduard Jaeger's Test-Types (Schrift-Scalen) and the Historical Development of Vision Tests", in: *Trans. Am. Ophthalmol. Soc.* 98 (2000), pp. 375–438.

Karl SABLIK, "Hering, Vintschgau und das Problem der Nachfolge Purkinjes", in: *Sudhoffs Archiv* 73 (1989), pp. 78–87.

Karl SABLIK, *Julius Tandler. Mediziner und Sozialreformer.* 2nd ed., Peter Lang, Frankfurt a. Main et al. 2010.

Moriz SACHS, "Über die transpalpebrale Eröffnung der vorderen Kammer", in: *Graefes Archiv* 105 (1921), pp. 376–383.

Moriz SACHS, "Bild und Wirklichkeit", in: *Wien. med. Wochenschr.* 71 (1921), cols. 1079–1081.

Johan SÆBØ, "Atrophia gyrata choroideae et retinae", in: *Brit. J. Ophthalmol.* 1948, pp. 824–847.

Ludwig von SALLMANN et al., "Ueber den Einfluß von Cortison auf Wundheilung, Makrophagozytose und Kapillarpermeabilität im Auge", in: *Wien. klin. Wochenschr.* 63 (1951), pp. 684–686.

Fritz SALZER, "Beiträge zur Keratoplastik IV. (Schlußbetrachtungen)", in: *Graefes Archiv* 105 (1921), pp. 469–490.
Maximilian SALZMANN, "Fall von Sarkom der Iris und des Ciliarkörpers", in: *Wien. klin. Wochenschr.* 6 (1893), pp. 166–167.
Maximilian SALZMANN, "Studien über das Myxosarkom des Sehnerven", in: *Graefes Archiv* 39/Abtheil. IV (1893), pp. 94–130.
Maximilian SALZMANN, *Anatomie und Histologie des menschlichen Augapfels im Normalzustande, seine Entwicklung und sein Altern.* Franz Deuticke, Leipzig and Vienna 1912.
Maximilian SALZMANN, "Die traumatische Cyclodialyse und ihre Diagnose am Lebenden", in: *Graefes Archiv* 105 (1921), pp. 551–566.
Maximilian SALZMANN, "Über Vererbung von Netzhautablösung", in: Wien. med. Wochenschr. 71 (1921), cols. 1082–1084.
Maximilian SALZMANN, "Ernst Fuchs †", in: *Zeitschr. Augenheilk.* 73 (1931), pp. 117–125.
Bernard SAMUELS, Adalbert FUCHS, *Clinical Pathology of the Eye. A Practical Treatise of Histopathology.* Paul B. Hoeber Inc. Medical Book Department of Harper & Brothers 1952.
A. H. SATTLER, "Hornhautfistel, herbeigeführt anscheinend durch Perforation einer zum Teil verkalkten Linse", in: Graefes Archiv 105 (1921), pp. 502–506.
Hubert SATTLER, "Behandlung der Keratitis", in: *Bericht d. Ophthalmol. Gesellsch. Heidelberg 1879*, pp. 140.
Hubert SATTLER, "Ferdinand von Arlt", in: *Klin. Monatsbl. Augenheilk.* 25 (1887), pp. 133–146.
Hubert SATTLER (ed.), "Albrecht von Graefe's grundlegende Arbeiten über den Heilwert der Iridektomie bei Glaukom", in: Karl Sudhoff (ed.), *Klassiker der Medizin.* Vol. 11. J. A. Barth, Leipzig 1911.
Hubert SATTLER, "Ein Beitrag zur Kenntnis der epibulbären Carcinome und ihrer Behandlung", in: *Graefes Archiv* 105 (1921), pp. 1207–1230.
Hubert SATTLER, "Über einen Fall von Neuritis nervi optici retrobulbaris als Frühsymptom der Basedowschen Krankheit", in: *Wien. med. Wochenschr.* 71 (1921), cols. 1084–1088.
W. SAUER, *Beitrag zur Casuistik der Irissarkome.* Med. Diss. Univ. Halle 1883.
Werner SAUER, *Österreichische Philosophie zwischen Aufklärung und Restauration. Beiträge zur Geschichte des Frühkantianismus in der Donaumonarchie* [= Richard HALLER (ed.), *Studien zur österreichischen Philosophie* vol. II]. Königshausen and Neumann, Würzburg 1982.
Anton SCHALLER, *Die Wertheim-Klinik. Eine Geschichte der II. Universitäts-Frauenklinik in Wien.* Maudrich, Vienna/Munich/Bern 1992.
Ferdinand SCHEMINZKY, Th. WENSE, *Die Geschichte des Physiologischen Institutes der Universität zu Innsbruck, in: Forschungen und Forscher der Tiroler Ärzteschule (1948–1950).* Vol II. Oberösterr. Landesverlag, Wels 1950.
Alfred SCHETT, "The Ophthalmoscope/Der Augenspiegel. Ein Beitrag zur Entwicklungsgeschichte bis zum Beginn des 20. Jahrhunderts/A Contribution to the History of its Development up to the Beginning of the 20th Century". Translated by Donald L. Blanchard, in: *Hirschberg History of Ophthalmology/Geschichte der Augenheilkunde. The Monographs/ Die Monographien.* Vol. 2/Bd. 2. Jean-Paul Wayenborgh, Oostende 1997.
F. SCHIECK, "Die Abhängigkeit des Verlaufs der tuberkulösen Prozesse am Auge von dem Stadium der Allergie des Gesamtorganismus", in: *Graefes Archiv* 105 (1921), pp. 257–270.
F. SCHIECK, A. BRÜCKNER (eds.), *Kurzes Handbuch der Ophthalmologie.* Vol. 5. Julius Springer, Berlin 1930.

J. SCHIEL, *System der deduktiven und induktiven Logik. Eine Darlegung der Principien wissenschaftlicher Forschung, insbesondere der Naturforschung von John Stuart Mill.* Friedrich Vieweg & Sohn. Braunschweig 1849.

J. SCHIEL, *Die Methode der inductiven Forschung als Methode der Naturforschung in gedrängter Darstellung hauptsächlich nach John Stuart Mill.* Friedrich Vieweg & Sohn, Braunschweig 1865.

Gregor SCHIEMANN, *Wahrheitsgewissheitsverlust. Hermann von Helmholtz' Mechanismus im Aufbruch der Moderne. Eine Studie zum Übergang von klassischer zu moderner Naturphilosophie.* Wissenschaftliche Buchgesellschaft 1997.

Gustav Adolph SCHIMMER, "Notizen über das Kärnthnerthor, die alte verschwundene Kärnthnervorstadt und die Vorstadt Wieden", in: *Das alte Wien. Darstellung der alten Plätze und merkwürdigsten jetzt größtenteils verschwundenen Gebäude Wiens.* Mit einem Vorwort zur Neuauflage von Isabella Wasner-Peter. Reprint der Hefte 1–12 nach den Originalausgaben der Jahre 1854–1856 aus dem Bestand der Wienbibliothek im Rathaus. Ed. Winkler-Hermaden, Schleinbach 2009.

Otto SCHIRMER, "Sympathische Augenentzündung". In: Theodor SAEMISCH (ed.), *Graefe-Saemisch Handbuch der gesammten Augenheilkunde.* 2nd ed., Part 2, vol. 6, VIII. Wilhelm Engelmann, Leipzig 1900.

Otto SCHIRMER, "Keratitis disciformis und Keratitis postvaccinolosa", in: Graefes Archiv 59 (1904), pp. 133ff.

Georgi SCHISCHKOFF (ed.), *Philosophisches Wörterbuch.* Founded by Heinrich Schmidt. 22. ed. Alfred Kröner, Stuttgart 1991 (= Kröners Taschenausgabe Vol. 13).

Wilhelm SCHLESINGER, "Erinnerung an Friedrich Jaeger", in: Wien. med. Wochenschr. 22 (1872), cols. 15–17.

K.-H. SCHMAUTZ, "Status dysraphicus und Heterochromiezyklitis", in: *Dt. Gesundh.-Wesen* 25 (1970), pp. 991–993.

A. SCHMIDL, *Wien wie es ist. Ein Gemälde der Kaiserstadt und ihrer nächsten Umgebungen in Beziehung auf Topographie, Statistik und geselliges Leben, mit besonderer Berücksichtigung wissenschaftlicher Anstalten und Sammlungen nach authentischen Quellen vorgestellt.* Carl Gerold, Wien, 1833.

Gabriela SCHMIDT, "Zur Entwicklung der Fächer Klinische Chemie und Laboratoriumsdiagnostik in der Wiener Schule", in: *Berichte zur Wissenschaftsgesch.* 14 (1991), pp. 231–239.

Gabriela SCHMIDT, "Eduard Albert and the Beginning of Human Nerve Grafting", in: *Acta chir. Austriaca* 25 (1993) 287–288.

Gabriela SCHMIDT, "Der Medizinhistoriker Max Neuburger und die Wiener medizinische Fakultät", in: *Wien. klin. Wochenschr.* 105 (1993), pp. 737–739.

Gabriela SCHMIDT, "Rokitansky als Pathophilosoph", in: *Sudhoffs Archiv* 89 (2005), pp. 170–195.

Gabriela SCHMIDT-WYKLICKY, "Ferdinand Karl Franz Ritter von Hebra (1816–1880)", in: Christoph LÖSER, Gerd PLEWIG (eds.), *Pantheon der Dermatologie.* Springer, Heidelberg 2008, pp. 417–432.

Gabriela SCHMIDT-WYKLICKY, Helmut GRÖGER, "Georg Josef Beer (1763–1821). Leben und Werk des Begründers der ältesten Universitäts-Augenklinik", in: *Spektrum Augenheilk.* 26 (2012), pp. 266–272.

Gabriela SCHMIDT-WYKLICKY, Helmut GRÖGER, "Die Gründung der weltweit ersten Universitäts-Augenklinik in Wien 1812 und ihre Erhebung zum Ordinariat 1818", in: *Spektrum Augenheilk.* 26 (2012), pp. 273–282.

Gabriela SCHMIDT-WYKLICKY, Helmut GRÖGER, "Anton von Rosas. Vorstand der Universitäts-Augenklinik in Wien 1821 bis 1855", in: *Spektrum Augenheilk.* 26/6 (2012), pp. 283–289.

Gabriela SCHMIDT-WYKLICKY, Helmut GRÖGER, "Ferdinand Ritter von Arlt. Vorstand der Universitäts-Augenklinik in Wien von 1856 bis 1883. Eine Würdigung zum 200. Geburtstag", in: *Spektrum Augenheilk.* 26 (2012), pp. 290–295.

Gabriela SCHMIDT-WYKLICKY, Helmut GRÖGER, "Die Gründung der II. Universitäts-Augenklinik in Wien 1883 und ihr erster Vorstand Eduard Jaeger von Jaxtthal 1883 bis 1884", in: Spektrum Augenheilk. 26 (2012), pp. 296–302.

Gabriela SCHMIDT-WYKLICKY, Helmut GRÖGER, **"**Carl Stellwag von Carion. Vorstand der I. UniversitätsAugenklink in Wien 1884 bis 1894", in: *Spektrum Augenheilk.* 26 (2012), pp. 303–308.

Gabriela SCHMIDT-WYKLICKY, Helmut GRÖGER, "Die Wiener Ophthalmologische Schule. Geist und Leistung der ersten 150 Jahre", in: *Spektrum Augenheilk.* 26 (2012), pp. 345–356.

Gabriela SCHMIDT-WYKLICKY, "Die Beziehungen des Graefe-Schülers Louis de Wecker (1832–1906) zur Wiener Ophthalmologischen Schule und zur österreichisch-ungarischen Monarchie", in: *Mitteilungen der Julius-Hirschberg-Gesellschaft zur Geschichte der Augenheilkunde* Vol. 14–2012 (2016), pp. 219–235.

Gabriela SCHMIDT-WYKLICKY, "Über die Ansätze zur Prävention und Pflege von Augenkrankheiten im Rahmen der Wiener Schule des 19. Jahrhunderts: Von der Volksaufklärung bis zur wissenschaftlichen Publizistik", in: *Mitteil. d. Julius-Hirschberg-Gesellsch. zur Geschichte d. Augenheilkunde* (forthcoming).

J. E. SCHMIDT, *Medical Discoveries Who and When. A dictionary of medical and related scientific discoveries in alphabetic order, giving in each case the name of the discoverer, his profession, nationality, and floruit, and the date of the discovery.* Charles Thomas, Springfield 1959.

Sigrid SCHMITZ, *Albert Neisser Leben und Werk auf Grund neuer, unveröffentlichter Quellen.* Triltsch Verlag, Düsseldorf 1968 (= *Düsseldorfer Arbeiten z. Geschichte d. Medizin* Vol. 29, at the same time Med. Diss., Univ. Düsseldorf 1967).

Georg SCHMORL, *Die pathologisch-histologischen Untersuchungsmethoden.* 16th rev. ed., ed. by P. Geipel, F. C. Vogel, Berlin 1934.

Isidor SCHNABEL, "Ueber Macularkolobom, physiologische Exkavation und angeborenen Conus", in: *Wien. med. Bl.* 7 (1884), cols. 161–166, 197–201, 229–232, and 259–261.

L. A. SCHNEIDER, "The Rockefeller Foundation, the China Foundation, and the development of modern science in China", in: *Soc. Sci. Med.* 16 (1982), pp. 1217–1231.

Maria SCHNEIDER, *Dr. med. Friedrich Jäger Ritter von Jaxtthal (1784–1871) – Augenarzt zu Wien und Leibarzt des Fürsten Metternich – Autobiographie mit Kommentar.* Diss. Techn. Univ. Munich 1988. [= *Medizin & Gesellschaft* Vol. 4]. Münster 1989.

Rudolf SCHNEIDER, "Zur Keratitis pustuliformis profunda", in: *Klin. Monatsbl. Augenheilk.* 69 (1922), pp. 238–241.

Rudolf SCHNEIDER, "Klinisches und Experimentelles zur Infektion mit Pyocyaneus und Bact. fluorescens liq. und zur Ringabszessbildung", in: *Klin. Monatsbl. Augenheilk.* 77/2 (1926), pp. 103–115.

Rudolf SCHNEIDER, "Zur Keratitis pustuliformis profunda", in: *Wien. klin. Wochenschr.* 64 (1952), p. 949.

Leopold SCHÖNBAUER, "Wenckebachs Verdienste um das Institut für Geschichte der Medizin", in: *Wien. klin. Wochenschr.* 67 (1955), No. 35/36.

Heinrich SCHOEPPE, "Das biologische Verhalten des Serums Altersstarkranker zum Linseneiweiß refraktometrisch untersucht in Anlehnung an die Mikro-Abderhalden-Reaktion", in: *Graefes Archiv* 105 (1921), pp. 251–256.

Joseph Ritter von SCHREIBERS, *Grundgesetze des Ackerbaues, nebst Bemerkungen über Gartenbau, Obstbaumzucht, Forst-Cultur und Holzpflanzung, von Sir John Sinclair, Gründer der königl. Gesellschaft des Ackerbaues in Großbritannien. Mit 9 Kupfern. Auf Veranlassung der k. k.Landwirthschafts-Gesellschaft in Wien aus dem Englischen übersetzt von Joseph Ritter v. Schreibers, Mitgliede der Gesellschaft.* Heubner, Vienna 1819.

Schriften des Vereins zur Verbreitung naturwissenschaftlicher Kenntnisse in Wien. Vol 1. Yr 1860/61. Carl Gerold's Sohn, Vienna 1862.

J. Michael SCHRÖDER, "Pathologie der Muskulatur", in: W. DOERR, G. SEIFERT, E. UEHLINGER, *Spezielle pathologische Anatomie.* Vol. 15. Springer-Verlag, Berlin/Heidelberg/New York 1982.

Gustav SCHUBERT, "Die Leistungen der Augenmuskeln und ihre Steuerung", in: *Wien. klin. Wochenschr.* 63 (1951), pp. 632–634.

Carl Heinrich SCHULTZ, *Natürliches System des Pflanzenreichs nach seiner inneren Organisation, nebst einer vergleichenden Darstellung der wichtigsten aller früheren künstlichen und natürlichen Pflanzensysteme.* August Hirschwald, Berlin 1832.

Paul SCHULZ, "Marginalien über die Wiener Revolution vom Jahre 1848 und ihre wichtigsten Folgen in der spätesten Zeit". W. Gerhard, Leipzig 1856, pp. 246; *Tageblatt der 32. Versammlung deutscher Naturforscher und Aerzte in Wien 1856.*

Theodor SCHWANN, "Ueber das Wesen des Verdauungsprocesses", in: *Arch. Anat. Physiol. wiss. Med.* Yr. 1836, pp. 90–138.

Theodor SCHWANN, "Vorläufige Mittheilung betreffend Versuche über die Weingährung und Fäulniss", in: *Ann. Phys. Chem.* 41 (1837), pp. 184–193.

Theodor SCHWANN, *Mikroskopische Untersuchungen über die Uebereinstimmung in der Struktur und dem Wachsthum der Thiere und Pflanzen.* Verlag d. Sander'schen Buchhandlung (G. E. Reimer), Berlin 1839.

Peter SCHWARZ, *Julius Tandler. Zwischen Humanismus und Eugenik.* Edition Steinbauer, Vienna 2017.

George Edmund de SCHWEINITZ," A Case of Retinitis circinata", in: *Ophthal. Rec.* 1900, pp. 1ff.

George Edmund de SCHWEINITZ, "Circinate Retinitis", in: *Ophthal. Rec.* 1901, pp. 160ff.

George Edmund de SCHWEINITZ, "Disappearance of the lesions in circinate retinitis", in: *Ophthal. Rec.* 1902.

Erasmo SCIMEMI, "Dermatolisia palpebrale (Blefarocalasi di Fuchs)", in: *Bollettino della Società tra i Cultori delle Scienze Mediche e Naturali,* Cagliari, Nr. 4 (1907), Special print.

B. SCOTT, J. Mc CLURE, J. A. W. WILDSMITH (eds.), *Reginal Anaesthesia 1884–1984. Centennial Meeting of Reginal Anesthesia. European Society of Regional Anaesthesia in Association with the American Association of Regional Anaesthesia.* Vienna, September 12–15, 1984.

Felicitas SEEBACHER, *"Freiheit der Naturforschung!" Carl Freiherr von Rokitansky und die Wiener Medizinische Schule. Wissenschaft und Politik im Konflikt,* in: *Schriftenreihe der Kommission für Geschichte der Naturwissenschaften, Mathematik und Medizin* 56. Verlag d. Österr. Akademie d. Wissenschaften, Vienna 2006.

Richard SEEFELDER, "Ein Beitrag zu den Geschwulstbildungen des retinalen Epithels der Regenbogenhaut", in: *Graefes Archiv* 105 (1921), pp. 271–278.

Richard SEEFELDER, "Klinische Beobachtungen über Pneumokokkenkonjunktivitis", in: *Wien. med. Wochensch.* 71 (1921), cols. 1088–1091.

Adalbert SELIGMANN, "Der Billroth'sche Hörsaal im Allgemeinen Krankenhause in Wien", in: *Wien. med. Wochenschr.* 77 (1927), p. 368.

Richard SEXAU, *Fürst und Arzt. Dr. med. Herzog Carl Theodor in Bayern. Schicksal zwischen Wittelsbach und Habsburg.* Styria, Graz/Vienna/Cologne 1963.

Ernst August SEYFARTH, Steven J. ZOTTOLI, "Ludwig Mauthner (1840–1894): neuroanatomist and noted ophthalmologist in Fin-de-Siècle Vienna", in: *Brain Behav. Evol.* 37 (1991), pp. 252–259.

David SHAVIT, *The United States in Asia. A Historical Dictionary.* Greenwood Press, New York/Westport/Connecticut/London 1990.

Paul D. SHERMAN, Colour Vision in the Nineteenth Century: The Young-Helmholtz-Maxwell-Theory. Institute of Physics Publishing 1981.

Harry SICHROVSKY, *Der Revolutionär von Leitmeritz: Ferdinand Blumentritt und der philippinische Freiheitskampf.* Österr. Bundesverlag 1983.

August SIEGRIST, "Atrophie der Sehnerven durch Gefäßdruck bei Hypophysistumor," in: *Graefes Archiv* 105 (1921), pp. 1069–1074.

Carl Ludwig SIGMUND, *Das k. k.chirurgische Operations-Institut in Wien. Darstellung der Geschichte so wie der innern Einrichtung des Institutes, und Übersicht aller darin bisher gebildeten Operateurs, der hinsichtlich derselben erflossenen Verordnungen und der Vorfälle in der chirurgischen Klinik der Wiener Hochschule während des Operations-Lehrcurses 1839–1841.* Braumüller und Seidel, Vienna 1841.

Sir John SINCLAIR, *The Code of Agriculture; Including Observations on Gardens, Orchards, Woods and Plantations; With an Account of all the Recent Improvements in the Management of Arable and Grass Land.* Sherwood, Neely & Jones, London 1817.

Sixteenth Annual Report of the Medical Superintendent of the Peking Union Medical College Hospital. For the Year Ending June 30, 1924. Peking 1924.

Manfred SKOPEC, "Anton Elfinger (1821–1864) – a forgotten medical illustrator", in: *Int. J. Dermatol.* 22/4 (1983), pp. 256–259.

Hans SLEZAK, "Zur Gründung der Ophthalmologischen Gesellschaft in Vienna (Wie alt ist diese Gesellschaft tatsächlich?)", in: Anton HOMMER, Stephan KAMINSKI (eds.), *100 Jahre Ophthalmologische Gesellschaft in Wien. Wien. med. Wochenschr.* 154 (2004), Suppl. 116, pp. 2–3.

(Joseph) Priestley SMITH, "Glaucoma", in: Ophth. Rev. Vol. X (1882), pp. 25–32.

(Joseph) Priestley SMITH, "Modes of Preserving and Drawing Ophthalmic Specimens", in: *Ophthalmic Review* II (1883), pp. 69–76.

Ronald E. SMITH, Robert A. NOZIK, *Uveitis.* Translated from American English and revised by Günther Grabner. Springer, Berlin/Heidelberg/New York/Tokyo 1986.

Herman SNELLEN, *Letterproeven, tot bepaling der gezichtsscherpte.* P. W. Van de Weijer, Utrecht 1862.

Charles SNYDER, "Alois Glogar, Karl Bräuer and Eduard Konrad Zirm", in: *Arch. Ophthalmol.* 74/6 (1965), pp. 871–874.

Charles SNYDER, *Our Ophthalmic Heritage.* Little, Brown & Comp., Boston 1967.

Souvenir de l'Exposition. Ed. Nels, Bruxelles, o. O., o. J.

Souvenir de Liège, n.p., n.d.

Franz SPÄTH, "Zur Geschichte der Chirurgie an der Karl-Franzens-Universität Graz", in: Walter HÖFLECHNER (ed.), *Publikationen aus dem Archiv der Universität Graz* Vol. 18. Graz 1986.

Karl STARGARDT, "Über Phlyktänen der Lidbindehaut des Auges," in: *Graefes Archiv* 105 (1921), pp. 528–537.

Statut des Operations-Institutes an der II. Augenklinik in Wien, n.d.

Kamila STAUDIGL-CIECHOWICZ, *Das Dienst-, Habilitations- und Disziplinarrecht der Universität Wien 1848–1918. Eine rechtshistorische Untersuchung zur Stellung des wissenschaftlichen Universitätspersonals* [= *Schriftenreihe des Archivs der Universität Vienna 22*]. Vienna University Press bei V&R unipress, Göttingen 2017.

Georg STEHLI, *Das Mikrotom und die Mikrotomtechnik. Eine Einführung in die Praxis der Mikrotomie,* Franckh'sche Verlagshandlung 1913.

Carl STELLWAG von CARION, *Die Ophthalmologie a naturwissenschaftlichen Standpuncte aus betrachtet.* Vol. 1, Herder, Freiburg 1853; Vol. 2/Parts 1 & 2. Enke, Erlangen 1855; Vol 2/ Parts 3 & 4, Enke, Erlangen 1858.

Karl STELLWAG von CARION, *Lehrbuch der praktischen Augenheilkunde.* Braumüller, Vienna 1861.

Carl STELLWAG von CARION, *Manuale di oculistica pratica. Prima versione italiana sulla seconda edizione tedesca per cura del dott. Antonio Quagliano.* Vallardi, Milano 1865.

Carl STELLWAG von CARION, *Treatise on the Diseases of the Eye, Including the Anatomy of the Organ.* Translated from the third German edition and edited by Charles E. Hackley and D. B. St. John Roosa with an appendix by the editors. Hardwicke, London; Wood, New York 1868.

Carl STELLWAG von CARION, *A gyakorlati szemészet tankönyve. A 3. jav. kiad. után forditotta Vidor Zsigmond.* Magyar Orvosi Könyvkiado Társulat, Pest 1868.

Karl STELLWAG von CARION, *Abhandlungen aus dem Gebiete der praktischen Augenheilkunde. Ergänzungen zum Lehrbuche.* Unter Mitwirkung der Herrn Prof. Dr. C. Wedl und Dr. E. Hampel. W. Braumüller, Vienna 1882.

Carl STELLWAG v. CARION, "Ueber eine eigenthümliche Form der Hornhautentzündung", in: *Wien. klin. Wochenschr.* 2 (1889), pp. 613–614.

Stenographisches Protokoll. Haus der Abgeordneten. IX. Session 409. Sitzung, am 10. März 1885, in: *Stenographische Protokolle über die Sitzungen des Hauses der Abgeordneten des österreichischen Reichsrathes.* Session IX. Vol. XIV. 400th–430th Meetings (pp. 13891 bis 15185.). K. K. Hof- und Staatsdruckerei, Vienna 1885, pp. 14270–14271.

Albert M. STEVENS, Frank C. JOHNSON, "A new eruptive fever associated with stomatitis and ophthalmia: report of two cases in children", in: Am. J. Dis. Children 24 (1922), pp. 526–533.

Dora STOCKERT-MEYNERT, *Theodor Meynert und seine Zeit.* Vienna/Leipzig 1930.

Rüdiger STOLZ, Joachim WITTIG, Günter SCHMIDT, *Carl Zeiss und Ernst Abbe: Leben, Wirken und Bedeutung.* Universitätsverlag, Jena 1993.

Erwin STRANSKY, "Erinnerungen an Heinrich Obersteiner", in: *Wien. klin. Wochenschr.* 69 (1957), pp. 537–538.

H. S. SUGAR, "Maximilian Salzmann. Ophthalmic pioneer and artist," in: *Surv. Ophthalmol.* 26 (1981), pp. 28–30.

Lambert M. SURHONE, Miriam T. TIMPLEDON, Susan F. MARSEKEN (eds), Adalbert Nikolaus Fuchs. Wieden, Kritzendorf, Technische Universität Wien, Ernst Fuchs, Schottengymnasium. βetascript publishing and Verlag Dr. Müller 2010.

Adolf Ritter von SZILY, "Der Conus nach unten", in: *Centralbl. prakt. Augenheilk.* 7 (1883), pp. 353ff.

Aurel v. SZILY, "Stereoskopische Versuche mit Schattenrissen", in: *Graefes Archiv* 105 (1921), pp. 964–972.

Josef TAPPEINER, "Ferdinand von Hebra und die Wiener Dermatologenschule", in: *Wien. med. Wochenschr.* 116 (1956).

Rudolf TERTSCH, "Über den Ringabscess der Cornea", in: *Graefes Archiv* 73/2 (1910), pp. 314–334.

Max TETZER, Lucian RYDEL, Otto BECKER, *Bericht über die Augenklinik der Wiener Universität. 1863–1865.* Unter Mitwirkung des Prof. Dr. Ferdinand Arlt. Wilhelm Baumüller, Vienna 1867.

Agostín Albarracín TEULÓN, "Die Stipendiaten des spanischen Rates für die wissenschaftliche Fortbildung und die Wiener Medizin des 20. Jahrhunderts", in: Erna LESKY (ed.), *Wien und die Weltmedizin*. Hermann Böhlaus Nachfolger. Vienna/Cologne/Graz 1974, pp. 219–224.

H. Stanley THOMPSON, Randy H. J. KARDON, "Irene E. Loewenfeld, PhD Physiologist of the pupil", in: *Neuroophthalmol.* 26/2 (2006), pp. 139–148.

Carl TOLDT, *Carl Toldt. O. ö. Professor der Anatomie an der Universität in Wien, gestorben am 13. November 1920. Autobiographie*. Urban & Schwarzenberg, Berlin/Vienna 1922.

F. T. TOOKE, "Dr. Edward Jackson – A Founder of the Section on Ophthalmology, College of Physicians of Philadelphia. The Personal Appreciation of Burton Chance", in: *Am. J. Ophthalmol.* 26 (1943), pp. 209–214.

Cristina Evangelista TORRES, *The Americanization of Manila, 1898–1921.* The University of the Philippines Press, 2010.

Paul TOWER, "Carl Wedl. Histopathology of the Eye in the Nineteenth Century", in: *Arch. Ophthalmol.* 63 (1960), pp. 756–760.

Karl Heinz TRAGL, *Chronik der Wiener Krankenanstalten*. Böhlau, Vienna/Cologne/Weimar 2007.

Edward TREACHER COLLINS, *In the Kingdom of the Shah*. T. F. Unwin, London 1896.

Edward TREACHER COLLINS, *The History and Traditions of the Moorfields Eye Hospital. One Hundred Years of Ophthalmic Discovery and Development*. H. K. Lewis and Co., London 1929.

Alois TROST (ed.), *Alt-Wiener Kalender für das Jahr 1919*. Kunstverlag Anton Schroll & Co., Vienna 1919.

Hans TUPPY, "Physiologie und Biochemie 1820–1930", in: Karl ACHAM (ed.), *Geschichte der österreichischen Humanwissenschaften*. Vol 2: *Lebensraum und Organismus des Menschen*. Passagen Verlag, Vienna 2001.

Twenty-Fourth Annual Report of the Medical Superintendent June 30, 1932. Peiping Union Medical College Hospital. Formerly the Peking Union Medical College Hospital. P. U. M. C. Press 1932, pp. 45–47.

Übersicht der akademischen Behörden, Professoren, Privatdocenten, Lehrer, Beamten etc. an der k. k.Universität zu *Wien für das Studienjahr 1877/78*. K. K. Hof- u. Staatsdruckerei, Vienna 1877.

Übersicht der akademischen Behörden, Professoren, Privatdocenten, Lehrer, Beamten etc. an der k. k.Universität zu *Wien für das Studienjahr 1896/97*. Adolf Holzhausen, Vienna 1896.

W. H. UHLAND, *Illustrirter Katalog der Pariser Weltausstellung von 1878*. Brockhaus, Leipzig 1880.

Wilhelm UHTHOFF, "Beiträge zur Klinik und Anatomie der degenerativen Veränderungen der Hornhaut und der Bindehaut", in: *Graefes Archiv* 105 (1921), pp. 205–220.

Joseph UNGER, *System des österreichischen allgemeinen Privatrechts*. Vol. 1. Breitkopf und Härtel, Leipzig 1856.

Universal-Lexicon der practischen Medicin und Chirurgie von Andral, Bégin, Blandin, Bouillaud, Bonvier, Cruveilhier, Cullerier, Devergie, Dugès, Dupuytren, Foville, Guibourt, Jolly, Lallemand, Londe, Magendie, Ratier, Rayer, Roche und Sanson. Frei bearbeitet sowie mit den allgemeinen und besonderen Grundsätzen und practischen Erfahrungen aus dem Gebiethe der Homöopathie bereichert von einem Vereine deutscher Aerzte. Vol. 3. Blepharoptosis – Cinae. H. Franke'sche Verlags-Expedition, Leipzig 1837.

"Université de Liége", in: R. KUKULA, K. TRÜBNER (eds.), *Minerva. Jahrbuch der gelehrten Welt.* 2nd yr 1892–1893. Verlag v. Karl J. Trübner, Strassburg 1893, pp. 399–403.

Constant VANLAIR, "Notice sur Voltaire Masius", in: Annuaire de l'Académie royale des Sciences, des Lettres et des Beaux-Arts de Belgique (1914), pp. 79–116.

Carl Graf VASQUEZ (ed.), *Polizey-Bezirk Alsergrund. Alsergrund, Breitenfeld, Michelbeurischergrund. Mit einem Grundrisse.* Vienna 1828.

Sabine VEITS-FALK, *Rosa Kerschbaumer-Putjata (1851–1923). Erste Ärztin Österreichs und Pionierin der Augenheilkunde. Ein außergewöhnliches Frauenleben in Salzburg.* (= Schriftenreihe des Archivs der Stadt Salzburg 23). Salzburg 2008.

Karl VELHAGEN, *Der Augenarzt.* Vol. IX. 2nd ed. Thieme, Leipzig 1983.

Philipp VERDERAME, "Über Infektionen des Auges durch den Bacillus pyocyaneus", in: *Centralblatt f. Bakteriologie, Parasitenkunde und Infektionskrankheiten* [= *Centralbl. Bakteriol. Parasitenk. Infektionskrankh.*] 58 (1911), pp. 302–317.

F. H. VERHOEFF, "A rare tumor arising from the pars ciliaris retinæ (terato-neuroma) of a nature hitherto unrecognized, and its relation to the so-called glioma-retinæ", in: *Transact. Am. Ophthalmol.* Soc. 10/2 (1904), p. 351–377.

Verordnungsbl. für d. Dienstbereich d. Ministeriums für Cultus u. Unterricht. Redigiert im k. k. Ministerium für Cultus u. Unterricht. Ausgegeben am 15. August 1882, Nr. 31, Verlag d. k. k.Ministeriums für Cultus u. Unterricht, Vienna 1882.

Ville de Liége. *Notice sur les curiosités à visiter. Nomenclature complète des Voies de Communication.* J. Claesen, Bruxelles 1905.

Maximilian v. VINTSCHGAU, "Physiologische Analyse eines ungewöhnlichen Falles partieller Farbenblindheit (Trichromasie des Spectrums)", in: *Arch. ges. Physiol.* 58 (1891), pp. 431–528.

Rudolf VIRCHOW, *Handbuch der speciellen Pathologie und Therapie.* Part. I. Ferdinand Enke, Erlangen 1854–1876.

Karl VOCELKA, *Verfassung oder Konkordat? Der publizistische und politische Kampf der österreichischen Liberalen um die Religionsgesetze des Jahres 1868* [= *Studien zur Geschichte d. österr.-ungar. Monarchie* Vol XVII]. Verlag der ÖAW, Vienna 1978.

Alfred VOGT, "Fehldiagnosen am Spaltlampenmikroskop, mit besonderer Berücksichtigung von Trugbildern", in: *Graefes Archiv* 105 (1921), pp. 507–527.

Richard von VOLKMANN, "Ueber den antiseptischen Occlusivverband und seinen Einfluss auf den Heilungsprocess der Wunden", in: *Sammlung klin. Vorträge* No. 96. Breitkopf & Härtel, Leipzig 1875.

Adolf VOSSIUS, "Über die Bestsche familiäre Maculadegeneration", in: *Graefes Archiv* 105 (1921), pp. 1050–1057.

G. WACHA, "Joseph Barth und die Schola anatomiae", in: Otto ZEKERT, *Kunst in Medizin und Pharmazie. HMW-Jahrbuch 1956.* Heilmittelwerke Wien 1956, pp. 57–59.

August WAGENMANN, "Über cystische Ektasie des Tränensacks durch Luft", in: *Graefes Archiv* 105 (1921), pp. 401–407.

J. F. WAGNER, *Orientirungs-Plan des Wiener k.k. allgemeinen Krankenhauses nebst Daten über dasselbe, über das Gebärhaus und die pathologisch-anatomische Anstalt in Wien.* Josef Šafář, Vienna 1886.

Julius WAGNER-JAUREGG, Ernst Fuchs 1851–1921, in: *Wien. klin. Wochenschr.* 34 (1921), No. 24.

Peter WALTER, Niklas PLANGE, *Basiswissen Augenheilkunde.* Springer, Berlin/Heidelberg 2017.

Philipp von WALTHER, Ectropium anguli externi, eine neue Augenkrankheit, und die Tarsoraphie eine neue Augenoperation, in: *J. Chir. Augenheilk.* 9 (1826), pp. 86–93.

Feliks WASIK, Albrecht SCHOLZ, Günther SEBASTIAN, Erinnerungen an Albert Neisser, in: *Der Hautarzt.* 31 (1980), pp. 328–333.

Peter G. WATSON, Sohan SINGH HAYREH, Scleritis and episcleritis, in: Brit. J. Ophthalmol. 60 (1976), pp. 163–191.

Jean-Paul WAYENBORGH, IBBO *International Biography and Bibliography of Ophthalmologists and Vision Scientists.* With the Co-operation of Saiichi Mishima and Charles Richard Keeler. (= *Hirschberg History of Ophthalmology. The Monographs* Vol. 7). Part 1 A–K, Oostende 2001; Part 2 L–Z. Oostende 2002.

Adolf WEBER, "Ueber Calabar und seine therapeutische Verwendung", in: *Graefes Archiv* 22 (1876), pp. 215–232.

Adolf WEBER, "Ueber die Wirkung des Pilocarpium muriaticum", in: *Centralbl. med. Wissensch.* 14 (1876), pp. 769–772.

Adolf WEBER, "Die Ursachen des Glaukoms", in: *Graefes Archiv* 23 (1877), pp. 1–91.

L. de WECKER, E. de JAEGER, *Traité des Maladies du Fond de l'Œil et Atlas d'Ophtalmoscopie.* Adrien Delahaye/Imprim. Impériale et Royale, Paris/Vienne 1870.

Louis de WECKER, "Notice nécrologique sur Frédéric Jaeger. Chevalier de Jaxtthal", in: *Ann. oculist.* 69 (1873), pp. 85–93.

Louis de WECKER, "Faut-il différencier la rétinite circinée, ou dégénérescence blanche, de la rétinite apoplectiforme", in: *Arch. d'opht.* 14 (1894), Special print.

Carl WEDL, *Grundzüge der pathologischen Histologie.* C. Gerold und Sohn, Vienna 1854.

Carl WEDL, *Atlas der pathologischen Histologie des Auges.* Unter Mitwirkung des Herrn Prof. Dr. Stellwag von Carion. Parts 1 & 2, Georg Wigand, Leipzig 1860. Parts 3 & 4, Georg Wigand, Leipzig 1861.

Carl WEDL, Emil BOCK, *Atlas zur Pathologischen Anatomie des Auges. XXXIII Tafeln in Lichtdruck.* K. K. Hof- und Staatsdruckerei, Vienna 1886.

Carl WEDL, Emil BOCK, *Pathologische Anatomie des Auges. Systematisch bearbeitet. Mit einem Atlas von XXXIII Tafeln.* K. K. Hof- und Staatsdruckerei. In Commission bei Carl Gerold's Sohn, Vienna 1886.

Eugen WEHRLI, "Zur Histologie der Keratitis punctata superficialis (FUCHS), Keratitis subepithelialis (ADLER)", in: *Klin. Monatsbl. Augenheilk.* 44/II (1906), pp. 224ff.

Georges WEILL, "Über Heterophthalmus", in: *Zeitschr. Augenheilk.* 11 (1904), pp. 165–176.

S. WEINBAUM, "Beitrag zur Kenntniss der Sarkomerkrankung der Augenhäute", in: *Graefes Archiv* 37/Abth. I (1891), pp. 185–202.

Joseph WELTERT, "Ein Fall von 'Retinitis circinata'", in: *Archiv Augenheilk.* 32 (1896), pp. 187–193.

Theodor WENSE, "Die Lehrkanzel für allgemeine und experimentelle Pathologie in Innsbruck und ihr Vorstand Prof. Dr. Gustav Bayer", in: *Forschungen und Forscher der Tiroler Ärzteschule (1948–1950).* Vol 2. Oberösterreichischer Landesverlag, Wels 1950.

Karl WESSELY, "Beiträge zu den Wachstumsbeziehungen zwischen dem Augapfel und seinen Nachbarorganen", in: *Graefes Archiv* 105 (1921), pp. 491–501.

Karl WESSELY, "Auge," in: Friedrich HENKE, Otto LUBARSCH (eds.), Handbuch der speziellen pathologischen Anatomie und Histologie. 11th vol. Julius Springer, Berlin Part 1 1928, Part 2 1931, Part 3 1937.

Maynard C. WHEELER, *The American Ophthalmological Society. The First Hundred Years.* University of Toronto Press 1964.

Johannes Wolfgang Cornelius WICHT, *Prof. Dr. Anton Freiherr von Eiselsberg. Leben und Wirken.* Diploma thesis. Med. Univ. Innsbruck 2011.

Hermann WILBRAND, Alfred SAENGER, *Die Neurologie des Auges.* Munich/Wiesbaden 1899–1927.

Heinrich R. v. WITTEK (ed.), *Festgabe zum 100jährigen Jubiläum des Schottengymnasiums gewidmet von ehemaligen Schottenschülern.* Wilhelm Braumüller, Vienna 1907.

Herwig WOLFRAM (ed.), *Österreichische Geschichte 1804–1914.* Ueberreuter, Vienna 1997.

M. WOLFRUM, A. BÖHMIG, "Zum Problem der Hornhautregeneration nebst Bemerkungen über den Keratokonus (Part 2)", in: *Graefes Archiv* 105 (1921), pp. 708–720.

Gregor WOLLENSAK, Holger VOGTEN, Herzog Carl Theodor in Bayern – ein adliger Ophthalmologe. In: Frank KROGMANN (ed.), Mitteilungen der Julius- Hirschberg-Gesellschaft zur Geschichte der Augenheilkunde Vol. 7 (2005). Königshausen & Neumann, Würzburg 2010, pp. 217–237.

Casey A. WOOD, "Blepharochalasis", in: *The American Encyclopedia And Directory of Ophthalmology.* Vol. II – B to Cataract, Incipient. Cleveland Press, Chicago 1913.

(Casey Albert WOOD), "Presentation to Dr. Ernst Fuchs". New York City, July 29, in: *Brit. J. Ophthalmol.* 13/9 (1929), p. 474.

(Würdigung zum 100. Geburtstag v. Leopold Schrötter R. v. Kristelli), in: *Monatsschr. f. Ohrenheilk. u. Laryngo-Rhinol.* 71 (1937), pp. 1131–1140.

Constant von WURZBACH, *Biographisches Lexikon des Kaiserthums Oesterreich, enthaltend die Lebensskizzen der denkwürdigen Personen, welche seit 1750 in den oesterreichischen Kronländern geboren wurden oder darin gelebt und gewirkt haben.* Verlag d. Univ.-Buchdruckerei L. C. Zamarski, Vienna 1856–1891 (60 vols).

Helmut WYKLICKY, "Von der Begründung der III. Medizinischen Fakultät in Innsbruck im Jahre 1869", in: *Wien. med. Wochenschr.* 119 (1969), col. 535.

Helmut WYKLICKY, "Der Anteil der Wiener medizinischen Schule an der Erforschung und Behandlung von Infektionskrankheiten", in: *Recipe* 4 (1979), pp. 7 ff.

Helmut WYKLICKY, *Zur Geschichte der Psychiatrie in Wien. Eine Bilddokumentation/Psychiatry in Vienna. An Illustrated Documentation.* Christian Brandstätter, Vienna 1983.

Helmut WYKLICKY, *Zur Geschichte der Augenheilkunde in Wien. Ophthalmology in Vienna. 100 Jahre II. Universitäts-Augenklinik in Wien.* Christian Brandstätter, Vienna 1984.

Helmut WYKLICKY, Manfred SKOPEC (eds.), *200 Jahre Allgemeines Krankenhaus in Wien.* Beiträge von Helmut LEITNER, Hellmut LORENZ, Georg MILLER-AICHHOLZ, Karl SABLIK, Manfred SKOPEC, and Helmut WYKLICKY. Jugend und Volk, Vienna/Munich 1984.

Helmut WYKLICKY, "Hundert Jahre Lokalanästhesie", in: *Wien. klin. Wochenschr.* 97 (1984), pp. 449–450.

Helmut WYKLICKY, Manfred SKOPEC, "Carl Koller (1857–1944) and his time in Vienna", in: D. B. SCOTT, J. Mc CLURE, J. A. W. WILDSMITH (Ed.), *Regional Anaesthesia 1884–1984. Centennial Meeting of Regional Anaesthesia. European Society of Regional Anaes-*

thesia in Association with the American Association of Regional Anaesthesia. Vienna, September 12–15, 1984, pp. 12–23.

Helmut WYKLICKY, "Zur Geschichte des Instituts für allgemeine und experimentelle Pathologie der Univ. Wien", in: *Wien. klin. Wochenschr.* 97 (1985), pp. 346 ff.

Helmut WYKLICKY, *Das Josephinum. Biographie eines Hauses. Die medicinisch-chirurgische Josephs-Akademie seit 1785. Das Institut für Geschichte der Medizin seit 1920.* Christian Brandstätter, Vienna 1985.

Helmut WYKLICKY, "Wiener Medizin um die Jahrhundertwende", in: Peter BERNER, Emil BRIX, Wolfgang MANTL (eds.), *Wien um 1900. Aufbruch in die Moderne.* Verlag für Geschichte und Politik, Vienna 1986, pp. 69–72.

Helmut WYKLICKY, "Ergänzungen zur Kenntnis des Stammvaters der medizinischen Schule von Galatasaray (Über unveröffentlichte Briefe Metternichs an Friedrich Jaeger)", in: Erwin LUCIUS, Arslan TERZIOGLU (eds.), Österreichisch-türkische medizinische Beziehungen. Berichte d. Symposions v. 28. u. 29. 4. 1986 in Istanbul. Istanbul 1987, pp. 78–86.

Helmut WYKLICKY, "Die Ophthalmologie in Wien vor und nach der Begründung der I. Universitäts-Augenklinik", in: *Spektrum Augenheilk.* 2/2A (1988), pp. 2–8.

Helmut WYKLICKY, "Die 'Wiener klinische Wochenschrift' von 1888–1970", in: *Wien. klin. Wochenschr.* 100 (1988), pp. 228–244.

Helmut WYKLICKY, "Theodor Billroth (1829–1894)", in: *Kunst des Heilens. Aus der Geschichte der Medizin und Pharmazie. Katalog der Niederösterreichischen Landesausstellung in der Kartause Gaming vom 4. Mai bis 27. Oktober 1991. Katalog des Niederösterreichischen Landesmuseums. N.F. 276.* – Wien: Amt der Niederösterreichischen Landesregierung, Kulturabteilung 1991, p. 651.

Helmut WYKLICKY, *Unbekanntes von Theodor Billroth. Eine Dokumentation in Fragmenten.* Verlag der Österreichischen Akademie der Wissenschaften, Vienna 1993.

A. L. WYMAN, "Baron de Wenzel, Oculist to King George III: His Impact on British Ophthalmologists", in: *Medical History* 35 (1991), pp. 78–88.

Thomas YOUNG, "The Bakerian Lecture: On the Theory of Light and Colours", in: *Phil. Transact. Royal Soc. London* 92 (1802) pp. 12–48.

Wilhelm v. ZEHENDER, "Friedrich Jäger, Ritter von Jaxttal," in: *Klin. Monatsbl. f. Augenheilk.* 10 (1872), pp. 177–181.

Wilhelm v. ZEHENDER (ed.), *Die Ophthalmologische Gesellschaft während der ersten fünfundzwanzig Jahre ihres Bestehens von 1863 bis 1888.* (= *Ausserordentliches Beilagenheft zu den Klinischen Monatsblätter für Augenheilkunde.* Yr. 26). Ferdinand Enke, Stuttgart 1888.

Carl ZEISS Optische Werkstaette Jena. *Mikroskope und mikroskopische Hilfsapparate.* No. 28, Jena 1889.

Carl ZEISS Optische Werkstaette Jena. *Mikroskope und mikroskopische Hilfsapparate.* 32nd ed. Jena 1902.

Hermann ZEISSL, *Grundriss der Pathologie und Therapie der Syphilis und der mit dieser verwandten venerischen Krankheiten.* Ferdinand Enke, Stuttgart 1876.

William ZENTMAYER, William Merrick SWEET, Arnold Herman KNAPP, Luther Crouse PETER (eds.), *An International Congress of Ophthalmology, Washington D. C., April 25, 26, 27, 28, 1922.*

Anton ZIEGLER, Carl Graf VASQUEZ (ed.), *Polizey-Bezirk Alsergrund. Alsergrund. Breitenfeld. Michelbeurischergrund. Mit einem Grundrisse.* Vienna 1828.

Eduard ZIRM, "Eine erfolgreiche totale Keratoplastik", in: *Graefes Archiv* 64/Abtheil. III (1906), pp. 580–593.

Eduard ZIRM, "Über Hornhautpfropfung", in: Wien. klin. Wochenschr. 28 (1907), pp. 61. (Demonstration in the Gesellsch. d. Ärzte in Wien).

Eduard ZIRM, "Über periodischen Exophthalmus und kongenitalen Enophthalmus, in: *Wien. med. Wochenschr.* 71 (1921), cols. 1091–1093.

Matthias E. ZIRM, Avi A. MANNIS, "Eduard Zirm (18863–1944)", in: Mark J. MANNIS, Avi MANNIS (eds.), *Corneal Transplantation: A History in Profiles*. Second Edition. Hirschberg History of Ophthalmology Volume Six. Wayenborgh Publications, Amsterdam 2018, pp. 129–141.

Maria ZOZOLOUL, Gregory TSOUCALAS, Marianna KARAMANOU, Konstantinos LAIOS, Ilias GEORGALAS, Athanasios DOUZENIS, George ANDROUTSOS, "The distinguished Austrian ophthalmologist Ernst Fuchs (1851–1930) and the 'sarcom des uveal-tractus'", in: *JBUO* 23 (2018), pp. 1563–1568.

Claudia ZRENNER, "The Discovery of the Lamina Basalis Choroideae by Carl Wilhelm Ludwig Bruch (1819–1884)", in: *Hist. Ophthal. Intern.* 3 (1984), pp. 213–260.

A. ZWIEAUER, "Ueber die Möglichkeit einer Behandlung von entzündlichen Erkrankungen des vorderen Abschnittes mit Tromoxan", in: *Wien. klin. Wochenschr.* 63 (1951), pp. 697–698.

II. Bibliography of Works about Ernst Fuchs in Chronological Order

Leopold KÖNIGSTEIN, "Das Sarkom des Uvealtraktus. Von Dr. Ernst Fuchs, Professor der Augenheilkunde in Lüttich", in: *Wien. med. Presse* 26 (1881), pp. 1611–1614.

(Ed.), " Ursachen und die Verhinderung (sic!) der Blindheit. Gekrönte Preisschrift von Dr. Ernst Fuchs, Professor der Augenheilkunde an der Universität Lüttich", in: *Wien. med. Presse* 26 (1885), pp. 1031–1033. (Review)

Hermann COHN, "Die Ursachen und die Verhütung der Blindheit. Gekrönte Preisschrift. Von Dr. Ernst Fuchs, ordentl. Prof. der Augenheilkunde an der Universität Lüttich. – Herausgegeben von der Society for the prevention of blindness. – Motto: Viribus unitis. Wiesbaden. Verlag J. F. Bergmann. 1885. Preis 2 M. 40 Pf.", in: *Dt. med. Wochenschr.* 11 (1885), pp. 240–241 and 257–258. (Review)

(Ed.), "Les causes et la prévention de la cécité, par M. le professeur Fuchs, traduit de l'allemand", in: *Bulletin de la clinique national ophtalmologique de l'hospice des Quinze-Vingts* 3 (1885), p. 148. (Review)

Review of *the Lehrbuch*, in: *Wien. klin. Wochenschr.* 3 (1890), pp. 256–257.

August REUSS, Review of the 2nd of the *Lehrbuch*, in: *Wien. klin. Wochenschr.* 4 (1891), p. 425.

Ludwig EISENBERG, *Das geistige Wien. Künstler- und Schriftsteller-Lexikon.* Vol. 2: *Medicinisch-naturwissenschaftlicher Theil. Mittheilungen über Wiener Fachschriftsteller und Gelehrte auf dem Gebiete der Medicin (nebst Thierheilkunde und Pharmacie) und Naturwissenschaften.* C. Daberkow, Wien 1893, p. 142.

Heinrich ADLER, Adolf KRONFELD, *Medicinische Chronik des XIX. Jahrhunderts.* 2nd ed. Moritz Perles, Wien 1901, p. 63.

Elin ELMGRÉN, Otteita Muistiinpanoista Köpenhaminen ja Wienin silmätautien klinikoilta". (Erinnerungen an die Kopenhagener und Wiener Augenkliniken), in: *Duodecim* No. 17, Helsinki 1901, pp. 194–200.

Julius Leopold PAGEL (ed.), *Biographisches Lexikon hervorragender Ärzte des 19. Jahrhunderts.* Urban & Schwarzenberg, Berlin/Vienna 1901(= Reprint Karger, Leipzig 1989), p. 566.

Carl HESZ (HESS), "Ernst Fuchs. (Zum 14. Juni 1911)", in: *Wien. klin. Wochenschr.* 24 (1911), pp. 833–834.

(Ed.), "La visita del Profesor Fuchs á México", in: *Anales de oftalmologia* 14 (1912), p. 130.

Julius HIRSCHBERG, "Geschichte der Augenheilkunde IX u. X. Die Reform der Augenheilkunde II". In: Theodor AXENFELD, Anton ELSCHNIG (ed.), *Handbuch der gesamten Augenheilkunde begründet von Albrecht Graefe und Theodor Saemisch, fortgeführt von Carl. Hess.* 2nd revised ed. Part II, Vol. XV, Ch. XXIII, Sect. 1. Julius Springer, Berlin 1918, pp. 429–433.

(Hallard R. BEARD), "Photomicrographs of Sections of the Eye, chosen by Prof. Ernst Fuchs as best illustrating his Lectures on the Pathological Anatomy of the Eye". Chicago n.d. (presum. 1921–1922, (typescript).

Oscar DIEM, Henry J. MINSKY, "Notes and Remarks on Professor Ernest Fuchs's Lectures on Histology and Pathology of the Eye. Revised by Prof. Fuchs". New York 1921. (typescript)

Festschrift zur Feier des siebzigsten Geburtstages Herrn Hofrat Prof. Dr. Ernst Fuchs in Wien gewidmet von Freunden und dankbaren Schülern, in: *Graefes Archiv* 105 (1921), pp. 1–1230. (73 original works by Rudolf Bergmeister, O. Purtscher, Fritz Rössler, E. Horniker, Julius Hirschberg, R. Greeff, C. v. Hess, A. Peters, W. Gilbert, Junius, W. Uhthoff, Harald G. Gjessing, Sigurd Hagen, Heinrich Schoeppe, F. Schieck, R. Seefelder, R. Deutschmann,

E. Lindgren, J. Meller, A. Fuchs, Moriz Sachs, Paul Kafka, J. Kyrle, A. Wagenmann, L. Heine, E. Hertel, A. Jess, M. Goldschmidt, Henning Rönne, Fritz Salzer, K. Wessely, C. H. Sattler, Alfred Vogt, Karl Stargardt, W. Koster., L. v. Liebermann, Maximilian Salzmann, Hans Lauber, Otto Marburg, A. Elschnig, Henning Rönne, G. F. Rochat, W. Reis, Josef Ingersheimer u. Walter Prinz, A. Birch-Hirschfeld, A. Bielschowsky, Albert von Plugk, M. Wolfrum u. A. Boehmig, J. W. Nordenson, K. Lindner, A. Pillat, F. Dimmer, Alfred Kestenbaum, A. Loewenstein, Viktor Hanke, Ernst Kraupa, J. van der Hoeve, V. Groenholm, Richard Cords, A. v. Szily, Andreas Rados, Ernst Bachstez, E v. Hippel, A. Vossius, E. Franke, A. Siegrist, Emil v. Grósz, Adolf Purtscher, Richard Krämer, Leonhard Koeppe, Fritz Ask u. J. van der Hoeve, Th. Axenfeld, H. Sattler (Wiedergabe d. Autorennamen entspr. d. Reihenfolge lt. Inhaltsverzeichnis).

Josef MELLER, "Hofrat Ernst Fuchs zum 70. Geburtstage", in: *Wien. med. Wochenschr.* 71 (1921), cols. 1041–1043.

Josef MELLER, "Rede bei der Übernahme des Marmorbildnisses von E. Fuchs am 14. 6. 1921. (Bericht aus den Verhandlungen der Ophthalmologischen Gesellschaft in Wien. Feier des 70. Geburtstages von Ernst Fuchs am 14. Juni 1921)", in: Josef MELLER, Ausgewählte Schriften und Reden. Wilhelm Maudrich, Wien 1935, pp. 75–78.

Julius WAGNER-JAUREGG, "Ernst Fuchs 1851–1921", in: *Wien. klin. Wochenschr.* 34 (1921), p. 287.

E. J. GOODWIN, "Prof. Fuchs in St. Louis", in: *Am J. Ophthalmol.* 5/1 (1922), p. 68.

(Ed.), "Feier des 70. Geburtstages Ernst Fuchs's am 14. Juni 1921 in Wien", in: *Zeitschr. Augenheilk.*47 (1922), pp. 47–63.

Adolph BARKAN, Arnold KNAPP, George S. DERBY, E.V.L. Brown, Joseph M. KELLER, "Ernst Fuchs Fund", in: Am. J. Ophthalmol. 10/7 (1927), p. 541.

(Ed.), in: *Boletín de informacion oftalmológica* 3 (1930), p. 2.

(Ed.), "Der berühmte Augenarzt Hofrat Fuchs gestorben", in: *Neue Freie Presse* No. 23776 (Evening paper), 22 November 1930, p. 3.

(Ed.), "Die letzten Säulen", in: *Neues Wiener Tagblatt* No. 23261, 23 November 1930.

Giuseppe GENTILINI, "Prof. Ernesto Fuchs", in: *Bollettino medici trentino* 9 (1930), pp. 3–8.

Viktor HANKE, "Ernst Fuchs", in: *Wien. med. Wochenschr.* 80 (1930), cols. 1575–1576.

Richard KRÄMER, "Ernst Fuchs – in memoriam. (Persönliche Erinnerungen)", in: *Med. Klinik* 26 (1930), pp. 1879–1880.

Hans LAUBER, "Ernst Fuchs †", in: *Klin. Monatsbl. f. Augenheilk.* 85 (1930), pp. 830–834.

Karl LINDNER, "Nachruf auf Prof. Ernst Fuchs gesprochen in der Sitzung der Gesellschaft der Ärzte vom 28. November 1930", in: *Wien. klin. Wochenschr.* 43 (1930), pp. 1517–1520.

Karl LINDNER, "Worte der Erinnerung an weiland Ernst Fuchs", in: *Wien. med. Wochenschr.* 80 (1930), cols. 1666–1667.

L. M., "Ernst Fuchs", in: *Annali di Ottalmologia e Clinica Oculistica* 58 (1930), pp. 1099–1101.

Josef MELLER, "Die wissenschaftliche Bedeutung des Hofrates Ernst Fuchs", in: *Neue Freie Presse* No. 23776 (Evening paper), 22 November 1930, p. 3.

Josef MELLER, "Ernst Fuchs †", in: *Wien. klin. Wochenschr.* 43 (1930), pp. 1493–1495.

F. MEZZATESTA, in: *Policlinico (sez. prat.)* 37 (1930), p. 1880.

August WAGENMANN, (Ernst Fuchs †), in: *Graefes Archiv* 125 (1930), 3rd issue (2 unpag. pages between pp. 312 and 313).

W. G. M. BYERS, in: *Canadian. Med. Assoc. J.* 24 (1931), p. 566–567.

Edward Treacher COLLINS, "Hofrat Professor Ernst Fuchs and his work", in: *Brit. J. of Ophthalmol.* 15 (1931), pp. 65–75.

Lawrence Webster FOX, "Professor Ernst Fuchs", in: *Am. J. Ophthalmol.* 14/2 (1931), pp. 166–167.

Jonas S. FRIEDENWALD, "The contributions of Professor Ernst Fuchs to ophthalmic pathology#, in: *Am. J. of Ophthalmol.* 14/2 (1931), pp. 138–140.

(Ed.), in: *Gaceta med. Española* 5 (1931), p. 5.

Harvey J. HOWARD, "Professor Ernst Fuchs", in: *Am. J. Ophthalmol.* 14 (1931), pp. 5–6.

Arnold KNAPP, "Obituary of Ernst Fuchs", in: *Bull. N. Y. Acad. Med.* 1931, Jan. 7 (1), pp. 68–69.

Arnold KNAPP, Bernard SAMUELS, "Ernst Fuchs, M. D. 1851–1930", in: *Arch. Ophthalmol.* 5/2 (1931), pp. 288–293.

Manuel MÁRQUEZ, Hans LAUBER, "El Profesor Fuchs", in: *Arch. de oftalmologia hispano-americanos* 31 (1931), pp. 2–9.

F. PARK LEWIS, Edward JACKSON, William Holland WILMER, George Franklin LIBBY, George Francis SUKER, William H. CRISP, Will Otto BELL, Harvey HOWARD, Hans BARKAN, Harry Searis GRADLE, Lawrence T. POST, Charles SWAB, "In Memory of Professor Ernst Fuchs", in: *Am. J. of Ophthalmol.* 14 (1931), pp. 1–7.

Karl LINDNER, Adolph BARKAN, "More about Ernst Fuchs. Interesting details of his life", in: Am. J. Ophthalmol. 14/4 (1931), pp. 335–338.

William Henry LUEDDE, "Ernst Fuchs (1851–1930) – An Appreciation", in: *Sight-Saving Rev.* 1 (1931), pp. 5–8.

S. H. M., "The Late Professor Fuchs", in: *Canad. Med. Assoc. J.* 24 (1931), p. 530.

Josef MELLER, "Ernst Fuchs. Worte der Erinnerung. (Gesprochen in der Gedächtnissitzung der Ophthalmologischen Gesellschaft in Wien am 15. Dezember 1930)", in: *Wien. med. Wochenschr.* 81 (1931), col. 41.

Josef MELLER, "Ernst Fuchs †", in: *Forschungen und Fortschritte. Korrespondenzblatt der deutschen Wissenschaft und Technik 7* (1931), p. 14.

Victor MORAX, "Ernst Fuchs 1851–1930", in: *Annales d'Oculistique* 168 (1931), pp. 821–826.

(Ed.), in: *Bull. New. York Acad. Med.*, Second Series, Vol. VII, January 1931, No. 1, p. 68.

Ludwig SALLMANN, "In memoriam Professor Ernst Fuchs, 1851–1930, visiting Professor of Ophthalmology to China in 1922", in: *Nat. Med. J. China* 17 (1931), pp. 1–5 and 123.

Maximilian SALZMANN, "Ernst Fuchs †", in: *Zeitschr. Augenheilk.* 73 (1931), pp. 317–325. (Gedächtnisrede, gehalten in der Trauersitzung der Ophthalmologischen Gesellschaft in Wien am 15. XII. 1930).

(Ed.), *Arch. d'Opht.* 48 (1931), pp. 52–54 (F. Terrien).

Julius WAGNER-JAUREGG, "Ernst Fuchs", in: *Akademie der Wissenschaften in Wien. Almanach* 81 (1931), pp. 191–200.

Constantin von ECONOMO, "(Nachruf, gesprochen in der Sitzung des Vereins für Psychiatrie und Neurologie in Wien vom 13. Januar 1931)", in: *Jb. Psych. Neurol.* 48 (1932), pp. 76–77.

Isidor FISCHER (ed.), *Biographisches Lexikon der hervorragenden Ärzte der letzten fünfzig Jahre.* Vol. 1. Urban & Schwarzenberg, Munich–Berlin 1932 (Reprints 1962 and 2004), pp. 461 (wrong date of death!)

Josef MELLER, "Ernst Fuchs (†)", in: *Die feierliche Inauguration des Rektors der Wiener Universität für das Studienjahr 1931/32. Am 17. November 1932.* Selbstverlag der Universität, Vienna 1932, pp. 25–27.

(Ed.), "Más sobre Ernesto Fuchs", in: *Arch. Oftalmol. Hispano-Americanos* 32 (1932), pp. 106–107.

Charles H. MAY, "Bronze plate of Professor Ernst Fuchs", in: *Am. J. Ophthalmol.* 16/1 (1933), p. 71.

Josef MELLER, *Über die Entwicklung der Lehre von der sympathischen Ophthalmie in der Wiener ophthalmologischen Schule.* (Erschienen in der Festschrift der Wiener klinischen Wochenschrift Nr. 20 zum 150jährigen Bestande des Wiener Allgemeinen Krankenhauses 1934), in: Josef MELLER, *Ausgewählte Schriften und Reden.* (Printed as a manuscript). Wilhelm Maudrich, Vienna 1935, pp. 171–208.

Lucien LEPLAT, "Ernest Fuchs (1882)", in: *Liber Memorialis. L'Université de Liège de 1867 à 1935. Notices biographiques.* Tome III. Faculté de Médecine. Rectorat de l'Université, Liège 1936, pp. 122–124.

Leopold SCHÖNBAUER, *Das Medizinische Wien. Geschichte/Werden/Würdigung.* 1st ed., Urban & Schwarzenberg, Berlin/Vienna 1944, pp. 385–386 and 2nd ed. 1947, pp. 416–417.

Jessie DOBSON, *Anatomical Eponyms.* Baillière, Tyndall & Cox. London 1946, p. 80.

B. CARRERAS DURÁN, "Profesor Ernesto Fuchs", in: *Archivios de la Sociedad Oftalmológica Hispano-Americana* (1951).

(Ed.), "Prof. Ernest Fuchs", in: *Revista brasileira de oftalmologia* 9 (1951), pp. 227–228.

Leopold ARZT, "Ernst Fuchs, dem Mitbegründer der Wiener klinischen Wochenschrift, zum 100. Geburtstag", in: *Wien. klin. Wochenschr.* 63 (1951), p. 613.

James E. LEBENSOHN, "Professor Ernst Fuchs (June 14, 1851–November 21, 1930)", in: *Am. J. Ophthalmol.* 34/5 (1951), pp. 772–774.

Karl LINDNER, "Zum 100. Geburtstage von Ernst Fuchs", in: *Wien. klin. Wochenschr.* 63 (1951), pp. 449–450.

Arnold PILLAT, "Der Beitrag der Wiener Schule zur Augenheilkunde", in: *Wien. klin. Wochenschr.* 63 (1951), pp. 614–617. (Address delivered to the Commemorative Meeting of the Gesellschaft der Ärzte Wien on the occasion of the 100th birthday of Ernst Fuchs, on 22 June 1951).

Arnold PILLAT, "The Contribution of the Vienna School to Ophthalmology", in: *Am. J. Ophthalmol.* 36 (1953), pp. 15–25.

Samuel J. KIMURA, Michael John HOGAN, P. THYGESON, "Fuchs's syndrome of heterochromic cyclitis", in: *Arch. Ophthalmol.* 54 (1955), pp. 179–186.

Alexander JOKL, "Ferdinand von Arlt and Ernst Fuchs: Two Representatives of the Vienna School of Ophthalmology", in: *Internat. Rec. Med.* 170 (1957), pp. 702–707.

Alexander JOKL, Ferdinand von Arlt and Ernst Fuchs: Two Representatives of the Vienna School of Ophthalmology, in: pp. A. Tydskrip vir Geneeskunde/South African Med. Journal 32 (1957), p. 301–303.

Karl LINDNER, "Ernst Fuchs. Ein weltberühmter Meister der Augenheilkunde", in: Fritz KNOLL (ed.), *Österreichische Naturforscher, Ärzte und Techniker.* Herausgegeben im Auftrage der Österreichischen Akademie der Wissenschaften. Verlag der Gesellschaft für Natur und Technik. Vienna 1957, pp. 122–124.

Österreichisches Biographisches Lexikon 1815–*1950.* Ed. by Österreichische Akademie der Wissenschaften under the aegis of Leo SANTIFALLER, rev. by Eva OBERMAYER-MARNACH. Vol. 1 (Inst. 4). Hermann Böhlaus Nachfolger, Graz/Cologne 1957, pp. 378.

Arnold PILLAT, "Ernst Fuchs", in: *Österreichische Ärzte als Helfer der Menschheit (Austrian Physicians in the Service of Mankind/Les Médecins autrichiens comme bienfaiteurs de l'humanité.* (= *Notring-Jahrbuch*). Notring der wissenschaftlichen Verbände Österreichs 1957, pp. 53–55.

Erna LESKY, "Aus dem Nachlaß Ferdinand von Arlts im Wiener medizinhistorischen Institut", in: *Klin. Monatsbl. f. Augenheilk.* 139 (1961), pp. 847–856.

Marlene JANTSCH, "Fuchs Ernst, Augenarzt", in: *Neue Deutsche Biographie.* Ed. by Bayerische Akademie der Wissenschaften. Vol. 5. Duncker & Humblot, Berlin 1961, pp. 677–678.

Gert A. ZISCHKA, *Allgemeines Gelehrten-Lexikon. Biographisches Wörterbuch zur Geschichte der Naturwissenschaften.* (= *Kröners Taschenausgabe* vol. 306). Alfred Kröner, Stuttgart 1961, pp. 229.

Alexander JOKL, "Ernst Fuchs (1851–1930)", in: N*eue Österreichische Biographie ab 1815. Große Österreicher.* Vol. XV. Amalthea, Vienna/Munich/Zürich 1963, pp. 142–150.

Peter C. KRONFELD, "Tribute to Ernst Fuchs", in: *Am. J. Ophthalmol.* 60/4 (1965), pp. 736–737.

Erna LESKY, Die Wiener Medizinische Schule im 19. Jahrhundert. Böhlau, Graz/Cologne 1965 (2nd ed. 1978), pp. 490–496.

Österreich Lexikon. Vol. 1. Österreichischer Bundesverlag und Verlag für Jugend und Volk, Vienna/Munich 1966, p. 360.

Allen G. DEBUS (Ed.), in: *World's Who's Who in Science. A Biographical Dictionary of Notable Scientists from Antiquity to the Present.* 1st ed. Marquis – Who's Who Inc., Chicago 1968, p. 617.

Marcel FLORKIN, "Apports viennois à la Faculté de médecine de Liege", in: Marcel Florkin, Léon-E. Halkin, *Chronique de l'Université de Liège.* Liège 1967, pp. 217–230.

Marcel FLORKIN, "Le 150e anniversaire de l'Université de Liège et l'histoire de sa Faculté de médecine". In: *Médecine et Hygiène* 25 (1967), pp. 537–538.

Irido-cyclitic Sympathica, in: James E. LEBENSOHN, *An Anthology of Ophthalmic Classics.* Williams & Wilkins Co. Baltimore 1969, pp. 254–261.

Reallexikon der Medizin und ihrer Grenzgebiete. Urban & Schwarzenberg. 3rd vol., Munich/Berlin/Vienna 1969, pp. 210–211.

Irene E. LOEWENFELD, H. Stanley THOMPSON, F"uchs's Heterochromic Cyclitis: A Critical Review of the Literature. I. Clinical Characteristics of the Syndrome", in: *Survey of Ophthalmol.* 17 (1973), pp. 394–414 and 415–457 (Bibliography); II. *Etiology and Mechanisms.* Ibid. 18 (1973), pp. 2–61.

Marcel FLORKIN, "Les Années de Professorat de Karl Gussenbauer, d'Alexander von Winiwarter et d'Ernst Fuchs à la faculté de médecine de Liège", in: Erna LESKY (ed.), *Wien und die Weltmedizin.* Hermann Böhlaus Nachfolger. Vienna/Cologne/Graz 1974, pp. 196–203.

M. J. HOGAN, I. WOOD, M. FINE, "Fuchs's Endothelial Dystrophy of the Cornea#, in: *Americ. J. Ophthalmol.* 78 (1974), pp. 363–383.

Peter KÄLIN, *Kurzbiographien von Ärzten des deutschen Sprachraums, die 1930 verstorben sind.* Zahnärztliche Dissertation, Universität Zürich 1977, pp. 56–60.

G. GODER, "Ernst Fuchs und sein Beitrag zur Ophthalmologie", In: Fol. Ophthalmol. 6 (1981), pp. 118–123.

Daniel G. VAUGHAN, "Peking Union Medical College: A Golden Age in Ophthalmology", in: *Transact. Pacific Coast Oto-Ophthalmol. Soc.* 62 (1981), pp. 1–15.

George GORIN, *History of Ophthalmology. Publish or Perish*, Wilmington 1982.

Wolfgang MÜNCHOW, "Geschichte der Augenheilkunde", in: Karl VELHAGEN (ed.), *Der Augenarzt.* Vol I.X. 2nd ed. Georg Thieme, Leipzig 1983.

B. STREIFF, "Ernst Fuchs (1851–1930) – Gedächtnisvorlesung Wien", 31 May 1984, in: *Klin. Monatsbl. Augenheilk.* 185 (1984), pp. 316–320.

Helmut WYKLICKY, *Zur Geschichte der Augenheilkunde in Wien/ Ophthalmology in Vienna. 100 Jahre II. Universitäts-Augenklinik.* Christian Brandstätter, Wien 1984.

Jens JESSEN, *Bibliographie der Selbstzeugnisse deutscher Mediziner, Erinnerungen, Tagebücher und Briefe.* Peter Lang, Frankfurt am Main/Bern/New York 1986, p. 34.

Jeremy M. NORMAN (ed.), Morton's Medical Bibliography. An Annotated Check-list of Texts Illustrating the History of Medicine (Garrison and Morton). Fifth Edition. Scolar Press. Aldershot 1991, pp. 925–926.

Daniel M. ALBERT, "Ernst Fuchs 1851–1930", in: *Men of Vision. Lives and Notable Figures in Ophthalmology.* The Classics of Ophthalmology Library/Gryphon Editions, New York 1993, pp. 381–392.

Felix CZEIKE, *Historisches Lexikon Wien in 5 Bänden.* Vol. 2, Kremayr & Scheriau, Wien 1993, pp. 428.

Ole Daniel ENERSON, http//www.whonamedit.com/1994–2001.

Daniel M. ALBERT, Edward NORTON, Reva HURTES, *Source Book of Ophthalmology.* Blackwell Science 1995, pp. 112–113.

Daniel M. ALBERT, Diane D. EDWARDS (ed.), *The History of Ophthalmology.* Blackwell Science, Cambridge 1996, pp. 87–89.

Jens JESSEN, Reiner VOIGT, *Bibliographie der Autobiographien.* Vol. 4. *Selbstzeugnisse, Erinnerungen, Tagebücher und Briefe deutschsprachiger Ärzte.* K. G. Saur. Munich/New Providence/London/Paris 1996.

Walther KILLY (ed.), *Deutsche Biographische Enzyklopädie.* Vol. 3. K. G. Saur. Munich/New Providence/London/Paris 1996, pp. 517–518.

Leslie T. MORTON, Robert J. MOORE, *A Chronology of Medicine and Related Sciences.* Scolar Press, Aldershot 1997, p. 241.

Gabriela SCHMIDT, *Sicherung musealer Gegenstände aus dem Alten Allgemeinen Krankenhaus. Endbericht zu dem Projekt des Bundesministeriums für Wissenschaft und Forschung GZ. 20.682/1–22/92.* Wien 1997, pp. 10 and 24–30. (Typescript, Bibliothek der Medizinischen Universität Wien/Abteilung Geschichte der Medizin).

Frank KROGMANN, "Streifzug durch die Geschichte der Augenheilkunde in Wien", in: *Mitteil. d. Österr. Gesellsch. f. Wissenschaftsgesch.* 18 (1998), pp. 125–152.

Anton SEBASTIAN, "Fuchs, Ernest (1851–1930)", in: *A Dictionary of the History of Medicine.* Parthenon Publishing Group New York/London 1999, p. 329.

Jan BEITING, "The Ophthalmology Hall of Fame", in: *EyeWorld (= Monthly Online J. Amer. Soc. Cataract Refract. Surg.)* http://www.eyewordorg/july00/0700p16.asp.

Jean-Paul WAYENBORGH, "Ernst Fuchs". In: IBBO *International Biography and Bibliography of Ophthalmologists and Vision Scientists.* Part 1 A–K. With the Co-operation of Saiichi Mishima and Charles Richard Keeler. (= *Hirschberg History of Ophthalmology. The Monographs* Vol. 7). Oostende 2001, pp. 270–271.

Diane ANGELUCCI, "Ernst Fuchs honored for advances in ophthalmology", in: *EyeWorld (= Monthly Online J. Amer. Soc. Cataract Refract. Surg.)*, http://www.eyeworldorg/apr01/0401p25.html.

Dietrich v. ENGELHARDT (ed.), *Biographische Enzyklopädie deutschsprachiger Mediziner.* Vol. 1. K. G. Saur, Munich 2002, p. 201.

"Ophthalmological Numismatics: Ernst Fuchs (1851–1930)", in: *Arch. Ophthalmol.* 120 (2002), p. 246.

Carlos LÓPEZ DE LETONA, "El Profesor Ernesto Fuchs y España (1931)", in: *Arch. Soc. Esp. Oftalmol.* 78/9 (2003), pp. 517–518.

Andreas MÜLLER, Charles N. J. Mc GHEE, "Professor Ernst Fuchs (1851–1930). A Defining Career in Ophthalmology", in: *Arch. Ophthalmol.* 121 (2003), pp. 888–891.

Jens Martin ROHRBACH, "Ophthalmopathology between yesterday and tomorrow", in: *Klin. Monatsbl. Augenheilk.* 221/2 (2004), pp. 87–91.

Rudolf VIERHAUS (ed.), *Deutsche Biographische Enzyklopädie*. 2nd rev. and enlarged ed. Vol 3. K. G. Saur, Munich 2006, p. 605.

Padmaja KRISHNAN, "Ernst Fuchs", in: *Kerala J. Ophthalm.* 20 (2008), p. 434–436.

Carl P. HERBORT, Moncef KHAIRALLAH, Editorial: "Fuchs's Uveitis: from Imperial Vienna to Global Appraisal", in: *Internat. Ophthalmol.* 30 (2010), pp. 449–452.

Gabriela SCHMIDT-WYKLICKY, Helmut GRÖGER, "Ernst Fuchs. Vorstand der II. Universitäts-Augenklinik in Wien 1885 bis 1915. Wien als weltweites Zentrum der Ophthalmopathologie", in: *Spektrum Augenheilk.* 26 (2012), pp. 312–318.

Maria ZOZOLOUL, Gregory TSOUCALAS, Marianna KARAMANOU, Konstantinos LAIOS, Ilias GEORGALAS, Athanasios DOUZENIS, George ANDROUTSOS, "The distinguished Austrian ophthalmologist Ernst Fuchs (1851–1930) and the 'sarcom des uvealtractus'", in: *JBUO* 23 (2018), pp. 1563–1568.

Gabriela SCHMIDT-WYKLICKY, "Ein ophthalmohistorischer Schatz: Die pathohistologische Sammlung von Ernst Fuchs in Wien", in: *Mitteilungen der Julius-Hirschberg-Gesellschaft* 16–2014 (2018), pp. 181–196.

III. Figures, Captions and Photo Credits

1–12: Autograph of the autobiography Ernst Fuchs wrote in 1926 at the behest of the Österreichische Akademie der Wissenschaften. Many thanks to Stefan Sienell, Archivist of the ÖAW.

13: Adalbert Fuchs (1779–1854), Ernst Fuchs's grandfather. Original in the Family Archive.

14: Adalbert Nikolaus Fuchs (1814–1886), Ernst Fuchs's father. Lithograph by L. Wallner 1856. Bildarchiv d. Österr. Nationalbibliothek.

15: Isabella Fuchs (1832–1902), née v. Schreibers. Ernst Fuchs's mother. Original in the Family Archive.

16: Ernst and his brother Wilhelm as children. Original photo in the Family Archive.

17: Wilhelm Fuchs (1853–1897) as a grownup. Original photo in the Family Archive.

18: Ernst Fuchs's enrolment at Vienna University in the winter semester of 1868/69. Archiv der Universität Wien. Photo C/O G.S.-W.

19: Ernst Fuchs as a student and assistant at the lab of physiologist Ernst Wilhelm Ritter von Brücke (1819–1892). Sammlungen der Medizinischen Universität Wien.

20: Ferdinand Ritter von Arlt (1812–1887). Director of the University Eye Clinic in Vienna. Lithograph byAdolf Dauthage 1859. Sammlungen der Medizinischen Universität Wien.

21: Record of Ernst Fuchs's graduation on 18 Feb. 1874). Archiv der Universität Wien.

22: Travelogue 1878. Handwritten report on Ernst Fuchs's study trip to Great Britain, France and the Netherlands. Archiv der Universität Wien. Page 1.

23: Lawrence Webster Fox (1853–1931). Original photo with handwritten dedication: "In grateful remembrance of Student days to Prof. E. Fuchs. L. W. Fox Philadelphia 1913." Family archive.

24: "Americans studying in the Fuchs ophthalmological Clinic Vienna 1909–10". "Course for Americans" at Vienna's 2nd University Eye Clinic. They were taught by the Fuchs assistants Maximilian Salzmann and Josef Meller (1st row, 3rd and 4th from left). Sammlungen der Medizinischen Universität Wien.

25: "Surgeons in Prof. Fuch[s]'s Ophthalmological Clinic Vienna – 1910". "Course for Americans" at Vienna's 2nd University Eye Clinic. The course was taught by Josef Meller (1st row, 2nd from right). Sammlungen der Medizinischen Universität Wien.

26: "Billroth im Hörsaal". Painting by Adalbert Franz Seligmann 1890. Belvedere, Vienna.

27: *Das Sarcom des Uvealtractus* (1882). Ernst Fuchs's "habilitation" thesis.

28: Advertisement of the publishing house Wilhelm Braumüller in Vienna with the portrait of Ernst Fuchs, who had his habilitation thesis printed at this publishers. Private collection; photo C/O G. S-W.

29: Appointment of Ernst Fuchs as Assoc Prof. and Director of the University Eye Clinic Liège 1881. Archive of Liège University Photo copy. With thanks to Liège University Archivist Marie-Élisabeth Henneau.

30: Julia-Rosina (called Julie) Fuchs, née May(e)r, Ernst Fuchs's wife. Original photo in the Family Archive.

31: Church marriage certificate. Ernst Fuchs and Julia-Rosina Mayr. Parish registery St. Rochus und Sebastian, 1030 Vienna. Marriage certificate. Marriage regiester Tom. 21, fol. 27, Pfarre Landstraße of 22 June 1882. Accessible online: http://www.matricula.online, Erzdiözese Wien. 03., Landstraße, St. Rochus.

32: Portrait of Ernst Fuchs on the occasion of his appointment as Full Professor at the University of Liège (February 1885). Lithograph by Florimond van Loo. Helmut WYKLICKY, Zur Geschichte der Augenheilkunde in Wien. Ophthalmology in Vienna. 100 Jahre 2nd University Eye Clinic. Christian Brandstätter, Wien 1984.
33: *Die Ursachen und die Verhütung der Blindheit* (1885). Preisschrift.
34: Georg Joseph Beer (1763–1821). Founder and first Director of Vienna's 1st University Eye Clinic (1812). Oil painting. Sammlungen der Medizinischen Universität Wien. Gabriela SCHMIDT-WYKLICKY, Helmut GRÖGER, "Georg Joseph Beer (1763–1821). Leben und Wirken des Begründers der ältesten Universitäts-Augenheilkunde". *Spektrum Augenheilk.* 26 (2012), pp. 266–272.
35: Eduard Jaeger Ritter von Jaxtthal (1818–1884). Founder and first Director of Vienna's 2nd University Eye Clinic (1884). Private collection; photo C/O G. S-W.
36: Building plan of the Allgemeines Krankenhaus in Wien. J. F. WAGNER, *Orientirungs-Plan des Wiener k. k.allgemeinen Krankenhauses.* Josef Šafář, Vienna 1886. Attachment: "Situationsplan des k. k.allgemeinen Krankenhauses in Wien". Detail with the numbered rooms of the 2nd University Eye Clinic.
37: Ernst Fuchs's appointment document as Full Professor and Director of Vienna's 2nd University Eye Clinic (30 July 1885). Archiv der Universität Wien.
38: "Antrittsvorlesung von Ernst Fuchs als Ordinarius und Vorstand der 2nd University Eye Clinic in Wien am 19. 10. 1885", in: *Wien. med. Bl.* 8 (1885), cols. 1301–1304.
39: Examination protocol for patients devised and made obligatory by Ernst Fuchs for the students of the 2nd University Eye Clinic. Private collection; photo C/O G. S-W.
40: The Professorial College of the Medical Faculty of Vienna University 1893. (Ernst Fuchs in the 2nd row, 5th from right behind his teacher Theodor Billroth). Private collection; photo C/O G. S-W.
41: Ernst Fuchs's visitor's card with handwritten message. Private collection; photo C/O G. S-W.
42: Main entrance of the old Allgemeines Krankenhaus (9th district, Alser Straße 4) ca. 1930. Original photo. Bildarchiv der Österreichischen Nationalbibliothek.
43: Outpatient card of the 2nd University Eye Clinic in Vienna's Allgemeines Krankenhaus, with a reminder of Prof. Fuchs's free daily one-hour surgery for indigent patients. Private collection; photo C/O G. S-W.
44: Prescription form for glasses from the 2nd University Eye Clinic with handwritten instructions to the Directorate of the Allgemeines Krankenhauses. Private collection; photo C/O G. S-W.
45: Mission Statement of the *Wiener klinische Wochenschrift* (1888). Title plage of the 1st issue 1, 5 April 1888.
46: Ludwig Mauthner (1840–1894). Monument by Rudolf Weyr (1898) in the Arcae Court of Vienna University (detail). Archiv der Universität Wien. Photo: C/O Franz Pfluegl. Freely accessible online: https://geschichte.univie.ac.at/de/bilder/ludwig-mauthner-1840-1894 (last accessed: 6 Sept. 2022).
47: Ernst Fuchs's statutes for the Operateur-Institut he initiated at 2nd University Eye Clinic in 1893.
48: Karl David Lindner (1883–1961). Ernst Fuchs's youngest assistant. Sammlungen der Medizinischen Universität Wien.
49: Karl David Lindner's handwritten notes, dated 14 Oct. 1909, on the diagnosis, treatment and the course the disease took in a trachoma patient. Lindner's personal notebook. Private collection; photo C/O G. S-W.

50: Ernst Fuchs with 17 assistants and with doctors from abroad visiting his Clinic ca. 1905/06. Original photo C/O Robert Thiele (Wien VIII., Alserstrasse 43) with the following signatures: 1st row: Richard Krämer, Rudolf Bergmeister, Tertsch, Maximilian Salzmann, Ernst Fuchs, Viktor Hanke, Guzmann, A. Sarafoff, A. Koenig; 2nd row: (2 illegible signatures), Wyler, Urmetzer, Josef Meller, Steidl, Trebiakowski, S. Korski, (illegible). Sammlungen der Medizinischen Universität Wien.

51: "Recipients of Honorary Degree of Fellowship of the Royal College of Physicians and Surgeons of England Aug. 6. 1913". Original photo, London 1913. (Ernst Fuchs and Anton Freiherr von Eiselsberg 1st row, centre). Sammlungen der Medizinischen Universität Wien.

52: Ernst Fuchs takes part in the meeting of the Section of Ophthalmology at the International Congress of Medicine, London 1913. Original photo (Ernst Fuchs row, 9th from right). Wellcome Collection, London (freely accessible on the internet).

53: "Letzte Fotographie mit den Herren der Klinik" [Last photo op with the gentlemen from the Clinic] (1915). Original photo with Ernst Fuchs's handwritten notes. Sammlungen der Medizinischen Universität Wien. 1st row.: 1st from left Josef Meller, 3rd from left Viktor Hanke, 2nd rwo.: 7th from left Ernst Fuchs, 9th from left Karl David Lindner.

54: Ernst Fuchs, *Lehrbuch der Augenheilkunde*. 1st ed. (1889). Private collection; photo C/O G. S-W.

55: Maximilian Salzmann (1862–1954). Christoph Wolfgang FASCHINGER, "Zum 150. Geburtstag von Maximilian Salzmann (1862–1954)", in: *Spektrum Augenheilk.* 27 (2013), pp. 153–156. Copyright: Springer Verlag, Vienna.

56: Ernst Fuchs's son, Adalbert Fuchs (1887–1973). Family archive.

57: *Text-Book of Ophthalmology*. First English edition of the *Lehrbuch*, translated by Alexander Duane (1892). Private collection; photo C/O G. S-W.

58: Alexander Duane (1858–1926), in: John WEEKS, Alexander Duane, M. D., D. Sc., in: *Transact. Am. Ophthalmol. Soc.* 24 (1926), pp. 18–20.

59: Edward Vail Lapham Brown (1876–1953). Peter C. KRONFELD, Edward Vail Lapham Brown, M. D., *Transact. Am. Ophthalmol. Soc.* 51 (1953), pp. 3–5.

60: *Diseases of the Eye*. 10th English edition of the *Lehrbuch* translated by E. V. L. Brown (1933). Private collection; photo C/O G. S-W.

61: *Manuel d'ophtalmologie*. 1st French edition of the *Lehrbuch* translated by C. Lacomte u. L. Leplat (1892). Private collection; photo C/O G. S-W.

62: *Tratado de enfermedades de los ojos*. 1st Spanish edition of the *Lehrbuch* translated by Victor Cebrián y Diez (1893). Private collection; photo C/O G. S-W.

63: Japanese edition of the *Lehrbuch* translated by Tatsushichiro Inouye (1895). Österreichische Nationalbibliothek.

64: Tatsushichiro Inouye (1869–1902). In: Jean-Paul WAYENBORGH, IBBO *International Biography and Bibliography of Ophthalmologists and Vision Scientists*. With the Co-operation of Saiichi Mishima and Charles Richard Keeler. (= *Hirschberg History of Ophthalmology. The Monographs* Vol. 7). Part 2 L–Z. Oostende 2002.

65: Japanese title page of the *Lehrbuch* 1895.

66: Giuseppe Cirincione (1863–1929) and Ernst Fuchs (2nd row centre to the right of Ernst Fuchs). Original photo, with Ernst Fuchs's handwritten note, "Passera Maggiore. Im Castello dei Cesari April 1921". Original photo. Family archive.

67: 2nd edition of Mario Pagani's Italian translation of the *Lehrbuch* (1932). Private collection; photo C/O G. S-W.

68: 2nd Russian translation of the *Lehrbuch* by E. P. Eberman and S. Kaplan (1910). Private collection; photo C/O G. S-W.

69: Chinese translation of the *Lehrbuch* by James Boyd Neal (1911). Private collection; photo C/O G. S-W.
70: James Boyd Neal (1855–1925). Original photo 1919. Freely accessible from Wikimedia Commons.
71: Colour photos of various changes of the fundus in the Chinese translation of the *Lehrbuch* (1911). Private collection; photo C/O G. S-W.
72: Examination of the eyes of a Chinese patient in the Chinese translation of the *Lehrbuch*. Private collection; photo C/O G. S-W.
73: Microscope (Zeiss, model: Stativ IIa) formerly owned by Ernst Fuchs.
74: Microscope (Zeiss, Modell: Stativ IIa) in: S. Czapski, Mittheilungen aus der Werkstatt von Carl Zeiss in Jena", in: *Zeitschr. wissenschaftl. Mikroskopie u. mikroskop. Technik* 4 (1887), pp. 289–292.
75: Cartoon: Ernst Fuchs with his "attributes": microscope, histological preparation and Atropin bottle. Buenos Aires 1927. Original drawing. Family archive.
76: Ring abscess. Histological preparation from Ernst Fuchs's collection of histological sections of normal and pathologically altered eyes.
77: Keratitis punctata superficialis dyed with fluorescein. 15th edition of the *Lehrbuch* as revised by Maximilian Salzmann 1926, Fig. 98, p. 354.
78: Aufhellungsstreifen [Absorption lines of the cornea]. 12th edition of the *Lehrbuch* (1910), p. 320.
79: Delle in der Hornhaut [Dellae in the cornea]. Histological preparation from Ernst Fuchs's collection of histological sections of normal and pathologically altered eyes.
80: Drawing of the histological changes brought about by keratitis disciformis in Josef MELLER, "Die histologischen Veränderungen des Auges bei der Keratitis disciformis", in: *Klin. Monatsbl. Augenheilk.* 43 (1905), pp. 335–352, plates VII-VII.
81: Knötchenförmige Hornhauttrübung [Nodular opacity of the cornea]. Histological preparation from Ernst Fuchs's collection of histological sections of normal and pathologically altered eyes.
82: Heterochromie. Original watercolour, signed and dated by Georg Joseph Beer (1791). In: *Lehrbuch*, edited by Adalbert Fuchs (1945), p. 486.
83: Endophthalmitis septica. Coloured drawing. Adalbert Fuchs, *Atlas der Histopathologie des Auges*. Franz Deuticke, Leipzig/Vienna 1923, Plate 15/1, p. 26.
84: Telegram sent by Guglielmo Marconi's wife, datedt 15 Oct. 1912. Original in the Family Archive.
85: Atrophia gyrata chorioideae et retinae. Ernst FUCHS, "Ueber zwei der Retinitis pigmentosa verwandte Krankheiten (Retinitis punctata albescens und Atrophia gyrata chorioideae et retinae)", in: *Archiv Augenheilk.* 32 (1896), pp. 111–116.
86: Retinitis circinata. Adalbert FUCHS, *Die Erkrankungen des Augenhintergrundes*. Franz Deuticke, Vienna 1943, Plate 19/1.
87: Schwarzer Fleck bei Myopie [Myopic black spot]. In: Ernst FUCHS, *Lehrbuch der Augenheilkunde*. 12th edition 1910, Fig. 188, p. 482.
88: Senile Opticusatrophie [Senile opticus atrophy]. In: (Hallard R. BEARD), Photomicrographs of Sections of the Eye, chosen by Prof. Ernst Fuchs as best illustrating his Lectures on the Pathological Anatomy of the Eye. Chicago n.d. (presum. 1920–1922), typescript, Figs. 47 and 48. Illinois College of Optometry Library, Chicago. Accessible online: https://www.worldcat.org/title/pathological-anatomy-of-the-eye-photomicrographs (last accessed: 20 July 2020).

89: Ernst Fuchs's storage container for histological preparations, detail. Sammlungen der Medizinischen Universität Wien.

90: Protokollbuch, Vol. 1. With a handwritten note of Ernst Fuchs on the inside of the cover. Private collection.

91: Handwritten catalogue of the Library of the former 2nd University Eye Clinic. 1. Band. Private collection.

92: Page 10 from the 1st volume of the handwritten catalogue of the 2nd University Eye Clinic's library. Private collection.

93: Ernst Fuchs's personal rubber stamp on an offprint Hermann Cohn had sent him. Private collection.

94: Rubber stamp of the library of the former 2nd University Eye Clinic. Private collection.

95: Folder for offprints of articles by Ernst Fuchs, with "Eigene Arbeiten 1876–1915" in Fuchs's own handwriting. Restored. Private collection.

96: 1903 outpatient statistic of his clinic compiled by Ernst Fuchs himself. Private collection; photo C/O G. S-W.

97: Marble relief of Ernst Fuchs in the Arcade Court of Vienna University's main building. Signed by J. Müllner 1921.

98a: Title page of the Festschrift presented to Ernst Fuchs on his 70th birthday on 14 June 1921.

98b: Portrait photograph of Ernst Fuchs on the back of the fly leaf of the Festschrift presented to him on his 70th birthday.

99: "Vor der Narkose" [Before anaesthesia]. Handwritten instructions by Ernst Fuchs. Sammlungen der Medizinischen Universität Wien, HS 1.569.

100a: Blepharorrhaphie nach Ernst Fuchs [Blepharorrhaphy according to Ernst Fuchs]. Anton ELSCHNIG, *Augenärztliche Operationslehre*. Vol 1, Julius Springer, Berlin 1922, Fig. 182, p. 162.

100b: Äussere Tarsorrhaphie nach Ernst Fuchs [External tarsorrhaphy according to Ernst Fuchs]. In: Josef MELLER, Josef BÖCK, *Augenärztliche Eingriffe. Eine kurzgefasste Operationslehre*. 5th edition, Springer, Vienna 1946, Fig. 90, p. 117.

101: Transfixio iridis nach Ernst Fuchs. Josef MELLER, Josef BÖCK, *Augenärztliche Eingriffe. Eine kurzgefasste Operationslehre*. 5th editiob, Springer, Wien 1946, p. 337, Fig. 220.

102: Schutzgitter für das linke Auge [Protective lattice for the left eye]. In: Ernst FUCHS, *Lehrbuch der Augenheilkunde*. 4th edition 1894, p. 750.

103: House number plate (with "Konskriptionsnummer") of Josef Leiter's workshop in Alsergrund (today: 9th District), Mariannengasse 11. Original: Endoskopie-Museum Wien. Many thanks to Dr. Helmut Gröger (Internationale Nitze-Leiter-Gesellschaft, Vienna).

104: Schutzgitter nach Ernst Fuchs für beide Augen [Protective lattice for both eyes according to Ernst Fuchs]. Katalog über ophthalmologische Instrumente und Apparate etc. der Firma Josef Leiter. Lieferant für die k. k.Universitäts-Kliniken. Wien 1906, Fig. 1114, S. 5.

105: Augenschutzklappe von Ernst Fuchs aus Aluminium [Protective eye cap according to Ernst Fuchs]. In: H. REINER, *Verzeichnis über Ophthalmologische Instrumente und Apparate etc*. Vienna 1909, No. 5970, p. 23.

106: Ophthalmoskop von Ernst Fuchs. In: H. REINER, *Verzeichnis über Ophthalmologische Instrumente und Apparate etc.* Vienna 1909, No. 5578, p. 6.

107: Kapselpinzette nach Ernst Fuchs [Capsule forceps according to Ernst Fuchs]. In: H. REINER, *Verzeichnis über Ophthalmologische Instrumente und Apparate etc.* Wien 1909, No. 5851, p. 17.

108: Kapselpinzette nach Ernst Fuchs in moderner Ausführung: Firma ReboPharm: einfach gebogen, 4x4 Zähne, Länge: 7 cm. Online accessible at: https://rebopharm24.de/shop/praxisbedarf/instrumente-und-geraete/pinzetten/111982/ (last accessed: 20 July 2020).

109: Passenger list of the steamer S. S. Amerika, on which Ernst Fuchs embarked for the USA for the first time on 29 June 1911 (Route Hamburg–New York). Source: Ernst Fuchs in the New York Passenger Lists, 1820–1957.
Year 1911; Arrival: New York. Microfilm Serial: T715, 1897–1957; Microfilm Roll: 1705; Line:10; Page Number: 48. Ernst Fuchs's name in line 10, below it, in line 11, the name of his wife, Julie, crossed out). Accessible online:
https://search.ancestry.com (last accessed: 27 June 2018).

110a: US immigration visa for Ernst Fuchs 1921. Front. Original in the Family archive.

110b: US immigration visa for Ernst Fuchs 1921. Back. Original in the Family archive.

111: Steamer S. S. Rijndam, on which Ernst Fuchs embarked on 27 September 1921 for the USA (Route: Rotterdam–New York). Source: Ernst Fuchs in the New York Passenger Lists, 1820–1957. Year 1921; Arrival: New York; Microfilm Serial: T715, 1897–1957; Microfilm Roll: 3033; Line: 13; Page Number: 106. Accessible online: https://search.ancestry.com (last accessed: 6 Sept. 2022).

112: "Curs in Houston Texas". Original photo with the inscription "Ernst Fuchs Society Houston Texas Jan 16-30-1922". Family archive.

113: "Kurs in St. Louis". Original photo with inscription on the back in Ernst Fuchs's handwriting. Names and countries of origin of 59 participants printed in lower margin. Sammlungen der Medizinischen Universität Wien.

114: "Curs in San Francisco". Original photo with inscription in Ernst Fuchs's handwriting. Family archive.

115a: Ministerial passport for Ernst Fuchs 1925. Front. Original in the Family Archive.

115b: Ministerial passport for Ernst Fuchs 1925. Back. Original in the Family Archive.

116: Leslie Dana Gold Medal. Sammlungen der Medizinischen Universität Wien.

117: "Honolulu: Dr. Fennel". Original photo with inscription in Ernst Fuchs's handwriting. Family archive.

118: "Tokio September 1922". Original photo with inscription in Ernst Fuchs's handwriting. Family archive.

119: "Tee im Hause Komoto's in Tokio". Original photo with inscription in Ernst Fuchs's handwriting. On the back handwritten dedication by Komoto: "Meinem verehrten Kollegen Herrn Prof. Dr. Fuchs zur freundlichen Erinnerung und in herzlicher Dankbarkeit Dr. Komoto. Tokio, 21. Sept. 1922" [To my revered colleague, Prof. Fuchs, in friendly commemoration and heartfelt gratitude Dr Komoto, Tokyo, 21 Sept. 1922]. Sammlungen der Medizinischen Universität Wien.

120: Ernst Fuchs paying a visit to the Eye Clinic of Nagoya University. Original photo with a handwritten dedication by the Director of the Clinic, Chuta Oguchi (1st row, to the left of Ernst Fuchs): "Seiner hochwohlgeboren Herr Professor Dr. E. Fuchs in freundlicher Erinnerung. Vorstand und Assistenten in der Augenklinik zu Nagoya, Japan". Sammlungen der Medizinischen Universität Wien.

121: Ernst Fuchs vor dem Eingang eines repräsentativen Gebäudes in westlicher Bauweise, vermutlich die Augenklinik an der Universität Kioto. Original photo with inscription on the back in Ernst Fuchs's handwriting: "Fotographie aus Kioto. Prof. Ishikawa der zweite links von mir" [Photo from Kyoto. Prof. Ishikawa second on my left]. Sammlungen der Medizinischen Universität Wien.

122: Ernst Fuchs paying a visit to the Eye Clinic of Kyoto University. Original photo with inscription in Ernst Fuchs's handwriting, "Kioto". Family archive.
123: Ernst Fuchs paying a visit to the Eye Clinic of Osaka University mit the handwritten dedication: "Herrn Geheimrat Prof. Dr. E. Fuchs von Dr. S. Miyashita und seinen Assistenten in Osaka Japan" [To Herr Geheimrat Prof. Dr. E. Fuchs, Dr. S. Miyashita and his assistants in Osaka Japan]. Original photo. Sammlungen der Medizinischen Universität Wien.
124: Ernst Fuchs lecturing at the University Eye Clinic Osaka. Original photo with inscription in Ernst Fuchs's handwriting, "Osaka" . Family archive.
125: Shigeru Kagoshima, Director of the University Eye Clinic Chiba paying a visit to Ernst Fuchs in Vienna on 27 Sept. 1924. Original photo with inscription in Prof. Kagoshima's handwriting: "Herr Hofrat Prof. Fuchs – Wien d. 27. Sept. 1924. Prof. S. Kagoshima. Augenklinik d. Universität zu Chiba Japan. Dr. W. Kichikawa. Director der Frauenklinik zu Oita Spital." Ernst Fuchs added, "Prof. Kagoshima". Family archive.
126: Tsing-Meu Li. Original photo with an inscription in Ernst Fuchs's handwriting. Family archive.
127: Harvey Howard (1880–1956). Original photo, dated "Dec. 1922", with a handwritten dedication to Ernst Fuchs: "To Professor Ernst Fuchs. In affectionate remembrance of him as our guest, our friend and inspiring teacher." Family archive.
128: Arnold Pillat (1891–1975). Original photo. Bildarchiv der Österreichischen Nationalbibliothek.
129: Ludwig von Sallmann (1892–1975). In: "Nachruf von Peter C. KRONFELD", in: *Trans. Am. Ophthalmol. Soc.* 74 (1976), pp. 8–11.
130: Peter C. Kronfeld (1899–1980). In: "Nachruf von Joseph HAAS", in: *Am. J. Ophthalmol.* 90/2 (1980), pp. 268–270.
131: The Dung Dai Med. School in Shanghai. Original photo of 115 persons (Ernst Fuchs 1st row, centre) in front of the Dung Dai Medical College and the Dung Dai Hospital. Inscription in Ernst Fuchs's handwriting. Sammlungen der Medizinischen Universität Wien.
132: José Rizal (1861–1896). Freely accessible internet version.
133: Ernst Fuchs (1st row, centre) and Sixto Y. Orosa e Ylagan (2nd row, behind Fuchs). Original photo with inscription in Ernst Fuchs's handwriting: "In Sulu. The Sulu Public Hospital. Neben mir Dr. Sixto Y. Orosa". Family archive.
134: Ernst Fuchs with F. W. Dudley and Fernando Calderon. Original photo with inscription in Ernst Fuchs's handwriting: "Dr. Calderon, Prof. Dudley (Antipolo bei Manila)." Family archive.
135: Ernst Fuchs's 1923 passport with the last stamps of his return to Austria Stempeln. Original in the Family Archive.
136: Ernst Fuchs's "Parte" [death notice]. Original in the Family Archive.
137: Funerary stele for Ernst and Julie Fuchs by Hans Bitterlich. Photo: Raimund Hofbauer.
138: Bronze plaque of Ernst Fuchs. Family archive. Photo: Raimund Hofbauer.
139: "Ernst Fuchs Award". Ophthalmology Hall of Fame 2001.
140: Portrait of Ernst Fuchs. Oil painting (detail) by Richard Bitterlich 1911.

IV. Index of Names

E

F

I

J

K

L

M

N

O

P

R

S

T

U